THE NURSE'S
DRUG HANDBOOK

THE NURSE'S DRUG HANDBOOK

SECOND EDITION

Suzanne Loebl

George Spratto, Ph.D.
Professor and Associate Head
Department of Pharmacology and Toxicology
Purdue University
Lafayette, Indiana

With comprehensive nursing implications by

Estelle Heckheimer, R.N., B.S., M.A.
Assistant Professor of Nursing
Fairleigh Dickinson University
Rutherford, New Jersey

A WILEY MEDICAL PUBLICATION
John Wiley & Sons
New York • Chichester • Brisbane • Toronto

Interior Design: Nancy Dale Muldoon
Cover Design: Wanda Lubelska
Production Editor: Eileen Tommaso

Library of Congress Cataloging in Publication Data:

Loebl, Suzanne.
    The nurse's drug handbook.

    (A Wiley medical publication)
    First ed. (©1977) entered under title.
    Bibliography: p.
    1. Chemotherapy—Handbooks, manuals, etc. 2. Drugs—
Handbooks, manuals, etc. 3. Nursing—Handbooks, manuals,
etc. I. Spratto, George, joint author. II. Heckheimer,
Estelle. III. Title. [DNLM: 1. Drug therapy—Nursing
texts. 2. Drugs—Nursing texts. QV55 N974]
RM262.L63 1980   615.5'8   80-15274
ISBN 0-471-06092-5
ISBN 0-471-06017-8 (pbk.)

Printed in the United States of America

10 9 8 7 6 5 4 3 2 1

To the memory of Dr. Hugo Bamberger
and to

Margaret Bamberger

Charles, Louis, and Anne Heckheimer

Lynne, Chris, Gregg, Rose, and Dominic Spratto

preface
to the second edition

Less than three years have passed since we put the finishing touches on the first edition of *The Nurse's Drug Handbook*. The instant popularity of this text-reference has convinced us that the manner in which we presented the increasingly complex pharmacological information was useful to nurses and others responsible for the safe administration of medications.

In the new edition, we have striven to strengthen the teaching aspect of *The Nurse's Drug Handbook*, while maintaining and improving its convenience as a reference book.

Emphasis again is placed on helping the nurse to make knowledgeable observations of the effects of drugs on patients. The nursing process for promoting compliance by patients with their medication regimens is stressed and includes specific educational material to teach patients and their families how to optimize drug therapy in the hospital and at home.

The second edition has some entirely new features. Laboratory test interference data about individual drugs were added where pertinent and available. A section explaining the mechanisms that may cause such interferences was added to Part One, which, as previously, provides basic information about drug administration.

Specific nursing implications for the administration of drugs by perfusion, central parenteral, inhalation, and intra-arterial techniques were also added to Part One.

Part One of the second edition also contains specific information on the administration of drugs to geriatric patients. Both physiological changes and patient-related problems (inadequate nutrition, use of many medications, lack of compliance, medication errors, and many other points) are discussed. A conveniently organized table that details the adverse effects that may occur in elderly patients from the use of specific agents is included. The information on the administration of drugs to children was also expanded.

Part Two of the first edition has been completely updated. Approximately 150 new drugs were added, and the dosages, indications, and interactions of all of the more than 1,000 drugs already in the book were revised to conform with the most up-to-date information and standards available. Drugs that have become obsolete or were withdrawn have been deleted.

Several entirely new chapters and sections were developed. The most important of these is a chapter on electrolytes, caloric agents, acidifying and alkalinizing agents. This addition was mandated by the rapid progress made in surgical techniques and in maintaining severely ill patients on total parenteral nutrition for prolonged periods of time.

Another new section contains information on local and general anesthetics. Emphasis is placed on that information of value to nurses who care for patients after they leave the operating room.

The chapter dealing with drugs affecting the central nervous system was revised. It now has separate sections on agents for Parkinsonism and minimal brain dysfunction. A separate section dealing with anti-inflammatory and remitting agents for the treatment of rheumatic diseases was also added. The fundamental principles underlying the drug therapy for each of these disease entities are summarized at the beginning of each section, and the very complete nursing implications contain an enormous amount of practical information. Emphasis on drug compliance and patient education were continued and strengthened in the belief that a patient who is well informed about his or her disease and its treatment often is an indispensable partner in the effort to achieve optimal results from drug therapy.

Current medical trends led us to add separate sections to the hormone chapter on ovarian stimulants used in the treatment of infertility and on abortifacients. These sections have especially comprehensive nursing implications because patients receiving these highly toxic and/or potent drugs must be monitored closely. A section on antiviral drugs was added to the chapter on anti-infectives. Data on sclerosing and pigmenting agents were also added.

The appendix was greatly expanded. Major new additions are:

1. Summary tables of the major clinically important drug interactions, arranged alphabetically by drug.
2. A summary table of laboratory test interferences, again arranged alphabetically by drug.
3. An alphabetic list of the combinations that appear in the list of the 200 most-prescribed drugs. The list gives the trade names of the combinations, the generic names of the components, the amount in which each is present, the pharmacological class of each component, the use of the preparation, and the dose usually prescribed.
4. The guide for intravenous administration of antibiotics and other pertinent drugs has been updated and greatly expanded. The stability of drugs at room temperature and in dextrose and saline solution is given, as well as the compatibility and incompatibility of the drugs with each other and with other agents that are commonly administered intravenously.

The table on poisons and their antidotes was expanded, information on the Federal Controlled Substance Act was added, and additional information on dosage computation was included. The Medic Alert System was also added.

Some of the changes incorporated in the second edition were mandated by new developments in pharmacology, some by the deepened perceptions of the authors, and some by suggestions from our readers. We would like to thank all those who took the trouble to share their thoughts about *The Nurse's Drug Handbook* with us, and we hope that the second edition will be even more useful than the first.

S.L.
E.H.
G.S.

preface
to the first edition

The Nurse's Drug Handbook is a clinically oriented combination text-reference book designed for both students and staff nurses. We have taken great care to provide a wide range of useful information for each drug in a handy and easily accessible form, yet we have also attempted to retain some of the features of a conventional pharmacology text.

Part One provides essential information about drugs in general, beginning with a section on how to use the handbook. Safety precautions in storing and preparing drugs are given, followed by detailed instructions on how to administer drugs to adults and children by all routes. The characteristics of common adverse reactions to drugs and the usual pathways of drug interactions are reviewed, and commonly used approximate equivalents and abbreviations are listed.

Part Two classifies drugs in a logical manner, either according to their nature or the medical condition they are intended to correct. Each group of drugs is introduced with a comprehensive review of the pharmaceutical agents, the mode of action, and advantages and drawbacks of that group of drugs. Within each section the drugs are listed alphabetically. We have attempted to be as complete as possible in listing the agents used for in-patient and out-patient care, giving more coverage to commonly used drugs than for those used rarely. Information on use, dosage, contraindications, and untoward reactions is presented in capsule form. Pediatric dosage is given when relevant.

A special feature of this handbook is the separate sections for each drug or group of drugs on nursing implications and on administration and storage with emphasis on helping the nurse recognize adverse effects of drugs early, before damage to the patient has occurred. Also, when relevant or known, drug interactions that may occur when two agents are administered concurrently are given. Practical ways of relieving or minimizing the inevitable discomforts associated with the administration of potent pharmaceuticals are indicated, and particular attention is given to the needs and reactions of older or debilitated patients.

Since ambulatory care is on the increase and potent drugs are used routinely by an ever-increasing number of people, the text emphasizes teaching the patient how to take medications at home and teaching him or her and responsible family members how to recognize adverse reactions that may occur and which should be reported to the physician. The nursing implications sections remind the nurse of any precautions the patient should take while using the drug, such as not operating machinery, eating or avoiding certain foods, and not taking certain over-the-counter drugs.

Even though this book is as simple and complete as we could make it, we have discouraged drug administration by rote. We have attempted throughout the text to explain why one drug may be preferred to another or why a certain course of action is to be followed. Also, although we have made every effort to ensure the accuracy of the text and dosages, some errors may nevertheless have escaped our notice. We thank in advance any readers who find errors and call them to our attention.

Administering drugs to patients has become one of the most important and complex aspects of nursing care. We hope that this handbook will be a valuable resource for the nurse and a guide to safer, easier, and more knowledgeable drug administration.

S.L.
E.H.
G.S.

acknowledgments

Any scientific text draws on work done by others in the same field. This is particularly true of a reference work in pharmacology, which of necessity contains a great quantity of detailed information. Additional information was obtained from discussing specific problems with scientists working with a particular group of pharmacologic agents.

The nursing implications presented in the text were derived from the nurse-author's clinical experience, from consultation with nurse colleagues, and from selected references.

A list of the most frequently consulted texts used in the writing of this book is presented in the bibliography. Our thanks and admiration go to all those on whose work ours is based.

We want to thank our colleagues at Fairleigh Dickinson and Purdue Universities for being patient with us during the year it took to revise *The Nurse's Drug Handbook* and for helping us by means of constructive criticism.

Thanks are also due to Dr. Ernest M. Loebl, professor of physical chemistry, Polytechnic Institute of New York, whose suggestions and reading of the manuscript were most helpful.

We want to thank Judy Loebl, Dianne Slac, and Judy Whitten for typing the manuscript. Their contribution was much greater than the simple word *typing* implies.

Last but not least we want to thank our families for their moral support and for the sacrifices they made while the first edition was being revised.

S.L.
E.H.
G.S.

contents

APPENDIX

PART ONE

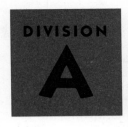

how to use this handbook

In writing this handbook the authors had to reconcile the sometimes conflicting demands of consistency, comprehensiveness, clarity, and ease of use for reference, while avoiding excessive length or redundancy. In view of these considerations the following format has been developed.

Part I provides general information regarding drug administration. Basic guidelines for nurses administering drugs are presented in Divisions A through M.

Division G contains a summary of the most important *untoward reactions* patients may exhibit when they react adversely to a drug. This section should be reread from time to time by all those involved in drug administration.

In addition to an untoward drug reaction, a specific *drug interaction* may result when two drugs are given concomitantly. This interaction may be desirable or, more often, undesirable. In either case, the nurse should be aware of its possible occurrence. The more common mechanisms that give rise to such drug interactions are detailed in Division H.

Material pertaining to laboratory test interference is detailed in Division I.

Special problems relating to the administration of drugs to pediatric and geriatric patients are discussed in Divisions E and F.

Mathematical conversion rules, formulas for calculating correct dosage, and commonly used abbreviations are presented in Divisions K, L, and M, respectively.

The major portion of the book, Part Two, discusses individual pharmacological agents. Since the manual is designed to serve both as a quick reference guide in busy clinics or on hospital floors and as a simple text in pharmacology, the material is arranged as follows:

Drugs that either belong to closely related families (e.g., penicillins, sulfonamides) or are used for the treatment of a particular disease (e.g., antimalarials) are grouped together.

Drugs that mainly affect one physiological system (e.g., cardiovascular) are grouped together in sections; these sections contain subsections that deal with specific conditions to be treated (e.g., hypertension, arrhythmias, convulsions).

Drugs affecting hormone balance (e.g., insulin, thyroid, antithyroid) are presented under appropriate headings.

Miscellaneous pharmacologic agents (e.g., gastrointestinal drugs, expectorants, cough suppressants) used for the treatment of common medical conditions are grouped together.

Drugs are arranged alphabetically within each group or subdivision with the generic name listed in bold type followed by the trade name(s).

This type of arrangement enables the nurse to locate an individual drug quickly and to find concise information about its safe administration (dosage, uses, contraindications, untoward reactions, and interactions). The handbook can also be used to obtain general information about the drugs themselves or the particular condition to be treated. The introduction to each section should be read carefully.

Depending on the agent or agents under consideration, information is given either for individual drugs or for an entire group. In the former case the material is cross-referenced.

Information for individual drugs is presented as follows:

Classification Defines type of drug unless this is self-evident.

General Statement Information about the type of drug, mode and duration of action, and why this agent may behave differently from other related drugs. When there is very little information to be presented under this heading, the heading is *Remarks*.

Use Indications for the particular agent.

Contraindications Outright contraindications for administration of the drug and circumstances under which it may be administered with special caution. The safe use of many of the newer pharmacologic agents during pregnancy or childhood has not been established. As a general rule, the use of drugs during pregnancy is contraindicated unless specified by a physician.

Untoward Reactions Discomforts the patient *may* experience while taking this particular agent.

Drug Interactions Drugs that may interact with one another are listed under this entry. The study of drug interactions is a rapidly expanding area of pharmacology. The compilation of such interactions is far from complete; therefore, listings in this manual are to be considered *only* as general cautionary guidelines.

As detailed in Division H of Part One, drug interactions may result from a number of different mechanisms (additive effects, interference with degradation of drug, increased speed of elimination). Such interferences may manifest themselves in a variety of ways; however, an attempt has been made throughout the text to describe these whenever possible as an increase ($\uparrow$) or a decrease ($\downarrow$) in the effect of the drug, followed by a brief description of the reason for the change.

It is important to realize that any side effects that accompany the administration of a particular agent may also be increased as a result of a drug interaction.

The reader should also be aware that the drug interactions are listed according to *groups* of drugs, under their generic names. For example, diuretics, thiazide, would include Diuril, which is widely used. The entry for salicylates includes aspirin. The trade name of a particular agent is given for clarity when the interaction is particularly important.

Laboratory Test Interferences These refer to the manner in which a drug may affect the laboratory test values of the patient. Some of these interferences are caused by the therapeutic or toxic effects of the drugs; others result from interference with the method itself. As detailed in Division I of Part One, interferences are described as false +, or (↑) values and as false −, or (↓) values. Many of the laboratory test interferences are also listed under the *Nursing Implications* of each drug.

Dosage The adult dose is always listed unless otherwise specified. The listed dosage is to be considered as a general guideline, since the exact amount of the drug to be given is determined by the physician. However, a nurse should question orders from the physician when dosages differ markedly from the accepted norm. We have tried to give complete data for drugs that are prescribed frequently. Pediatric dosages are listed whenever relevant.

Administration/Storage This information provides specific pointers on how to administer and store particular agents. When in doubt, consult the extensive data given in Part One, Division C.

Nursing Implications Designed to assist the nurse with situations that may arise when administering the drug under consideration. The nurse must also observe the patient for the *Untoward Reactions* listed under that heading. If severe, these must be reported to the physician. Severe untoward reactions are sometimes cause for discontinuation of the drug.

The nursing implications emphasize the nurse's role in teaching the patient. This is especially important for drugs that must be taken by the patient at home for a prolonged period of time.

Patient Compliance and Education Detailed, general guidelines on how to promote compliance of patients with their drug therapy regimen are provided in Part One, Division J. In addition, specific information on patient education is provided in the *Nursing Implications* for each drug. The proper teaching of patients is one of the most challenging aspects of nursing, but the instructions must be tailored to the needs, awareness, and sophistication of each patient.

The previous points are covered for all drugs. When drugs are presented as a group rather than individually, the points may only be covered once for each group. In this case the nurse must look for the appropriate entry at the beginning of the group.

For example, the Contraindications, Untoward Reactions, Drug Interactions, Administration, and Nursing Implications for all the penicillins are so similar that they are only listed once at the beginning.

The names of the drugs (both generic and trade), dosage, some remarks, and length of action differ from agent to agent. Such information is given either in tabular form (used when little additional information is required) or as individual *drug entries*, when the amount of necessary material would make tabular presentation too unwieldy.

Information relevant to a particular drug, and not to the whole group, is listed under appropriate headings such as *Additional Contraindications*, or *Additional Nursing Implications*. Such entries are *in addition* to and not *instead* of the regular entry, which must also be consulted.

The Appendix section contains the following tables and information:

1. Commonly used normal physiological values
2. Parenteral Drug therapy for antibiotics and other drugs commonly administered intravenously
3. Poisoning
   General measures
   Toxic agents and their antagonists
   General agents useful in treating overdosage and poisoning
4. Selected clinically important drug interactions (alphabetic)
5. Effects of drugs on laboratory values
6. Commonly prescribed combination drugs
7. Federal Controlled Substances Act
8. Medic alert emblems
9. Glossary
10. Bibliography

You are now ready to use *The Nurse's Drug Handbook*. We hope that it will be a trustworthy friend.

Even though the material presented may at first seem overwhelming, remember that the effective drugs now at the disposal of the entire health team are the key to today's better, more effective medical care.

To quote Dr. Victor R. Fuchs, a leading student of present-day medicine: "The great power of drugs is a development of the twentieth century—many would say of the past forty years. Our age has been given many names—atomic, electronic, space, and the like—but measured by the impact on people's lives it might just as well be called the 'drug age'."

The administration of drugs and the monitoring of their effects on the patient is a crucial part of the nursing process.

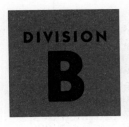

nursing implications for drug therapy

Nursing implications refer to the actions and precautions that must be observed by the nurse when administering a particular drug. The nurse is not merely a drug dispenser blindly following the physician's orders; rather, the nurse is a professional utilizing knowledge of physiology, pathology, sociology, nursing, psychology, and pharmacology to participate in a team approach to disease prevention and drug therapy.

Reports from the patient, nursing assistants, and family, as well as from the physician, are considered when making nursing decisions. Observing and reporting to the physician both therapeutic and untoward reactions to drugs are meaningful and essential functions of the professional nurse. The initiation of appropriate nursing intervention significantly influences the success of drug therapy.

The following nursing implications are related to all drug therapy. They will be repeated selectively in the discussion of particular drugs to reinforce the importance of specific nursing procedures related to a classification of drugs or to an individual drug.

1. Check the medication card with the physician's written order for patient's name, date of order, drug dosage, route, time of administration, and diet.
2. Check whether the patient is scheduled for any diagnostic procedures that contraindicate administration of medications (e.g., gastrointestinal series, F.B.S.). Withhold medication and check with physician if indicated.
3. Check in *Drug Handbook* for physiological action, therapeutic use, untoward effects, contraindications, drug interactions, nursing implications, and recommended dosage for those drugs not already known. Use other references such as the *Formulary Service* or *PDR* if necessary.
4. Select the specific drug ordered by the physician. Substitutes are neither acceptable nor legal.
5. Check that the dosage of the drug is within normal limits. If the dosage is not within normal limits, withhold the drug and discuss the safety of the dosage prescribed with the physician.
6. Prepare the specific dose ordered by the physician. If the strength of the solution or tablet on hand is not suitable for exact measurement, check with the pharmacist about the availability of another strength. If a more appropriate strength is not available, notify the physician, who may adjust the dosage so that medication may be measured carefully.

7. If a suitable strength tablet is unavailable, and unless contraindicated, the nurse may crush a soluble tablet and dissolve it in a small, measured amount of water. The desired fraction of the solution is then given to patient. This is not a method of choice.

8. Unless contraindicated, soluble tablets may be crushed and dissolved in a small amount of fluid and given to patients unable to swallow the tablet. Alternatively, an elixir may be provided by the pharmacy. Syrups and elixirs should not be given to diabetic patients.

9. When preparing and administering drugs, take into account the patient's name, age, sex, diagnosis, social background, religious preferences, diet, and medical history.

10. Before drug administration, identify the patient. Evaluate his emotional and physical state to determine his ability to receive the medication by the prescribed route. If the patient (e.g., a child) cannot or will not tolerate the drug by the route indicated, withhold the drug and consult with the physician, who may reduce the dosage, withdraw the drug, change the route of administration, or order another drug.

11. Take into consideration laboratory test interferences when selecting a method of testing and when using test results as a guide for administration of medication.

12. Consider the rate of excretion of drugs and the need to maintain blood levels when scheduling times for administration (e.g., penicillin, insulin).

13. Administer drugs as close to the designated time as possible. The recommended limits are one-half hour before or one-half hour after the designated time. Drugs ordered a.c. should usually be given 20 minutes before the meal. Schedule drugs and administer them at times that will maximize their therapeutic effectiveness while minimizing their untoward reactions (e.g., diuretics in the morning so that diuresis will be completed before bedtime).

14. Chart fluids taken with drugs if patient is on intake and output. Provide only liquids allowed on the diet.

15. Stay with the patient until oral drugs have been swallowed.

16. Use your knowledge of desired effects, undesired effects, and drug interactions to observe the patient for positive and negative results. Report these observations. Untoward reactions may necessitate withholding the drug or emergency action.

17. Chart the administration of drugs and related observations immediately after administration (or if drug is withheld) to prevent duplication and errors resulting from omissions in communication.

18. Having consulted with other members of the health team, the nurse or pharmacist should teach the patient and the family the techniques and information necessary for successful administration of any drugs to be continued after discharge. This teaching is essential to promote drug compliance.

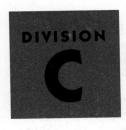

safety precautions for preparation and storage of medications

1. Work with adequate lighting.
2. Be very attentive.
3. Check labels three times: (1) when taking medication from storage; (2) when preparing medication; and (3) when replacing medication in storage.
4. Check expiration date, and discard medication if expiration date has passed.
5. Do not use discolored medication or medication with unexpected precipitate unless specifically directed otherwise (e.g., directions for administration may indicate that for a certain medication a change in color does not interfere with the safety of the drug).
6. Pour oral liquids from the bottle on the opposite side of the label.
7. Wipe the bottle after pouring a liquid.
8. Hold the medicine cup at eye level to pour medication. The meniscus (the lower curve of the liquid) should be at the calibration line indicating the proper dosage.
9. Pour tablets or capsules into the cap of the bottle and then empty the cap into the medication cup. Tablets or capsules are not to be poured into the nurse's hand.
10. Administer only those medications that you have prepared personally.
11. Once poured, do not return medications to the storage container.
12. Use sterile equipment and sterile technique to prepare parenteral medications.
13. Use recommended diluent for parenteral medications; follow directions for proper concentration and speed of administration of the medication.
14. Discard needles and syringes in appropriate containers.
15. Discard ampules with unused portions of medication.
16. Store drugs as recommended.
17. Return bottles with damaged labels to pharmacy.
18. Do not leave medicine cabinets unlocked or medications unattended.
19. Complete a narcotic count at the end of every shift.

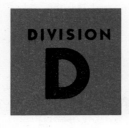

DIVISION D

nursing implications for the administration of medications by different routes

ADMINISTRATION OF ORAL MEDICATION

1. Administer irritating drugs with meals or snacks to minimize their effect on the gastric mucosa.
2. If food interferes with the absorption of the drug, or if digestive enzymes destroy a significant portion of the medication, administer between meals or on an empty stomach.
3. If patient is vomiting, withhold medication and report to physician.

Tablets/ Capsules

1. Unless a tablet is scored, it should not be broken to adjust dosage. Breaking may cause incorrect dosage, gastrointestinal (GI) irritation, or destruction of drug in an incompatible pH. *Scored tablets* may be broken with a file.
2. *Time release capsules, and enteric-coated tablets* should not be tampered with in any way. Instruct the patient to swallow whole and not to chew.
3. *Sublingual tablets* are to be placed underneath tongue. Instruct the patient not to swallow or chew such tablets and not to drink water, all of which will interfere with effectiveness of medication.
4. *Buccal tablets* should be placed between gum and cheek (next to upper molar). Instruct the patient to avoid disturbing tablet during absorption.

Liquids

1. **Emulsions.** May be diluted with water.
2. **Suspensions.** Shake well until there is no apparent solid material.
3. **Elixirs.** Do not dilute. Diluent may cause precipitation of drug.
4. **Salty Solutions.** Unless contraindicated because of patient's diet, mix with water or fruit juice to improve taste.

ADMINISTRATION BY INHALATION

Nursing Implications Applicable for All Methods of Administration by Inhalation

1. Administer only one medication at a time through nebulizer, unless specifically ordered to the contrary. Several drugs used together may cause undesirable reactions, or they may inactivate each other.
2. Measure medication precisely with a syringe. Dilute medication as ordered, and place in nebulizer. For home administration ascertain that the patient has equipment necessary for preparation of medication and is able to measure accurately.
3. Discard medication left in nebulizer from previous administration.
4. Teach patient to assemble, disassemble, and clean equipment.
5. Emphasize need to clean mouthpiece and nebulizer after each administration. Other tubing is to be cleaned each day.
6. Seat patient comfortably or place in semi-Fowler position to permit greater diaphragmatic expansion.

Additional Nursing Implications Applicable for Inhalation Therapy by Nebulization

1. Types of nebulizers:
   a. Commercial metered-dose hand nebulizers.
   b. Hand nebulizers filled with diluted medication.
   c. Nebulizer connected by rubber tubing to a source of compressed air or oxygen. Midway in the rubber tubing, a Y tube is inserted; one end of the Y tube is open, and the other end is connected by more rubber tubing to the nebulizer.
2. *Test equipment* before initiating therapy:
   a. Place medication in nebulizer.
   b. Turn on either compressed air or oxygen as ordered.
   c. Occlude open end of Y tube with finger. If the equipment is working properly, a fine spray will be seen leaving the nebulizer.
3. Teach patient self-administration of medication by nebulization utilizing the following directions:
   a. Place medication in nebulizer.
   b. First exhale slowly through pursed lips.
   c. Position nebulizer in mouth, but do not seal lips to it.
   d. Take a deep breath through the mouth and at the same time to squeeze the bulb of the nebulizer or close the end of the Y tube.
   e. Hold breath for 3 to 4 seconds at full inspiration.
   f. Exhale slowly through pursed lips to create more pressure in the air passages, which will carry medication through the bronchial tree.
   g. Repeat cycle for the number of times ordered to utilize medication in nebulizer, depending on instructions for particular medication.

Additional Nursing Implications Applicable for Inhalation Therapy by Intermittent Positive Pressure Breathing (IPPB)

1. Select the inspiratory flow rate ordered by medical supervision. Initial treatment is often started at 5 cm of water pressure to help patient adjust to using the machine correctly; then pressure is gradually increased to the most effective level, which is usually 15 to 20 cm of water pressure for a 15-minute treatment 3 to 4 times a day.
2. Encourage a slow respiratory rate, diaphragmatic breathing, and prolonged expiration through pursed lips.
3. Advise patient to take several deep breaths and to exhale as fully as possible.
4. Encourage coughing effectively several times during treatment, if clearance of secretions is the goal.
5. Administer at least 1 hour after meals to prevent nausea and vomiting.
6. Mist therapy should be provided as ordered either before or after IPPB.

Evaluate the extent of improvement after therapy by having patient breathe after all air has been pushed out. Assess respiratory rate and effort and describe any secretions that are produced.

Additional Nursing Implications After Administration of Medication by Inhalation

1. Assist patient with postural drainage or clapping and vibrating as ordered.
2. Evaluate the extent of improvement after therapy. Have patient push all air out and then breathe. Assess respiratory rate and effort, and describe any secretions that are produced.
3. Cleanse equipment thoroughly at least once daily by soaking in 1:3 solution of white vinegar and water, rinsing thoroughly, and air drying.

ADMINISTRATION BY IRRIGATIONS AND GARGLES

1. Throat irrigations should not be warmer than 120° F so that they do not destroy or damage tissue.
2. Warn the patient that gargling with full strength antiseptic solution may destroy normal defenses of the mouth and pharynx.

ADMINISTRATION OF NOSE DROPS

1. Have paper tissue available.
2. Nasal passages should be cleared before nose drops are instilled.
3. Have patient tilt head over the side of the bed, or place a support under neck so that it is hyperextended.
4. Insert dropper about ⅓ of an inch into the nares and instill the drops.
5. Avoid touching the external nares with the dropper since this may cause sneezing.
6. Instruct patient to maintain position for 1 to 2 minutes until the medication is absorbed.
7. Vasoconstrictor drops should not be administered for more than 3 consecutive days or a rebound effect may occur.

8. To prevent cross-contamination, each patient should have his/her own dropper and medication bottle. If only one bottle is available, use individual droppers.

ADMINISTRATION OF EYE DROPS

1. Instruct the patient to lie down or sit with head tilted back.
2. Have a separate paper tissue available for each eye.
3. Draw only the amount of solution needed for administration into eye dropper.
4. Wipe the lids and eyelashes clean prior to instillation.
5. Hold the dropper close to the eye but do not touch eyelids or lashes with the dropper so that the patient will not be startled.
6. Expose the lower conjunctival sac.
7. Allow the prescribed number of drops to fall into the center of the exposed sac. Avoid having drops fall on cornea; this is unpleasant for patient and may cause tissue damage.

ADMINISTRATION OF EYE OINTMENT

Follow the same precautions and instructions as for the administration of eye drops. The warmth of the body melts the ointment and spreads the medication over the area to be treated.

ADMINISTRATION OF EAR DROPS

1. Warm drops to body temperature.
2. Have the patient lie on side with the ear to be treated facing up.
3. For instillation in adults, pull the cartilagenous part of the pinna (the external part of the ear) back and up. Point the dropper in the direction of the eardrum, and allow the drops to fall in the direction of the external canal.
4. For instillation of drops in children under 3 years of age, pull the pinna back and down. Point the dropper in the direction of the eardrum and allow the drops to fall on the external canal.
5. Have the patient remain on side for a few minutes after instillation to allow medication to reach eardrum and be absorbed.
6. Never pack a wick tightly into the ear. On occasion, a loose cotton wick is inserted into the ear by the physician so that the medication will bathe the eardrum continuously. The wick should be changed when it appears nonabsorbent or soiled.

ADMINISTRATION OF DERMATOLOGIC PREPARATIONS

Medications can be applied to the skin by rubbing, patting, spraying, painting, or by iontophoresis (medication is driven into skin by means of an electric current).

1. Use sterile technique if there is a break in the skin.
2. Cleanse skin before medication is applied. The cleansing agent should be specified by the physician.
3. Remove ointment from jar with a tongue depressor and not with fingers.
4. If medication is to be rubbed in, apply using firm strokes.
5. Apply only a thin layer of medication unless specified otherwise.
6. Solutions should be painted on with applicator.
7. If medication stains, warn patients so that they can take adequate precautions (use old sheets or plastic cloth).
8. Moist dressings or compresses are prepared by soaking sterile towels in solution ordered, wringing them out, and applying them to the area to be treated. Sterile gloves should be worn if sterile solution is to be applied.

RECTAL ADMINISTRATION

Retention Enemas

1. In order to avoid peristalsis, administer retention enemas slowly, using a small amount of solution (no more than 120 ml) and a small rectal tube.
2. Instruct the patient to lie on left side and to breathe through mouth to relax the rectal sphincter.
3. Retention enemas containing medication should be administered after a bowel movement to promote maximum absorption of medication in the empty rectum.
4. Have patient remain flat for 30 minutes after administration of enema.

Suppositories

1. As a rule, suppositories should be refrigerated since they tend to soften at room temperature.
2. Use finger cot to protect the finger used for insertion (index finger for adults, fourth finger for infants). Instruct patient to lie on left side and to breathe through mouth to relax the sphincter. Gently insert the suppository beyond the internal sphincter.
3. Have patient remain on side for 20 minutes after insertion of suppository.
4. If indicated, teach the patient how to self-administer enema or suppository. Observe self-administration to ensure that procedure is being done correctly.

VAGINAL ADMINISTRATION

1. Arrange douche containing medication so that container hangs just above the patient's hip. In this manner the force of the liquid does not drive the solution through the cervical os.
2. Vaginal and genitourinary suppositories can be inserted with applicators.

3. If indicated, instruct the patient on how to self-administer vaginal medication. Observe self-administration to check whether procedure is done properly.
4. Instruct patient to remain in bed at least 20 minutes after administration to ensure that medication bathes the area being treated.

ADMINISTRATION OF PARENTERAL MEDICATION

Intradermal or Intracutaneous Injections

These injections are made into the dermis and produce local effects. The techniques are used mainly for anesthesia and sensitivity tests.

After injection, observe the patient for local reactions, such as redness and swelling.

Intrasynovial or Intra-articular Injection

Used for the relief of pain or the local application of medication. Be aware that local discomfort is usually intensified for several hours before palliative effect sets in.

Hypodermoclysis

This technique is primarily used in patients who require parenteral fluids but whose veins do not permit IV infusion.

During the procedure, a large amount of fluid is slowly injected subcutaneously into the loose tissues on the outer side of the upper body or, more often, into the anterior aspect of the thigh.

An IM 20- or 22-gauge needle, 1½ in long, is recommended for children; a 19-gauge, 2½–3-in needle is satisfactory for adults.

Hyaluronidase, an enzyme that breaks down the main constituents of intracellular connective tissue, is sometimes added to the medication so that the fluid will be absorbed rapidly and cause less discomfort.

Subcutaneous (SC) and Intramuscular (IM) Injections

For more detailed instructions about SC and IM injections, see pages 16–17 and your textbook on nursing techniques.

1. Use sterile technique.
2. In selecting the proper gauge and length of needle for injection, consider age, weight, condition of patient, and physical properties of medication.
3. In order to promote absorption of medication and minimize pain after IM injection, palpate potential site. Choose a site that is not tender to patient and where tissue does not become firm on palpation. Alternate the sites of injection, and chart the sites used. For example, RD for right deltoid, RGM for right gluteus medius. (See Figure 1.)
4. Cleanse site selected for injection using a circular motion. Begin at the point of injection and move outward and away from the point of insertion.
5. For SC injection, pick up tissue in selected area and hold firmly until needle has been inserted at a 45° angle.
6. For IM injection, stretch the skin if patient is in a normal state of nutrition. If the patient is emaciated, pinch the tissue to form a

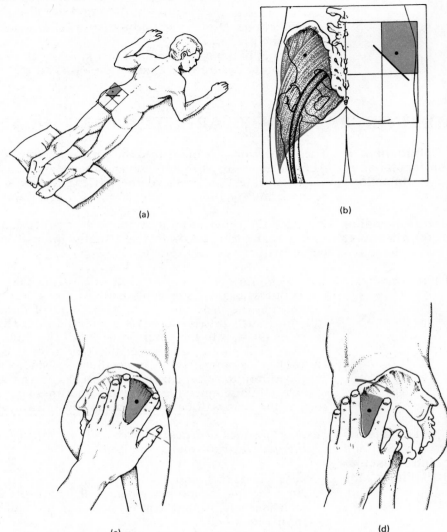

Figure 1. *Intramuscular injection sites.* (a) *position for administration into gluteus maximus area;* (b) *detailed administration into gluteus maximus;* (c) *area for administration of IM into right ventrogluteal area;* (d) *area for administration of IM into left ventrogluteal area.*

       muscle bundle to ensure that the medication is injected into the muscle. Insert needle at a 90° angle.

7. Leave a margin of needle at least ½ in from hub to prevent its complete disappearance in case of breakage.

8. When preparing for SC and IM injections include a small bubble of air in syringe (0.2–0.3 ml) in addition to medication. The air bubble

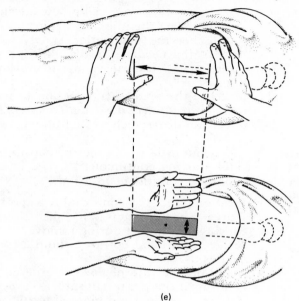

(e)

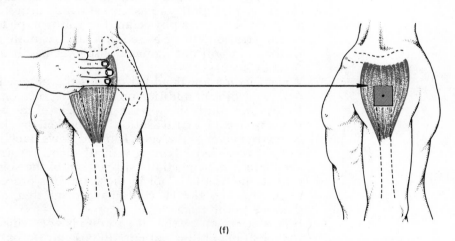

(f)

Figure 1 continued. (e) area for administration of IM into vastus lateralis: top, length of area, bottom, breadth of area; and (f) area for administration of IM into the deltoid.

will help expel all solution from the needle so that irritating solutions will not leak into the tissues as the needle is withdrawn.
9. Insert the needle quickly to minimize pain. After insertion, aspirate to be sure that the needle is not in a blood vessel. If blood returns into the syringe, withdraw the needle and discard the medication.

Prepare another dose using new sterile equipment, select another site, and start the injection again.

10. Administer the medication slowly to allow for absorption, and remove the needle quickly while pressing down at the point of insertion with a sterile sponge to prevent bleeding. Apply a Bandaid if necessary.

11. Massage the area after injection to increase circulation and promote absorption of the drug. This step is contraindicated in the case of certain drugs such as Bicillin where absorption should be slow.

Intravenous Injections (Direct or via Continuous Infusion)

The physician usually assumes responsibility for direct IV administration and starting continuous IV. The following nursing implications apply only to continuous infusion.

1. Position patient as comfortably as possible and explain procedure.
2. If area to be injected is hairy, shave it to prevent adhesive tape from causing discomfort during removal.
3. Attach additional bottles of fluid as ordered and label number of bottles used.
4. Maintain the rate of flow as ordered. Check the rate of flow by counting drops per minute at least every 30 minutes or more often if patient is restless and moves limb where IV is inserted. Count flow rate even if infusion pump is in use.
5. Check amount of fluid administered at least hourly.
6. Check hospital policy to ascertain which drugs a nurse may add to an IV on order by a physician. For volutrol (pedometer, piggyback) administration, dilute as required and regulate the flow so that the medication will not damage tissue yet be absorbed before loss of potency occurs.
7. When medication is added, record the name of the drug, dosage, date, and time of addition on the bottle, bag, or volutrol container.
8. In some hospitals the correct placement of the needle in the vein or the absence of extravasation is checked by lowering the bottle below the level of the vein. If blood flows back into the needle and tubing, the needle is in a vein. If blood returns very slowly, the needle may have partially slipped out of the vein. If blood does not return, the needle is not in the vein. This procedure is not recommended when the IV contains a drug that may cause necrotic damage to the tissue.
9. If flow stops, check that the tubing is not "kinked" or occluded by the position of the patient. If possible, reposition the patient's extremity to reestablish flow.
10. Prevent air embolism by
    a. removing the infusion before the bottle and tubing are completely empty of solution.
    b. checking that all connections in intravenous are tight.
    c. clamping off the first bottle that is empty in a Y-type set (parallel hookup) to prevent air from the empty bottle being drawn into vein.
    d. following instructions very carefully for blood-pumping type of equipment.

     e. positioning the extremity receiving the infusion below the level of the heart to prevent negative pressure, venous collapse, and sucking of air into tubing.

     f. positioning the clamp regulating the flow preferably no lower than the level of the heart and no higher than 4 in above the level of the heart to prevent the formation of negative pressure in the tubing below.

     g. allowing the tubing to fall below the level of the extremity to help prevent air from entering the vein should the infusion bottle empty before the IV is discontinued.

11. Recognize an air embolism by the occurrence of sudden vascular collapse, cyanosis, hypotension, tachycardia, venous pressure rise, and loss of consciousness.

12. Be prepared to assist with treatment should an air embolism occur. Position patient on left side and administer oxygen and other supportive measures.

13. Prevent "speed shock" by checking the rate of flow frequently and observing for untoward symptoms associated with the drug being administered.

14. Check for symptoms of extravasation into tissue characterized by pain, edema, and coolness at site of insertion and reduction in the rate of flow. If the IV is infiltrating, stop the flow and report.

15. Do not flush a clogged IV. The flow might have been stopped by an embolus that should not be moved into the circulation. Report the situation to physician.

16. Chart intake and output.

17. Check for symptoms of phlebitis, such as pain, tenderness, and redness along the path of the vein. Patients receiving IV for more than 24 hours are especially prone to phlebitis.

18. Remove the IV when ordered by the physician. Clamp off tubing before removing the IV so as to prevent extravasation into subcutaneous tissues. Press down with a sterile sponge at site of needle or plastic tube while it is moved to prevent bleeding. Apply bandage to former injection site to prevent bleeding and infection.

CENTRAL PARENTERAL ADMINISTRATION

1. Explain total protein regimen and the procedure for central parenteral administration to the patient.

2. Assist with catheter insertion.

     a. Use strict surgical asepsis (gown, mask, and gloves).

     b. Place patient in Trendelenburg position to raise venous pressure.

     c. Have local anesthetic available if ordered.

     d. Place a rolled towel lengthwise under patient's back to make the subclavian vein more prominent.

     e. Shave area of insertion and prep with acetone and Betadine.

     f. Instruct the patient to bear down (Valsalva maneuver) when the needle is inserted to prevent air from entering the vein and causing an air embolism.

    g. Assist as catheter is sutured to skin to prevent dislodgement.

    h. Assist with application of antibiotic ointment and dry sterile dressing at site of insertion.

    i. Check that patient is x-rayed to verify position of tube before TPN is initiated.

3. Control sepsis.

    a. Use sterile technique in changing dressing q 48 hr.

    b. Provide skin care at site of catheter insertion when dressing is changed. Use antibiotic ointment ordered.

    c. Use sterile technique in changing infusion tubing and piggyback q 24 hr.

    d. Use sterile technique in handling bottle of TPN solution.

    e. Observe solution for clouding, growth, or matter in the bottle. If contamination is observed, hang a new bottle and return contaminated one to pharmacy for culture.

    f. Use 5% D/W if bottle of TPN must be removed and another bottle of TPN is not readily available.

    g. Assess body temperature q 4 hr for elevation indicating infection.

    h. After hanging a new bottle, monitor for a temperature spike that would indicate contamination.

    i. If patient has chills or fever and other signs of sepsis, replace bottle and tubing and send equipment for culture. Further tests such as blood, urine, sputum, x-rays, and physical exam are done to locate foci of infection. Should the cause of the infection be undetermined and the fever continues for 12 to 24 hours, assist with removal of catheter and with insertion of catheter on the other side.

4. Maintain the rate of flow.

    a. Preferably use an infusion pump or an alarm system.

    b. Use an infusion pump when an 0.22 micron filter is used. The flow with an 0.45 micron filter will continue by gravity drip so that an infusion pump is not essential.

    c. Count the drip rate at least every half hour if an infusion pump is not available.

    d. Calculate and maintain a uniform flow rate for 24 hours.

    e. Check for kinks and position tube meticulously.

5. Make assessments.

    a. Assess for signs of overload such as prominence of neck, arm, and hand veins (early symptoms), lassitude, headache, nausea, twitching, hypertension, mental fuzziness, somnolence, and convulsions.

    b. Assess for infiltration by noting pain and swelling in shoulder, neck, or face.

    c. Report a wet dressing indicating improperly placed, slipped, or broken catheter or a leak at the tubing union.

    d. Check fractional urines q 6 hr for glycosuria. Use Tes-Tape to check urine of patient receiving cephalosporins to prevent false positives.

    e. Measure and record daily intake and output.

    f. Weigh daily and expect a weight gain of approximately 12 oz for an adult and 20–35 gm for an infant daily.

    g. Check lab reports for electrolyte balance and renal and liver function.

    h. Compute and chart a caloric count of daily oral intake.

ADMINISTRATION BY INTRA-ARTERIAL INFUSION

Administration by intra-arterial infusion involves insertion of a teflon catheter by a surgeon under fluroscopy into the artery leading directly into the area to be treated. The arteries commonly used are the brachial, axillary, carotid, and femoral. The drug is then pumped steadily through the catheter. The tumor receives a high concentration of the chemotherapeutic agent before it is distributed to the rest of the body. The drug may be administered at varying intervals of time. Intra-arterial infusion may be performed on an ambulatory basis with a portable infusion pump, but the patient must be taught how to monitor the apparatus.

1. Observe tissue in local area for reaction, such as erythema, mild edema, blistering, and petechiae.
2. Describe observations completely when charting and report to doctor.
3. Report pain since it may be indicative of severe injury to normal tissue, vasospasm, or intravasation.
4. Maintain rate of pump as ordered.
5. Do not permit infusion fluid to run through completely, because air will then enter the tubing. Add fluid as needed.
6. Clamp tubing if an air bubble is noted and call doctor.
7. **Do not** *Disconnect the Tubing Between the Pump and the Patient to Release the Air Bubble Because Hemorrhage will Occur.*
8. Apply pressure if hemorrhage occurs from the artery.
9. Check tubing for kinks and prevent compression of tubing.
10. Vital signs should be checked periodically (q 15 minutes) when therapy is initially instituted until BP is stabilized.
11. Observe site of infusion for infection.
12. Monitor intake and output to detect renal failure.

ADMINISTRATION BY PERFUSION (EXTRA-CORPOREAL OR ISOLATION PERFUSION)

Perfusion technique involves the administration of large doses of highly toxic drugs to an isolated extremity, organ, or region of the body. For perfusion in the lower extremity, the iliac, femoral, and popliteal arteries and veins are used; for upper extremity perfusion, the axillary artery and vein are injected. The abdominal aorta and vena cava are used for pelvic perfusion. The actual perfusion is accomplished in the operating room where, by means of a pump oxygenator, the patient's blood is circulated in a closed system for the part of the body involved. Efforts are made by the use of a tourniquet or ligature to prevent seepage of the concentrated drug into the systemic circulation. Seepage of the drug results in destruction of normal tissue.

PREOPERATIVELY

1. Explain procedure to patient, answer questions, and provide emotional support.
2. Weigh patient because dosage of chemotherapeutic agent and heparin are calculated on the basis of body weight.
3. Be certain that hematologic tests, urinalysis, and x-rays have been done.

POSTOPERATIVELY

1. Assess for tanning, erythema, or blistering of skin over area perfused. Symptoms resemble toxic reaction to radiation.
2. Assess local tissue for thrombosis and phlebitis.
3. Ascertain if hematologic tests have been made and evaluated for depression of bone marrow function, which is due to seepage of concentrated drug into systemic circulation.
4. Assess for signs of infection, such as fever and malaise, since septicemia may occur.
5. Assess extremity perfused for color and warmth and report untoward symptoms.
6. Assess patient for pain, which may be indicative of severe tissue damage.
7. Assess for hemorrhage, hypotension, fibrillation, arrhythmia, sudden chest pain, and pulmonary edema, all of which may be precipitated by perfusion.
8. Continue to provide comprehensive nursing care, including physical and emotional support.

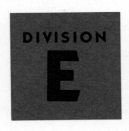

DIVISION E drug response of the pediatric patient

GENERAL CONSIDERATIONS

The administration of drugs to children presents several specific problems. The pediatric patient has a different pharmacodynamic sensitivity than the adult. Furthermore, there often is a long delay between the marketing of a drug for adults and the establishment of a rational therapeutic regimen for pediatric patients.

Many of the problems encountered in the pediatric administration of drugs are due to age and development related to differences in the distribution of drugs in the body and in the rates at which drugs are absorbed and eliminated.

Absorption The pH of the GI tract is higher in infants than in adults. Therefore, drugs that are absorbed in acid environment are absorbed more slowly in children (slower onset of action) than in adults. Conversely, drugs that are destroyed by acid have a longer half life (longer activity) in children than in adults.

Topical absorption is usually faster in pediatric patients, because their epidermis is thinner.

Distribution Throughout the Body A much larger proportion of body weight is water in children than in adults; the converse is true for fat. Thus, drugs that are water soluble are distributed in a smaller volume (are more concentrated) in adults than in children. Drugs that are fat soluble are more concentrated in children than in adults.

Plasma Protein Binding The plasma protein binding of drugs is usually less extensive in children, especially in neonates, than it is in adults because of lower percentage of plasma protein. This results in a greater concentration of free drugs (bioavailability) in children than in adults.

Hepatic Degradation and Renal Excretion Both the liver and the kidneys of neonates and infants are immature compared with adults. The liver, for instance, has a lower concentration of the enzymes that participate in the degradation of drugs; drugs, like phenytoin, that are metabolized by the liver as a rule, are broken down more slowly in infants than in adults.

Renal excretion, on the other hand, which represents a complex balance between elimination and reabsorption, often is faster in infants than in adults (shorter duration of action).

All these factors are taken into consideration when a pediatric dosage is established. The administration of drugs to pediatric patients also involves many practical considerations that are detailed below.

Special Nursing Implications for the Administration of Pediatric Medications

1. Try to gain the child's cooperation by using techniques and an approach appropriate to the level of development.
2. Indicate to the child in a firm but friendly manner that it is time to take the medication.
3. If the child cannot, or will not, cooperate so that parenteral medication can be administered, restrain him with the help of other personnel, as necessary, and then administer medication.
4. Crush pills for infants or children under 5 years of age, and dissolve them in syrup, water, or nonessential foods (e.g., applesauce).
5. Do not force oral medications since aspiration pneumonia is a threat. Report to the physician if the child consistently refuses or

spits out the medication so that another drug or another form of the medication can be ordered.

6. When using a plastic dropper or plastic syringe to administer medication, direct the tip toward the inner aspect of the cheek of the mouth to avoid aspiration and stimulation of the cough reflex.

7. When administering PO medication to an infant, hold the child securely against your body with one arm around the child support-

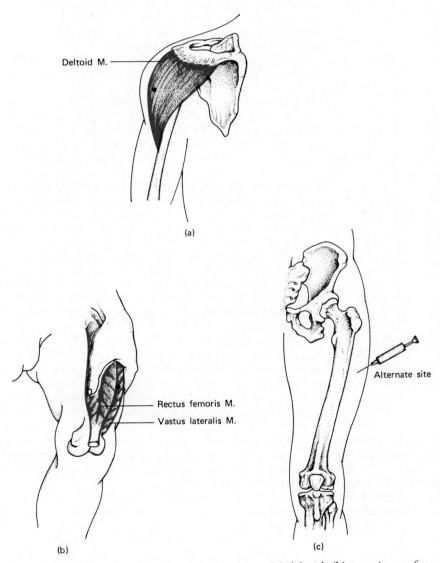

Figure 2. Pediatric intramuscular injection sites: (a) deltoid; (b) anterior surface of midlateral thigh; and (c) anterolateral surface of upper thigh.

ing his head and neck and your other hand holding his free arm while administering the medication. Elevate the infant's head to prevent aspiration.

8. Wake the child before administering medication.

9. Utilize diversional techniques when giving medications to a child. For example: suggest the child count or recite the alphabet while receiving a parenteral injection or suggest that the child lie on his abdomen and turn his toes in to help relax the gluteal muscles. For a child who is quite young, play a music box or set a toy in motion and talk with the patient.

10. When administering ear drops to a child under 3 years of age, pull the pinna of the ear back; for a child over 3 years of age, pull the pinna of the ear back and up.

11. Children under 2 years of age should receive IM injections into the vastus lateralis or rectus femoris (Figure 2), since gluteal muscles are as yet too underdeveloped to be utilized for IM administration and damage to the sciatic nerve is likely to occur.

12. Recognize a child's negative feelings and demonstrate empathy. Do not shame the child. Compliment him on positive aspects of cooperative behavior and demonstrate acceptance and liking even though the child may not have cooperated.

13. When possible, explain to the child the benefits of medication. Realize that hospitalization and medication are regarded as punishment by some children.

14. After medication offer juice or water and verbal praise. Do not offer bribes such as candy, lollipops, or special privileges. These suggest that medications are bad and reward is necessary for an activity that the child should learn to understand is helpful to him/her.

15. On the pediatric floor, the medication cart and drugs should be constantly under the eyes of the nurse. She must always be alert to the possibility that children may take medications that are not theirs or may tamper with them in some way. Syringes and needles must never be left with a child to use as a toy after the nurse has left.

16. If a child does not have a name tag, identification must be made according to hospital policy before medication is administered.

17. Before beginning to pour medications the nurse should be aware of the floor plan of the ward and of the age, weight, and diagnosis of the children who are to receive the various medications.

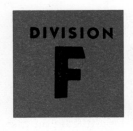

F drug response of the geriatric patient

GENERAL CONSIDERATIONS

Although little concrete data are available, it generally is believed that the aged population is more sensitive to both the therapeutic and toxic effects of many drugs. A comprehensive discussion of the many factors which might influence the response of the elderly patient to drugs is beyond the scope of this text; however, several points are worthy of consideration.

1. **Chronic Disease States.** Diabetes, heart disease, hypertension, chronic respiratory disease, and "senility" are diseases which require chronic drug therapy. Some of these diseases may result in an increase, while others may result in a decrease in drug response. For example, presence of chronic respiratory disease is known to exaggerate the respiratory depression observed with central nervous system depressants.

2. **Physiological and Psychological Change As a Function of Age.** These changes result in a decrease in the functional capacity of the body leading to an alteration of drug response due to changes in absorption from the GI tract, distribution of the drug in the body (as a result of changes in blood flow or composition of body mass), biotransformation of drugs in the liver (i.e., drug-metabolizing enzymes are decreased), excretion of the drug or its metabolites (due to decreased ability of the kidney to filter or actively secrete drugs), and changes in organ or receptor sensitivity. It also is known that serum albumin decreases with age. Thus, since free drug concentration determines drug distribution and elimination, a decrease in binding of drugs to plasma proteins (or other body tissues) could result in altered responses in the elderly patient. For example, a decreased percentage of protein-bound warfarin will lead to a greater pharmacological effect of the drug. On the other hand, reduced protein binding of phenytoin results in a greater amount of the drug available for excretion leading to a reduced pharmacological effect and a shorter duration of action.

3. **Nutrition and Diet.** For many reasons, the elderly population often manifests dietary deficiencies either due to lack of a balanced diet or to low food intake. The resultant vitamin deficiencies or inadequate food intake may alter the response to drugs.

4. **Use of Many Medications.** It is estimated that because of the increased incidence of chronic illnesses in the elderly, this population uses more than two and one-half times as much medication as the rest of the population. As the number of different drugs used

increases, the risk of drug interactions or adverse drug reactions increases.

5. **Lack of Compliance and Medication Errors.** It has been estimated that as much as 60% of the elderly population either fails to take their medication or takes it incorrectly. Reasons for this include (a) impaired mental capacity (patient forgets to take the medication); (b) problems with sight, hearing, or mobility, which result in failure to take the medication or errors in taking the medication; (c) complicated dosing schedules, which confuse the patient so that he/she fails to understand what medication to take or when to take it; (d) alteration of drug regimen based on the personal judgment of the patient, resulting in overdosage or underdosage; and (e) unavailability of medication because the patient is unable to afford it, or because the supply has been used up prior to appointment with the physician.

Thus, it is important for the nurse to ensure that the geriatric patient fully understands how and when to take medication and to monitor carefully drug response in the elderly. The nurse must also be aware of specific symptoms caused by an altered drug response.

Table 1 lists some of the more common drugs or drug classes that warrant special monitoring in the geriatric patient, the reasons for the concern, and the symptoms that may indicate an altered response.

Special Nursing Implications for the Administration of Geriatric Medications

1. Assess the geriatric patient for adverse drug reactions, recognizing that the earliest manifestation of drug toxicity in the elderly is mental confusion. For example, the initial symptoms of digitalis toxicity in the elderly are not necessarily nausea and vomiting, as in younger patients, but rather are changes in mental status due to decreased cerebral perfusion and decreased cardiac output due to secondary arrhythmias.

2. Assess whether failure to thrive in the elderly, characterized by insidious and progressive physical deterioration, deteriorating social competence, loss of appetite, and diminishing concentration, is the result of adverse drug reactions.

3. Assess whether acute brain syndrome characterized by disorientation to person, place, or time, memory impairment for both remote and recent past, impairment of intellectual function, and emotional lability is the result of adverse drug reactions. If so, syndrome may be reversed by withdrawing medications.

4. Recommend and/or provide, as necessary, good oral hygiene before and after administration of medication to promote ingestion and to prevent an unpleasant aftertaste.

5. Provide sufficient fluids to permit easy swallowing and to help movement of medication through the GI tract. Assist patient into a position that prevents aspiration and promotes swallowing of medication.

6. Examine oral cavity of debilitated patient to ensure that medication has not adhered to mucous membranes and, in fact, has been swallowed.

TABLE 1   DRUGS AND DRUG CLASSES WHICH WARRANT SPECIAL MONITORING IN THE GERIATRIC PATIENT

Drug/Drug Class	Age-Induced Changes	Symptoms
Antacids	Increased chance of decreased GI absorption of various drugs	Lack of or reduced response to drug
	Antacids with high sodium content may aggravate renal or cardiac insufficiency	Edema; intensification of congestive heart failure
Barbiturates	Intensification of action of the drug	Increased CNS depression, disorientation, delirium, forgetfulness
	Paradoxical stimulant effects	Excitement, apprehension, CNS stimulation
Digitalis preparations	Enhanced drug toxicity due to changes in body mass, obesity, etc. Also serum half-life is prolonged	Early signs of digitalis toxicity: changes in mental status, anorexia, blurred vision, halos (white or yellow) around bright objects, cardiac palpitations, nausea, vomiting
Methylphenidate	Methylphenidate-induced decrease in hepatic metabolism of phenytoin, phenothiazines, tricyclic antidepressants, coumarin anticoagulants	Intensification of drug response
Narcotic analgesics	Mental confusion and an increase of co-existing mental impairment	Morphine: respiratory depression Codeine: constipation, urinary retention Meperidine: nausea, hypotension, respiratory depression
Penicillin	Enhanced central nervous system toxicity due to decreased renal elimination	CNS Stimulation. Possibility of seizures, coma.
Phenothiazines	Increased incidence of orthostatic hypotension	Dizziness, light-headedness when arising from a sitting or lying position; fainting
	Increased chance of Parkinson-like symptoms and extrapyramidal effects	Twitching, lip smacking, pill-rolling of fingers, restlessness, sudden jerking movements of hands and legs
	Increased anticholinergic side effects	Aggravation of glaucoma, urinary retention
	Cholestatic jaundice	Abdominal pain, hyperpigmentation, pruritis, prolonged fever
	Aggravation of epilepsy or mental depression	
Phenylbutazone	Increased frequency of agranulocytosis, aplastic anemia, and sodium retention	Unusual fatigue, cardiac palpitations, exertional dyspnea, recurrent high fever, skin rash, ulcers of the mouth, prolonged sore throat, edema

TABLE 1   DRUGS AND DRUG CLASSES WHICH WARRANT SPECIAL MONITORING IN THE GERIATRIC PATIENT (*Continued*)

Drug/Drug Class	Age-Induced Changes	Symptoms
Phenytoin	Increased incidence of neurologic and hematologic toxicity in patients with hypoalbuminemia or renal disease	Intensification of the effects of phenytoin
	Increased chance of folate deficiency	Skin pallor, tiredness, glossitis, nausea and anorexia—signs of megaloblastic anemia
Propranolol	Increased incidence of adverse reactions	Bradycardia, dizziness, headache, drowsiness, heart block, hypotension
Reserpine	Increased incidence of adverse reactions	Peptic ulcer, bradycardia, increased parasympathomimetic activity, mental depression (abnormal irritability, frequent early morning awakening and/or nightmares)
Sulfonamides	Increased chance of a hypoglycemic reaction especially if used with oral hypoglycemics	Signs of hypoglycemia: hunger, weakness, sweating, tremors
Thiazide diuretics	Increased chance of hypoglycemic reactions especially if used with oral hypoglycemics	Signs of hypoglycemia: hunger, weakness, sweating, tremors
	Alteration of urinary elimination of uric acid	Gout-like attacks
	More troublesome orthostatic hypotension	Light-headedness, dizziness, fainting when arising from sitting or prone position
	Increased incidence of cardiac arrhythmias especially if patient is also digitalized; hypokalemia more frequent	Signs of potassium depletion: tiredness, leg cramps, muscle weakness, dehydration, constipation
Tricyclic anti-depressants	Increased incidence of anticholinergic side effects	Aggravation of glaucoma, urinary retention, dry mouth
	Increased incidence of confusion	Restlessness, agitation, sleep disturbances, disorientation, delusions, forgetfulness
Warfarin	Enhanced anticoagulant effect due to decrease in plasma protein binding	Bleeding, hemorrhage

7. Crush tablets too large to swallow and mix with small amount of applesauce.
8. Do not break open capsules that are too large to swallow, because they are very unpleasant to taste. Check if another form of the drug may be prescribed by the doctor or compounded by the pharmacist.

9. Combine bitter preparations, such as vitamin, mineral, and electrolyte preparations, with foods, such as applesauce or juice, to make medication more palatable and to prevent gastric irritation. Geriatric patient often loses tastebuds for sweetness and may perceive medication as bitter.

10. Tell patients that you are administering medication, even though it may seem to them that they are only receiving food. Patients should know when they are receiving medication.

11. Remain with patient receiving a suppository until drug is absorbed. Because of the reduced body temperature of the elderly patient, it may take longer for a suppository to melt in the bowel and vagina than in younger patients.

12. Encourage patient to retain suppository. The desire to expel the suppository may be strong because of the extended length of time needed to dissolve medication.

13. Check with doctor whether another route may be used, if patient has difficulty retaining suppository.

14. Alternate injection sites and apply a small dry sterile dressing with pressure after an injection, since the geriatric patient tends to bleed after an injection because of the loss of elasticity of tissue.

15. Avoid injection into immobile limb, if possible, because inactivity of limb will reduce rate of absorption.

16. Inspect site of injection of medication since reduction in cutaneous sensation may prevent patient being aware of pain, infection, intravasation, or other trauma.

17. Assist patient to maintain a nutritious diet to prevent dietary deficiencies, which would result in body dysfunction and may alter response to medications.

18. Assess patient for signs of fluid overload, such as dyspnea, cough, increased respirations, and edema due to cardiac and renal dysfunction, which is more common in the elderly and alters response to drugs.

19. Anticipate that if half-life of a medication is increased by deficient renal function, the drug may be administered less frequently or in smaller doses.

20. Assess and report to doctor whether a patient continues to manifest symptoms indicating need for continuous drug therapy or whether patient is compensating and may require less medication. Reduction in strength and number of medications, thereby minimizing adverse reactions and interactions, is a major goal of successful drug therapy in the aged.

21. Administer one dose of medication each day to ensure better drug compliance, unless it is essential to use divided dose schedule.

22. Request doctor to order a slower acting diuretic for the geriatric patient if the stress of a rapid acting diuretic, such as furosemide (Lasix), is causing incontinence.

23. Administer tricyclic drugs at bedtime to minimize patient experiencing dry mouth.

24. Discourage continuous use of hypnotics, since they are of little

value if taken repeatedly. Provide warm milk and backrub at bedtime, rather than medication.

25. Assess patient on insulin and oral antidiabetics for mild hypoglycemic reactions, characterized by speech disorders, confusion, and disorientation, rather than by the restlessness, tachycardia, and profuse perspiration which occur in the younger patient. Since periodic mild hypoglycemic reactions causing permanent brain damage may result from medication and patient's inability to ingest recommended dietary intake, confer with doctor regarding advisability of continued therapy.

26. Prevent drug-induced immobility since this leads to perceptual changes, dehydration, and decubitus ulcer formation.

27. Assess tongue for signs of dehydration, characterized by furrows. Turgidity or fullness of tongue indicates hydration. Since the mucous membranes of the mouth may be chronically dry because of mouth breathing, an absence of subcutaneous fat, and the presence of atropic epidermal changes that make checking for elasticity useless, assessment of the tongue is the best indication of the hydration state of the elderly patient.

28. Encourage patient to discard drugs no longer part of the medication regimen to prevent self-medication and confusion of drugs.

29. Encourage patient to confer with doctor if he/she feels that medication is no longer required rather than to discontinue treatment.

30. Monitor drug compliance very closely in patient taking more than five medications, since this increases the number of adverse reactions, and interactions. See section on *Nursing Process for Promoting Patient Compliance with Medication Regimen.*

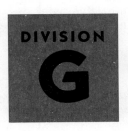

drug toxicity (untoward reactions)

OVERDOSAGE

Too large a dose of prescribed medication results in an exaggerated response. For example, if a patient becomes lethargic and drowsy from a drug administered for its tranquilizing effects, the response is caused by excessive primary action of the drug. Relative overdosage may be seen in patients who for some reason do not metabolize or excrete a particular drug rapidly enough or who are particularly sensitive to the effects of the drug. Overdosage effects can usually be controlled by reducing dosage and/or by increasing the intervals between administration.

Elderly or debilitated patients often require smaller dosages.

SIDE REACTIONS

Many drugs have other known actions besides the primary ones. The effect of these so-called secondary actions is predictable. For example, an antihistamine administered to reduce allergic manifestations causes drowsiness as a secondary or untoward reaction. This effect should be kept at a minimum in order not to interfere with the patient's normal functioning. If the drowsiness becomes excessive, the dosage of the antihistamine may have to be reduced or the physician may substitute another drug with fewer side effects.

DRUG POISONING

Drug poisoning results from a large overdose either accidental or intentional (suicide). The patient may also be excessively susceptible to the pharmacologic agent or fail to eliminate it at the normal rate because of hepatic or renal damage. Poisoning with a drug may lead to collapse and death, if the drug is not withdrawn and adequate treatment instituted. The nurse is responsible for prevention of accidents by teaching the care and storage of drugs, for observing and reporting signs of toxicity, for provision of first aid, and for providing emergency drugs and equipment needed for treatment while assisting the physician (see table of antidotes in *Appendix 3* for treatment of poisoning). Regardless of whether the poisoning is due to an attempted overdose or is accidental, the family members need emotional support at this time.

DRUG ALLERGIES (HYPERSENSITIVITY)

Allergic responses to drugs, which occur in some patients and not in others, can take many different forms. They closely resemble the more familiar types of allergies to foreign proteins.

Allergic (hypersensitivity) reactions occur when the body has been previously in contact with a particular drug (sensitization) and then, on later exposure to the same drug, has an allergic response. The response may be an *immediate reaction* involving antigen (in this case the drug or part thereof) and antibody, resulting in the release of histamine. In mild cases the reaction is limited to urticaria, wheals, and itching of the skin. In severe cases, there is an *anaphylactic reaction* characterized by circulatory collapse or asphyxia due to swelling of the larynx and occlusion of the bronchial passages. Many patients are hypersensitive to penicillin, for example. The hypersensitivity response may also be a *delayed reaction*, occurring several days or even weeks after the drug has been administered. Delayed reactions are characterized by drug fever, swelling of the joints, and reactions involving the blood-forming organs and the kidneys.

DRUG IDIOSYNCRASIES

Idiosyncratic reactions are believed to occur in patients who have an inborn inability to handle certain types of chemicals and who therefore manifest an abnormal or unusual response to the drug. The response may be excessive or unusual. For example, in some patients a tranquilizing drug causes excitement rather than sedation.

Since there is no clear distinction between delayed hypersensitivity reactions and idiosyncratic reactions, the manifestations of these untoward reactions are considered together in the following paragraphs.

GENERAL UNTOWARD REACTIONS

Dermatologic Reactions

The skin is frequently involved in drug reactions. Although all drugs may cause dermatologic disturbances in some patients, certain pharmacologic agents are more prone to do so than others (i.e., penicillin, sulfonamides, bromides, iodides, arsenic, gold, quinine, thiazides, and antimalarials).

The dermatologic manifestations may range from pruritis and mild urticaria to all types of exanthematous eruptions, maculopapular rash, angioedema, pustular eruptions, granulomas, erythema nodosum, photosensitivity reactions, and alopecia.

In general, the administration of a drug is discontinued when the patient manifests even a mild skin reaction. The most serious types of reactions are extensive urticaria, angioedema, and those accompanied by systemic manifestations.

Some of the more serious, drug-induced skin reactions are detailed below:

1. **Exfoliative Dermatitis.** An obstinate, itchy, scaling of the skin, frequently accompanied by loss of hair and nails. Initial symptoms are a patchy or erythematous eruption accompanied by fever and malaise. Gastrointestinal symptoms are noted occasionally and are possibly caused by a similar lesion of the GI epithelium. Skin color changes from pink to dark red. The characteristic flaking begins after about 1 week. The skin remains smooth and red. New scales form as the old ones peel off. Relapses occur frequently, and death occasionally occurs as a result of secondary infection.

2. **Erythema Multiforma.** An acute or subacute eruption of the skin characterized by macules, papules, wheals, vesicles, and sometimes bullae. The lesions involve mostly the distal portions of the extremities, the face, and the mucous membranes. The condition is often accompanied by generalized malaise, arthralgia, and fever. The condition may recur and each attack usually lasts 2 to 3 weeks.

   The most serious type of erythema multiforma is the *Stevens-Johnson syndrome*. The bullous, blistery rash extends to the mucosa of the mouth, pharynx, and anogenital region. The syndrome is accompanied by high fever, severe headache, stomatitis, conjunctivitis, rhinitis, urethritis, and balanitis. It is often fatal.

3. **Photosensitivity.** A wide variety of unusual skin reactions characterized by dermatitis, urticaria, erythema multiformalike lesions, and thickened and scaling patches may occur in some patients after a few minutes of exposure to sunlight.

Blood Dyscrasias

The bone marrow of certain patients is particularly sensitive to drugs. This may result in the insufficient manufacture of platelets, white blood cells, or red blood cells.

In principle, all drugs may cause blood dyscrasias in a particularly susceptible patient, but drugs such as the antineoplastics, certain antibiotics (including chloramphenicol), and phenylbutazone do so more frequently.

Patients who receive a drug that may cause bone marrow depression are monitored closely by frequent blood counts.

Some of the frequently observed blood dyscrasias are listed below.

1. **Agranulocytosis:** A complete absence of granulocytes associated with a marked reduction in circulating leukocytes is the most common blood dyscrasia to occur as an untoward effect of drug therapy. Early clinical signs are symptoms of infection, such as a sore throat, skin rash, fever, or jaundice.
2. **Aplastic Anemia:** Occurs when the bone marrow is damaged and blood-forming cells are replaced by fatty tissue. The result is pancytopenia, a reduction in all formed elements of blood. Aplastic anemia is usually fatal. Symptoms include anemia, leukopenia, and thrombocytopenia.
3. **Hemolytic Anemia:** Occurs when circulating red blood cells are destroyed either because of an antigen-antibody reaction or when a patient sensitive to certain chemicals has an idiosyncratic reaction. For instance, certain members of the black race or individuals originating from certain regions of the Mediterranean inherit a sex-linked enzyme deficiency (glucose-6-phosphate dehydrogenase) which makes their red blood cells particularly sensitive to hemolysis by certain "oxidizing" drugs (including aspirin). Ingestion of these agents may cause acute intravascular hemolysis marked by hematuria. Treatment involves withdrawal of drug.
4. **Thrombocytopenia:** Platelet deficiency may result from destruction of the circulating platelets by pharmacologic agents or by depression of the platelet-forming elements of the bone marrow. The latter is the more serious manifestation. Severe thrombocytopenia is characterized by purpura followed by hemorrhage.

Hepatotoxicity (Liver Damage)

1. **Biliary Obstruction.** Some drugs affect the lining of the bile channels, causing them to narrow. Bile may back up into the bloodstream, and the patient appears jaundiced.
2. **Hepatic Necrosis.** Drug-induced damage of liver cells characterized by nausea, vomiting, and abdominal pain followed by jaundice.

Nephrotoxicity (Kidney Damage) Drug-induced degeneration of renal tubules which may interfere with further excretion of the drug. This results in increased drug toxicity. Nephrotoxicity is characterized by hematuria, anuria, casts in urine, edema, proteinuria, and uremia.

Ototoxicity (Ear Damage) Results in damage to the vestibular and/or auditory portion of the eighth cranial nerve.

1. **Vestibular Damage.** Characterized by vertigo (sensation of turning and falling) and nystagmus (rapid, rhythmic, side-to-side movement of the eyeballs).
2. **Auditory Damage.** Characterized by tinnitus (ringing in the ears or a roaring sound) and progressive hearing loss. This effect may be caused by certain antibiotics (kanamycin, neomycin) and diuretics (ethacrynic acid, furosemide).

Central Nervous System Toxicity Such toxicity is characterized by poor motor coordination, loss of judgment, depression of consciousness, or overstimulation including convulsions. Symptoms of depression are most likely to occur with barbiturates, other sedative-hypnotics, antianxiety agents, and alcohol.

Certain drugs also interfere with the transmission of nerve impulses at the myoneural junction. This causes muscle weakness and reduced ankle and knee reflexes. Gradually this untoward reaction can lead to apnea and cardiac arrest.

Tardive dyskinesia, characterized by the impairment of the power of voluntary movement resulting in fragmentary or incomplete movements, has been observed after long-term administration of antipsychotic drugs.

Gastrointestinal Disturbances Drug-induced nausea, diarrhea, and vomiting may result from either local irritation or systemic effects.

Drug Interactions See section H.

Drug Dependence Although not exactly an untoward reaction, drug dependence may be considered one of the problems associated with the administration of drugs.

The term "drug dependence" was developed to encompass both *psychological (psychic) dependence*, that is, drive or craving to take the drug for relief of tensions, discomfort, or for pleasure, and *physical dependence*, characterized by the appearance of physical symptoms when the administration of the drug is discontinued.

Psychological Dependence May be mild or severe. In *mild dependence* the person is accustomed to taking a drug that gives him a sense of well-being; for example, caffeine in coffee or nicotine in cigarettes. Such a person is said to be habituated and will not readily give up the drug. He/she tends to feel uneasy when deprived of it. Yet, if he/she so desires it, the habituated person can usually, of his/her own accord, give up the drug without resort to professional help. In *severe dependence* the person craves the feeling that the drug provides and will use compulsive efforts to obtain the drug (e.g., the use of heroin or amphetamines). Severe psychological dependence on drugs seems to occur in people who, once having experienced a feeling from a drug that is particularly satisfying, will continue to compulsively seek out the drug. Nurses should note patients who are asking for drugs more frequently than most patients with similar conditions. The names of such patients should be brought to the attention of the physician.

Physical Dependence The continued ingestion of certain drugs (narcotics and depressants) results in an alteration in the body such that the drug is now required for the individual to function "normally." This is referred to as physical dependence. Discontinuation of a drug on which the patient is physically dependent may lead to *withdrawal symptoms*. These may vary with the particular drug. The withdrawal from narcotics results in increased autonomic nervous system activity and increased central nervous system (CNS) excitability (see general statement on *Narcotics*, page 352). Withdrawal from depressants (barbiturates, sedative-hypnotics, antianxiety agents) also results in increased excitability of certain regions of the CNS, notably those controlling motor and mental functions. The patient becomes tremulous and may suffer grand mal seizures, confusion, disorientation, and psychotic reactions.

Drugs in Pregnancy
Most of the drugs taken by a pregnant woman pass the placental barrier and may affect the embryo and fetus. The embryo appears to be particularly sensitive to the effect of drugs during the first trimester of pregnancy when organogenesis is occurring.

As a rule, a woman who is pregnant or attempting to become pregnant should not take any *pharmacologic agent* unless specifically so ordered, or permitted, by her physician.

Thus, *all drugs are contraindicated in pregnancy unless the benefit derived outweighs the risk of fetal malformation.*

This warning also applies to over-the-counter drugs, and the nurse should explain this to pregnant patients.

Drugs in Childhood
The safe use of many of the newer pharmacologic agents in childhood has not yet been established. In case of doubt, it is wise to ask the physician whether a particular agent is suitable for pediatric patients.

Pediatric dosage is listed whenever relevant and/or available. The pediatric dosage can also be computed from the adult dosage by means of Young's, Clark's, or Fried's rules (see *Division L*, pp. 45–48).

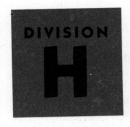

drug interactions: general considerations

Because many patients now receive more than one pharmacologic agent, drug interactions are a potentially major clinical problem. Indeed, in addition to having their intended, specific therapeutic effect, drugs may also influence other physiological systems. The likelihood is high that two concomitantly administered agents influence some of the same pathways.

In most cases it is nevertheless possible to administer two interacting agents concurrently, provided that certain precautions, such as dosage adjustments, are taken. Moreover, drug interactions are not always adverse. They are sometimes taken advantage of therapeutically. For example, probenecid may be administered with penicillin to decrease the excretion rate of the penicillin and therefore result in higher blood levels.

The study of drug interactions is rapidly becoming a complex subspeciality of pharmacology. An attempt has been made throughout the text to reduce the complex explanation of drug interactions to the simplest possible terms.

A brief review of the major mechanisms that give rise to drug interactions are reviewed in this section. This may enable the nurse to anticipate similar situations with other drug combinations.

It is important to remember that interactions apply not only to the intended therapeutic action of the drugs but also to their side effects.

It is also to be noted that the drug does not have to be a prescription one. Salicylates (aspirin) are an important interactant, as are common cathartics and constipating agents. Beverages like alcohol, and foods like tyramine-rich cheese may also play an important role.

Drug interactions often require an adjustment in dosage of one or both agents or discontinuation of one. Common major drug interactions are summarized alphabetically by drug in the Appendix, Section 4.

DRUGS WITH OPPOSING PHARMACOLOGIC EFFECTS

The therapeutic effects of either or both agents may be cancelled, decreased, or abolished. An example is the combination of pilocarpine, a cholinergic drug prescribed for glaucoma, and an anticholinergic or atropine-like drug.

The interaction is usually described as "decreased effect" in the text. Correction could involve administration of only one agent, adjustment in time of administration, or increase in dosage of one or both agents.

SIMILAR PHARMACOLOGIC EFFECTS

When two drugs have similar pharmacologic effects, their combined use may result in an effect equal to or even larger than the sum of that obtained if either agent were used separately. This interaction is described as "increased effect." The terms "additive," or "potentiation," might also be used to describe this interaction. An example of this interaction is the concomitant use of agents with CNS depressant actions such as alcohol, antianxiety agents, hypnotics, and antihistamines.

CHANGE IN THE AMOUNT OF AVAILABLE DRUG

Change in Absorption from the GI Tract

The absorption of most drugs from the stomach or GI tract is pH dependent. The concomitant use of an agent that alters the pH can change the rate of absorption, and thus either increase (↑) the effect or decrease (↓) the effect of the drug.

For example, the use of antacids that increase the pH of the stomach will result in a decrease in the absorption of aspirin, which is more rapidly absorbed at a lower pH.

The absorption of drugs is also affected by how long they reside in the GI tract. Drugs that affect the motility of the GI tract also affect drug absorption. The net effect of a cathartic usually is decreased absorption [decreased (↓) effect] since the drug to be absorbed in the GI tract stays there for a shorter period of time. Constipating agents, on the other hand, often result in increased absorption [increased (↑) effect].

The presence of food may also affect the absorption of drugs from the GI tract. For example, the absorption of tetracyclines is inhibited in the presence of dairy products (e.g., milk, cheese) since the calcium present in such foods complexes with the drug.

Alteration of Urinary Excretion

Closely related to the rate at which drugs are absorbed from the GI tract is the rate at which they are eliminated in the urine or reabsorbed from the glomerular filtrate. Drugs that are eliminated more slowly because of another concomitantly administered agent stay in the body longer; thus the effect of the drug is increased.

Drugs that are eliminated faster, or are reabsorbed less, because of another concomitantly administered agent result in a decrease in the effect of the drug.

As in the case of absorption from the GI tract, elimination by the kidney is pH dependent. The pH of the urine is sometimes altered purposely by the administration of an alkalinizing agent (sodium bicarbonate) or an acidifying agent (ammonium chloride). Whether a drug will be excreted faster or more slowly with a change in pH depends on the drug. The alkalinization of the urine, for example, is sometimes taken advantage of with drugs like the sulfonamides. These agents are more soluble at a higher pH, and thus the possibility of crystallization in the kidney is reduced.

DISPLACEMENT OF DRUGS FROM PROTEIN-BINDING SITE

Several types of drugs bind to plasma protein. The resulting protein-bound drug is less active than the free drug.

Protein binding is considered when dosage is established so that a given amount of drug will have the desired pharmacologic effect. This relationship however, may be altered when another agent, which also binds to protein, is added to the therapy. If the attraction of drug B for the protein is greater than that of drug A, drug A will be displaced (or released) from the protein-binding site. This, then, will result in a greater amount of drug A available, and thus the effect of drug A will be increased. One such example is the coumarin-type anticoagulants, which are bound to protein but can be displaced by a variety of agents. A greater than expected amount of anticoagulant can have severe effects, including fatal hemorrhages.

CHANGES IN DRUG METABOLISM

1. Most drugs are degraded in the liver by specific enzymes (drug-metabolizing enzymes). A change in the activity of an enzyme results in a change in the availability of the drug. Often such an interaction results in inhibition of the enzyme and hence longer bioavailability (increased effect) of the drug.

   However, certain drugs may stimulate the activity of enzymes involved in the breakdown of another pharmacologic agent. The barbiturates, for example, appear to stimulate certain drug-metabolizing enzymes in the liver. This results in a more rapid disappearance of the drugs normally degraded by such enzymes (e.g., steroid hormones including estrogen and progesterone, and coumarin-type anticoagulants).

2. The pharmacologic mode of action of certain drugs, such as the monoamine oxidase (MAO) inhibitors or disulfiram, consists of inhibiting a particular enzyme. An interaction may occur when this inhibited enzyme system is called upon to degrade another drug or food product.

   For example, the above mechanism plays a role in the much publicized interaction of the MAO inhibitors and tyramine-rich foods like cheese. The tyramine cannot be degraded (as usual) by monoamine oxidase since the enzyme is inhibited. Tyramine accumulates and may cause severe hypertension.

   Such an interaction is also taken advantage of in the treatment of alcoholics with disulfiram (Antabuse). The latter interferes with the metabolism of alcohol, leading to the accumulation of acetaldehyde, which has such unpleasant physiological effects that the patient will refrain from alcohol ingestion while on disulfiram.

ALTERATION OF ELECTROLYTE LEVELS

Drugs that promote the loss (e.g., potassium) or retention (e.g., calcium) of electrolytes may cause the heart to become particularly sensitive to the toxic effects of digitalis. Such an interaction has been noted in the concomitant use of thiazide diuretics (which cause potassium loss) and digitalis.

ALTERATION OF GASTROINTESTINAL FLORA

Antibiotics and other antimicrobial agents often kill the intestinal flora that synthesize vitamin K. A decrease in vitamin K concentration, which is involved in blood coagulation, increases the effect of anticoagulants and may result in hemorrhage.

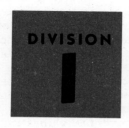

DIVISION
I

laboratory test interferences

Laboratory tests play a crucial role in diagnosis and medical care. During drug therapy, they are used to monitor the therapeutic efficacy and the side effects of a particular drug. Such tests may or may not be related to the condition for which the drug is prescribed. Thus, penicillins given for an infection may affect the urine glucose determination performed for other reasons.

Drugs, however, can also interfere with the actual measurement on which the diagnostic test is based (methodological interference). Such interferences may result in false positive (false +) or abnormally high (↑) values, as well as false negative (false −) or abnormally low (↓) values. It is often difficult to distinguish between the real changes due to the therapeutic agent and interference with the method itself. Furthermore, since a particular drug may affect one method of performing a given laboratory procedure and not another, it is important to consider the specific testing method used in each particular instance.

The interference with laboratory tests can be subdivided as follows:

Physical Interference For example, coloration of urine is affected by the excretion of a drug or its metabolite, which, in turn, may mask abnormal colors contributed by bile, blood or porphyrins, and interfere with tests based on fluorometric, colorimetric and photometric determinations. For example, tetracyclines interfere with the fluorometric methods for porphyrin determination.

Biological Interferences For example, the drug or its metabolites may stimulate or suppress the enzyme system on which the test is based.

Chemical Interference For example, there may be interference with the oxidation-reduction reactions that are the basis of Benedict's urinary glucose tests.

Most laboratory interferences give rise to false positive results. Altered liver function tests often are grouped together, and they may include one or several of the following: *False + or ↑ values* —serum alkaline phosphatase, serum bilirubin (icterus index), serum BSP, serum cephalin flocculation, SGOT, SGPT, thymol turbidity, urinary bilirubin. *False − or ↓ values* —blood glucose and serum cholesterol. Most methodological errors can be avoided when tests are performed on a sample taken 12 to 24 hours after withholding all medication or food, or by switching to another test. However, this is not always possible. There also still is some inconsistency in the reports by experts on the effects of various drugs on laboratory tests. Therefore, the listings of *Laboratory Test Interferences* should be used only as a general guide.

As in the case of the drug interactions, laboratory tests may be affected by all the drugs a patient is taking, including non-prescription agents.

The agents that most often interfere with laboratory test values are: the *anticoagulants, anticonvulsants, antihypertensives, antiinfectives, oral hyperglycemics, hormones,* and *central nervous system drugs.*

The uncovering of laboratory test interferences is a relatively new field, and new "errors" are constantly being discovered. A few of the major interferences are listed in section 5 of the appendix. Some of the better known *Laboratory Test Interferences* are listed in the specific drug entries either as part of the *Nursing Implications* or as separate entries.

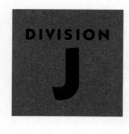

DIVISION J

nursing process for promoting compliance with medication regimen

ASSESSMENT

Assess patient's personality, personal motivation, experiential background, ability to learn, and willingness to change by examining four factors influencing teaching and learning.

1. **Physical.** Appraise weakness, immobility.
2. **Psychological.** Discuss understanding and acceptance of condition and therapy.
3. **Socio-cultural.** Explore priorities and values, class, life style.
4. **Environmental.** Evaluate physical surroundings, family members.

PLANNING

Use assessment in all planning to promote drug compliance.

1. Set up mutually agreed goals with the patient. For example, the doctor's order is for Lente Insulin 30 units o.d. before breakfast. A mutual goal might be for the patient to be able to administer his/her own insulin.
2. Develop a teaching plan to promote compliance.
   a. Identify behavioral objectives for the teaching-learning process. State what the patient should be able to do after the teaching-learning process. For example, after the teaching-learning process the patient will be able to administer insulin to himself/herself.
   b. Select appropriate methodology for teaching and promoting compliance (e.g., one-to-one, lecture discussion, movies, slides).

IMPLEMENTATION

1. *Do Not Rush Patient.* Allow patient to learn at his/her rate.
2. Select an area without distractions where teaching can be effective.
3. Emphasize the reward of maintained health status or improved health status to be achieved by taking medications as ordered, since motivation is of primary importance in achieving drug compliance.

4. Provide patient with clear, simple verbal and written directions. (Written directions must be large enough to be legible for patient.)
5. Provide clear, legible cards with information about name of drug, reason for use, untoward reactions, dosage, frequency of administration, and appropriate action to be taken for untoward reaction.
6. Provide a checkoff calendar for patient indicating day and time medication is to be taken.
7. Encourage patient to associate taking medication with daily events; for example, medication after meals.
8. Provide small containers and label for hours of day patient is to take medications. Teach patient to stock each container with appropriate medication once a day so that he/she will have medications organized for the entire day. This technique is particularly helpful for patients with poor memory.
9. Provide containers for each day of the week, and put in medications to be taken on specific days for patient who has difficulty organizing or handling medications.
10. Arrange for financial assistance if patient is financially unable to purchase medication or equipment needed.
11. Use equipment that may be easily purchased and replaced.
12. Use equipment that is easy to handle and adaptable to home use.
13. Note number of tablets/capsules or amount of solution that patient receives from pharmacist.
14. Teach technique for administration of medication.
15. Observe return demonstration by patient. Preferably, a family member or significant other person should be present during this return demonstration.
16. Include a family member or significant other person as part of the support system for helping a patient achieve compliance with a medical regimen.

EVALUATION

1. At regular intervals, arrange patient follow-up.
   a. Observe patient for attitude toward self, illness, and medication regimen.
   b. Listen to verbalization regarding compliance.
   c. Assess for possible therapeutic effects.
   d. Assess for possible untoward reactions.
   e. Count number of tablets/capsules or amount of solution remaining and compare to original amount issued to ascertain correct usage.
   f. Observe a return demonstration by patient. Preferably have a family member or significant other person present at this return demonstration.
2. Praise patient for compliance with medication regimen when success is demonstrated.
3. Refer to a home health agency, for further intervention by a community health nurse, those clients who appear to lack motivation or ability to carry out regimen as prescribed.

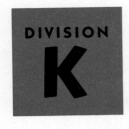

DIVISION K
commonly used approximate equivalents

VOLUME

Metric	Apothecary	Household	Sign
1 ml	15 minims		
4 ml	1 dram	1 scant teaspoon	ℨ
5 ml	1¼ drams	1 teaspoon	
15 ml	4 fluid drams	1 tablespoon	
30 ml	1 fluid ounce	2 tablespoons	℥
250 ml	8 fluid ounces	1 measuring cup (240 ml)	
500 ml	1 pint		
1000 ml	1 quart (32 ounces)		

WEIGHT

Metric	Apothecary
1000 μg = 1 mg	1/65 grain
65 mg	1 grain
1 gm	15.4 grains
4 gm	60 grains (1 dram) (approximate)
29.5 gm	1 ounce
1000 gm = 1 kg	2.2 pounds

RULES FOR CONVERSION OF CENTIGRADE AND FAHRENHEIT

To convert Centigrade to Fahrenheit:

$$\frac{9 \times C}{5} + 32 = F$$

To convert Fahrenheit to Centigrade:

$$(F - 32) \times 5/9 = C$$

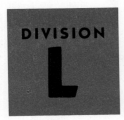
formulas for calculating dosage for administration of medications and IV flow rate

1. $$\frac{D \text{ (dose required)}}{X \text{ (units to be administered)}} = \frac{H \text{ (dose available)}}{\text{(no. units containing dose available)}}$$

Example: The physician orders 16 mg of elixir of phenobarbital. The dose on hand is 4 mg/4 ml. How many millimeters should be administered?

$$\frac{16}{X} = \frac{4}{4}$$
$$4X = 64$$
$$X = 16 \qquad \text{Ans. 16 ml}$$

Example: The physician orders prednisone 20 mg. The tablets on hand are 5 mg each. How many tablets should be administered?

$$\frac{20}{X} = \frac{5}{1}$$
$$5X = 20$$
$$X = 4 \qquad \text{Ans. 4 tablets}$$

2. *Clark's rule* used for computation of pediatric dosage:

$$\frac{\text{Weight in pounds} \times \text{adult dose}}{150} = \text{safe dosage for individual child}$$

3. *Fried's rule* used for computation of pediatric dosage for infant or child up to 2 years of age:

$$\frac{\text{Child's age in months} \times \text{adult dose}}{150} = \frac{\text{safe dosage for individual}}{\text{infant or child}}$$

4. *Young's rule* used for computation of pediatric dosage for child over 2 years of age:

$$\frac{\text{Age in years} \times \text{adult dose}}{\text{Age in years} + 12} = \text{safe dosage for child}$$

TABLE 2 BODY SURFACE AREA OF ADULTS*

Nomogram for determination of body surface area from height and weight

Height	*Body surface area*	*Weight*

Source: From the formula of Du Bois and Du Bois, *Arch. intern. Med.*, **17**, 863 (1916):
$S = W^{0.425} \times H^{0.725} \times 71.84$, or $\log S = \log W \times 0.425 + \log H \times 0.725 + 1.8564$
(S = body surface in cm², W = weight in kg, H = height in cm).
Reproduced from Documenta Geigy Scientific Tables, 7th Edition.
Courtesy CIBA-GEIGY Limited, Basle, Switzerland

* A straight edge is placed from the patient's height in the left column to his/her weight in the right column and this intersect on the body surface area column indicates his/her body surface area.

TABLE 3 BODY SURFACE AREA OF CHILDREN*

Nomogram for determination of body surface area from height and weight

Source: From the formula of Du Bois and Du Bois, *Arch. intern. Med.*, **17**, 863 (1916):
$S = W^{0.425} \times H^{0.725} \times 71.84$, or $\log S = \log W \times 0.425 + \log H \times 0.725 + 1.8564$
(S = body surface in cm², W = weight in kg, H = height in cm).
Reproduced from Documenta Geigy Scientific Tables, 7th Edition.
Courtesy CIBA-GEIGY Limited, Basle, Switzerland

* A straight edge is placed from the patient's height in the left column to his/her weight in the right column and this intersect on the body surface area column indicates his/her body surface area.

5. Formula using *Surface Area of Child* (see Table 3, p. 47) for computation of pediatric dosage for child:

$$\frac{\text{Surface area of child (in square meters)} \times \text{adult dose}}{1.7} = \text{safe dosage for individual child}$$

6. Formula based on *Recommended Pediatric Dosage per Kilogram of Body Weight:*

    Milligrams × kilograms of child's body weight = safe dosage for 24 hour

Example: John weighs 88 lb. The recommended pediatric dosage for Chlor-trimeton is 2 mg/kg/24 hr. What would be a safe dose for John for the total 24 hours?

    88 lb/2.2 lb/kg = 40 kg
    40 kg × 2 mg/kg = 80 mg = safe dosage for 24 hours for John

Total doses for 24 hours are to be divided and administered at appropriate intervals as indicated by the physician.

Note: Safe dosage for adrenal steroids, digitalis, and antineoplastics are not computed by mg/kg/24 hr since these drugs have a wide dosage range and specialized usage.

7. Formula for calculation of IV flow rate:

$$\frac{\text{Total volume infused} \times \text{drops/ml}}{\text{Total time for infusion in minutes}} = \text{drops/minute}$$

Check the directions with the IV set for the number of drops/ml it delivers because different brands and types vary.

Example: The order reads, "Give 240 ml of 5% D/W in 4 hours." What would be the rate of flow?

    The directions on the set indicate that the number of drops/ml is 15.

$$X = \frac{240 \times 15}{4 \times 60}$$
$$X = \frac{60 \times 1}{1 \times 4}$$
$$X = 15$$

Ans. The rate of flow = 15 drops/minute

Example: The order reads, "Ampicillin 0.5 gm IV." After adding the reconstituted Ampicillin, the Volutrol chamber has 30 ml of fluid. Directions on the ampicillin vial indicate that the medication must be given in 1 hour. What would the rate of flow be for this medication to be received in one hour?

$$X = \frac{30 \times 60}{1 \times 60}$$
$$X = 30$$

Ans. The rate of flow = 30 drops/minute

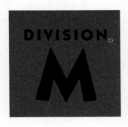

DIVISION M

commonly used abbreviations

aa	of each	o.n.	every night
a.c.	before meals	O.S.	left eye
ad lib.	freely, as desired	os	mouth
b.i.d.	two times a day	oz	ounce
c̄	with	p.c.	after meals
caps.	capsule	PO	by mouth
d.	day	PR	by rectum
dr.	dram	PRN	when required
elix.	elixir	q	every
ext.	extract	q.d.	every day
gm	gram	q.h.	every hour
gr.	grain	q.i.d.	four times daily
gtt	a drop	q.o.d.	every other day
hr	hour	q.s.	as much as required
h.s.	hour of sleep, bedtime	s.	without
IM	intramuscular	SC	subcutaneous
IV	intravenous	s.o.s.	one dose if necessary
m.	minim	sp.	spirits
mcg or μg	microgram	ss	one-half
mEq	milliequivalent	stat	immediately
ml	milliliter	tab.	tablet
o.d.	every day	t.i.d.	three times a day
O.D.	right eye	tr.,	tinct., tincture
o.h.	every hour	ung.	ointment

PART TWO

1

ANTI-INFECTIVES

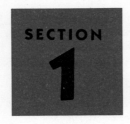

SECTION 1
antibiotics

Penicillins	Amoxicillin	Oxacillin Sodium
	Ampicillin	Penicillin G Benzathine, Oral
	Ampicillin Sodium	Penicillin G, Benzathine and Procaine
	Carbenicillin Disodium	Sterile Penicillin G Benzathine
	Carbenicillin Indanyl Sodium	Suspension
	Cloxacillin Sodium Monohydrate	Penicillin G Potassium
	Dicloxacillin Sodium Monohydrate	Penicillin G Sodium
	Hetacillin	Penicillin G, Procaine, Aqueous
	Hetacillin Potassium	Phenoxymethyl Penicillin
	Methicillin Sodium	Phenoxymethyl Penicillin Potassium
	Nafcillin Sodium	Ticarcillin Disodium
Erythromycins	Erythromycin	Erythromycin Gluceptate
	Erythromycin Estolate	Erythromycin Lactobionate
	Erythromycin Ethylsuccinate	Erythromycin Stearate
Tetracyclines	Chlortetracycline Hydrochloride	Oxytetracycline
	Demeclocycline Hydrochloride	Oxytetracycline Calcium
	Doxycycline Hyclate	Oxytetracycline Hydrochloride
	Doxycycline Monohydrate	Tetracycline
	Methacycline Hydrochloride	Tetracycline Hydrochloride
	Minocycline Hydrochloride	Tetracycline Phosphate Complex
Cephalosporins	Cefaclor	Cephaloglycin Dihydrate
	Cefadroxil Monohydrate	Cephaloridine
	Cefamandole Nafate	Cephalothin Sodium
	Cefazolin Sodium	Cephapirin Sodium
	Cefoxitin Sodium	Cephradine
	Cephalexin	
Chloramphenicol and Derivatives	Chloramphenicol	Chloramphenicol Sodium Succinate
	Chloramphenicol Palmitate	
Clindamycin and Lincomycin	Clindamycin Hydrochloride Hydrate	Clindamycin Phosphate
	Clindamycin Palmitate Hydrochloride	Lincomycin Hydrochloride Monohydrate
Polymyxins	Colistimethate Sodium	Polymyxin B Sulfate
	Colistin Sulfate	
Aminoglycosides	Amikacin Sulfate	Neomycin Sulfate
	Gentamycin Sulfate	Streptomycin Sulfate
	Kanamycin	Tobramycin Sulfate
Miscellaneous Antibiotics	Bacitracin	Spectinomycin Hydrochloride
	Novobiocin Calcium	Pentahydrate
	Novobiocin Sodium	Troleandomycin
	Paromomycin Sulfate	Vancomycin Hydrochloride

General Statement Originally, all antibiotics were chemical substances produced by microorganisms (bacteria, fungi) that suppress the growth of, and often kill, other microorganisms. Today, many antibiotics are either partially or entirely prepared synthetically.

Antibiotics interfere with the metabolism of the infectious agent. In particular, the antibiotics interfere with protein synthesis and/or formation of the cell wall of microorganisms.

Antibiotics vary in their effectiveness. Some affect only a few types of microorganisms. They are referred to as narrow-spectrum antibiotics; others affect many different types of microorganisms and are called broad-spectrum antibiotics.

Antibiotics also vary in potency. Some are bacteriostatic, that is, they only inhibit the growth of an infectious agent. Others are bactericidal and kill the infectious agent outright. The bacteriostatic or bactericidal action of a particular agent is also affected by its concentration at the site of infection.

Uses Antibiotics, as a group, are effective against most bacterial pathogens, as well as against some of the rickettsias and a few of the larger viruses. They are ineffective against viruses that cause influenza, hepatitis, and the common cold.

The choice of the antibiotic depends on the nature of the illness to be treated, the sensitivity of the infecting agent, and the patient's previous experience with the drug. Hypersensitivity and allergic reactions (see p. 32) may preclude the use of the agent of choice.

In addition to their use in acute infections, antibiotics are given prophylactically in the following instances:

1. To protect persons exposed to a known specific organism.
2. To prevent secondary bacterial infections in acutely ill individuals suffering from infections unresponsive to antibiotics.
3. To reduce risk of infection in patients suffering from various chronic illnesses.
4. To inhibit spread of infection from a clearly defined focus—as after accidents or surgery.
5. To "sterilize" the bowel, or other areas of the body in preparation for extensive surgery.

Instead of using a single agent, the physician may sometimes prefer to prescribe a combination of antibiotics.

Contraindications Hypersensitivity reactions to certain antibiotics are common and may preclude the use of a particular agent.

Untoward Reactions The antibiotics have few direct toxic effects. Kidney and liver damage, deafness, and blood dyscrasias are occasionally observed.

The following undesirable manifestations, however, occur frequently.

1. Antibiotic therapy often suppresses the normal flora of the body, which in turn keeps certain pathogenic microorganisms, such as

Candida albicans, *Proteus*, or *Pseudomonas* from causing infections. If the flora is altered, *superinfections* (monilial vaginitis, enteritis, urinary tract infections), which necessitate the discontinuation of therapy or use of other antibiotics, can result.

2. Incomplete eradication of an infectious organism. Casual use of these agents also favors the emergence of *resistant* strains insensitive to a particular drug. Resistant strains often are either mutants of the original infectious agents that have developed a slightly different metabolic pathway and can exist in spite of the antibiotic, or are variants that have developed the ability to release a chemical substance—for instance, the enzyme penicillinase—which can destroy the antibiotic.

In order to minimize the chances for the development of resistant strains, antibiotics are usually given for a prescribed length of time after acute symptoms have subsided. Casual use of antibiotics is discouraged for the same reasons.

Laboratory Tests   The bacteriological sensitivity of the infectious organism to the antibiotic should be tested by the laboratory prior to the initiation of therapy and during treatment.

Administration/ Storage

1. Check expiration date on container.
2. Check for recommended method of storage for the drug and store accordingly.
3. Clearly mark the date of dilution and strength of solutions of all drugs. Note the length of time that the drug may be stored after dilution.
4. Complete the administration of antibiotics by volutrol before the drug loses potency.

Nursing Implications

1. Check with patient to determine if he/she has had an allergic reaction to the antibiotic in the past.
2. Report any history of allergy to an antibiotic to the physician. Conspicuously mark the chart and the patient's bed railing, and notify the patient that he/she is not to have the drug at any future time unless the doctor specifically allows him/her to do so after having reviewed history of allergic reaction to the drug.
3. Observe all patients after administration of antibiotics for an allergic reaction such as anaphylactic shock, skin rash, or urticaria. Report a reaction of this type immediately to the physician.
4. Have oxygen and epinephrine immediately available for use in case of an allergic reaction.
5. Withhold drug and check with doctor when two or more antibiotics that cause similar toxic reactions, such as neuro- or nephrotoxicity, are ordered for a patient.
6. Observe patient for therapeutic response, such as reduction of fever, increased appetite, and increased sense of well-being.
7. Observe the patient for superinfections, particularly those fungal in nature, demonstrated by black furred tongue, nausea, and diarrhea.

8. Emphasize to patient that the prescribed course of therapy must be completed even after discharge from hospital and even if he/she is feeling well.
9. Teach the patient that antibiotics should be used only with medical supervision and that antibiotics remaining after the course of therapy has been completed should be discarded.
10. Ensure that the order for an antibiotic is reviewed by medical supervision at least every 5 to 7 days and have the order either renewed or cancelled.
11. Antibiotic effectiveness depends on maintaining adequate blood levels. Space the time of drug administration evenly throughout each 24 hours (e.g., t.i.d. means every 8 hours around the clock).

PENICILLINS

General Statement
These antibiotic substances were originally produced by the penicillium mold. These penicillins were acid-sensitive and could be destroyed in the stomach. Penicillin is maximally active at the pH of blood.

Today, many semisynthetic penicillins are available. These have the advantage of being resistant to penicillinase, an enzyme produced by certain bacteria that destroys penicillin, and are effective after oral administration.

Depending on the concentration of the drug, penicillin is either bacteriostatic or bactericidal.

Penicillin interferes with the formation of the bacterial cell wall. The drug is most effective against young, rapidly dividing organisms and has little effect on mature resting cells.

Penicillin is distributed throughout most of the body and passes the placental barrier. It also passes into synovial, pleural, pericardial, intraperitoneal, and spinal fluids and into the fluids of the eye. Although normal meninges are relatively impermeable to penicillin, the drug is better absorbed by inflamed meninges.

The renal, cardiac, and hematopoietic function, as well as the electrolyte balance, of patients receiving penicillin should be monitored at regular intervals.

Uses
Penicillins are used for pneumonia, meningitis, gonorrhea, otitis media, sinus infections, urinary tract infections, beta-hemolytic streptococcus infections, syphilis, anthrax, yaws, diphtheria, gas gangrene, tetanus, rat-bite fever, and Vincent's stomatitis, and as a prophylactic for patients with rheumatic fever.

Contraindications
Hypersensitivity to penicillin and cephalosporin. To be used with caution in patients with a history of asthma, hayfever, or urticaria.

Untoward Reactions
Penicillins are potent sensitizing agents, and it is estimated that 15% of the American population is presently allergic to the antibiotic. Hypersensitivity reactions are reported to be on the increase in pediatric practice.

Parenteral injection of penicillin is more hazardous than oral administration. Sensitivity onset is often delayed in that patients may have been able to take penicillin for years before allergic reactions develop.

Allergic reactions are characterized by skin rashes, acute exfoliative dermatitis, exudative erythema multiforma, eosinophilia, fever, joint pains, and pruritus. Reactions may be *immediate* (within 20 minutes) or *delayed* (as long as days or weeks after initiation of therapy).

More severe reactions include angioedema, serum sickness, anaphylaxis, Arthus phenomenon (local edema, severe inflammation, swelling, redness, pain, and necrosis after injection of sensitizing agent) and Stevens-Johnson syndrome.

For **emergency treatment** of severe allergic or anaphylactic reactions, epinephrine (0.3–0.5 ml of a 1:1000 sol. SC or IM or 0.2–0.3 ml diluted in 10 ml saline, given slowly by IV), corticosteroids, and other supplies should be on hand.

Kidney damage has been observed after penicillin administration. Except for methicillin, the manifestation is a sensitization reaction. Clinical manifestations may include proteinuria, hematuria, fever, eosinophilia, and acute renal failure. Pyuria has been observed occasionally. Symptoms usually disappear when the drug is stopped, but fatalities have been reported.

Massive IV doses of penicillin G potassium can cause hyperkalemia.

In those instances where penicillin is the drug of choice, the physician may decide to use it even though the patient is allergic, adding medication to the regimen to control the allergic response.

Other untoward reactions may include pain, sterile abcesses, phlebitis and thrombophlebitis near injection site, and superinfections.

Drug Interactions	*Interactant*	*Interaction*
	Antacids	↓ Effect of penicillins due to ↓ absorption form GI tract
	Antibiotics Chloramphenicol Erythromycins Neomycin Tetracyclines	↓ Effect of penicillins
	Anticoagulants	Penicillins may potentiate pharmacologic effect
	Aspirin	↑ Effect of penicillins by ↓ plasma protein binding
	Phenylbutazone	↑ Effect of penicillins by ↓ plasma protein binding
	Probenecid	↑ Effect penicillins by ↓ excretion

Laboratory Test Interference   Massive Doses: False + or ↑ urinary glucose, protein and turbidity.

Dosage   Penicillin is available for oral, parenteral, inhalation, and intrathecal administration. Dosages for individual drugs are given in drug entries.

Long-acting preparations are frequently used.

Oral doses must be higher than IM or SC because a large fraction of penicillin given orally may be destroyed in the stomach.

Administration Intramuscular and intravenous administration of penicillin causes a great deal of local irritation. These antibiotics are thus injected slowly.

IM injections are made deeply into the gluteal muscle. IV injections are usually made over a period of 5 to 10 minutes through the tubing of an IV infusion.

The penicillins (diluted with additional diluent) are also given by IV drip at a rate of 100 to 150 drops a minute.

Nursing Implications Also see *Nursing Implications* under general statement for *Antibiotics*, page 56.

1. Observe for allergic reactions and have epinephrine and oxygen available.
2. Anticipate that allergic reactions are most common in patients with history of asthma, hayfever, or atopic dermatitis.
3. Observe for superinfections.
4. Administer oral penicillin on an empty stomach because food inhibits absorption of drug. It should be given 1 hour before meals or 2 to 3 hours after meals.
5. Do not administer long-acting type of penicillin intravenously.
6. Do not massage repository (long-acting) types of penicillin after injection.
7. Teach the patient that he/she must return for repository penicillin injections.
8. Teach the patient to finish the entire prescribed course of treatment even though he may feel well.
9. Teach the patient to refrain from self-medication with leftover antibiotics.
10. Treatment with penicillin should continue until all the medication prescribed by the physician is gone unless the physician specifically stops the medication.
11. Treatment of patients with alpha-hemolytic strep should be continued with penicillin for a minimum of 10 days in order to prevent development of acute rheumatic fever or glomerulonephritis.

AMOXICILLIN AMOXIL, LAROTID, POLYMOX, ROBAMAX, SUMOX, TRIMOX, UTIMOX, VAN-MOX, WYMOX

Remarks Semisynthetic penicillin closely related to ampicillin. Drug is destroyed by penicillinase and does not offer any great advantage over penicillin G. Amoxicillin is acid resistant and 50% to 80% of oral dose is absorbed from the GI tract. Peak serum levels are reached 2 hours after oral administration.

Additional Uses Genitourinary tract infections. Respiratory infections by *H. influenzae*. Skin and soft tissue infections by nonpenicillinase-producing organisms.

Dosage **PO only:** 250–500 mg q 8 hr; **pediatric under 20 kg:** 20–40 (or more) mg/kg, daily in 3 equal doses. *Gonorrhea:* 3 gm, as single dose.

Administration/ Storage Dry powder is stable at room temperature for 18 to 30 months. Reconstituted suspension is stable for 1 week at room temperature and for 2 weeks at 2°–8° C.

AMPICILLIN A-CILLIN, AMCILL, OMNIPEN, PENBRITIN, PENSYN, POLYCILLIN, PRINCIPEN, SK-AMPICILLIN, TOTACILLIN, OTHERS

AMPICILLIN SODIUM AMCILL-S, OMNIPEN-N, PEN A/N, PENBRITIN-S, POLYCILLIN-N, PRINCIPEN/N, SK-AMPICILLIN-N, TOTACILLIN-N, OTHERS

Remarks Synthetic, broad-spectrum antibiotic suitable for gram-negative bacteria. Acid resistant, destroyed by penicillinase. Absorbed more slowly than other penicillins.

Additional Uses Infections of respiratory, GI, and genitourinary tract caused by *Shigella, Salmonella, E. coli, H. influenzae, Proteus* strains, and *Enterococcus.* Also, otitis media in children, bronchitis, meningitis, rat-bite fever, and whooping cough.

Dosage **Ampicillin, PO; Ampicillin Sodium, IV, IM.** *Respiratory tract and soft tissue infections,* **IM, IV, body weight 40 kg or more:** 250–500 mg q 6 hr; **less than 40 kg:** 25–50 mg/kg/day in equally divided doses. **PO, 20 kg or more:** 250 mg q 6 hr; **less than 20 kg:** 50 mg/kg/day in equally divided doses. *Gastrointestinal and genitourinary tracts,* **IV, IM, body weight of 40 kg or more:** 500 mg q 6 hr; **less than 40 kg:** 50 mg/kg/day in equally divided doses. **PO, 20 kg or more:** 500 mg q 6 hr; **less than 20 kg:** 100 mg/kg/day in equally divided doses. *Urethritis (due to gonorrhea),* **IM, IV,** 2 doses of 500 mg each at intervals of 8 to 12 hr; may be repeated. **PO:** 3.5 gm with 1 gm probenecid (given SC) simultaneously as a single dose. *Bacterial meningitis,* **IM and/or IV, adults and children:** 150–200 mg/kg/day in divided doses q 3 to 4 hr. *Septicemia,* **adults and children:** 150–200 mg/kg/day, IV for first three days, then IM q 3 to 4 hr.

Administration/ Storage
1. After reconstitution for IM or direct IV administration, the solution of sodium ampicillin must be used within the hour.
2. IV injections of reconstituted sodium ampicillin should be given slowly; 2 ml should be given over a period of at least 3 to 5 minutes.
3. Administration by IV drip: original solution reconstituted may be added to sodium chloride injection, dextrose injection, invert sugar, or one-sixth molar lactate. Check product information for the length of time that drug retains potency in a particular solution.
4. Ampicillin chewable tablets should not be swallowed whole.
5. Give oral dosage at least 2 hours after or 1 hour before a meal.

Additional Nursing Implications

Observe skin closely for rashes as they occur more often with this drug than with other penicillins.

CARBENICILLIN DISODIUM GEOPEN, PYOPEN

Remarks

This semisynthetic penicillin provides high urine levels that make it especially suitable for urinary tract infections. The drug is acid labile and must be injected.

Carbenicillin disodium attains peak blood levels after 1 hour and is rapidly eliminated (low or absent after six hours). Urinary excretion rates can be slowed by concurrent administration of probenecid.

Additional Uses

Urinary tract and systemic infections caused by *Pseudomonas aeruginosa*, *Proteus* species, *E. coli*, and *Neisseria gonorrhea*.

Additional Contraindications

Pregnancy. Use with caution in patients with impaired renal function.

Additional Untoward Reactions

Neurotoxicity in patients with impaired renal function. Superinfections, furry tongue, dry mouth, vaginitis, increased SGOT levels, hyperkalemia. IM: pain at injection site. IV: vein irritation, phlebitis.

Dosage

IM or **IV,** *Urinary tract uncomplicated:* 1–2 gm q 6 hr; *severe:* 200 mg/kg/day by IV drip. *Systemic severe:* 30–40 gm daily IV in divided doses or by IV drip. *Gonorrhea:* single 4 gm IM injection divided between 2 sites (1 gm probenecid PO is administered 30 minutes prior to injection); **Pediatric,** *Urinary tract,* **IM** or **IV:** 50–200 mg/kg/day in divided doses q 4 to 6 hr. Do not give probenecid to children under 2 years of age. *Systemic, Proteus and E. coli:* 250–500 mg/kg/day IV in divided doses or by continuous drip. **Pseudomonas:** 400–500 mg/kg/day IV in divided doses or by continuous drip.

Reduce all dosages in case of renal insufficiency.

Administration/ Storage

1. Minimize pain at site of deep intramuscular injection by reconstituting medication with 0.5% lidocaine (without epinephrine) or bacteriostatic water for injection containing 0.9% benzyl alcohol. Obtain a written order to use lidocaine or benzyl alcohol for dilution.
2. Do not administer more than 2 gm in any one IM injection.
3. Read directions carefully on package insert for IM and IV administration because drug is very irritating to tissue.
4. Unused reconstituted drug should be discarded after 24 hours when stored at room temperature, and should be discarded after 72 hours when refrigerated. Label with date and time when reconstituting drug.

Nursing Implications

1. Observe patient with impaired renal function for (a) neurotoxicity manifested by hallucinations, impaired sensorium, muscular irritability, and seizures, and (b) hemorrhagic manifestations, such as ecchymosis, petechiae, and frank bleeding of gums and/or rectum.

2. Observe patient with impaired cardiac function for edema, weight gain, and respiratory distress that may be precipitated by sodium in carbenicillin.
3. Observe patient for reaction to probenecid if it is administered with carbenicillin.

CARBENICILLIN INDANYL SODIUM GEOCILLIN

Remarks This semisynthetic penicillin is indicated only for urinary tract infections or prostatitis. The drug, which is acid stable, provides high blood and urinary tract levels after 1 hour. The drug is rapidly eliminated (low or absent after 6 hours).

Uses Urinary tract infections by susceptible organisms.

Additional Contraindications Pregnancy. Safe use in children not established. Use with caution in patients with impaired renal function.

Additional Untoward Reactions Neurotoxicity in patients with impaired renal function, superinfections, furry tongue, dry mouth, vaginitis, increased SGOT levels, hyperkalemia.

Unpleasant taste, nausea, vomiting, diarrhea, flatulence, abdominal cramps.

Additional Drug Interactions When used in combination with gentamicin or tobramycin for pseudomonas infections, effect of carbenicillin may be enhanced.

Dosage **PO:** 382–764 mg q.i.d.

Administration/ Storage
1. Protect from moisture.
2. Store at temperature of 30° C or less.

Nursing Implications See *Nursing Implications* for Carbenicillin Disodium. Provide good mouth care to try and minimize nausea and unpleasant aftertaste.

CLOXACILLIN SODIUM MONOHYDRATE CLOXAPEN, TEGOPEN

Remarks More resistant to penicillinase than penicillin G. Well absorbed from GI tract.

Additional Uses Infections caused by penicillinase-producing staphylococci, streptococci and pneumococci, excluding enterococci. Osteomyelitis.

Dosage **PO:** 250–500 mg q.i.d.; **pediatric up to 20 kg:** 50–100 mg/kg daily in 4 equal doses. Older children receive adult dose.

Administration/ Storage	1. Add amount of water stated on label in 2 portions and shake well after each addition. 2. Shake well before pouring each dose. 3. Refrigerate reconstituted solution and discard unused portion after 14 days.
Additional Nursing Implications	Observe closely for wheezing and sneezing since they are more likely to occur with this drug.

DICLOXACILLIN SODIUM MONOHYDRATE DYCILL, DYNAPEN, PATHOCIL, VERACILLIN

Remarks	Not destroyed by penicillinase. Not indicated for meningitis.
Additional Use	Resistant staphylococcus infections.
Dosage	**PO (capsules or suspensions):** 125–250 (or more) mg q 4 to 6 hr; **pediatric under 40 kg:** 12.5–25 mg/kg in 4 equal doses; children weighing more than 40 kg receive adult dose. Dosage not established for newborn.
Administration/ Storage	1. To prepare oral suspension, shake container to loosen powder, measure water for reconstitution as indicated on label, add half of the water and immediately shake vigorously because usual handling may cause lumps. Add the remainder of the water and again shake vigorously. 2. Shake well before pouring each dose. 3. Refrigerate reconstituted solution and discard after 14 days. 4. Give at least 1 hour before meals or no sooner than 2 to 3 hours after a meal.
Additional Nursing Implications	Anticipate possible difficulty when administering suspension, particularly with children because the medication has an unpleasant taste.

HETACILLIN VERSAPEN

HETACILLIN POTASSIUM VERSAPEN-K

Remarks	This broad-spectrum antibiotic is inactive until converted, in the body, to ampicillin. The characteristics of hetacillin are, thus, identical with ampicillin. Peak serum levels are attained in 2 to 3 hours and decrease slowly over 8 hours. Prolonged and intensive therapy at higher doses than recommended may be necessary for GI and urinary tract infections.

Additional Uses Infections of the respiratory, GI, genitourinary tract and of the middle ear caused by *Shigella, Salmonella, E. coli, H. influenzae, Proteus strains, Micrococcus pneumoniae, Group A beta-hemolytic-streptococcus, Enterococcus,* and non-penicillinase-producing *Staphyloccus aureus.*

Dosage **PO, IM, IV:** Varies with condition treated. **Patients weighing 40 kg or more:** 225–450 mg q.i.d.; **patients weighing less than 40 kg:** 22.5–45 mg/kg daily in 4 equally divided doses.

Administration/ Storage
1. Reconstitute pediatric drops by adding water in 2 portions and shaking thoroughly with cap on after each portion of water is added. Add amount of water specified on the label.
2. Refrigerate PO suspension after reconstitution and discard remaining portion after 14 days.
3. The parenteral injection premixed with lidocaine is *only* for IM administration.
4. Discard unused parenteral solution 6 hours after reconstitution.

Nursing Implications Administer at least 2 hours after or 1 hour before a meal.

METHICILLIN SODIUM AZAPEN, CELBENIN, STAPHCILLIN

General Statement A semisynthetic salt unaffected by penicillinase; particularly suitable for soft tissue and penicillin G-resistant infections. Used for resistant staphylococcus infections. Use with caution in patients with renal failure. Safe use in neonates has not been established. Periodic renal function tests are indicated for long-term therapy.

Additional Uses Infections by penicillinase-producing staphylococci; osteomyelitis, septicemia, enterocolitis, bacterial endocarditis.

Dosage **IM or IV:** 1 gm (or more) q 4 to 6 hr; **pediatric, IM only:** 25 mg/kg (or more) q 6 hr.

Administration/ Storage
1. Do not use dextrose solutions for diluting methicillin because their low acidity may destroy antibiotic.
2. Inject medication slowly. Methicillin injections are particularly painful.
3. Inject deeply into gluteal muscle.
4. To prevent sterile abscesses at injection site, include 0.2–0.3 ml of air in syringe before starting injection so that when the needle is withdrawn the irritating solution will not leak into tissue.
5. Methicillin is very sensitive to heat when dissolved. Therefore, solutions for IM administration must be used within 24 hours, if standing at room temperatures, or within 4 days, if refrigerated. Solutions for IV use must be used within 8 hours.
6. In order to prevent destruction when given by IV infusion, drug

should be administered as intermittent doses into the IV tubing rather than by being dissolved all at once into the IV fluid package.

Additional Nursing Implications
1. Do not mix methicillin with any other drug in the same syringe or IV solution.
2. Watch for pain along the course of the vein into which the drug was administered and check for redness or edema at site of injection.
3. Observe for hematuria and casts in urine.
4. Observe for pallor, ecchymosis, or bleeding.

NAFCILLIN SODIUM NAFCIL, UNIPEN

Remarks Used for resistant staphylococcus infections. Parenteral therapy is recommended initially for severe infections.

Additional Uses Infections by penicillinase-producing staphylococci; also certain pneumococci and streptococci.

Additional Untoward Reactions Sterile abscesses and thrombophlebitis occur frequently, especially in the elderly.

Dosage **PO:** 250–1000 mg q 4 to 6 hr; **pediatric:** 25–50 mg/kg body weight daily in 4 divided doses; **neonates:** 10 mg/kg body weight 3 to 4 times daily. **IM:** 500 mg q 6 hr; **pediatric:** 25 mg/kg daily in 2 doses; **neonates:** 10 mg/kg daily in 2 doses. **IV:** 500–1000 mg q 4 hr; **older children:** 50 mg/kg in 6 equal doses.

Administration/ Storage
1. Reconstitute for oral use by adding powder to bottle of diluent, replacing cap tightly. Then **shake thoroughly until all powder is in solution.** Check carefully for undissolved powder at bottom of bottle. Solution must be stored in refrigerator and unused portion discarded after 1 week.
2. Reconstitute for parenteral use by adding required amount of sterile water. Shake vigorously. Date bottle. Refrigerate after reconstitution and discard unused portion after 48 hours.
3. For direct IV administration, dissolve powder in 15–30 ml of sterile water for injection or isotonic sodium chloride solution and inject over 5- to 10-minute period into the tubing of flowing IV infusion. For IV drip, dissolve the required amount in 100–150 ml of isotonic sodium chloride injection and administer by IV drip over a period of 15 to 90 minutes.

Additional Nursing Implications
1. Observe patient for GI distress.
2. Administer IM by deep intragluteal injection.
3. Do not administer IV to newborn infants.
4. Observe for pain along the course of the vein and for redness or edema at site of IV injection.

OXACILLIN SODIUM BACTOCILL, PROSTAPHLIN

Remarks   Resistant to penicillinase. Used for resistant staphylococci infections. Relatively acid stable.

Additional Uses   Infections caused by penicillinase-producing staphylococci; also certain pneumococci and streptococci.

Additional Untoward Reactions   GI disturbances after PO administration are frequent; also, pain and swelling at IM injection site; thrombophlebitis after IV administration.

Dosage   Primarily given **PO** but may be given **IM** and **IV. All routes:** 500–1000 mg q 4 to 6 hr; **pediatric less than 40 kg:** 50 mg/kg q 4 hr; **neonates:** 25 mg/kg daily in divided doses. Drug should be given for a minimum of 5 days.

Administration/ Storage
1. Administer IM by deep intragluteal injection.
2. Reconstitution: Add sterile water for injection in amount indicated on vial. Shake until solution is clear. For parenteral use, reconstituted solution may be kept for 3 days at room temperature or 1 week in refrigerator. Discard outdated solutions.
3. IV administration (two methods):
   a. For rapid, direct administration, add an equal amount of sterile water or isotonic saline to reconstituted dosage and administer over period of 10 minutes.
   b. For drip method, add reconstituted solution to either dextrose, saline, or invert sugar solution and administer over a 6-hour period, during which time drug remains potent.

Additional Nursing Implications
1. Observe for GI distress.
2. Observe for pain, redness, and edema at the site of IV injection and along the course of the vein.
3. Observe for pain and swelling at IM injection site.

PENICILLIN G BENZATHINE, ORAL BICILLIN

STERILE PENICILLIN G BENZATHINE SUSPENSION BICILLIN LONG-ACTING SUSPENSION, PERMAPEN

Remarks   This is a very long-acting (repository) form of penicillin in an aqueous vehicle. It is administered most often as a sterile suspension. Rare instances of renal damage occur as with all forms of penicillin G.

Additional Uses   Most gram-positive (streptococci, staphylococci, pneumococci) and some gram-negative (gonococci, meningococci) organisms. Syphilis. Prophylaxis of glomerulonephritis, surgical infections, secondary infections following tooth extraction, tonsillectomy, rheumatic fever, and syphilis.

Dosage   **PO, adult:** 400,000–600,000 units q 4 to 6 hr. *Rheumatic fever prophylaxis:* 200,000 units b.i.d.; **pediatric under 12:** 25,000–90,000 units/kg in 3 to 6 divided doses/day. **IM,** *Streptococcus,* **adult:** single dose of 1.2 million units; **older children:** 900,000 units; **children under 60 lb:** 300,000–600,000 units. *Rheumatic fever prophylaxis:* 1.2 million units q 4 weeks. *Syphilis:* one dose of 2.4 million units.

Administration/ Storage

1. Shake multiple dose vial vigorously before withdrawing the desired dose, since medication tends to clump on standing. Check that all medication is dissolved and that there is no residue at bottom of bottle.
2. Use a 20-gauge needle and do not allow medication to remain in the syringe and needle for long periods of time before administration because the needle may become plugged and syringe "frozen."
3. Inject deeply into the muscle and *do not massage* injection site.
4. Before injection of medication, aspirate needle to ascertain needle is not in a vein.
5. Rotate and chart site of injections.
6. *Do not administer IV.*

Additional Nursing Implication   Explain to patient why he/she must return for repository penicillin injections.

PENICILLIN G, BENZATHINE AND PROCAINE   BICILLIN C-R

Remarks   This drug is intended for moderately severe infections and is for IM use only.

Use   Streptococcal infections (A, C, G, H, L, and M), without bacteremia, of the upper respiratory tract, skin, and soft tissues. Scarlet fever, erysipelas, pneumococcal infections, and otitis media.

Dosage   **IM,** *Streptococcal infections,* **adults and children over 60 lb:** 2,400,000 units, given at a single session using multiple injection sites or alternately in divided doses on days 1 and 3; **children 30–60 lb:** 900,000–1,200,000 units; **infants and children under 30 lb:** 600,000 units. *Pneumococcal infections, except meningitis:* 1,200,000 units; **pediatric:** 600,000 units q 2 to 3 days until temperature is normal for 48 hours.

PENICILLIN G POTASSIUM   GENECILLIN-400, K-CILLIN-500, PENTIDS, PFIZERPEN G, SK-PENICILLIN G, SUGRACILLIN, OTHERS

PENICILLIN G SODIUM

Remarks   Because of its low cost, penicillin G is still first choice for treatment of many infections. Rapid onset makes it especially suitable for fulminating infections. Destroyed by acid and penicillinase.

Additional Uses   Most gram-positive (streptococci, staphylococci, pneumococci) and some gram-negative (gonococci, meningococci) organisms. Also syphilis, fulminating infections, and congenital syphilis.

Additional Untoward Reactions   Rapid IV administration may cause hyperkalemia and cardiac arrhythmias. Renal damage occurs rarely.

Dosage   **PO, adults and children over 12:** 600,000–3,000,000 units daily; **children under 12:** 25,000–90,000 units/kg/day in 3 to 6 divided doses. **IM, IV, adults:** 1–20 million units daily (doses as high as 60 million units daily may be required); **children:** 300,000–1,200,000 units daily (doses as high as 10 million units may be necessary); **infants:** 600,000 units daily in 2 divided doses. For *prophylaxis in rheumatic fever*, **adults and children, PO:** 400,000 units twice daily.

Administration/ Storage
1. Use sterile water, isotonic saline USP or 5% D/W and mix with volume recommended on label for desired strength.
2. Loosen powder by shaking bottle prior to addition of diluent.
3. Hold vial horizontally and rotate slowly while directing the stream of the diluent against the wall of the vial.
4. Shake vigorously after addition of diluent.
5. Solutions may be stored at room temperature for 24 hours, or in refrigerator for 1 week. Discard remaining solution.
6. Use 1% to 2% lidocaine solution as diluent for IM if ordered by doctor to lessen pain at injection site. Do not use procaine as diluent for aqueous penicillin.
7. Note the long list of drugs that should *not* be mixed with penicillin during IV administration:

Aminophylline	Metaraminol	Sodium bicarbonate
Amphotericin B	Novobiocin	Sodium salts of
Ascorbic acid	Oxytetracycline	barbiturates
Chlorpheniramine	Phenylephrine	Sulfadiazine
Chlorpromazine	Phenytoin	Tetracycline
Gentamicin	Polymyxin B	Tromethamine
Heparin	Prochlorperazine	Vitamin B complex
Hydroxyzine	Promazine	Vancomycin
Lincomycin	Promethazine	

Additional Nursing Implications
1. Drug should be ordered specifying sodium or potassium salt.
2. Observe patient for GI disturbances which may lead to dehydration. Dehydration decreases the excretion of the drug by the kidneys and may raise the blood level of penicillin G to dangerously high levels that can cause kidney damage.

PENICILLIN G, PROCAINE, AQUEOUS CRYSTICILLIN A.S., DURACILLIN A.S., PFIZERPEN-A.S., TU-CILLIN, WYCILLIN

Remarks   Long-acting (repository) form in aqueous or oily vehicle. Destroyed by penicillinase. Because of slow onset, a soluble penicillin is often administered concomitantly for fulminating infections.

Additional Uses   Penicillin-sensitive staphylococci, pneumococci, and streptococci. Gonorrhea, all stages of syphilis. *Prophylaxis:* rheumatic fever, pre- and postsurgery.

Dosage   **IM only, usual:** 600,000–1,000,000 units daily. *Syphilis/Gonorrhea:* 4.8 million units total.

**Administration/
Storage**
1. Note on package whether medication is to be refrigerated, since some brands require this to maintain stability.
2. Shake multiple dose vial thoroughly to ensure uniform suspension before injection. If the medication is clumped at the bottom of the vial, it must be shaken until clump dissolves.
3. Use a 20-gauge needle and aspirate immediately after withdrawing medication from the vial; otherwise needle may become clogged and syringe may "freeze."
4. Aspirate needle to ensure that the needle is not in a vein.
5. Inject deep into muscle at a slow steady rate.
6. Rotate and chart injection sites.

**Additional
Nursing
Implications**   Observe for wheal or other skin reactions at site of injection that may indicate a reaction to procaine as well as to penicillin.

PHENOXYMETHYL PENICILLIN PENICILLIN V, V-CILLIN

PHENOXYMETHYL PENICILLIN POTASSIUM BETAPEN VK, COCILLIN V-K, LEDERCILLIN VK, PENAPAR VK, PENICILLIN VK, PENICILLIN V POTASSIUM, PEN-VEE K, PFIZERPEN VK, REPEN-VK, ROBICILLIN VK, RO-CILLIN VK, SK-PENICILLIN-VK, UTICILLIN VK, V-CILLIN K, VEETIDS

**General
Statement**   These preparations are closely related to penicillin. They are acid-stable and resist inactivation by gastric secretions. They are well absorbed from GI tract and not affected by foods.
  Periodic blood counts and renal function tests are indicated during long-term usage.

Additional Uses   Penicillin-sensitive staphylococci, pneumococci, streptococci, gonococci. *Prophylaxis:* rheumatic fever, pre- and postsurgery.

**Additional Drug
Interaction**   Neomycin may cause ↓ absorption of phenoxymethyl penicillin potassium.

Dosage   **PO only.** Range: 125 mg t.i.d. to 625 mg 6 times/day; **children under 12:** 15–50 mg/kg in 3 to 6 divided doses; **children over 12:** adult dose.

Administration   May be administered after meals since food does not affect absorption.

TICARCILLIN DISODIUM TICAR

Remarks   Parenteral semisynthetic antibiotic with an antibacterial spectrum resembling carbenicillin. Primarily suitable for treatment of gram-negative organisms, but also effective for mixed infections. Combined therapy with gentamicin or tobramycin is sometimes indicated for treatment of *Pseudomonas* infections. The drugs *should not* be mixed during administration because of gradual mutual inactivation. Peak serum levels are attained after 1 hour, and elimination is virtually complete after 6 hours.

Uses   Bacterial septicemia, skin and soft tissue infections, acute and chronic respiratory tract infections caused by susceptible strains of *Pseudomonas aeruginosa*, *Proteus* species, and *E. coli*.

Genitourinary tract infections caused by above organisms and *Enterobacter* and *Streptococcus faecalis*. For infections when immunologic mechanisms are impaired. For patients on hemodialysis.

Additional Contraindications   Pregnancy. Use with caution in presence of impaired renal function and for patients on restricted salt diets.

Additional Untoward Reactions   GI disturbances including nausea, vomiting. Neurotoxicity and neuromuscular excitability, especially in patients with impaired renal function. Superinfections. Pain and induration at injection site, phlebitis, hypokalemia, elevated alkaline phosphatase, SGOT, and SGPT values.

Additional Drug Interaction   Effect of carbenicillin may be enhanced when used in combination with gentamicin or tobramycin for *Pseudomonas* infections.

Dosage   *Systemic infections*, **adults, children, IV** *infusion:* 200–300 mg/kg body weight in divided doses q 3 to 6 hr. *Systemic, pediatric,* **IM** or **IV** infusion, **Neonates less than 2 kg: initial,** 100 mg/kg; **then,** 75 mg/kg q 8 hr during first week after birth, **then** increase to 75 mg/kg q 4 to 6 hr; **neonates weighing over 2 kg: initial,** 100 mg/kg; **then** 75 mg/kg q 4 to 6 hr during first 2 weeks; **then** 100 mg q 4 hr. *Uncomplicated urinary tract infections:* **IM** or **IV adults and children over 40 kg:** 1 gm q 6 hr; **children under 40 kg:** 50–100 mg/kg/day in individual doses q 6 to 8 hr. *Complicated urinary tract infections* **adults and children:** 150–200 mg/kg daily in divided doses by intermittent IV infusion every 4 to 6 hr.

Patients with renal insufficiency should receive a loading dose of 3 gm **(IV)** and subsequent doses as indicated by creatinine clearance.

Administration/ Storage   1. Discard unused reconstituted solutions after 24 hours when stored at room temperature, and after 72 hours when refrigerated.
2. Reconstitute with 1% lidocaine HCl (without epinephrine) or with bacteriostatic water for injection containing 0.9% benzyl alcohol to prevent pain and induration.
3. Use dilute solution of 50 mg/ml or less for IV use, and administer slowly to prevent vein irritation and phlebitis.
4. Do not administer more than 2 gm of the drug in each IM site.

Nursing Implications
1. Observe for signs of hemorrhagic manifestations, such as petechiae, ecchymosis, or frank bleeding.
2. Observe patients with cardiac history for edema, weight gain, or respiratory distress precipitated by sodium in drug.

ERYTHROMYCINS

General Statement

The erythromycins are produced by strains of *Streptomyces erythreus* and have bacteriostatic and occasionally bactericidal activity. The agents interfere with protein synthesis.

The erythromycins are absorbed from the upper part of the small intestine. Erythromycin for oral use is coated with an acid-resistant material to avoid destruction by gastric juice.

Erythromycin diffuses into body tissues, the peritoneal, pleural, ascitic and amniotic fluids, the saliva, the placental circulation, and across the mucous membrane of the tracheobronchial tree. It diffuses poorly into the spinal fluid.

Uses

Erythromycins are preferred for respiratory tract infections, rheumatic fever prophylaxis, and the treatment of syphilis in penicillin-sensitized patients.

They are the drug of choice in *Mycoplasma pneumoniae*, and effective in infections caused by *Neisseria*, some strains of *H. influenzae*, *Pasteurella*, *Brucella*, *C. diphtheriae*, *Clostridia*, *Listeria*, *Treponema*, and rickettsia.

Erythromycins are effective in the management of diseases produced by streptococci, including the beta-hemolytic strains, and staphylococci. Excellent results have been obtained in the treatment of staphylococcal pneumonia, bacteremia, endocarditis, intestinal amebiasis, osteomyelitis, meningitis, furuncles, carbuncles, wound infections, diphtheria—particularly the carrier state—and acute and chronic intestinal amebiasis. Also for Legionnaire's Disease.

The drug is also indicated for prophylaxis before tooth extraction or surgery in patients with a long history of rheumatic fever or congenital heart disease.

Many erythromycins are available in ointment and solutions for ophthalmic, otic, and dermatological use.

Contraindication

Hypersensitivity to erythromycin.

Untoward Reactions

Nausea, vomiting, abdominal distress, and diarrhea. Skin eruptions, urticaria. Superinfections due to eradication of normal bacterial flora. IM injections of doses above 100 mg often produce painful reactions at injection site. IV infusions often cause thrombophlebitis. Periodic liver function tests and blood counts during long-term therapy are indicated.

TABLE 4 ERYTHROMYCINS

Drug	Main Uses	Dosage	Remarks
Erythromycin (E-Mycin, Erythrocin, Ilotycin, Robimycin, RP-Mycin)	Respiratory infections, beta-hemolytic streptococci, amebiasis	**PO:** usual, 250 mg q 6 hr, can increase to 4 gm/day; **pediatric:** 30–50 mg/kg/day in 3 to 4 divided doses. *Primary Syphilis:* 20–40 gm in divided doses over a period of 10 to 15 days.	Food does not affect absorption.
Erythromycin estolate (Ilosone)	Sensitive staphylococci, pneumococci, and streptococci in penicillin-sensitized patients	**Adults and children over 23 kg, PO:** 250–500 mg q 6 hr; **children 4.5–11.5 kg:** 11 mg/kg q 6 hr; **children 11.5–23 kg:** 125 mg q 6 hr.	Most active form of erythromycin with relatively long-lasting activity. Special contraindications: cholestatic jaundice or preexisting liver dysfunction; not recommended for treatment of chronic disorders such as acne and furunculosis or for prophylaxis of rheumatic fever *Additional Untoward Reactions* Jaundice, cholestiasis—usually after 10–14 days of therapy, alteration of certain laboratory tests. *Administration/Storage* Shake oral suspension well before pouring Do not store suspension longer than 2 weeks at room temperature Chewable tablets must be chewed or crushed
Erythromycin ethylsuccinate (E.E.S., Pediamycin, Wyamycin)	Sensitive staphylococci, pneumococci and streptococci in penicillin-sensitized patients. Topical: skin infections by susceptible organisms	**Adults and older children, PO:** 400 mg q 6 hr; **pediatric:** 30–50 mg/kg/day in 3 to 4 divided doses. *Primary Syphilis:* 48–64 gm in divided doses over 10 to 15 days. *Dysenteric Amebiasis:* 400 mg q.i.d. for 10 to 14 days. Prior to surgery to prevent *alpha-hemolytic streptococci-induced endocar-*	The injectible form contains 2% butylbenzocaine and is contraindicated in patients allergic to the "caine" (procaine, benzocaine, etc.) type of local anesthetic *Administration/Storage* Inject into large muscle mass Rotate site of injections Do not administer to infants as muscle mass is too small

Drug	Uses	Dose	Remarks
		ditis: 800 mg before procedure and 400 mg q 6 to 8 hr for 4 doses after procedure.	Do not mix with other medications in same syringe Avoid accidental IV administration Refrigerate aqueous suspensions and store for maximum of 1 week Chewable tablets must be chewed or crushed
Erythromycin gluceptate (Ilotycin Gluceptate IV)	Primarily for unconscious, vomiting, or gravely ill patients with serious infections of gram-positive bacteria, especially hemolytic streptococci, pneumococci or staphylococci	**Adults and children, IV only:** 250–1000 mg q 6 hr. *Acute pelvic inflammatory disease caused by gonorrhea:* 500 mg q 6 hours for 3 days followed by 250 mg erythromycin stearate PO q 6 hrs for 7 days.	*Drug Interactions* Drug for IV administration is incompatible with many drugs including: carbenicillin, chloramphenicol, cephalothin, phenytoin, heparin, barbiturates, streptomycin, tetracycline, vitamin B complex *Administration/Storage* Follow directions on vial for dilution Concentrate, which must be diluted futher before administration, will remain stable in refrigerator for 7 days Administer slowly over period of 20 to 60 min or infuse IV over 24 hours
Erythromycin lactobionate (Erythrocin Lactobionate IV)	For seriously ill or vomiting patients suffering from infections by susceptible organisms	**Adults and children:** 15–20 mg/kg/day up to 4 gm/day in severe infections. *Acute pelvic inflammatory disease caused by gonorrhea:* 500 mg q 6 hr for 3 days followed by 250 mg erythromycin stearate. **PO:** q 6 hr for 7 days.	Change to oral therapy as soon as possible. *Drug Interactions* Incompatible for IV administration with aminophylline ascorbic acid, carbenicillin, cephalothin, chloramphenicol, colistimethate, heparin, metaraminol, tetracycline, vitamin B complex
Erythromycin stearate (Bristamycin, Erypar, Erythrocin Stearate, Ethril, Pfizer-E, Romycin, SK-Erythromycin, Wyamycin)	Sensitive staphylococci, pneumococci, and streptococci in penicillin-sensitized patients	**PO buffered tablets:** 250–500 mg q 6 hr; **Pediatric:** 30–50 mg/kg daily in 4 to 6 equally divided doses.	Drug causes more allergic reactions, such as skin rash and urticaria, than other erythromycins *Administration* Do not administer with meals because food decreases absorption.

73

Drug Interactions

Interactant	Interaction
Acetazolamide	↑ Effect of erythromycin in urine due to alkalinization
Lincomycin	↓ Effect of erythromycin
Penicillin	Effect ↓ by erythromycins
Sodium bicarbonate	↑ Effect of erythromycin in urine due to alkalinization

Laboratory Test Interference

+ or ↑ False values of urinary catecholamines, urinary steroids and SGOT and SGPT values.

Dosage

PO and **IM** (painful); some preparations can be given **IV**. (See Table 4, p. 72.)

Nursing Implications

See also *Nursing Implications* under *Antibiotics* (p. 56).

1. Observe for allergic response; have emergency equipment available.
2. Observe for superinfections characterized by black furry tongue, nausea, and diarrhea.
3. Observe patient for positive therapeutic response, such as reduction of fever, increased appetite, and increased sense of well-being.
4. Observe for GI disturbances.
5. Inject deep into muscle mass. Injections are painful and irritating.
6. Do not administer with or immediately prior to fruit juice or other acid drinks because acidity may decrease activity of drug.
7. Do not routinely administer PO medication with meals because food decreases the absorption of most erythromycins. However, physician may order medication to be given with food to reduce GI irritation.
8. Erythromycins are often administered in combination with sulfonamides. In that case, observe all the precautions indicated for both groups of drugs.

Nursing Implications for Erythromycin Antibiotic Ointments

1. Report skin reactions to physician and discontinue use.
2. Medications can be stored at room temperature for 1 week and under refrigeration for several weeks.
3. Clean affected area before applying ointment.

Nursing Implications for Ophthalmic Solutions

Observe for mild reaction which, though usually transient, must be reported to physician.

Nursing Implications for Otic Solutions

1. Instill at room temperature.
2. Pull pinna of ear down and back for children under 3 years of age, and up and back for patients over 3 years of age.

TETRACYCLINES

General Statement
These broad-spectrum antibiotics are obtained by chemical modification of substances produced by *Streptomyces aureofaciens* and *rimosus*. Their effect is mostly bacteriostatic. They interfere with the protein synthesis of the infectious organism and thus halt its growth and reproduction.

Tetracyclines are well absorbed from the stomach and upper small intestine. They are well distributed throughout all tissues and fluids and diffuse through the placental barrier and noninflamed meninges.

Uses
Mostly used for bacterial, various rickettsial, and mycoplasmic infections.

Because the tetracyclines easily promote the emergence of resistant strains, they are usually not the first choice for infections responding to penicillin or streptomycin. However, they are indicated for patients hypersensitive to penicillin or other antibiotics.

Tetracyclines are the antibiotic of choice in certain venereal infections, such as lymphogranuloma venereum, granuloma inguinale, and chancroid.

They are also used for nonvenereal infections of the genitourinary tract, shigellosis, hemolytic anemia, pinworm infestations, as an adjunct for amebic infections, brucellosis, psittacosis, *Trichimonas vaginalis*, Rocky Mountain spotted fever, typhus, cholera, relapsing fever, and meningitis caused by *H. influenzae*. Acute trachoma and inclusion conjunctivitis respond well to topical application.

Contraindications
Hypersensitivity; avoid drug during tooth development stage (last trimester of pregnancy, neonatal period, and early childhood) because tetracyclines interfere with enamel formation and dental pigmentation.

Use with caution and at reduced dosage in patients with impaired kidney function.

Never administer intrathecally.

Untoward Reactions
Minor GI disturbances, such as bulky loose stools and diarrhea. Allergic reactions, superinfections, fever, liver damage, dizziness, and hoarseness, increased azotemia, and sodium excretion with renal insufficiency. Increased intracranial pressure in young infants. Photosensitivity.

Parenteral tetracyclines may cause severe liver damage, especially in pregnant women and in patients with diminished renal function. They may cause death if given during last trimester of pregnancy.

They may cause bone lesions or staining and deformity of teeth in children up to 8 years old and in newborns whose mothers had received the drug.

The administration of deteriorated tetracyclines may result in Fanconi like syndrome characterized by nausea, vomiting, acidosis, proteinuria, glycosuria, aminoaciduria, polydipsia, polyuria, hypokalemia.

Drug Interactions

Interactant	Interaction
Antacids, oral	↓ Effect of tetracyclines due to ↓ absorption from GI tract
Anticoagulants, oral	IV tetracyclines ↑ hypoprothrombinemia
Diuretics	Concomitant therapy cause ↑ BUN levels especially with previous renal impairment
Heparin	Tetracyclines ↓ activity of heparin
Iron preparations	↓ Effect of tetracyclines due to ↓ absorption from GI tract
Methoxyflurane	↑ Risk of kidney toxicity
Penicillins	Tetracyclines may mask bactericidal effect of penicillins
Sodium bicarbonate	↓ Effect of tetracyclines due to ↓ absorption from GI tract

Laboratory Test Interference

False + or ↑ urinary catecholamines, urinary protein (degraded), coagulation time. False − or ↓ urinary urobilinogen glucose tests (see *Nursing Implications*).

Prolonged use or high doses may change liver function tests, and white blood counts.

Dosage

PO, IM, IV, and topical. (For details see Table 5, p. 77.)

Nursing Implications

1. Observe for allergic reactions; have epinephrine and oxygen readily available for emergency use.
2. Observe for superinfections so that adequate therapy may be instituted.
3. Check expiration date of drug since use of outdated or deteriorated drugs has resulted in Fanconilike syndrome (see *Untoward Reactions*).
4. Discard unused capsules to prevent use of medication that has deteriorated.
5. Administer on an empty stomach. Withhold antacids, dairy foods, and other foods high in calcium for at least 2 hours following PO administration. Milk is not to be administered with medication.
6. Report gastric distress to doctor, who may order a light meal with the medication or reduce the individual dose of the medication and increase the frequency of administration.
7. Administer IM into a large muscle mass to avoid extravasation into SC or fat tissue. Administer slowly to minimize pain.
8. Check intake and output because renal dysfunction may result in accumulation of the drug and toxicity.
9. Observe for symptoms of enterocolitis, such as diarrhea, pyrexia, abdominal distention, and scanty urine. These symptoms may necessitate discontinuation of drug and substitution, by the doctor, of another antibiotic. Fluid electrolyte balance must be maintained.
10. Observe patient for sore throat, dysphagia, fever, dizziness, hoarseness, and inflammation of mucous membranes of body.
11. Prevent or treat pruritus ani by cleansing of the anal region with water several times a day and after each BM.

TABLE 5 TETRACYCLINES

Drug	Dosage	Remarks
Chlortetracycline hydrochloride (Aureomycin)	**PO and IV, usual:** 250–500 mg q 6 to 12 hr; **pediatric:** 10–20 mg/kg daily in divided doses	Single oral doses above 250 mg are not well absorbed. Topical route should be avoided due to the danger of hypersensitization
Demeclocycline hydrochloride (Declomycin)	**PO:** 600 mg daily in 2 to 4 divided doses; **pediatric:** 6–12 mg/kg daily in 2 to 4 divided doses. *Gonorrhea:* 3 gm in divided doses over a 4-day period.	Causes photosensitivity more frequently than other tetracyclines. May cause increased pigmentation of skin. Antihistamines and corticosteroids may be useful in treatment of hypersensitivity
Doxycycline hyclate (Doxychel, Vibramycin Hyclate) Doxycycline monohydrate (Doxychel, Vibramycin, Monohydrate)	**PO:** 1st day, 100 mg q 12 hr; **maintenance:** 100 mg daily in single or divided doses; **pediatric:** 1st day, 4.4 mg/kg in divided doses; **maintenance:** 2.2 mg/kg/day in single or divided doses. *Syphilis:* 300 mg/day in divided doses for 10 days. *Gonorrhea:* 300 mg first day followed by 200 mg/day for 3 days.	More slowly absorbed, and thus more persistent than other tetracyclines. Preferred for patients with impaired renal function for treating infections outside urinary tract. *Administration/Storage* Powder for suspension has expiration date of 12 months from date of issue. Solution stable for 2 weeks when stored in refrigerator
Methacycline hydrochloride (Rondomycin)	**PO:** 600 mg daily in 2 to 4 divided doses; **pediatric:** 6–12 mg/kg daily in 2 to 4 divided doses *Gonorrhea:* **initially,** 900 mg; **then** 300 mg q.i.d. for a total of 5.4 gm. *Syphilis:* 18–24 gm in divided doses over 10 to 15 days.	Pediatric dosage should not be administered with milk formulas or calcium-containing foods
Minocycline hydrochloride (Minocin, Vectrin)	**PO, initial:** 200 mg; **maintenance:** 100 mg q 12 hr; not to exceed 400 mg/24 hr; **pediatric, initial:** 4 mg/kg; **maintenance:** 2 mg/kg q 12 hr.	Absorption less affected by milk or food than other tetracyclines

(Continued)

TABLE 5 TETRACYCLINES (*Continued*)

Drug	Dosage	Remarks
Oxytetracycline (Terramycin)	**IV, IM, PO:** 250–500 mg q 6 to 12 hr; **Pediatric:** 10–20 mg/kg/day in divided doses.	Do not give with food or antacid. Pediatric dosage should not be administered with milk or calcium-containing foods. Check dilutions for IV administration
Oxytetracycline calcium (Terramycin-calcium) Oxytetracycline hydrochloride (Oxlopar, Oxy-Tetrachel, Terramycin Hydrochloride, Tetramine, Uri-Tet)	Same as Oxytetracycline	
Tetracycline (Achromycin V, Panmycin, Retet–S, Robitet, Sumycin, SK-Tetracycline, Tetracyn, others) Tetracycline hydrochloride (Achromycin V, Panmycin, Robitet, Sumycin, Tetracyn, Tetrex-S) Tetracycline phosphate complex (Tetrex)	**PO (all forms):** usual, 250–500 mg q 6 hr; **pediatric:** 25–50 mg/kg. **IM** (hydrochloride, phosphate complex): 200–800 mg daily in 2 to 3 divided doses; **pediatric:** 15–25 mg/kg up to maximum of 250 mg daily. **IV** (hydrochloride only): 250–500 mg q 6 to 12 hr up to maximum of 2 gm daily; **pediatric:** 12 mg/kg daily in divided doses.	Dosage always expressed as the hydrochloride salt. Administer IV very slowly. Rapid administration may cause thrombophlebitis. Do not administer the phosphate complex intravenously.

12. Observe patient on IV therapy for redness, swelling, and pain along vein.
13. Observe patient for nausea, vomiting, chills, fever, and hypertension, resulting from too rapid IV administration or an excessively high dose.
14. Observe for bulging fontanel in young infants, which may be caused by increased intracranial pressure.
15. Observe patients with impaired hepatic or renal function for impairment of consciousness or other CNS disturbances because drug may interfere with respiration of brain tissues.
16. Observe patients with impaired kidney function for azotemia, hyperphosphatemia, acidosis, weight loss, anorexia, nausea, vomit-

ing, and dehydration even when such patients receive standard doses of tetracyclines. Continue observations after cessation of therapy because symptoms may appear later.

17. Observe patients on long-term therapy for blood dyscrasias.
18. Observe patients on large IV doses or on simultaneous maximum doses by more than one route for hepatic failure and pancreatic damage.
19. Advise patient to avoid direct or artificial sunlight that may cause a severe sunburnlike reaction.
20. Observe for onycholosis (loosening or detachment of the nail from nailbed).

CEPHALOSPORINS

General Statement The cephalosporins are semisynthetic antibiotics derived from cultures of *Cephalosporium acremonium*. They resemble the penicillins both chemically and pharmacologically. Their action is primarily bactericidal and results from their interfering with the formation of the bacterial cell wall. Like the penicillins, the cephalosporins are most effective against young, rapidly dividing organisms.

Some cephalosporins are rapidly absorbed from the GI tract and quickly reach effective concentrations in the urinary, GI, and respiratory tracts except in patients with pernicious anemia or obstructive jaundice. The drugs are eliminated rapidly in patients with normal renal function.

The cephalosporins are broad spectrum antibiotics, more effective against gram-positive than gram-negative bacteria. Their spectrum includes: *A. beta-hemolytic streptococci, staphylococci* —including penicillinase-producing strains—*Streptococcus pneumoniae, E. coli, Proteus mirabilis, Klebsiella* species, and *H. influenzae*. The antibiotics can be destroyed by cephalosporinase.

Uses Infections of the respiratory tract, skin, soft tissue and genitourinary tract, and otitis media. The drugs are occasionally used for septicemia, acute endocarditis, syphilis, gonorrhea, bone and joint infections. It is always desirable to determine the susceptibility of the organism to a particular cephalosporin before instituting therapy.

Contraindications Hypersensitivity to cephalosporins. Patients hypersensitive to penicillin may occasionally cross-react to cephalosporins. The safe use of cephalosporins in pregnancy and lactation has not been established.

Use with caution in the presence of impaired renal or hepatic function or together with other nephrotoxic drugs. Creatinine clearances should be performed on all patients with impaired renal function who receive cephalosporins.

Untoward Reaction *Nephrotoxicity*, especially in patients over 50 and under 3 years of age. *GI disturbances:* nausea, vomiting, diarrhea. *Superinfections:* vaginitis, oral candidiasis, glossitis, vaginal and anal pruritus. *Blood dyscrasias:*

neutropenia, leukopenia, thrombocytopenia, agranulocytosis, anemia. *Hepatic dysfunction:* slightly elevated SGOT and SGPT values. Also headaches, malaise, dizziness, fatigue, dyspnea, paresthesia.

Parenteral administration of cephalosporins can cause phlebitis, pain and induration at IM injection site, and sterile abscesses.

Drug Interactions

Interactant	*Interaction*
Anticoagulants	Cephalosporins ↑ prothrombin time
Colistin	↑ Renal toxicity of cephalosporins
Ethacrynic Acid	↑ Renal toxicity of cephalosporins
Furosemide (Lasix)	↑ Renal toxicity of cephalosporins
Gentamicin	Additive renal toxicity
Probenecid (Benemid)	↑ Effect of cephalosporins by ↓ excretion by kidney

Laboratory Test Interference

False + for urinary glucose with Benedict's solution, Fehling's solution or Clinitest. Enzyme tests (Clinistix, Tes-Tape) are unaffected. False + Coomb's test.

Administration

Can be administered without regard to meals.

Nursing Implications

1. Observe patients with a history of hypersensitivity reaction to penicillins for cross-reactivity to cephalosporins.
2. Observe for hypersensitivity reactions manifested by anaphylaxis or by milder reactions characterized by maculopapular rash, urticaria, and eosinophilia.
3. Use Tes-Tape to evaluate for glycosuria because false-positives may be obtained with Benedict's solution, Clinitest tablets, or Fehling's solution.
4. Recognize that medication may cause a positive direct Coombs test. This would be of concern if patient is being cross-matched for transfusion or in newborns whose mothers had cephalosporins during pregnancy.
5. Observe for superinfection due to overgrowth of non-susceptible organisms, such as *Pseudomonas* and *Candida.* Emphasize need for good preventive hygienic measures.
6. Observe for impaired renal function demonstrated by casts, proteinuria, reduced output, increased BUN, or increased serum creatinine.
7. Anticipate that dosage will be lowered for patients who already have renal impairment.

CEFACLOR CECLOR

Remarks

Cefaclor is well absorbed following oral administration with peak serum levels reached within one hour. Approximately 60–85 percent of the drug is excreted unchanged in the urine within eight hours.

Use

Otitis media caused by susceptible strains of *H. influenzae, S. pneumoniae,* staphylococci, or group A beta-hemolytic streptococci; bronchitis and pneumonia caused by susceptible strains of *S. pneumoniae, H. influenzae,* or group A beta-hemolytic streptococci.

Additional Untoward Reactions Pruritis, urticaria, vaginitis; slight elevation in BUN or serum creatinine.

Dosage **Adult:** 250 mg q 8 hr. Dose may be doubled in more severe infections or those caused by less susceptible organisms. Total daily dose should not exceed 4 gm; **children:** 20 mg/kg/day in divided doses q 8 hr. Dose may be doubled in more serious infections, otitis media, or for infections caused by less susceptible organisms. Total daily dose should not exceed 1 gm. Safety for use in infants less than one month of age not established.

CEFADROXIL MONOHYDRATE DURICEF

Remarks Safe use in children (and during pregnancy) not established. Creatinine clearance determinations must be carried out in patients with renal impairment.

Uses Urinary tract infections caused by *E. coli, Proteus mirabilis,* and *Klebsiella* species.

Dosage **PO:** 1 gm b.i.d. **For patients with creatinine clearance rates below 50 ml/min: initial,** 1 gm; **maintenance,** 500 mg at following dosage intervals: q 36 hr for creatinine clearance rates of 0–10 ml/min; q 24 hr for creatinine clearance rates of 10–25 ml/min; q 12 hr for creatinine clearance rates of 25–50 ml/min.

CEFAMANDOLE NAFATE MANDOL

Remarks Cefamandole nafate has a particularly broad spectrum of activity, including even some gram-negative organisms; *Citrobacter freundii,* numerous species of *Enterobacter,* indole positive *Proteus* and *Providencia stuartii.*

Uses Serious infections by susceptible organisms of the lower respiratory and urinary tract, peritonitis, septicemia, skin and skin structure infections.

Dosage **IV or deep IM injection** (in gluteus or lateral thigh to minimize pain): usual 0.5–1 gm q 4 to 8 hr. *Severe infections:* Up to 2 gm q 4 hr; **infants and children:** 50–100 mg/kg/day in equally divided doses q 4 to 8 hr. *Severe:* Up to 150 mg/kg/day (not to exceed adult dose) divided as above. *Impaired renal function: initial,* 1–2 gm, then a maintenance dosage is given, depending on creatinine clearance according to schedule provided by manufacturer.

Administration/
Storage
1. Consult package insert for details on how to reconstitute drug.
2. Reconstituted solutions of cefamandole nafate are stable for 24 hours at room temperature, and 96 hours when stored in refrigerator. Cefamandole solutions reconstituted with dextrose or sodium chloride are stable for 6 months when frozen immediately after reconstitution.
3. Carbon dioxide gas forms when reconstituted solutions are kept at room temperature. This gas does not affect the activity of the antibiotic and may be dissipated or used to aid in the withdrawal of the contents of the vial.
4. Use separate IV fluid containers and separate injection sites for each drug when cefamandole is administered concomitantly with another antibiotic such as an aminoglycoside.

CEFAZOLIN SODIUM ANCEF, KEFZOL

Remark   Parenteral cephalosporin.

Use   Severe infections of the respiratory and urinary tracts by susceptible organism. Recommended by USPHS for treatment of gonorrhea during pregnancy in patients allergic to penicillin.

Dosage   **IM** or **IV:** 250 mg q 8 hr to 1 gm q 6 hr. Doses up to 6 gm have been given for various serious infections such as endocarditis. *Gonorrhea;* **IM:** 2 gm, together with 1 gm **(PO)** of probenecid; **pediatric over 1 month:** 25–50 mg/kg in 3 to 4 divided doses/day. Dosages are decreased in patients with impaired renal function.

Administration
1. Dissolve the solute by shaking vial.
2. Discard reconstituted solution after 24 hours at room temperature and after 96 hours when refrigerated.

CEFOXITIN SODIUM MEFOXIN

Remarks   Cefoxitin is a cephalosporin with a particularly broad spectrum. It is penicillinase- and cephalosporinase-resistant and is stable in the presence of beta lactamases.

Dosage   **IM** or **IV:** 1–2 gm q 6 to 8 hr. In very severe infections, 12 gm have been given/day. Reduce dosage in presence of renal dysfunction.

Administration/
Storage
1. Do not mix with other antibiotics during administration.
2. Reconstituted solutions are stable for 24 hours at room temperature, one week in refrigerator, and 26 weeks when frozen.
3. Store drug vials below 30°C.
4. Reconstituted solutions are white to light amber. Color does not affect potency.

5. For IM injections lidocaine hydrochloride 0.05% (without epinephrine) may be used as diluent, by doctor's order, to reduce pain at injection site.
6. Do not administer cefoxitin rapidly because it is irritating to veins.

Nursing Implications
1. Monitor intake and output and withhold medication and report to doctor if there is transient or persistent reduction of urinary output.
2. Assess site of infusion for pain and redness because medication causes thrombophlebitis.

CEPHALEXIN KEFLEX

Remarks Cephalosporin for PO administration.

Uses Respiratory tract infections caused by *D. pneumoniae* and group A beta-hemolytic streptococci; skin and soft tissue infections caused by staphylococci; and acute infections of the urinary tract.

Dosage **PO:** 250 mg q 6 hr up to 4 gm daily; **pediatric:** 25–50 mg/kg daily in 4 equally divided doses. Dosage may have to be reduced in patients with impaired renal function or increased for very severe infections. Action of drug can be prolonged by the concurrent administration of oral probenecid (Benemid).

Administration/ Storage After reconstitution the drug should be refrigerated and the unused portion discarded after 14 days.

CEPHALOGLYCIN DIHYDRATE KAFOCIN

Remarks Acid-stable cephalosporin for PO administration.

Uses Acute and chronic urinary tract infections, including cystitis, pyelitis, and pyelonephritis. However, when an oral cephalosporin is indicated for urinary tract infection, cephalexin is preferred.

Dosage **PO:** 250–500 mg 4 times daily. In case of severe infection, therapy may be initiated with a parenteral cephalosporin; **pediatric:** 25–50 mg/kg daily in divided doses.

Administration May be given without interference of food.

Additional Nursing Implications Administer with caution to patients with peptic ulcer.

CEPHALORIDINE LORIDINE

Remarks Cephalosporin for parenteral use. This compound is particularly nephrotoxic and has largely been displaced by other cephalosporins.

Additional Contraindications Impaired renal function.

Laboratory Test Interference Large doses may produce false positive results in urinary protein tests which use sulfosalicylic acid. Cephaloridine may also prolong prothrombin times.

Dosage **IM** and **IV:** 250 mg–1 gm 2 to 4 times a day up to an absolute maximum of 4 gm. *Gonorrhea;* **IM:** 2 gm (single dose); **pediatric in children older than 1 month:** 30–50 mg/kg daily in divided doses.

Administration/ Storage
1. Do not expose to light.
2. Do not mix with other antibiotics.
3. Do not use a diluent containing parabens preservative.
4. Warm diluent and ampule in hand, and shake to help dissolution of medication.
5. Warm ampule in hand and shake if recrystallization occurs before IM injection.
6. Store the straw-colored solution no longer than 4 days in the refrigerator.

CEPHALOTHIN SODIUM KEFLIN NEUTRAL

Remarks This cephalosporin is poorly absorbed from GI tract and must be given parenterally. Cephalothin sodium has a low nephrotoxicity, ototoxicity, and neurotoxicity, which makes it suitable for the treatment of patients with impaired renal function.

Additional Uses Osteomyelitis, and occasionally endocarditis.

Laboratory Test Interference Large doses may produce false + results in urinary protein tests which use sulfosalicylic acid. Cephalothin may also falsely elevate urinary 17-ketosteroid values.

Dosage **IM** or **IV:** 0.5–1.0 gm q 4 to 6 hr, regardless of route. For severe infections doses up to 12 gm daily have been prescribed; **pediatric:** 80–160 mg/kg daily in divided doses. **Peritoneal dialysis:** 6 mg/100 ml dialysis fluid.

Administration/ Storage
1. Dilute according to directions on package insert.
2. Discard reconstituted solution after 12 hours at room temperature and after 96 hours when refrigerated.
3. Dissolve precipitate by warming in hand and shaking. Do not overheat.
4. Retain for use slightly discolored solution.
5. Replace medication and IV solution after 24 hours.
6. For direct IV administration use a small needle into larger veins.

CEPHAPIRIN SODIUM CEFADYL

Remarks Cephalosporin for parenteral administration. The compound is virtually excreted within 6 hours.

Dosage **IM** or **IV:** 0.5–1 gm q 4 to 6 hr, up to 12 gm/day for very serious infections; **pediatric, children older than 3 months:** 40–80 mg/kg daily in 4 equally divided doses. Reduce dosage for patients with renal impairment.

Administration 1. Discard after 12 hours when kept at room temperature and after 10 days when refrigerated at 4°C.
2. Retain for use slightly discolored solutions.

CEPHRADINE ANSPOR, VELOSEF

Remarks This cephalosporin can be administered both orally and parenterally. In severe infections, therapy is usually initiated parenterally. The drug is rapidly absorbed from GI tract or IM injection site (30 minutes to 2 hours) and 60% to 90% of the drug is excreted after 6 hours. The drug is very similar to cephalexin.

Contraindications Safe use in children under 1 year of age and pregnancy has not been established.

Dosage **PO:** 250–500 mg or more q 6 hr. **IM (deep)** or **IV:** 0.5–1 gm or more q.i.d. up to maximum of 8 gm/day; **pediatric over 9 months, PO:** 25–50 mg/kg daily in 4 equally divided doses. *Otitis media* caused by *H. influenzae,* 75–100 mg/kg or more in 4 equally divided doses up to maximum of 4 gm. **IM** or **IV, children older than 1 year:** 50–100 mg/kg in 4 equally divided doses. 300 mg/kg have been used for severely ill infants and children but total pediatric dose should never exceed adult dose.

Administration/ Storage 1. Dilute according to directions on package insert.
2. Do not mix with Lactated Ringer's Injection.
3. Discard reconstituted solution after 10 hours at room temperature and after 48 hours when refrigerated at 5°C.
4. Retain for use slightly yellow solution.
5. Be especially careful to inject IM into muscle since sterile abscesses from accidental subcutaneous injection have occurred.
6. Protect before and after reconstitution from excessive heat and light.
7. Replace medication in prolonged IV administration after 10 hours.
8. Administer PO medication without regard to meals.

CHLORAMPHENICOL AND DERIVATIVES

CHLORAMPHENICOL AMPHICOL, CHLOROMYCETIN, MYCHEL

CHLORAMPHENICOL PALMITATE CHLOROMYCETIN PALMITATE

CHLORAMPHENICOL SODIUM SUCCINATE CHLOROMYCETIN SODIUM SUCCINATE, MYCHEL-S

General Statement

This antibiotic was originally isolated from *Streptomyces venezuellae* and is now produced synthetically. Its activity is mostly bacteriostatic. Chloromycetin appears to inhibit protein synthesis in susceptible organisms and is rapidly absorbed from the GI tract.

Uses

Not to be used for trivial infections, for diseases that can be treated with other agents, or for prophylaxis. Treatment of choice for typhoid fever. Also used for other systemic salmonella infections, *Bacteroides* infections, rickettsial disease, infections caused by lymphogranuloma, psittacosis, mycoplasma, cystic fibrosis, and meningitis caused by *H. influenzae*, as well as urinary infections caused by *P. vulgaris, K. pneumoniae, H. influenzae*, and *P. aeruginosa*.

Contraindications

Hypersensitivity to chloramphenicol; pregnancy, especially near term and during labor; nursing mother. Avoid simultaneous administration of other drugs that may depress bone marrow.

Untoward Reactions

Blood dyscrasias (aplastic anemia), irreversible and reversible bone marrow depression, anemia, gastrointestinal as well as macular and vesicular skin eruptions, fever, pancytopenia, leukopenia, thrombocytopenia. Optic and general neuritis, superinfection, oropharyngeal candidiasis, staphylococcal enteritis, hemorrhage of the skin as well as of the mucosal and serosal areas of the mouth, bladder, and intestine. In neonates, chloramphenicol may cause "the gray syndrome," characterized by rapid respiration, ashen gray color, vomiting, loose green stools, progressive abdominal distension, progressive pallid cyanosis, vasomotor collapse and death. This syndrome can be reversed when the drug is discontinued.

Remarks

Neonates should be observed particularly closely because the drug accumulates in the bloodstream, and the infant is thus subject to greater hazards of toxicity.

Bone marrow depression occurs occasionally. Each patient, therefore, should have daily hemoglobin determinations, WBCs, and differential counts over 24–48 hours. Therapy must be discontinued if the WBCs fall below 4000 and granulocytes below 40%.

Serum iron should be determined occasionally since an increase in serum iron is an early sign of toxicity.

Drug Interactions	*Interactant*	*Interaction*
	Alcohol, ethyl	"Antabuselike" reaction possible
	Anticoagulants, oral	Chloramphenicol potentiates pharmacological effect
	Antidiabetics, oral	Chloramphenicol potentiates pharmacological effect due to ↓ breakdown in liver
	Iron preparations	Chloramphenicol ↓ response to iron therapy
	Phenytoin	Chloramphenicol potentiates pharmacological effect due to ↓ breakdown in liver
	Vitamin B_{12}	Chloramphenicol ↓ response to vitamin B_{12} therapy

Dosage Chloramphenicol, chloramphenicol palmitate **PO, IV, adults and children:** 50 mg/kg daily in 4 equally divided doses q 6 hr. Can be increased to 100 mg/kg daily in very severe infections; **children:** 50 mg/kg/day in 4 divided doses; **neonates and children with immature metabolic function:** 25 mg/kg daily in 4 equally divided doses q 6 hr.

Chloramphenicol sodium succinate—**IV,** same dosage as above; switch to **PO** as soon as possible.

Chloramphenicol ophthalmic ointment 1%—small amount of ointment placed in lower conjunctival sac q 3 hr (or more frequently), day and night, for a minimum of 48 hours.

Chloramphenicol ophthalmic solution 0.5%– 1 to 2 drops 2 to 4 times daily (or more often) day and night for a minimum of 48 hours.

Administration/ Storage Administer IV as a 10% solution over at least a 60 second interval.

Nursing Implications See *Nursing Implications* under *Antibiotics*

1. Administer only to hospitalized patients.
2. Administer only as long as necessary and avoid repeated courses of therapy with chloramphenicol.
3. Anticipate reduction in dosage in patients with impaired renal function, hepatic function, and in newborn infants.
4. Observe for bone marrow depression characterized by weakness, fatigue, sore throat, and bruising.
5. Avoid concomitant administration of drugs that cause bone marrow depression.
6. Observe for optic neuritis, characterized by bilaterally reduced visual acuity which is an indication for immediate discontinuation of drug.
7. Observe for peripheral neuritis, characterized by pain and disturbance of sensation, indications for immediate discontinuation of the drug.
8. Observe premature and newborn infants for the "gray syndrome" characterized by rapid respirations, failure to feed, abdominal distention with or without vomiting followed by progressive pallid cyanosis and vasomotor collapse.
9. Observe for GI side effects, neurotoxic reactions, and jaundice.

CLINDAMYCIN AND LINCOMYCIN

CLINDAMYCIN HYDROCHLORIDE HYDRATE CLEOCIN HYDROCHLORIDE

CLINDAMYCIN PALMITATE HYDROCHLORIDE CLEOCIN PEDIATRIC

CLINDAMYCIN PHOSPHATE CLEOCIN PHOSPHATE

Classification   Clindamycin and lincomycin.

General Statement   This semisynthetic antibiotic is related to lincomycin. It interferes with the protein metabolism of infectious agents and is both bacteriostatic and bactericidal. Antibacterial spectrum is similar to that of erythromycin and includes a variety of gram-positive, particularly staphylococci, streptococci, and pneumococci, and some gram-negative organisms. The drug is rapidly absorbed from the GI tract and widely distributed in body tissues and fluids, including bone.

Uses   Infections of the respiratory, genital, and urinary tracts, skin and soft tissue infections, actinomycosis, septicemia, and osteomyelitis, as well as an adjunct to the treatment of dental infections.

Contraindications   Hypersensitivity to clindamycin. Use with caution in patients with renal disease and with a history of asthma or allergies.

Untoward Reactions   Abdominal pain, diarrhea, anorexia, nausea and vomiting, bloody or tarry stools, and excessive flatulence. Skin rashes and urticaria occur infrequently. Hyperbilirubinemia, leukopenia, eosinophilia, and alterations in some blood enzyme concentrations.

Drug Interaction   Clindamycin should not be given concurrently with erythromycin. Also, clindamycin may enhance effect of neuromuscular blocking agents.

Laboratory Test Interference   ($\uparrow$) levels of SGOT, SGPT, NPN, bilirubin, BSP retention and ($\downarrow$) platelet counts.

Dosage   Clindamycin hydrochloride hydrate, clindamycin palmitate hydrochloride. **PO only:** 150–450 mg q 6 hr; **pediatric:** 8–16 mg/kg daily in 3 to 4 divided doses; **children less than 12.5 kg:** 37.5 mg t.i.d. is the minimum dose.

Clindamycin phosphate, **IM** or **slow IV infusion:** 600–1200 mg daily in 2, 3, or 4 divided doses. *Life-threatening infections:* up to 4.8 gm daily; **pediatric:** 15–25 mg/kg daily in 3 to 4 divided doses up to 25–

40 mg/kg/day in divided doses. Dosage should be reduced in case of severe renal impairment.

Administration
1. Give parenteral clindamycin only to hospitalized patients.
2. Dilute to maximum concentration of 6 mg/ml.
3. Administer IV over a period of 20 to 60 minutes.

Nursing Implications

See *Nursing Implications* under *Antibiotics*.

1. Observe for toxic GI disturbances, such as abdominal pain, diarrhea, anorexia, nausea, vomiting, bloody or tarry stools, and excessive flatulence.
2. Observe for jaundice and decrease in white blood count.
3. Anticipate that patients with renal disease will usually receive a reduced dosage.
4. Monitor intake and output.
5. Do not administer to infants under 1 month unless physician reaffirms order.

LINCOMYCIN HYDROCHLORIDE MONOHYDRATE LINCOCIN

Classification
Clindamycin and lincomycin.

General Statement
Antibiotic isolated from *Streptomyces lincolnensis.* Its antibacterial spectrum resembles that of the erythromycins. It interferes with protein synthesis of infectious agent and is mostly bacteriostatic. Patients with preexisting monilial infections should receive antimonilial therapy. Total blood counts and liver function tests should be done periodically during long-term therapy.

Uses
Lincomycin is not a first-choice drug in the treatment of any infection but is used most often in patients allergic to penicillin. It is effective against group A beta-hemolytic streptococci, pneumococci, and some strains of staphylococci. Useful for the treatment of respiratory tract, urinary tract, and skin and soft tissue infections caused by susceptible organisms. Also used for osteomyelitis and septicemia and, in conjunction with diphtheria antitoxin, in the treatment of diphtheria.

Contraindications
Hypersensitivity to lincomycin. Not indicated in the treatment of viral and minor bacterial infections. Use with caution, and in reduced dosages, in patients with impaired renal and liver function and with endocrine and metabolic diseases.

Untoward Reactions
Severe persistent diarrhea, occasionally with blood and mucus in the stools (observed more frequently with oral drug). Nausea, vomiting, abdominal cramps, heartburn, glossitis, stomatitis, and general discomfort. Hypersensitivity reactions and superinfections. Skin rashes. Cardiac arrest has occurred in conjunction with rapid IV infusion in patients with endocarditis.

Drug Interactions

Interactant	Interaction
Erythromycin	↓ Effect of both drugs
Cyclamate	↓ Effect of lincomycin due to ↓ absorption from GI tract
Kaolin-pectin (Kaopectate)	↓ Effect of lincomycin due to ↓ absorption from GI tract
Neuromuscular Blocking Agents	↑ Effect of blocking agents

Dosage   **PO, adults:** 500 mg t.i.d.-q.i.d.; **children over 1 mo of age:** 30–60 mg/kg/day in 3–4 divided doses depending on severity of infection. **IM, adults:** 600 mg q 12–24 hr; **children over 1 mo of age:** 10 mg/kg/day q 12–24 hr depending on severity of infection. **IV, adults;** 0.6–1.0 gm q 8 to 12 hours up to 8 gm, depending on severity of infection; **children over 1 mo of age:** 10–20 mg/kg/day depending on severity of infection. **Subconjunctival injection:** 0.75 mg.

Administration
1. Prepare drug for administration as directed on package insert.
2. Administer on an empty stomach between meals and not with a sugar substitute, such as sodium or calcium cyclamate.
3. Administer slowly IM to minimize pain.

Nursing Implications
1. Observe and report severe persistent diarrhea with blood and mucus in stools. This necessitates discontinuation of drug.
2. Observe and report generalized aches and pains.
3. Observe and report transient flushing and a sensation of warmth and cardiac disturbances, which may accompany IV infusions. Monitor pulse before, during, and after infusion until stable at levels normal for patient.

POLYMYXINS

COLISTIMETHATE SODIUMCOLY-MYCIN M

COLISTIN SULFATECOLY-MYCIN S

Classification   Antibiotic, polymyxin.

General Statement   This antibiotic is derived from *Bacillus polymyxa* var. *colistinus*. It is both bactericidal and bacteriostatic. It is not absorbed from the GI tract.

Uses   Primarily for urinary tract infections caused by susceptible strains of *Pseudomonas aeruginosa* and other susceptible gram-negative organisms. Also useful for septicemia, wounds, burns, and respiratory tract infections. Indicated PO for acute bacterial diarrhea in infants and children.

Contraindications   Hypersensitivity to the drug. Minor infections.

Untoward Reactions   Nephrotoxicity. Neurotoxic effects: abnormal sensations around the mouth and tongue (circumoral or lingual paresthesia). Visual disturbances, vertigo, neuromuscular blocking effect, and apnea. These effects are not reversed by neostigmine but may be reversed by IV calcium gluconate or calcium chloride.

Fever, GI disturbances, rashes, and occasional pain at site of injection have also been reported.

Dosage   Colistimethate **IV** or **deep IM injection, adults and children:** 1.5–5 mg (maximum)/kg daily in 2 to 4 divided doses.
Colistin sulfate—**PO:** 5–15 mg/kg daily in 3 divided doses. Reduce dosage in patients with renal impairment.

Administration/ Storage
1. Prepare both the solution for injection and the suspension for PO administration according to instructions on package insert.
2. Refrigerate reconstituted medications and discard after 7 days.
3. Administer IM medications deep into the muscle.
4. Protect solution from light.
5. Oral suspensions of the drug are stable for 2 weeks, if refrigerated.

Nursing Implications   See also *Nursing Implications* under *Antibiotics.*

1. Observe for nephrotoxicity demonstrated by albuminuria, hematuria, anuria, casts, edema, and uremia.
2. Monitor intake and output.
3. Instruct patient to report tingling sensation about mouth and tongue, visual and speech disturbances, pruritis, and ototoxic effects.
4. Warn patients to avoid hazardous tasks, since drug may cause speech disturbances, dizziness, vertigo, and ataxia.
5. Have oxygen and calcium chloride for parenteral injection available in case of apnea.

POLYMYXIN B SULFATE (INJECTABLE) AEROSPORIN

Classification   Antibiotic, polymyxin.

General Statement   Polymyxin B sulfate is derived from the spore-forming soil bacterium *Bacillus polymyxa*. It is bactericidal against most gram-negative organisms; rapidly inactivated by alkali, strong acid, and certain metal ions; it is virtually nonabsorbed from the GI tract except in newborn infants. After parenteral administration, polymyxin B seems to remain in the plasma.

Uses   PO: nonsystemic intestinal infections, such as enteritis caused by *Shigella, Pseudomonas,* or gram-negative organisms.

Parenteral: severe resistant *Pseudomonas* infections, such as septicemia, and meningitis (for latter, also given intrathecally). Also useful in infections caused by *E. coli*, *A. aerogenes*, *K. pneumoniae*, or *H. influenzae*, and pulmonary infections due to *Pseudomonas aeruginosa*.

Topical: infections of skin, mucous membranes, ear (external otitis), and eye (corneal ulcers due to *P. aeruginosa*).

Contraindications

Hypersensitivity. Polymyxin B sulfate is a potentially toxic drug to be reserved for the treatment of severe, resistant infections in hospitalized patients. The drug is not indicated for patients with severely impaired renal function or nitrogen retention.

Untoward Reactions

Nephrotoxicity (acute tubular necrosis): transient albuminuria, cellular casts, azotemia, proteinuria, hematuria, and nitrogen retention. Neurologic disturbances (peripheral neuropathy): dizziness, transient blurring of vision, irritability, weakness, and paresthesias (numbness) of mouth and face. High dosage may cause ataxia and dysarthria. Pain at injection site. Superinfections. Nausea, vomiting, diarrhea, and abdominal cramps after large oral doses, noncompetitive neuromuscular blockade, and respiratory insufficiency (apnea). Respiratory paralysis is not antagonized by neostigmine but may sometimes be reversed by calcium gluconate.

Drug Interactions

Interactant	Interaction
Cephalosporins	↑ Renal toxicity
Skeletal muscle relaxants (surgical)	↑ Muscle relaxation
Succinylcholine	
d-Tubocurarine	
Aminoglycoside antibiotics	Additive toxic effects
Gentamicin	
Kanomycin	
Neomycin	
Streptomycin	

Laboratory Test Interference

False + or ↑ levels of urea nitrogen, and creatinine. Casts and RBC in urine.

Dosage

IM, IV, adults and children: 15,000–25,000 (maximum) units/kg daily in divided doses q 6 hr; **infants:** up to 40,000 units/kg/day. **Intrathecally** (*meningitis*), **adults and children over 2 years:** 50,000 units once daily for 3–4 days, **then** 50,000 units every other day until 2 weeks after cultures are negative. **Inhalation, adults and children:** 1–2 ml of a solution containing 1–10 mg/ml 4 to 6 times daily, up to maximum of 2.5 mg/kg/day. **Topical:** For eye and ear, concentration depends on use.

Administration/ Storage

1. Store and dilute as directed on package insert.
2. Pain on IM injection can be lessened by reducing drug concentration as much as possible. It is preferable to give drug more frequently in more dilute doses. If ordered, procaine hydrochloride (2.0 ml of a 0.5% to 1.0% solution per 5 units of dry powder) may be used for mixing the drug for IM injection.

3. *Never use preparations containing procaine hydrochloride for IV or intrathecal use.*

Nursing Implications

See *Nursing Implications* under *Antibiotics.*

1. Do not administer with other nephrotoxic or neurotoxic agents.
2. Observe for nephrotoxicity characterized by albuminuria, casts, nitrogen retention, and hematuria. Monitor intake and output.
3. Observe for drug fever and neurologic disturbances, demonstrated by dizziness, blurred vision, irritability, circumoral and peripheral numbness and tingling, weakness, and ataxia. Usually, these symptoms disappear within 24 to 48 hours after the drug is discontinued.
4. Observe for muscle weakness, an early sign of muscle paralysis and impending apnea. Withhold drug when signs of muscle weakness appear. Be prepared to assist respiration and have calcium gluconate on hand for emergency use in case of respiratory difficulties.
5. Use safety precautions for ambulatory or bedridden patients with neurologic disturbances.
6. Anticipate a prolonged regimen of topical application of polymyxin B solution, since drug is not toxic when used in wet dressings, and the physician may wish to avoid emergence of resistant strains.

AMINOGLYCOSIDES

General Statement

The aminoglycosides are broad spectrum antibiotics, primarily used for the treatment of serious gram-negative infections caused by *Pseudomonas, E. coli, Proteus, Klebsiella,* and *Enterobacter.* The mechanism of action of the antibiotics is the inhibition of protein synthesis of the infecting microorganism.

Because they are poorly absorbed from the GI tract, the aminoglycosides are usually administered parenterally, the only occasional exception being some enteric infections of the GI tract and prior to surgery. The aminoglycosides are rapidly absorbed after IM injection; peak blood levels occur within 1 to 2 hours. The average half-life in normal adults is 2 to 3 hours. It is longer in young infants, the elderly, and in the presence of impaired renal function.

Aminoglycoside antibiotics are distributed in the extra-cellular fluid, cross the placental barrier, but not the blood-brain barrier. Penetration of the cerebrospinal fluid is increased when the meninges are inflamed.

The aminoglycosides are excreted, largely unchanged, in the urine. This makes the drugs suitable for urinary tract infections. Concomitant administration of bicarbonate (alkalinization of urine) improves treatment of such infections. There is considerable cross-allerginicity between the individual aminoglycosides. The aminoglycosides are powerful antibiotics that can induce serious side effects. They should not be used for minor infections. Except for streptomycin, resistance of the organisms to aminoglycosides develops slowly. Whenever possible, the sensitivity of the infectious agent should be determined before instituting therapy.

Uses Septicemia, bacteremia, infected surgical wounds, burns, and severe infections of the skin and soft tissues, including respiratory and selected urinary tract infections caused by susceptible organisms.

Orally, some of the drugs are suitable for preoperative intestinal antisepsis, nonsystemic GI infections as an adjunct for the mechanical cleansing of the big bowel, and for cirrhotic patients with hepatic coma.

Contraindications Hypersensitivity of aminoglycosides, long-term therapy (except streptomycin for tuberculosis). Use with extreme caution in patients with impaired renal function or pre-existing hearing impairment. Safe use in pregnancy and during lactation not established.

Untoward Reactions **Ototoxicity** Both auditory and vestibular damage have been noted. The risk of ototoxicity and vestibular impairment is increased in patients with poor renal function and the elderly. Loss of hearing, sometimes preceded by tinnitus and vertigo, can occur several weeks after discontinuation of drugs.

Renal impairment This may be characterized by cylindria, oliguria, proteinuria, increased BUN, NPN or creatinine. Rarely, some of the aminoglycosides cause neuromuscular blockade and apnea which may be reversed by IV neostigmine or calcium gluconate. Also, other types of neurotoxicity: numbness, tingling of skin, optic neuritis, peripheral neuritis, arachnoiditis, encephalopathy, muscle twitching, and convulsions; increased SGOT, SGPT and serum bilirubin; transient hepatomegaly, decreased serum calcium, splenomegaly, changes in blood counts, fever, rash, itching, urticaria, generalized burning, joint pain, laryngeal edema; nausea, vomiting, headache, increased salivation, lethargy, anorexia, weight loss, pulmonary fibrosis, changes in blood pressure, superinfections. Intestinal lesions may increase systemic absorption of the drugs and increase toxicity. Local irritation or pain at IM injection site. Renal, auditory, and vestibular functions should be assessed regularly during drug administration.

Drug Interaction

Interactant	*Interaction*
Anticoagulants, oral	Gentamicin potentiates pharmacological effect
Carbenicillin	Inhibits activity of gentamicin
Cephalosporins	Additive renal toxicity
Ethacrynic acid	Additive ototoxicity
Ether	↑ Muscle relaxation
Other aminoglycoside antibiotics	↑ Chance of ototoxicity and renal toxicity
Kanamycin	
Neomycin	
Streptomycin	
Skeletal muscle relaxants (surgical)	↑ Muscle relaxation
Succinylcholine	
d-Tubocurarine	

Laboratory Tests Interferences ↑ BUN, BSP retention, creatinine, SGOT, SGPT, bilirubin. ↓ Cholesterol values.

Dosage See individual agents.

Administration
1. Inject drug deep into muscle mass to minimize transient pain.
2. Administer for only 7 to 10 days and avoid repeating course of therapy unless serious infection is present that does not respond to other antibiotics.

Nursing Implications
1. Obtain patient's body weight for correct calculation of dosage.
2. Observe for nephrotoxicity.
   a. Assess closely patients with renal dysfunction because they are more susceptible to developing toxicity. Ascertain that a pretreatment audiogram is done and repeated during therapy, if administration of aminoglycosides is to exceed 5 days.
   b. Assess for presence of cells or casts in urine, oliguria, proteinuria, lowered specific gravity, or increasing BUN, NPN, or creatinine.
   c. Maintain intake and output.
   d. Hydrate patient well unless contraindicated.
3. Observe for signs of ototoxicity.
   a. Assess patient for tinnitus and vertigo, signs of vestibular injury more common with gentamycin and streptomycin.
   b. Assess for subjective hearing loss or loss of high tones on the audiometer, indicating auditory damage more common with kanamycin and neomycin.
   c. Protect patient with vestibular dysfunction by supervising ambulation and providing side rails if necessary.
   d. Continue monitoring ototoxicity because the onset of deafness may occur several weeks after therapy when aminoglycoside has been discontinued.
4. Observe for neuromuscular blockade leading to apnea when aminoglycoside is administered together with a muscle relaxant or after anesthesia. Have calcium gluconate or neostigmine available to reverse blockade.
5. Withhold medication and check with medical supervision if signs of toxicity are noted. Doctor will either reduce dosage or discontinue medication.
6. Do not administer concurrently or sequentially with a topical or systemic nephrotoxic or ototoxic drug; for example, potent diuretics, such as ethacrynic acid or furosemide.
7. Assess closely premature infants, neonates, and older patients receiving aminoglycosides because they are particularly sensitive to their toxic effects.

AMIKACIN SULFATE AMIKIN

Classification Antibiotic, aminoglycoside

Remarks Amikacin is derived from kanamycin. Its spectrum is somewhat broader than that of other aminoglycosides, including *Gerratia* and

Acinetobacter species, as well as certain *Staphylococci* and *Streptococci.* Amikacin is effective against both penicillinase and non-penicillinase producing organisms.

Additional Uses Neonatal sepsis, infections of the CNS system, including meningitis; intra-abdominal infections, including peritonitis; post-operative infections, including post-vascular surgery.

Dosage **IM** (preferred) and **IV, adults, children, and older infants:** 15 mg/kg/day in 2 to 3 equally divided doses q 8 to 12 hr, **maximum daily dose:** 15 mg/kg. *Uncomplicated urinary tract infections* 250 mg b.i.d.; **newborns:** loading dose of 10 mg/kg followed by 7.5 mg/kg q 12 hr. *Impaired renal function:* normal loading dose of 7.5 mg/kg; **then** administration should be monitored by serum level of amikacin (35 μg/ml max) or creatinine clearance rates.

Administration/ Storage for IV Administration
1. Add 500 mg vial to 200 ml of sterile diluent, such as normal saline or 5% D/W.
2. Administer over a 30 to 60 minute period for children and adults.
3. Administer to infants in the amount of fluid ordered by the doctor. The IV administration to infants should be 1 to 2 hours.
4. Store colorless liquid at room temperature no longer than 2 years.
5. Potency is not affected if the solution turns a very light yellow.

GENTAMICIN SULFATE GARAMYCIN

Classification Antibiotic, aminoglycoside.

Remarks The drug can be used concurrently with carbenicillin for the treatment of serious *Pseudomonas* infections. However, the drugs should not be mixed in the same flask because the latter will inactivate the antibiotic.

Additional Uses Gentamicin is the drug of choice for hospital-acquired gram-negative sepsis. Also, intrathecally for *Pseudomonas meningitis.* Primary and secondary skin infections, such as impetigo, insect bites, furunculosis, skin cysts, or abscesses caused by susceptible organisms, respond well to topical treatment with gentamicin cream or ointment.

Additional Drug Interaction With carbenicillin, gentamicin may result in increased effect when used for Pseudomonas infections.

Dosage **IM or IV infusion, adults with normal renal function:** 1–1.5 mg/kg q 8 hr; **children:** 2–2.5 mg/kg q 8 hr; **infants and neonates:** 2.5 mg/kg q 8 hr. This dose should be administered only if creatinine clearance is equal to or in excess of 10 ml/min/m^2 body surface. **Adults with impaired renal function:** use formula—serum creatinine (mg/100 ml) × 8 to calculate interdose interval (in hr).

Administration of Cream or Ointment
1. Remove the crusts of impetigo contagiosa before applying ointment to permit maximum contact between antibiotic and infection.
2. Apply ointment gently and cover with gauze dressing if desirable.
3. Avoid further contamination of infected skin.

KANAMYCIN KANTREX

Classification Antibiotic, aminoglycoside.

Remarks The activity of kanamycin resembles that of neomycin and streptomycin.

Additional Drug Interaction Procainamide. ↑ Muscle relaxation.

Dosage **PO and IM, intraperitoneally, by inhalation, direct instillation into abscessed cavity, adults and children, IM:** 15 mg/kg/day in 2 to 4 equally divided doses. **Maximum daily dose:** 1.5 gm regardless of body weight. **Dose for impaired renal function:** use formula, serum creatinine (mg/100 ml) × 9 = dosage interval (in hr). **IV:** maximum of 15 mg/kg/day injected slowly. **IP:** 500 mg diluted in 20 ml distilled water. **PO:** *Suppression of intestinal bacteria:* 8–12 gm/day in divided doses. **Inhalation:** 250 mg 2 to 4 times/day.

Administration
1. Do not mix with other drug medication in IV bottle. Administer IV slowly and at concentrations not exceeding 2.5 mg/ml.
2. Unopened vials may change color, but this does not affect potency of drug.
3. Do not mix with other drugs in same syringe for IM injection.
4. Inject deep into large muscle mass to minimize pain and local irritation. Rotate sites of injection. Local irritation may occur with large doses.
5. IV administration is rarely used and must not be used for patients with renal impairment.
6. Drug should not be administered for more than 12 to 14 days.

NEOMYCIN SULFATE MYCIFRADIN SULFATE, NEOBIOTIC

Classification Antibiotic, aminoglycoside.

Additional Uses **PO:** Hepatic coma, bacterial diarrhea, sterilization of gut prior to surgery. Therapy of intestinal infections due to pathogenic strains of *E. coli* primarily in children. **Topical:** widely used for infections of the skin, eyes, and ears, including skin wounds and ulcers.

Additional Contraindication Intestinal obstruction (PO).

Additional Untoward Reactions

Muscle relaxation, respiratory depression and arrest. Oral neomycin sulfate has a laxative effect. Skin rashes after topical or parenteral administration.

Additional Drug Interactions

Interactant	Interaction
Penicillin V	↓ Effect of penicillin due to ↓ absorption from GI tract
Procainamide	↑ Muscle relaxation produced by neomycin

Dosage

PO (preoperatively): 1.0 gm q hr 4 times; **then** 1.0 gm q 4 hr for 24 to 72 hr; **other:** 30–60 mg/kg daily in divided doses. **IM:** 10–15 mg/kg daily in 3 to 4 divided doses up to a maximum of 1.0 gm. **Not recommended for use in children or infants.**

Maximum course of therapy is 10 days. The drug is also administered by instillation in case of emergency abdominal surgery or peritonitis.

Topical Application Neomycin alone or in combination with other antibiotics (bacitracin or gramicidin) and/or an anti-inflammatory agent (corticosteroid) is used for a variety of topical infections.

Ophthalmic A small amount of a 0.5% ointment is instilled into the conjunctival sac one or more times daily. 1 to 2 drops of a 0.1% to 0.5% solution is instilled into the eye 2 to 4 times daily. **Severe infections.** A 4.0% solution may be used safely 2 to 4 times daily, or a weaker solution may be applied more frequently.

Otic For external otitis, chronic otitis media, and various dermatoses of the external auditory canal. Instill 3 to 5 drops 3 to 4 times daily. Alternately, a gauze wick moistened with the preparation may be loosely inserted into the external canal.

Dermatologic Used for itching, burning, inflamed skin conditions that are threatened by, or complicated by, a secondary bacterial infection. Apply cream to affected area 2 to 3 times daily.

Additional Nursing Implications

1. Have on hand neostigmine to counteract renal failure, respiratory depression and arrest, which may occur when neomycin is administered intraperitoneally.
2. Anticipate a slight laxative effect produced by oral neomycin. Withhold the drug and consult with physician in case of suspected intestinal obstruction.
3. For preoperative disinfection, patient should receive a low-residue diet and, unless contraindicated, a cathartic immediately preceding PO administration of neomycin sulfate, 1.0 gm q 1 to 4 hours for 24 to 72 hours.
4. Apply ointment or solution of neomycin after cleaning the affected area. Solution is apparently more effective than ointment and is used in wet dressings.

STREPTOMYCIN SULFATE

Classification	Antibiotic, aminoglycoside.
Remarks	Like other aminoglycoside antibiotics, streptomycin is rapidly distributed throughout most tissues and body fluids including necrotic tubercular lesions.
Additional Uses	Tuberculosis in conjunction with other antitubercular agents. Emergence of resistant strains has greatly reduced the usefulness of streptomycin; also tularemia, glanders (*Actinobacillus mallei*), bubonic plague (*Pasteurella pestis*), brucellosis, cholera, and bacterial endocarditis caused by *H. influenzae*.
Additional Contraindications	Hypersensitivity, contact dermatitis, and exfoliative dermatitis. Do not give to patients with myasthenia gravis.
Additional Untoward Reactions	Peripheral neuritis, neuromuscular blockade, and apnea with parenteral administration are reversible by neostigmine.
Dosage	**IM only, individualized:** usually 1–4 gm daily in divided doses. Single dose should not exceed 1.0 gm; **pediatric:** 10–20 mg/kg b.i.d. *Tuberculosis* (adjunct): 1.0 gm 2 to 3 times weekly for 4 months; **pediatric:** 20 mg/kg daily. Older, debilitated patients usually receive lower dosages.

Administration/ Storage

1. Protect hands when preparing drug. Wear gloves if drug is prepared often because it is irritating.
2. In a dry form, the drug is stable for at least 2 years at room temperature.
3. Aqueous solutions prepared without preservatives are stable for at least 1 week at room temperature and for at least 3 months under refrigeration.
4. Use only solutions prepared freshly from dry powder for intrathecal and intrapleural administration because commercially prepared solutions contain preservatives harmful to tissues of the central nervous system and pleural cavity.
5. Commercially prepared, ready-to-inject solutions are for IM use only. These solutions are prepared with phenol and are stable at room temperature for prolonged periods of time.
6. Administer deep into muscle mass to minimize pain and local irritation.
7. Solutions may darken after exposure to light, but this does not necessarily cause a loss in potency.
8. When injection into the subarachnoid space is required for treatment of meningitis, only solutions made freshly from the dry powder should be used. Commercial solutions may contain preservatives toxic to the CNS.

TOBRAMYCIN SULFATE NEBCIN

Classification   Antibiotic, aminoglycoside.

Remarks   This aminoglycoside is very similar to gentamicin and can be used concurrently with carbenicillin.

Dosage   **IM** (preferred) and **IV, adults, children and older infants:** 3 mg/kg/day in 3 equally divided doses q 8 hr, 5 mg/kg/day in 3 to 4 equal doses have been used for seriously ill patients; **neonates 1 week of age or less:** up to 4 mg/kg/day in 2 equal doses q 12 hr. Dosage is to be reduced and monitored by creatinine clearance rate (see package insert for formula) in patients with impaired renal function.

Administration/ Storage
1. Prepare IV solution by diluting calculated dose of tobramycin with 50–100 ml of IV solution.
2. Infuse over 20 to 60 minutes.
3. Use proportionately less diluent for children than for adults.
4. Do not mix with other drugs for parenteral administration.
5. Store drug at room temperature—no longer than 2 years.
6. Discard solution of drug containing up to 1 mg/ml after 24 hours at room temperature.

MISCELLANEOUS ANTIBIOTICS

BACITRACIN BACIQUENT

Classification   Antibiotic, miscellaneous.

General Statement   Antibiotic produced by *Bacillus subtilis*. Bactericidal for many gram-positive organisms and *Neisseria*. Not absorbed from the GI tract. When given parenterally, drug is well distributed in pleural and ascitic fluids.

Bacitracin has a very high nephrotoxicity. Its systematic use is restricted to infants (see uses). Renal function must be carefully evaluated prior to and daily during use.

Uses   Bacitracin is used locally during surgery for cranial and neurosurgical infections caused by susceptible organisms.

As an ointment (preferred) or solution, bacitracin is prescribed for superficial pyodermalike impetigo and infectious eczematoid dermatitis, for secondary infected dermatoses (atopic dermatitis, contact dermatitis), and for superficial infections of the eye, ear, nose, and throat by susceptible organisms.

Parenteral use is limited to the treatment of staphylococcal pneumonia and staphylococci-induced empyema in infants.

Contraindication   Hypersensitivity or toxic reaction to bacitracin. Pregnancy.

Untoward Reactions   Nephrotoxicity, renal failure, renal tubular necrosis, toxic reactions, nausea, vomiting.

Dosage   **Topical:** apply directly to affected areas once or twice daily. Ointment contains 500 units/gm. Solution to be applied as wet dressing should contain 250–1000 units/ml. **IM, infants, 2.5 kg and below:** 900 units/kg/day in 2 to 3 divided doses; **over 2.5 kg:** 1,000 units/kg/day in 2 to 3 divided doses.

Administration   1. Do not mix bacitracin with glycerin or other polyalcohols that cause drug to deteriorate. Bacitracin unguentin base is anhydrous, consisting of liquid and white petrolatum.
2. Cleanse area before applying bacitracin as a wet dressing or ointment.
3. Adequate fluid intake must be maintained with parenteral use.

Nursing Implications   1. Check that renal function tests have been done prior to initiating therapy and daily during therapy.
2. Monitor intake and output.
3. Maintain adequate fluid intake and output with parenteral use of the drug.
4. Test pH of urine daily because it should be kept at 6 or greater to decrease renal irritation.
5. Have available sodium bicarbonate or another alkali to administer should pH drop below 6.
6. Do not administer concurrently or sequentially with a topical or systemic nephrotoxic drug.
7. Withhold drug and consult with doctor when fluid output is inadequate.

NOVOBIOCIN CALCIUM ALBAMYCIN CALCIUM

NOVOBIOCIN SODIUM ALBAMYCIN SODIUM

Classification   Antibiotic, miscellaneous.

General Statement   Novobiocin is derived from *Streptomyces niveus* and is primarily bacteriostatic. It is readily absorbed from the GI tract and diffuses well into pleural, joint, and ascitic fluids.

Oral use of drug is to be avoided if possible.

Drug is to be given in doses high enough to prevent resistant strains.

Frequent total and differential blood counts and liver function tests should be performed during prolonged therapy.

Jaundice, hyperbilirubinemia, or sulfobromophthalein retention is an indication for discontinuation of drug.

Uses Infections by susceptible strains of staphylococci and *Proteus*. Indicated for the treatment of enteritis, postoperative wound infections, cellulitis, abscesses and ulcers, and resistant urinary tract infections.

Contraindications Hypersensitivity to novobiocin. Avoid use in newborn or premature infants. Because of the frequency of toxic effects associated with oral use, novobiocin is not recommended for the treatment of minor infections.

Untoward Reactions Novobiocin is a potent sensitizing agent and can cause skin rash, urticaria, fever, pruritus, swollen joints, and blood dyscrasias, which can be fatal. Liver damage, jaundice, nausea, vomiting, anorexia, abdominal distress, and lightheadedness have also been reported. The drug may also cause superinfections and favors the emergence of resistant strains, particularly staphylococci. It can cause neonatal hyperbilirubinemia.

Drug Interaction Tetracyclines diminish effectiveness of novobiocin.

Dosage **PO, IM, and IV:** 250–500 mg q 6 to 12 hr. Maximum is 2.0 gm daily; **pediatric:** 15–45 mg/kg daily in divided doses.

Administration
1. For IM administration, dissolve 500 mg as indicated on package insert in 5 ml of accompanying diluent.
2. Administer deep into muscle mass.
3. Divide IM dose into 2 sites to reduce pain.
4. Rotate sites of injection.
5. IV administration is less painful than IM administration. For IV, dilute solution further as indicated on package insert.
6. Inject IV over a period of 5 to 10 minutes to prevent venous irritation and thrombophlebitis.

Nursing Implications See also *Nursing Implications* under *Antibiotics*.

1. Observe for allergic reactions, since drug is a potent sensitizing agent. Have emergency equipment available.
2. Observe for symptoms of blood dyscrasias, such as anemia, purpura, paleness, and bleeding.
3. Observe newborn infants for jaundice, which may lead to kernicterus and subsequent brain damage. Withhold drug if jaundice is noted.
4. Observe whether patient is able to tolerate oral intake, and report to physician so that drug may be ordered PO as soon as possible.

PAROMOMYCIN SULFATE HUMATIN

Classification Antibiotic, miscellaneous.

General Statement Paromomycin is obtained from *Streptomyces rimosus forma paromomycina*. Its spectrum of activity resembles that of neomycin and kanamycin. The drug is poorly absorbed from the GI tract and is ineffective against systemic infections when given orally.

Uses   Enteric bacterial infections caused by susceptible organisms such as *Salmonella, Shigella, Proteus,* acute and chronic intestinal amebiasis, and bacillary dysentery. Also effective for preoperative suppression of intestinal flora and as an adjunct in the treatment of hepatic coma.

Contraindications   Intestinal obstruction. To be used with caution in the presence of GI ulceration because of possible systemic absorption.

Untoward Reactions   Diarrhea or loose stools. Nausea, abdominal cramps, heartburn, emesis, headache, skin rash, and pruritus ani. Superinfections, especially by monilia.

Drug Interaction   Penicillin is inhibited by paromomycin.

Dosage   **PO;** *Hepatic coma.* 4 gm daily in divided doses. *Intestinal amebiasis,* **adults and children:** 25–35 mg/kg daily in 3 to 4 divided doses for a minimum of 5 days.

Administration   1. Do not administer parenterally.
2. Administer before or after meals.

Nursing Implications   See also *Nursing Implications* under *Antibiotics.*

Observe and report diarrhea, dehydration, and general weakness.

SPECTINOMYCIN HYDROCHLORIDE PENTAHYDRATE TROBICIN

Classification   Antibiotic, miscellaneous.

General Statement   Spectinomycin is produced by *Streptomyces spectabilis.* The antibiotic interferes with protein synthesis, is mainly bacteriostatic, and is effective against a wide variety of gram-negative and gram-positive organisms, including those causing gonorrhea. It is ineffective against syphilis, and this is why it is a poor choice of drug when mixed infections are present.

Spectinomycin is not absorbed from the GI tract and is only given IM.

Uses   Acute gonorrhea in infections resistant to penicillin or in patients allergic to penicillin.

Contraindication   Sensitivity to drug.

Untoward Reactions   A single dose of spectinomycin has caused soreness at the site of injection, urticaria, dizziness, nausea, chills, fever, and insomnia.

Multiple doses have caused a decrease in hemoglobin, hematocrit, and creatinine clearance and an increase in alklaline phosphatase, blood urea nitrogen, and serum glutamic pyruvic transaminase (SGPT)

Dosage   **IM:** 2 gm. In areas where antibiotic resistance is known to be prevalent, give 10 gm divided between 2 gluteal injection sites.

Administration/ Storage
1. Powder is stable for 3 years.
2. Use reconstituted solution within 24 hours.
3. Inject deeply into the upper outer quadrant of the gluteus muscle.
4. Injections may be made in two sites for patients requiring 4 gm.

Nursing Implications   Advise patients treated with spectinomycin and suspected of having syphilis to return for serologic tests monthly for at least 3 months.

TROLEANDOMYCIN TAO

Classification   Antibiotic, miscellaneous.

General Statement   Troleandomycin is a broad spectrum antibiotic salt prepared from cultures of *Streptomyces antibioticus*. Its spectrum of activity resembles that of erythromycin, being bacteriostatic and effective against gram-negative bacteria. Troleandomycin is widely distributed in body tissues and fluids but not in spinal fluid unless the meninges are inflamed.

Periodic liver function tests are indicated. Troleandomycin may alter some liver function tests for periods of up to 5 weeks. When used for acute gonococcal infection in patients with suspected lesions of syphilis, dark field examination should precede initiation of therapy and serologic tests should be made at monthly intervals for 3 months.

Uses   Severe, acute infections by susceptible staphylococci, streptococci, pneumococci, clostridium, and corynebacterium. Single doses of troleandomycin are effective against acute gonococcal urethritis.

Contraindications   Hypersensitivity to drug. Liver dysfunction or known sensitivity toward hepatotoxic drugs. Not recommended for prophylaxis or therapy for longer than 10 days. Occasional cross-sensitivity with erythromycin.

Untoward Reactions   Hepatotoxicity: hyperbilirubinemia and jaundice. Superinfections. Local irritation at site of injection. Nausea, vomiting, esophagitis, rectal burning, diarrhea, headache, and skin rash. Rarely, anaphylactoid reactions.

Dosage   **PO:** 250–500 mg q 6 hr. Single 1.0 gm dose for acute gonococcal urethritis in males; **pediatric:** 6.6–11 mg/kg q 6 hr.

Nursing Implications   Also see *Nursing Implications* under *Antibiotics*.

Observe for jaundice as drug should be discontinued at first signs of hepatotoxicity.

VANCOMYCIN HYDROCHLORIDE VANCOCIN HYDROCHLORIDE

Classification   Antibiotic, miscellaneous.

General Statement   This antibiotic, derived from *Streptomyces orientalis*, inhibits cell wall synthesis. It is bactericidal and bacteriostatic. It diffuses in pleural, pericardial, ascitic, and synovial fluids after parenteral administration. Auditory and renal function tests are indicated before and during therapy.

Uses   Agent should be reserved for life-threatening infections for patients allergic to penicillin or staphylococcus resistant to penicillin. Also, endocarditis, osteomyelitis, pneumonia, and septicemia. Oral administration is useful in treatment of enterocolitis.

Contraindications   Hypersensitivity to drug. Minor infections. Use with extreme caution in the presence of impaired renal function or previous hearing loss.

Untoward Reactions   Ototoxicity (may lead to deafness), nephrotoxicity (may lead to uremia), nausea, chills, fever, hypersensitivity, skin rashes, anaphylaxis, tinnitus. Thrombophlebitis at site of injection. Deafness may progress after drug is discontinued.

Drug Interactions   Never give with other ototoxic or nephrotoxic agents.

Dosage   **IV, PO:** 0.5–1 gm q 6 hr up to 4 gm/day; **children** 45 mg/kg/day in divided doses.

Administration/ Storage

1. Mix as indicated on package insert.
2. Intermittent diffusion is the preferred route, but continuous IV drip may be used.
3. Avoid rapid IV administration as this may result in nausea, warmth, and generalized tingling.
4. Avoid extravasation during injections.
5. Reduce risk of thrombophlebitis by rotating injection sites or adding additional diluent.
6. Dilute one 500 mg vial in 1 ounce of water for oral administration. Patient may drink solution or it may be administered by nasogastric tube.
7. Aqueous solution is stable for 2 weeks.
8. Once rubber stopper is punctured, ampule should be refrigerated to maintain stability.

Nursing Implications   See also *Nursing Implications* under *Antibiotics* at the beginning of this section.

1. Observe for ototoxicity demonstrated by tinnitus, progressive hearing loss, dizziness, and/or nystagmus.
2. Observe for nephrotoxicity demonstrated by albuminuria, hematuria, anuria, casts, edema, and uremia.
3. Monitor intake and output.

antifungal agents

Amphotericin B	Griseofulvin Ultramicrosize
Flucytosine	Miconazole
Griseofulvin	Nystatin

Several types of fungi or yeasts are pathogenic for humans. Some fungal infections are systemic, and others are limited to the skin, hair, or nails. A third group infects mostly moist mucous membranes, including the GI tract and vagina. *Candida* organisms belong to this last group.

Drug therapy depends both on the infectious agent and on the type of infection. An accurate diagnosis of the infection, prior to therapy, is most important for the choice of the therapeutic agents.

As in other infections, it is important that drug therapy be continued until the infectious agent has been completely eradicated to avoid the emergence of resistant strains.

AMPHOTERICIN B FUNGIZONE I.V.

Classification Antibiotic, antifungal.

General Statement This antibiotic is produced by *Streptomyces nodosus* and is the drug of choice for deep infections. It can be administered IV, instilled into cavities (intrathecally), and used topically. Amphotericin B is fungistatic rather than fungicidal. It is effective against most pathogenic fungi, including North American blastomycosis.

The drug is very toxic and should only be used for patients under close medical supervision with a relatively certain diagnosis of deep mycotic infections. IV administration is usually reserved for life-threatening disease.

Uses Disseminated North American blastomycosis, cryptococcosis, and other systemic fungal infections, including coccidioidomycosis, paracoccidioidomycosis, histoplasmosis, aspergillosis, disseminated candidiasis, and monilial overgrowth resulting from oral antibiotic therapy. Topical: cutaneous and mucocutaneous infections of *Candida* (*Monilia*) infections.

Contraindication Hypersensitivity to drug.

Untoward Reactions Few, when applied topically. IV: rise in BUN (above 40 mg/100 ml), NPN (above 10 mg/100 ml), and elevated creatinine levels, which may dictate intermittent use of drug. Fever, chills, tremor, anorexia, nausea, vomiting, sweating, chest pain, muscle weakness (due to hypokalemia), and transitory vestibular disturbances. Also rash, weight loss, generalized pain, and local inflammation at injection site.

Prophylactic administration of antipyretics and/or antihistamines and corticosteroids reduce adverse reactions. Should such reactions recur, drug should be discontinued.

Drug Interactions

Interactant	Interaction
Corticosteroids Corticotropin	↑ K depletion caused by amphotericin B
Digitalis glycosides	↑ K depletion caused by amphotericin B, ↑ incidence of digitalis toxicity
Skeletal muscle relaxants (surgical) Succinylcholine d-Tubocurarine	↑ Muscle relaxation

Laboratory Test Interference: ↑ SGPT, SGOT, alkaline phosphatase, creatinine, BUN, NPN, BSP retention values.

Dosage **Slow IV infusion, initial:** 250 μg/kg daily. Increase gradually by 100–200 μg/kg up to maximum dose of 1.0 mg/kg/day. **Never exceed:** 1.5 mg/kg/day. Treatment is usually continued for 2 to 4 months. **Intrathecal, initial:** 100 μg daily. Increase to maximum of 750 μg every other day. **Topical:** amphotericin B comes as lotion, cream, or ointment which is liberally applied to affected areas 2 to 4 times/day.

Administration/ Storage

1. Follow directions on vial for dilution. Only use distilled water without a bacteriostatic or 5% dextrose as diluent in order to avoid precipitation of drug.
2. Strict aseptic technique must be used in preparation as there is no bacteriostatic agent in the medication.
3. Use sterile needle every time entrance is made into the vial.
4. Do not use saline solution or distilled water with bacteriostatic agent as a diluent since a precipitate may result.
5. Do not use the initial concentrate if there is any precipitate.
6. Do not use a membrane filter in the IV line since the drug forms a colloidal solution and particles may be filtered out.
7. Protect from light during administration and storage.
8. Minimize local inflammation and danger of thrombophlebitis by administering the solution below the recommended dilution of 100 μg/ml.
9. Initiate therapy in the most distal veins.
10. Have on hand 200 to 400 units of heparin sodium since it may be ordered for the infusion to prevent thrombophlebitis.
11. Administer the IV for 6 hours.
12. Amphotericin may be stored in DW for 24 hours in a dark room or in a refrigerator for 1 week without significant loss of potency.
13. Use dilutions of 0.1 mg/ml immediately after preparation.

Nursing Implications

1. Interrupt IV and notify physician should patient develop adverse reaction during administration.
2. Ascertain whether physician wants patient to have antipyretics, antihistamines, or antiemetics prior to IV therapy.
3. Check that weekly BUN, NPN, and potassium levels have been determined. Ascertain that the physician is aware of any untoward results.
4. Observe for muscle weakness, a sign of hypokalemia.
5. Have potassium chloride available to administer if needed.
6. Monitor vital signs every half hour during IV administration and at least daily while patient is on therapy.
7. Monitor intake and output and report reduction in urine output and blood sediment, or cloudiness in the urine.
8. Weigh patient twice weekly and be alert to signs of malnutrition and dehydration.
9. Observe and report sensory loss or foot drop in patients receiving intrathecal amphotericin as inflammation of the spinal roots may occur.

Creams and Lotions:
1. Rub into lesion.
2. Reassure patient that drug does not stain the skin when it is rubbed into the lesion.
3. Advise patient that any discoloration of fabrics caused by cream or lotion may be removed by washing with soap and water.
4. Advise patient that any discoloration caused by ointment may be removed by a standard cleaning fluid.

FLUCYTOSINE ANCOBON

Classification   Antibiotic, antifungal.

General Statement   This synthetic antifungal agent is indicated only for serious systemic fungal infections. The drug is less toxic than amphotericin B. Liver, renal system, and hematopoetic system must be closely monitored.

Uses   Systemic infections by susceptible strains of *Candida* or *Cryptococcus*.

Contraindications   Hypersensitivity to drug. Use with extreme caution in patients with kidney disease or history of bone marrow depression.

Untoward Reactions   Nausea, vomiting, diarrhea, rash, anemia, leukopenia, thrombocytopenia; increase in BUN, creatinine levels, and certain enzymes. Adverse CNS manifestations have been reported.

Dosage   **PO, adult and children:** 50–150 mg/kg daily in 4 divided doses. Patients with renal impairment receive lower dosages.

Administration   Reduce or avoid nausea by administering the tablets a few at a time over a 15-minute period.

Nursing Implications
1. Before administering first dose, check that culture has been taken.
2. Ascertain that weekly cultures are taken to determine that strains have not become resistant. Strain is considered resistant if MIC (minimal inhibitory concentration) value is greater than 100.
3. Monitor input and output. Report reduction in urine output as well as blood, sediment, or cloudiness in the urine.

GRISEOFULVIN FULVICIN-U/V, GRIFULVIN V, GRISACTIN, GRISOWEN

GRISEOFULVIN ULTRAMICROSIZE FULVICIN-P/G, GRIS-PEG

Classification Antibiotic, antifungal.

General Statement Griseofulvin is a natural antibiotic derived from a species of *Penicillium*. It is the only oral drug effective against dermatophytic (tinae ringworm) infections. When taken systemically, the drug is deposited in the newly formed skin and nails, which are then resistant to reinfection by the tinae. The drug is not effective against *Candida*. Susceptibility of the infectious agent should be established before treatment is begun.

Uses Tinae (ringworm) infections of skin including athlete's foot, and infections of the scalp, groin, and nails.

Contraindications Porphyria or history thereof, hepatocellular failure, and hypersensitivity to drug.

Untoward Reactions Headache, vertigo, angioneurotic edema, skin rash, GI discomfort, monilial overgrowth, allergic reactions. Rarely photosensitization and transient loss of hearing. Cross-reactivity with penicillin occurs rarely.

Drug Interactions

Interactant	Interaction
Alcohol, ethyl	Tachycardia and flushing with griseofulvin
Anticoagulants, oral	↓ Effect of anticoagulants due to ↓ breakdown in liver
Barbiturates	↓ Effect of griseofulvin due to ↓ absorption from GI tract

Laboratory Test Interferences ↑ SGPT, SGOT, alkaline phosphatase, BUN, and creatinine level values.

Dosage **PO:** 500 mg daily in single or divided doses; **pediatric:** 11 mg/kg/day. Give after meals. Length of treatment varies from 1 month to 1 year.

Nursing Implications
1. Advise patient to eat a diet high in fat, since this enhances absorption of griseofulvin from the intestines.
2. Encourage patient to take all medication prescribed to prevent recurrence of infection.

3. Advise patient of need for body hygiene to prevent reinfection.
4. Warn patient to avoid exposure to intense natural or artificial light since photosensitivity reaction may occur.
5. Instruct patient to report fever, sore throat, and malaise, symptoms of leukopenia.
6. Inform patient that he/she will be considered cured when repeated cultures and scrapings of affected site are negative.

MICONAZOLE MONISTAT I.V.

Classification   Antifungal agent.

General Statement   Miconazole is a broad-spectrum fungicidal agent which acts by altering the permeability of the cell membrane. The drug is metabolized rapidly in the liver; excretion of the drug is unaltered in patients with renal insufficiency, including patients on hemodialysis.

Uses   Systemic fungal infections caused by coccidioidomycosis, candidiasis, cryptococcosis, paracoccidioidomycosis, chronic mucocutaneous candidiasis. When used for the treatment of either fungal meningitis or urinary bladder infection, IV infusion must be supplemented with intrathecal administration or bladder irrigation of the drug. *Investigationally:* As ointment for treatment of athletes foot, and vaginal infections.

Untoward Reactions   *General:* pruritis, rash, fever, flushing, drowsiness. *Gastrointestinal:* nausea, vomiting, diarrhea, anorexia. *Hematologic:* thrombocytopenia, aggregation of erythrocytes, rouleau formation on blood smears. Transient decrease in hematocrit. *Cardiovascular:* transient tachycardia or arrhythmias in patients following rapid administration of undiluted drug. Transient decrease in serum sodium values. The vehicle for the drug (PEG 40 Castor Oil) may cause hyperlipidemia.
 Safe use in pregnancy and in children under 1 year of age has not been established.

Drug Interaction   Miconazole may increase the anticoagulant effect of coumarin anticoagulants.

Dosage   **IV infusion, adults:** 200–3600 mg/day in divided doses depending on the specific organism, **pediatric:** total daily dose, 20–40 mg/kg in divided doses; a dose of 15 mg/kg/infusion should not be exceeded. **Intrathecal:** 20 mg/dose of the undiluted solution as an adjunct to **IV** therapy. **Bladder instillation:** 200 mg of diluted solution as adjunct treatment of fungal infections of urinary bladder.

Administration   1. IV therapy may be required from 1 to more than 20 weeks depending on the organism.
2. For IV infusion, the drug should be diluted in at least 200 ml of either

0.9% sodium chloride or 5% dextrose solution and administered over a period of 30 to 60 minutes.

3. Succeeding intrathecal injections should be alternated between lumbar, cervical, or cisternal punctures every 3 to 7 days.

Nursing Implications
1. Provide symptomatic treatment for nausea, vomiting, diarrhea, dizziness, and pruritus.
2. Observe for redness and pain at site of IV infusion.

NYSTATIN MYCOSTATIN, NILSTAT

Classification Antibiotic, antifungal.

General Statement This natural antifungal antibiotic is derived from *Streptomyces noursei* and is both fungistatic and fungicidal against all species of *Candida*. The drug is too toxic for systemic infections. It can be given PO for intestinal moniliasis infections but is not absorbed from the GI tract. These infections, however, occur rarely.

Uses *Candida albicans* infections of the skin, mucous membranes, GI tract, vagina, and mouth (thrush).

Untoward Reactions Large oral doses may cause epigastric distress, nausea, vomiting, and diarrhea. *Note:* Nystatin is combined with tetracycline to prevent fungal superinfections from the latter. Examples are the products Achrostatin V, Comycin, Declostatin, and Terrastatin.

Dosage **Vaginal tablets:** 100,000–200,000 units daily inserted in vagina. **PO:** 500,000–1,000,000 units t.i.d. to decrease possibility of reinfection from intestine. *Thrush;* **Oral suspension,** 400,000–600,000 units q.i.d. (½ dose in each side of mouth and retained as long as possible before swallowing); **infants:** 200,000 units q.i.d.; **premature or low birth weight:** 100,000 units q.i.d. **Ointment, cream, and dusting powder** (contains 100,000 units/ml or gm): use as directed on package.

Administration/ Storage
1. Protect drug from heat, light, moisture, and air.
2. Do not mix oral suspension in foods since the medication will be inactivated.
3. The suspension can be stored for 7 days at room temperature or for 10 days in the refrigerator without loss of potency.
4. Apply nystatin ointment to mycotic lesions with a swab.
5. Drop 1 ml of oral suspension in each side of mouth or apply with a swab to treat oral moniliasis. Instruct patient to keep medication in mouth as long as possible before swallowing.
6. Insert vaginal tablets high in vagina with an applicator.

Nursing Implications
1. Instruct patient to continue using vaginal tablets even when menstruating since the treatment should be continued for 2 weeks.
2. Advise patient to discontinue medication and report to physician should vaginal tablets cause irritation.

3. Continue administration of medication for at least 48 hours after symptoms have disappeared. Anticipate that vaginal tablets may be continued in the gravid patient for 3 to 6 weeks before term to reduce incidence of thrush in the newborn.

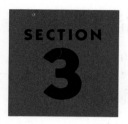

sulfonamides

Mafenide Acetate
Phthalylsulfathiazole
Silver Sulfadiazine
Sulfacetamide Sodium
Sulfachlorpyridazine
Sulfacytine
Sulfadiazine
Sulfadiazine Sodium
Sulfamerazine
Sulfameter

Sulfamethazine
Sulfamethizole
Sulfamethoxazole
Sulfamethoxypyridazine
Sulfapyridine
Sulfasalazine
Sulfisoxazole
Sulfisoxazole Acetyl
Sulfisoxazole Diolamine
Sulfonamide Combinations

General Statement

These drugs are synthetic, bacteriostatic agents with a wide range of antimicrobial activity against gram-positive and gram-negative organisms. At high concentrations, some are bactericidal.

Sulfonamides are poorly soluble, weak acids. They form salts with bases. The sodium salts are very soluble in water.

The sulfonamides interfere with the utilization of para-aminobenzoic acid (PABA), required by bacteria for growth; thus sulfonamides halt multiplication of bacteria but do not kill fully formed microorganisms.

The various sulfonamides are absorbed and excreted at widely differing rates. This has an important bearing on their therapeutic use. For instance agents that are poorly absorbed from the GI tract are particularly indicated for intestinal infections because they remain localized in the intestine for a long time.

Agents that are rapidly absorbed and rapidly excreted are referred to as *short-acting sulfonamides*. Those that are excreted slowly are *long-acting sulfonamides. Intermediate-acting sulfonamides* fall in between.

Long-acting sulfonamides are potentially more dangerous than short-acting preparations because the drug persists in the body for several days after untoward symptoms are noted and administration has been discontinued. Thus, long-acting sulfonamides should be used only rarely and cautiously.

Sulfonamides are absorbed into the bloodstream and distributed throughout all tissues, including the cerebrospinal fluid where concentrations attain 50% to 80% of that found in the blood.

It is always desirable to determine the susceptibility of the pathogen before, or soon after, initiation of therapy.

Sulfonamides have the advantage of being relatively inexpensive.

Uses   The range of usefulness of the sulfonamides has been greatly reduced by the emergence of resistant strains of bacteria and the development of more effective antibiotics.

They are still extremely useful (sometimes the drug of first choice), however, for the treatment of certain conditions, including acute bacillary dysentery caused by *Shigella* organisms, ulcerative colitis, cholera, trachoma and inclusion conjunctivitis, chancroid, norcardiosis, and toxoplasmosis.

Because of their rapid renal excretion, sulfonamides are useful for the treatment of episodic nonobstructive urinary tract infections by susceptible organisms.

The drugs are still sometimes used for the suppression of intestinal flora prior to and following intestinal surgery.

Contraindications   Except for hypersensitivity reactions, there are few absolute contraindications. Sulfonamides, however, are potentially dangerous drugs and cause a 5% overall incidence of major and minor untoward reactions.

Sulfonamides should be used with caution, and in reduced dosage, in patients with impaired liver or renal function, intestinal or urinary tract obstructions, blood dyscrasias, allergies, asthma, and hereditary glucose-6-phosphate dehydrogenase deficiency.

Sulfonamides may cause mental retardation and should never be administered during the third term of pregnancy to nursing mothers or infants under 2 months of age, except for the treatment of congenital toxoplasmosis (a serious parasitic disease that can cause brain inflammation) or in life-threatening situations.

Untoward Reactions   Blood dyscrasias, including acute hemolytic anemia, agranulocytosis (10 to 14 days after initiation of therapy), thrombocytopenia, and aplastic anemia.

Impairment of renal function (crystalluria, hematuria, oliguria, acidosis), purpura hemorrhagica, drug fever, jaundice, or severe dermatitis.

Long-acting sulfonamides can induce Stevens-Johnson syndrome, a nonspecific reaction involving the skin, mucous membranes, and other organ systems. The condition is characterized by a high fever, headaches, and rash and is fatal in 25% of the cases.

Sulfonamides also can cause various benign skin and mucous membrane manifestations such as scarlitinal, urticarial, and petechial exfoliative dermatitis. The presence of such rashes requires immediate withdrawal of drug.

Dizziness, headache, fatigue, mental depression, psychosis, restlessness, irritability, nausea, vomiting, ataxia, peripheral neuritis, and drowsiness occur frequently.

Prolonged therapy may produce overgrowth of nonsusceptible organisms.

By killing the intestinal flora, the sulfonamides also reduce the bacterial synthesis of vitamin K. This may result in hemorrhage. Administration of vitamin K to patients on long-term sulfonamide therapy is recommended.

Drug Interactions

Interactant	Interaction
Alcohol, ethyl	Toxicity ↑ by sulfonamides
Anesthetics, local	↓ Effect of sulfonamides
Antacids	↓ Effect of sulfonamides due to ↓ absorption from GI tract
Anticoagulants, oral	↑ Effect of sulfonamides due to ↓ plasma protein binding
Antidiabetics, oral	↑ Hypoglycemic effect due to ↓ in plasma protein binding
Barbiturates	↑ Effect of barbiturates due to ↓ in plasma protein binding
Indomethacin (Indocin)	↑ Effect of sulfonamides by ↑ blood levels
Methenamine (Mandelamine)	↑ Chance of sulfonamide crystalluria due to acid urine
Mineral oil	↓ Effect of nonabsorbable sulfonamides in GI tract
Oxacillin	↓ Effect of oxacillin due to ↓ absorption from GI tract
Paraldehyde	↑ Chance of sulfonamide crystalluria
Phenylbutazone (Butazolidin)	↑ Effect of sulfonamide by ↑ blood levels
Phenytoin (Dilantin)	↑ Effect of phenytoin due to ↓ breakdown in liver
Probenecid	↑ Effect of sulfonamides by ↓ in plasma protein binding
Salicylates	↑ Effect of sulfonamides by ↑ blood levels

Laboratory Test Interference

False + or ↑ liver function tests (amino acids, bilirubin, BSP), renal function (BUN, NPN, creatinine clearance), blood counts, prothrombin time, Coombs test. Urine glucose: copper reduction methods such as Benedict's or Clinitest, protein, urobilinogen.

Dosage

See Table 6, page 115. Sulfonamides are usually given PO. Dosage is adjusted individually. An initial loading dose is usually recommended. Short-acting compounds must be given every 4 to 6 hours.

Topical application of sulfonamides is rarely ordered today except for Sulfamylon (mafenide), which is used as a 10% ointment to treat burn infections.

Creams of triple sulfa or sulfisoxazole are used for vaginitis.

When sulfonamides are given as adjuncts to GI surgery, medication is usually started 3 to 5 days prior to surgery, and for 1 to 2 weeks postoperatively, after peristalsis has resumed.

TABLE 6 SULFONAMIDES

Drug	Main Use	Dosage	Remarks
Mafenide acetate (Sulfamylon Acetate)	Prophylactic, topical application in the treatment of burns (prevention of infections)	**Cream:** $1/16$ in. thick film applied over entire surface of burn b.i.d. for 60 days	Do not use for already established infections. Unlike other sulfonamides, mafenide is not inhibited by pus or body fluids
			Additional Untoward Reactions Burns treated with Sulfamylon are to be covered only with a thin dressing. Causes pain on application.
Phthalylsulfathiazole (Sulfathalidine)	Adjunct for treatment of ulcerative colitis during acute attacks; GI surgery	*Ulcerative colitis,* **PO:** 50–100 mg/kg daily in 3 to 6 equally divided doses. *Surgery:* 125 mg/kg daily in 3 to 6 equally divided doses for 3 to 5 days prior to and 1–2 weeks after surgery, *after peristalsis has returned to normal.* **Maximum daily dose: 8 gm**	After 3 to 5 days, produces soft, tenacious, stringy stools with decreased coliform count.
			Additional Contraindications Intestinal obstruction. May increase pre- and postoperative bleeding.
			Additional Nursing Implications Observe and report signs of intestinal obstruction characterized by vomiting, reverse peristalsis, and abdominal distention. Observe for preoperative and excessive postoperative bleeding due to vitamin K deficiency.
Silver sulfadiazine (Silvadene)	Topically for prevention and treatment of sepsis in second and third degree burns	Same as mafenide acetate	*Administration* With a sterile glove apply $1/16$ inch layer to all debrided, cleansed, burned areas 1–2 times daily or when ung. is accidentally removed. Dressings are not required. Continue application until healing occurs. The drug is absorbed from burn areas; thus, plasma concentration may reach therapeutic levels.

(Continued)

115

TABLE 6 SULFONAMIDES (*Continued*)

Drug	Main Use	Dosage	Remarks
Sulfacetamide sodium (Cetamide, Isopto Cetamide, Sebizon, Sodium Sulamyd, Sulfacel-15 Ophthalmic, Others)	Topically for ophthalmic infections; dermatoses	1–2 drops of 10%, 15%, or 30% solution in conjunctival sac several times daily, 10% ophthalmic ointment t.i.d.– q.i.d. in conjunctival sac. For dermatoses, apply lotion (10%) to affected area b.i.d.– q.i.d.	
Sulfachlorpyridazine (Nefrosul, Sonilyn)	See General Uses	**PO, initial:** 2–4 gm initially; **then,** 2–4 gm daily in 3 to 6 equally divided doses; **pediatric infants older than 2 months, initial:** 75 mg/kg; **maintenance:** 150 mg/kg in 4 to 6 equally divided doses. Up to maximum of 6 gm daily	Short-acting. Well absorbed from GI tract.
Sulfacytine (Renoquid)	Only used for acute non-obstructive urinary tract infections	**PO initial:** 500 mg; **maintenance:** 250 mg q.i.d. for 10 days	Short-acting. Protect tablets from heat, light, and moisture. Do not use in children under 14 years.
Sulfadiazine (Microsulfon) Sulfadiazine Sodium	Urinary tract infections. Bacillary dysentery. Rheumatic fever prophylaxis	**PO, initial:** 2–4 gm; **maintenance:** 2–4 gm daily in 3 to 4 divided doses; **pediatric over 2 months:** 75 mg/kg/day; **maintenance:** 150 mg/kg/day in 4 to 6 divided doses. **IV, SC, initial:** 50 mg/kg/day; **maintenance:** 100 mg/kg/day in 3 divided doses **SC** or by slow **IV** infusion. *Rheumatic fever prophylaxis,* **under 30 kg:** 0.5 gm/day; **over 30 kg:** 1 gm/day	Short-acting. Often combined with other anti-infectives. *Additional Nursing Implications* Maintain adequate fluid intake. Prevent extravasation into SC or fat tissue as drug may cause necrosis of tissue around blood vessel. Observe for redness, swelling and pain along vein after IV administration. For parenteral administration the concentrate must be diluted so as to contain 50 mg/ml. Sterile water for injection is preferred diluent.

Sulfamerazine	Rarely used other than in combination with other sulfonamides	**PO, initial:** 3–4 gm; **maintenance:** 3–4 gm daily in 3 to 6 equally divided doses; **pediatric 3 to 10 year,** 1.5 gm initially; **then** 1 gm q 12 hr; **infants 6 months to 3 years:** 1 gm initially; **then** 0.5 gm q 12 hr; **infants under 6 months:** 0.5 gm initially; **then** 0.25 gm q 12 hr	Intermediate-acting
Sulfameter (Sulla)	Only used for urinary tract infections	**PO, initial:** 1.5 gm; **maintenance:** 500 mg daily as single dose	Long-acting. Photosensitivity may occur. Therapy should be discontinued unless favorable clinical effects are noted within first 14 days. Continuous therapy should not exceed 18 days. *Additional Contraindications* Children below 12 years, pregnant women, nursing mothers, patients weighing less than 100 pounds or with renal or hepatic dysfunction. Should be administered with caution to patients receiving oral hypoglycemics of the sulfonylurea type. *Additional Nursing Implications* Caution patients against excessive exposure to sunlight or ultraviolet light to prevent photosensitivity. Observe for photosensitivity (sunburn-like appearances). Administer drug after breakfast. Provide adequate fluid intake for at least 48 hours after drug has been discontinued. Intermediate-acting. Use of this agent alone for treatment of infections is at present uncommon. *(Continued)*

TABLE 6 SULFONAMIDES (*Continued*)

Drug	Main Use	Dosage	Remarks
Sulfamethazine	Rarely used other than in combination with other sulfonamides		Short-acting. Use of this agent alone for treatment of infections is at present uncommon.
Sulfamethizole (Bursul, Microsul, Proklar, Sulfstat Forte, Thiosulfil, Unisul, Urifon)	Urinary tract infections	**PO, adults:** 0.5–1 gm t.i.d.-q.i.d.; **pediatric over 2 months:** 30–45 mg/kg/day in 4 divided doses.	Short-acting
Sulfamethoxazole (Gantanol, Gantanol DS)	Urinary and upper respiratory tract infections	**PO, initial:** 2 gm; **maintenance:** 1 gm 2 to 3 times daily; **pediatric, initial:** 50–60 mg/kg; **maintenance:** 25–30 mg/kg b.i.d. Maximum dose not to exceed 75 mg/kg/day.	Intermediate-acting
Sulfamethoxypyridazine (Midicel)	Systemic and urinary tract infections, trachoma, chronic infections, prophylaxis in rheumatic fever patients, acne vulgaris, otitis media.	**PO, initial:** 1–2 gm; **maintenance:** 0.5 gm daily or 1 gm q 2 days; **adults under 60 kg, maintenance:** 250 mg daily; **children and infants over 2 months, initial:** 30 mg/kg; **maintenance:** 15 mg/kg. *Prophylaxis of streptococcus:* 2–3 gm/wk in a single dose	Long-acting, rapidly absorbed from GI tract. Therapy for trachoma: 40–120 days. *Additional Contraindications* Pregnancy. Administer immediately after a meal.
Sulfapyridine	Dermatitis herpetiformis	**PO, initial:** 500 mg q.i.d., when improvement is noted, decrease by 500 mg daily at 3-day intervals, until symptom-free maintenance is achieved. Increase dosage if symptoms return	Intermediate-acting. Slowly and incompletely absorbed from GI tract. More toxic than other sulfonamides; seldom used
Sulfasalazine (Azulfidine, Sulcolon, S.A.S.-500)	Ulcerative colitis	**PO, initial:** 3–4 gm daily in divided doses; **maintenance:** 500 mg q.i.d.; **pediatric, initial:** 40–60 mg/kg daily in 4 equally divided doses. **Maintenance:** 30 mg/kg daily in 4 equally divided doses	Intermittent therapy (2 wk on/2 wk off) is recommended. Drug does not affect microflora *Additional Contraindications* Children below 5 years, persons with marked sulfonamide and

Drug	Indications	Dosage	Remarks
Sulfisoxazole (Gantrisin, J-Sul, Rosoxol, SK-Soxazole, Sulfalar) Sulfisoxazole Acetyl (Gantrisin)	Urinary tract infections, topical and ophthalmic infections	**PO, initial:** 2–4 gm; **maintenance:** 4–8 gm daily in 3 to 6 divided doses; **pediatric over 2 months, initial:** 75 mg/kg/day. **Maintenance:** 150 mg/kg/day in 4 to 6 doses. Maximum of 6 gm/day. **Vaginal cream:** 250–500 mg (2.5–5 ml) into vagina b.i.d. for 2 weeks. Course may be repeated. **Ophthalmic:** 1–2 gtt of 4% solution t.i.d.–q.i.d.	Short-acting
Sulfisoxazole diolamine (Gantrisin Diolamine)	Urinary tract infections.	**IM or slow IV. SC** when necessary. **All ages, initial:** 50 mg/kg, **maintenance:** 100 mg/kg daily in 3 to 4 divided doses	Switch to PO administration as soon as possible. For SC administration, dilute commercial solution containing 400 mg/ml with sterile water for injection, to obtain solution containing 50 mg/ml
Combinations of sulfonamides Sulfacetamide, Sulfadiazine, Sulfamerazine (Buffonamide, Trizyl)	See individual drugs	**PO:** 3–4 gm initially, **then** 1 gm q 6 hour; **children and infants over 2 months:** ½ calculated dose initially, **then** 150 mg/kg daily in 4 to 6 divided doses	Produces higher blood levels of sulfonamide. Incidence of crystalluria is reduced
Sulfadiazine Sulfamerazine Sulfamethazine (Gelazine, Neotrizine, Quadetts, Sulfaloid, Sulfazem, Sulfose, Terfonyl, Triosulf, Triple Sulfa, Trisem, Trisureid)	See individual drugs	**PO, adults:** 3–4 gm initially; **then** 1 gm q 4 hour; **pediatric over 2 months:** 75 mg/kg initially; **then** 150 mg/kg/day in 4 to 6 divided doses	See above
Sulfathiazole Sulfacetamide Sulfabenzamide (Sultrin)	Prophylaxis or treatment of cervical and vaginal infections	One vaginal tablet at bedtime and on arising for 10 days. Or, one applicatorful of cream b.i.d. for 4 to 6 days; **then** reduce dosage to ¼–½	Available as cream or vaginal tablets

Nursing Implications

See also *Nursing Implications* under *Antibiotics*, page 56.

1. Observe patient for the following untoward reactions that require the withdrawal of drug:
   a. Skin rash.
   b. Blood dyscrasias characterized by sore throat, fever, pallor, purpura, jaundice, or weakness.
   c. Serum sickness characterized by eruptions of purpuric spots and pain in limbs and joints. Serum sickness may develop 7 to 10 days after initiation of therapy.
   d. Early symptoms of Stevens-Johnson syndrome characterized by high fever, severe headaches, stomatitis, conjunctivitis, rhinitis, urethritis, and balanitis (inflammation of the tip of the penis).
   e. Jaundice, which may indicate hepatic involvement, 3 to 5 days after initiation of therapy.
   f. Renal involvement characterized by renal colic, oliguria, anuria, hematuria, and proteinuria.
   g. Echymosis and hemorrhage caused by decreased synthesis of vitamin K by intestinal bacteria.
2. Test pH of urine once a day with Labstix. Excess acidity, or administration of a particularly insoluble sulfonamide, may require alkalinization of urine. The drug of choice for this purpose is sodium bicarbonate.
3. Encourage adequate fluid intake to prevent crystalluria. Measure intake and output. Minimum output of urine should be 1500 ml daily. For long-acting sulfonamides, adequate fluid intake must be maintained 24 to 48 hours after discontinuation of drug.
4. Question patient as to what other drugs are taken since numerous drug interference reactions have been reported.
5. Question unusual order for long-acting sulfonamides.
6. Teach patient to report side effects and untoward symptoms, to take drug on time, to remain under medical supervision, and that certain sulfonamides may color the urine orange-red.

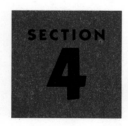

SECTION 4

sulfones

Dapsone   Sulfoxone Sodium

General Statement

The sulfones are synthetic agents with mycobacteriostatic activity in particular against *Mycobacterium leprae* (Hansen's bacillus) and *M. tuberculosis*. The sulfones are used mostly for the treatment of leprosy.

All sulfones are related to dapsone (4,4'-diaminodiphenylsulfone), which is often referred to as the "parent sulfone."

The sulfones interfere with the metabolism of the infectious organism and are bacteriostatic.

Sulfones are widely distributed throughout the body.

Uses Lepromatous and tuberculoid types of leprosy, dermatitis herpetiformis, and malaria.

Contraindication Advanced amyloidosis of kidneys.

Untoward Reactions Anemia. Hemoglobin levels, however, usually return to normal levels with usage.

Methemoglobinemia (cyanosis) but usually does not necessitate discontinuation of therapy.

Lepra reaction (erythema nodosum leprosum) characterized by malaise, fever, and appearance of painful areas of inflammatory enduration, which may necessitate discontinuation of drug.

Arthralgia, iritis, iridocyclitis, neuritis, lymphadenitis, orchitis, swelling of the hands and feet, and hepatosplenomegaly.

Leukopenia, dermatitis, hypersensitivity reactions, GI disturbances, anorexia, nausea, vomiting, headaches, nervousness, insomnia, blurred vision, drug fever, and psychosis.

Sulfones are excreted very slowly and untoward reactions consequently are cumulative.

Dosage Therapy should be initiated with small amounts and increased gradually in the absence of toxic symptoms (see individual drugs).

Regular rest periods are suggested for long-term therapy.

Arrested cases may receive low-dose therapy for life.

Drug Interaction

Interactant	Interaction
Probenecid	↑ Effect of sulfones due to inhibition of renal excretion

Laboratory Test Interference Altered liver function tests.

Nursing Implications
1. Observe for improvement of inflammation and ulceration of the mucous membranes during the first 3 to 6 months of therapy. Lack of response may indicate need of other therapy.
2. Dosage is increased slowly during initiation period.
3. Observe patient particularly closely when dosage is increased.
4. Observe for anemia.
5. Check whether doctor wishes patient to receive hematinics.
6. Use strict medical asepsis because patient may have leukopenia.
7. Observe patient for cyanosis and degree of anoxemia.
8. Observe for allergic dermatitis, which usually appears before the tenth week of therapy during which time dose is increased. Allergic

dermatitis may not necessarily necessitate discontinuation of treatment.

9. Observe for psychoses, GI disturbances, Lepra reaction, headaches, dizziness, lethargy, severe malaise, tinnitus, paresthesias, deep aches, neuralgic pains, and ocular disturbances.

10. May be administered during pregnancy and lactation without harm to fetus or infant.

11. Reassure nursing mothers that the blue color of the skin of the nursing baby is transitory and harmless.

12. Observe patients with other concurrent chronic conditions particularly closely and anticipate reduction in dosage of sulfones.

DAPSONE AVLOSULFON

Remarks   See General Statement, p. 120. Drug of choice. Most widely used sulfone because it is the least expensive. Observe nursing infants who may develop transient bluish tinge. Twice weekly dosage is preferred.

Additional Uses   Leprosy and tuberculoid-type leprosy.

Dosage   **Weekly schedule for** *uncomplicated lepromatous leprosy:* weeks 1 to 4, 25 mg a week; weeks 5 to 8, 50 mg 2 times a week; weeks 9 to 12, 75 mg 2 times a week; weeks 13 to 16, 100 mg 2 times a week; weeks 17 to 20, 100 mg 3 times a week; weeks 21 to 24, 100 mg 4 times a week. A 1-week rest period every 2 months is indicated; **children:** ¼ – ½ adult dose. *Uncomplicated tuberculoid leprosy:* maximum dose should not exceed 200 mg/week. *Uncomplicated dimorphous leprosy:* maximum dose should not exceed 300 mg/week.

Additional Nursing Implication   Observe for toxic effects before increasing therapy.

SULFOXONE SODIUM DIASONE SODIUM

Remarks   See page 120. Metabolized to dapsone.

Additional Uses   Leprosy, tuberculoid types of leprosy, and dermatitis herpetiformis.

Dosage   *Leprosy,* **PO, initial:** Weeks 1 to 2, 330 mg 2 times weekly; weeks 3 to 4, 330 mg 4 times a week, thereafter, 330 mg daily for 6 days of each week; **pediatric over 4 years:** ½ adult dose.

Dermatitis herpetiformis, **initial:** 330 mg daily for 1 week; the dose may be increased to 660 mg daily, if necessary; **maintenance:** 330 mg daily.

Rest periods of 2 weeks to 2 months are recommended, though this may not be possible without recurrence of symptoms in dermatitis herpetiformis.

Additional Nursing Implications

1. Observe for toxic symptoms before increasing dosage.
2. Do not divide enteric coated tablets because gastric irritation may result.

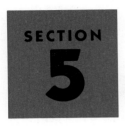

SECTION

5

anthelmintics

Diethylcarbamazine Citrate
Hexylresorcinol
Mebendazole
Piperazine Citrate
Piperazine Phosphate

Pyrantel Pamoate
Pyrvinium Pamoate
Quinacrine Hydrochloride
Tetrachloroethylene
Thiabendazole

General Statement

Helminthiasis, or infestation of the body by parasites, is a very common affliction. About 20 million Americans are said to harbor pinworms, for instance. Therefore, anthelmintics are very important drugs; their purpose is to rid the body of parasitic worms, eggs, and larvae.

Humans can become infested by a great variety of worms. Some of the more common worms are given below.

Filaria This infestation is transmitted by mosquitoes. The parasite is a very tiny roundworm that migrates into the lymphatic system and bloodstream. Living and dead worms can obstruct the lymphatics, causing elephantiasis. Mosquito control is the chief means of combating this infestation. **Drug Treatment:** Results are poor. The drugs used are antimony potassium tartrate and diethylcarbamazine.

Hookworm Infestation with hookworm is quite common. These worms cause debilitation resulting in iron-deficiency anemia, characterized by fatigue, lassitude, and apathy. Several variants of hookworm exist. **Drug Treatment:** Tetrachloroethylene, thiabendazole, hexylresorcinol, and bephenium hydroxynaphthoate.

Pinworms These infestations are common in school-age children. Complications are rare, although heavy infestations may cause abdominal pain, weight loss, and insomnia. **Drug Treatment:** Piperazine citrate, pyrvinium pamoate, pyrantel pamoate, thiabendazole.

Roundworms Cause a serious parasitic infestation because the worms can penetrate other tissues. They can obstruct the respiratory and gastrointestinal tracts as well as the bile duct or appendix. **Drug Treatment:** Piperazine, hexylresorcinol, pyrantel pamoate, thiabendazole, mebendazole.

Schistosomiasis The parasitic infestation of the liver occurs most often in Asia and some parts of Africa. Called schistosomiasis or bilharziasis, it is transmitted by certain species of snails and is very difficult to eradicate. **Drug Treatment:** Trivalent antimony compounds, hexylresorcinol.

Tapeworm The tapeworm consists of a scolex or head that hooks into a segment of intestine. The body is that of a segmented flatworm, sections of which are found in the stools. Tapeworm infestations are difficult to eradicate but have few side effects. **Drug Treatment:** Quinacrine.

Threadworms This parasite infests the upper GI tract. Heavy infestations can cause malabsorption syndrome, diarrhea, and general discomfort. **Drug Treatment:** Thiabendazole, hexylresorcinol (for heavy infestations only—PO and retention enemas), pyrvinium pamoate.

Whipworm This threadlike parasite lodges in the mucosa of the cecum. **Drug Treatment:** No reliable drug treatment; bephenium hydroxynaphthoate, thiabendazole, mebendazole and hexylresorcinol have been used.

Trichinosis These parasites are transmitted by the consumption of raw or inadequately cooked pork. The infection is serious; larvae burrow into the bloodstream and form cysts in skeletal muscle. No effective therapeutic agent exists that will eradicate the larvae. **Drug Treatment:** Corticosteroids to control the inflammation caused by systemic infestation; thiabendazole.

Parasites that infest only the intestinal tract can be eradicated by locally acting drugs. Other parasites enter tissues and must be treated by drugs that are absorbed from the GI tract.

Accurate diagnosis is extremely important before treatment is started because its success depends on selecting the drug best suited for the eradication of a specific infestation.

Since many parasitic infestations are transmitted by persons sharing bathroom facilities, the physician may wish to examine the entire household for parasitic infestation. Treatment is often accompanied or followed by repeated laboratory examinations to determine whether the parasite has been eradicated.

Untoward Reactions Since the anthelmintics do not belong to any one chemical group, their untoward reactions are related to specific compounds. However, nausea, vomiting, cramps, and diarrhea are common to most.

Nursing Implications 1. Provide the patient or family with written instructions regarding diet, cathartics, enemas, medications, and follow-up tests when treatment is to be carried out at home.

2. Review these instructions with patient or family member to be sure they are understood by the person responsible for the patient's treatment and care.
3. Emphasize the need for follow-up examinations to check the results of treatment.

Good hygienic practices reduce the incidence of helminthiasis.

Pinworms

1. Instruct responsible family member how to prevent infestation with pinworms:
   a. Wash hands after toileting and before meals.
   b. Keep nails short.
   c. Wash ova from anal area in the morning.
   d. Apply antipruritic ointment to anal area to reduce scratching, which transfers pinworms.
2. Alert family that physician may wish all members to be examined for pinworms.
3. After the end of the treatment course, swab the perianal area each morning with Scotch tape until no further eggs are found on microscopic examination for 7 consecutive days.

Roundworms Two to three weeks after therapy have microscopic stool examination to determine fecal egg count. Stools must be examined daily until no further roundworm ova are found.

Hookworm/Tapeworm After the administration of medication, cathartics, and enema, examine the results of the enema for the head of the worm, which will appear bright yellow.

DIETHYLCARBAMAZINE CITRATE HETRAZAN

Remarks Diethylcarbamazine apparently damages the threadlike microfilaria and their larvae so that they are readily destroyed by the defense systems of the body. Adult worms of most species are killed. The drug is readily absorbed from the GI tract and rapidly distributed throughout the body fluids and tissues.

Uses Systemic parasitic disease caused by filaria, especially of the *Wucheria bancrofti, W. malayi,* and *Loa loa* types. These infections are transmitted by certain mosquitoes.

Contraindications and Cautions Patients with onchocerciasis—the filial worm infestation—have violent reactions, including an allergic eye inflammation, within 15 hours.

Untoward Reactions Transient headache, general malaise, weakness, joint pain, anorexia, nausea, and vomiting.

Dosage   *Filariasis, Onchocerciasis, Loiasis:* 2–4 mg/kg t.i.d. for 3 to 4 weeks. *Ascariasis,* **adults:** 13 mg/kg/day for 7 days; **children,** 6–10 mg/kg t.i.d. for 7 to 10 days.

Additional Nursing Implications

1. Anticipate that the concomitant administration of antihistamines and corticosteroids may be ordered for the treatment of onchocerciasis.
2. Have hydrocortisone eyedrops, 5% solution, on hand in case of ocular complications.
3. Administer drug after meals.

HEXYLRESORCINOL

Remarks   This compound is one of the less toxic, more versatile anthelmintics.

Uses   Roundworms, hookworms, threadworms, whipworms, dwarf tapeworms, and schistosomes (flukes).

Contraindications   Gastroenteritis, peptic ulcer.

Untoward Reactions   Irritation and ulceration of the oral mucosa. Frequent use may cause GI, hepatic, or cardiac damage.

Drug Interactions

Interactant	Interaction
Alcohol	↓ Effect of hexylresorcinol
Mineral oil	↓ Effect of hexylresorcinol

Dosage   **Adults and older children:** 1 gm; **pediatric 8 to 12 years:** 800 mg; **6 to 8 years:** 600 mg; **under 6 years:** 400 mg. Treatment may be repeated after 1 week.

Administration

1. Give saline cathartic night before treatment.
2. Give in the morning on empty stomach.
3. Tablets should be swallowed whole to avoid irritation of buccal mucous membranes.
4. Give indicated number of tablets in 1 dose with a glass of water.
5. No food should be taken for minimum of 4 hours after administration.
6. Give saline cathartic 24 hours after administration of drug to remove worms from bowel.

MEBENDAZOLE VERMOX

Classification   Anthelmintic.

Remarks   Mebendazole exerts its anthelmintic effect by blocking the glucose uptake of the organisms, thereby depleting their energy until death results.

Uses Whipworm, pinworm, roundworm, common and American hookworm infections; in single or mixed infections.

Contraindications Hypersensitivity to mebendazole. Pregnancy. Use with caution in children under 2 years of age.

Untoward Reactions Transient abdominal pain and diarrhea.

Dosage *Whipworm, roundworm, and hookworm,* **PO, adults and children:** 1 tablet morning and evening on 3 consecutive days. *Pinworms:* 1 tablet, 1 time. All treatments can be repeated after 3 weeks.

Administration 1. Tablet may be chewed, crushed and/or mixed with food.
2. No prior fasting, purging or other procedures required.

PIPERAZINE CITRATE ANTEPAR CITRATE, MULTIFUGE, VERMIZINE

PIPERAZINE PHOSPHATE PIPERAVAL

Remarks The drug is believed to paralyze the muscles of parasites; this promotes their elimination. The drug is readily absorbed from the GI tract.

Uses Pinworm (oxyuriasis) and roundworn (ascariasis) infestations. Particularly recommended for pediatric use.

Contraindications Nephritis.

Untoward Reactions Piperazine has a low toxicity. Rare side effects include nausea, vomiting, diarrhea, and headache. Excessive dosage may cause neurological disturbances and muscular weakness.

Drug Interactions Concomitant administration of piperazine and phenothiazines may result in an increase in extrapyramidal effects caused by phenothiazines.

Laboratory Test Interference False − or ↓ uric acid values.

Dosage *Pinworms,* **PO, adults and children:** 50–65 mg/kg body weight for 7 days up to a maximum daily dose of 2.5 gm. *Roundworms,* **adults:** 1 dose of 3.5 gm/day for 2 consecutive days; **children:** 1 dose of 75 mg/kg/day for two consecutive days; maximum daily dose: 3.5 gm.

Administration Administer drug after breakfast or in 2 divided doses.

Additional Nursing Implication Advise patient to keep pleasant-tasting medication out of reach of children.

PYRANTEL PAMOATE ANTIMINTH

Remarks The anthelmintic effect is attributed to the neuromuscular blocking effect of this agent.

Uses Pinworm and roundworm infestations.

Contraindications Use with caution in presence of liver dysfunction.

Untoward Reactions GI effects (most frequent): anorexia, nausea, vomiting, cramps, diarrhea. Transient elevation of SGOT.
CNS reactions: headache, dizziness, drowsiness, insomnia.
Skin rashes.

Dosage **PO, adults and children:** 1 dose of 11 mg/kg (maximum). **Maximum total dose:** 1.0 gm.

Administration 1. Drug may be taken without regard to food intake.
2. Purging not necessary prior to or during treatment.
3. May be taken with milk or fruit juice.

PYRVINIUM PAMOATE POVAN

Remarks The drug appears to inhibit respiration of parasitic worms. Not absorbed to any great extent from GI tract.

Uses Pinworm infestations.

Contraindications Intestinal obstruction, acute abdominal disease, and other conditions in which there might be GI absorption. To be used with caution in patients with renal or hepatic disease.

Untoward Reactions Nausea, vomiting, cramping, diarrhea, hypersensitivity.

Dosage **PO:** 1 dose of 5 mg/kg body weight. Dose may be repeated in 2 to 3 weeks.

Administration 1. Instruct patient to swallow tablet whole to prevent staining of teeth.
2. Administer tablets rather than liquid because this reduces the chance of emesis.

Additional Nursing Implications 1. Pour liquid medication carefully because it stains materials.
2. Advise patients and parents that the drug stains teeth, underclothing, stools, and vomitus a bright red.

QUINACRINE HYDROCHLORIDE ATABRINE HYDROCHLORIDE

Uses Effective against beef, pork, fish, and dwarf tapeworms. Used for giardiasis. Antimalarial.

Contraindications Patients with a history of psychosis. Pregnancy. To be used with extreme caution in patients with psoriasis or those receiving the antimalarial primaquine.

Untoward Reactions Headaches, mild gastrointestinal symptoms, psychotic attacks, dermatitis, and temporary discoloration of skin.

Drug Interaction The side effects of alcohol are increased in patients receiving quinacrine due to the increased accumulation of acetaldehyde.

Laboratory Test Interference False + or ↑ values for diagenex blue (gastric function test).

Dosage *Beef, Pork, Fish Tapeworm,* **PO, adults:** 4 doses of 200 mg 10 minutes apart with sodium bicarbonate (600 mg with each dose); **pediatric 5 to 14 years:** 400–500 mg in 3 to 4 divided doses 10 minutes apart with sodium bicarbonate (300 mg with each dose). *Giardiasis,* **adults:** 100 mg daily for 5 to 7 days; **children:** 7 mg/kg/day in 3 divided doses after meals for 5 days. *Antimalarial,* **adults and children over 8 years:** 200 mg with 1 gm sodium bicarbonate every 6 hr for 5 doses; **then,** 100 mg t.i.d. for 6 days; **children 4 to 8 years:** 200 mg 3 times the first day, **then** 100 mg 2 times daily for 6 days; **children 1 to 4 years:** 100 mg 3 times the first day, **then** 100 mg daily for 6 days. *Suppression of malaria,* **adults:** 100 mg/day; **children:** 50 mg/day. Drug should be taken for 1 to 3 months.

Administration
1. Maintain patient on low fat diet for 24 to 48 hours before medication to minimize systemic absorption.
2. Omit lunch and supper on day before drug is given.
3. Administer a saline cathartic on evening before medication.
4. Administer quinacrine hydrochloride with 600 mg of sodium bicarbonate to minimize nausea and vomiting.
5. Administer a saline cathartic 1 hour after medication is given.
6. Follow by a soap suds enema to be sure the bright yellow head of the tapeworm is expelled.
7. Administer the drug through a duodenal tube, if ordered, to reduce gastric irritation.

TETRACHLOROETHYLENE

General Statement This chemical, with anesthetic properties, is used as an anthelmintic for the treatment of hookworms. Its anesthetic properties are assumed to release the grip of worms on the intestinal wall. Since tetrachloroethylene may stimulate migration of roundworms, patients who harbor both roundworms (*ascaris*) and hookworms should *first* be treated with hexylresorcinol, which affects both worms, and then with tetrachloro-ethylene.

Use

Hookworm infestations, especially by *Necator americanus*.

Contraindications

Fatty degeneration of liver. Small or severely ill children. Dehydrated patients.

Untoward Reactions

GI effects: burning sensation of stomach, abdominal cramps, nausea, vomiting.
  CNS effects: headaches, dizziness, inebriation, loss of consciousness (rare).

Dosage

PO: 1 dose of 5 ml; **pediatric:** 0.12 ml/kg to a maximum of 5 ml. Treatment is often repeated after interval of 4 days.

Administration/ Storage

1. Do not expose solution to air.
2. Discard exposed solution and broken gelatin capsules.

Additional Nursing Implications

1. Advise patient to avoid fats and alcohol on the day before adminis-tration of the drug because they tend to aid in the absorption of the drug.
2. Instruct patient to eat a light evening meal on the day prior to treatment.
3. Administer a saline cathartic on the evening prior to administration of the drug to increase contact between drug and parasites.
4. Omit breakfast on the day of treatment and give gelatin capsules on an empty stomach.
5. Administer a purgative dose of magnesium sulfate within 2 hours after administration of the drug.
6. Keep patient at rest for 4 hours after ingestion of drug to minimize CNS effects and protect patient from injury.
7. Have bedpan readily available for patient.

THIABENDAZOLE MINTEZOL

Remarks

The drug interferes with the metabolism of several helminths. It is readily absorbed from the GI tract.

Uses

Cutaneous larva migrans, pinworms, threadworms, large roundworms, hookworms, and whipworms. Particularly useful for the treatment of mixed infestations.

Contraindications

To be used with caution in patients with hepatic disease or impaired hepatic function.

Untoward Reactions

GI disturbances, including nausea, vomiting, diarrhea, and constipa-tion. The drug may also affect the CNS, cause hyperglycemia, a decrease in pulse rate and blood pressure.

Dosage **PO:** 25 mg/kg body weight b.i.d. up to a maximum of 3.0 gm. Treatment consists of 1- or 2-day courses, as ordered, on consecutive days or, for pinworms, at 1-week intervals.

Administration Administer drug preferably after meals.

Additional Nursing Implications Caution patient and a responsible family member about the CNS disturbances and loss of mental alertness that can be caused by the drug. The patient should not go to school or operate machinery after taking the drug.

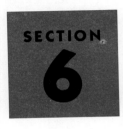

SECTION 6 antitubercular agents

Aminosalicylate Calcium
Aminosalicylate Potassium
Aminosalicylate Sodium
Aminosalicylic Acid
Capreomycin Sulfate
Cycloserine

Ethambutol Hydrochloride
Ethionamide
Isoniazid
Pyrazinamide
Rifampin
Streptomycin Sulfate

General Statement Tuberculosis is rarely treated by a single drug because this usually leads to the emergence of resistant strains. However, when only one drug is used, the drug of choice is isoniazid.

The primary agents for the treatment of tuberculosis are isoniazid, streptomycin, ethambutol, and para-aminosalicylic acid (PAS). A combination of isoniazid–streptomycin–ethambutol is presently favored by many clinicians for advanced cavitary pulmonary tuberculosis. For noncavitous disease, ethambutol has replaced PAS as the drug of first choice.

Nursing Implications See also *Nursing Implications* under *Antibiotics* (p. 56).

1. Anticipate that more than one antitubercular agent will be given concomitantly to prevent the emergence of a resistant strain.
2. Do not administer concomitantly antitubercular agents that are highly ototoxic.
3. Assess for nephrotoxicity, ototoxicity, and some hepatotoxicity. These are caused by most antitubercular agents.
4. Protect the patient manifesting vestibular difficulties during ambulation to prevent falls and injury.
5. Teach patient the importance of taking drugs as ordered.

AMINOSALICYLATE CALCIUM PAS CALCIUM, TEEBACIN CALCIUM

AMINOSALICYLATE POTASSIUM TEEBACIN KALIUM

AMINOSALICYLATE SODIUM PAMISYL SODIUM, PARASAL SODIUM, PAS SODIUM, PASDIUM, TEEBACIN

AMINOSALICYLIC ACID PARA-AMINOSALICYLIC ACID, PAS, TEEBACIN ACID

Classification   Primary antitubercular agent.

Remarks   Bacteriostatic agent. Drug is absorbed from the GI tract and diffuses freely into most tissues.

Uses   Adjuvant to other tuberculostatic agents in the treatment of pulmonary and extrapulmonary tuberculosis. Often used concurrently with isoniazid and/or streptomycin.

Contraindications   Hypersensitivity to PAS. To be administered with caution to patients with impaired renal function.

Untoward Reactions   Mild GI disturbances, hypersensitivity, hepatic damage, crystalluria, mild renal irritation, and transient goiter. Hypersensitivity reaction may be characterized by a gradual rise in body temperature to 102°–104° F (39°–40° C) in previously afebrile patients.

Drug Interactions

Interactant	Interaction
Ammonium chloride	↑ Chance of aminosalicylic acid crystalluria
Anticoagulants, oral	Additive effect on prothrombin time
Ascorbic acid	↑ Chance of aminosalicylic acid crystalluria
Isoniazid	↑ Effect of isoniazid due to ↓ metabolism
Para-aminobenzoic acid (PABA)	Inhibits activity of aminosalicylic acid
Phenytoin	↑ Effect of phenytoin
Probenecid	↑ Effect of aminosalicylic acid by ↓ excretion by kidney
Pyrazinamide	↓ Pharmacological effect of pyrazinamide
Rifampin	↓ Effect of rifampin due to ↓ absorption from GI tract
Salicylates	Possible ↑ effect of PAS due to ↓ excretion by kidney or ↓ plasma protein binding

Laboratory Test Interference   Discolors urine. False + acetoacetic acid test.

Dosage   *Aminosalicylate calcium or sodium,* **PO:** 12–15 gm/day in 2 to 3 divided doses; **children:** 200–300 mg/kg/day in 3 to 4 divided doses. *Aminosalicylate potassium:* 250–375 mg/kg/day. *Aminosalicylic acid:* 10–12 gm/day in 3 to 4 divided doses; **children:** 200–300 mg/kg/day in 3 to 4 divided doses.

Administration/ Storage

1. Store in a light-resistant dry jar at a cool temperature.
2. Solutions for oral administration should be used within 24 hours and under no circumstances if color is darker than that of a freshly prepared solution.
3. Reduce GI disturbance by administering the drug after meals or with 5–10 ml of aluminum hydroxide, as ordered by the physician.

Additional Nursing Implications

See also *Nursing Implications* under *Antibiotics* (p. 56) and those at the beginning of this section.

1. Observe for GI distress, which usually disappears after several days of therapy. Persistence may require cessation of therapy.
2. Observe for hypersensitivity reaction characterized by rise in body temperature (102°–104° F; 39°–40° C) in previously afebrile patients.
3. Observe for goiter and hypothyroidism. Anticipate physician ordering thyroid therapy if conditions appear.
4. Use Tes-Tape to evaluate glycosuria since a false-positive reaction may be obtained with Benedict's solution, Clinitest tablets, or Fehling's solution.

CAPREOMYCIN SULFATE CAPASTAT SULFATE

Classification   Secondary agent, antitubercular.

Remark   Antibiotic agent.

Uses   Resistant-type tubercle bacillus. Usually given in combination with ethambutol and isoniazid. Also used in initial treatment.

Contraindications   Hypersensitivity to drug. Never use together with streptomycin.

Untoward Reactions   Hearing loss, tinnitus, pain at injection site, eosinophilia, transient proteinuria, cylinduria, and nitrogen retention. Hypokalemia. Severe renal failure is rare.

Dosage   **IM:** 1.0 gm daily for 60 to 120 days followed by 1.0 gm every 2 to 3 weeks.

Administration/ Storage

1. Reconstituted solutions are stable for 48 hours at room temperature and for 14 days when refrigerated.
2. Capreomycin sulfate injections may develop a pale straw color and darken, but this does not affect the efficacy of the product.
3. Administer deep into large muscle mass to minimize pain, induration, excessive bleeding, and sterile abscesses at site of injection.

Additional Nursing Implications

1. Observe for ototoxicity manifested by damage to vestibular and auditory portion of eighth cranial nerve, tinnitus, deafness, dizziness, ataxia.
2. Protect patient with vertigo or ataxia during ambulation.
3. Observe for symptoms of nephrotoxicity evidenced by decreasing renal function. If decreased, patient must be evaluated and the drug either reduced or discontinued.

CYCLOSERINE SEROMYCIN

Classification

Secondary antitubercular agent.

General Statement

Broad-spectrum antibiotic produced by a strain of *Streptomyces orchidaceus* or *Garyphalus lavendulae*. It is a secondary antitubercular agent believed to interfere with formation of bacterial wall. It is readily absorbed from the GI tract.

Uses

Active pulmonary and extrapulmonary tuberculosis. Indicated only when primary therapy with streptomycin, isoniazid, and para-aminosalicylic acid cannot be used. Also useful in the treatment of acute urinary infections caused by susceptible organisms, especially *E. coli* and *Aerobacter aerogenes*.

Contraindications

Hypersensitivity to cycloserine, epilepsy, depression, severe anxiety, psychosis, severe renal insufficiency, and alcoholism.

Untoward Reactions

CNS neurotoxicity: drowsiness, dizziness, headache, mental confusion, tremor, lethargy, allergic dermatitis, photosensitivity, psychotic reactions, anxiety, convulsions (petit and grand mal seizures), liver damage, and peripheral neuropathy.

Neurotoxic effects depend on blood levels of cycloserine. Hence, frequent determinations of cycloserine blood levels are indicated, especially during the initial period of therapy.

Drug Interaction

Ethionamide potentiates the CNS toxicity of cycloserine.

Dosage

Tuberculosis: 250 mg q 12 hr for the first 2 weeks. If no adverse reactions occur, dose may be increased to 250 mg q 8 hr. (Blood levels of the drug should be maintained at 20–30 μg/ml.) Some patients may require 250 mg q.i.d. *Urinary tract infection:* for patient with normal renal function, 250 mg q 12 hr.

Additional Nursing Implications

1. Observe for sudden development of congestive heart failure in patients receiving high doses of cycloserine.
2. Observe for untoward reactions, especially neurologic, as these will necessitate withdrawing the drug at least for a short period of time. Have emergency equipment available for convulsions (pyridoxine, anticonvulsants, sedatives, oxygen, IV, gastric lavage, respirator, means of maintaining body temperature, mouth gag, and rails).

3. Caution patient against operating any machinery as the drug promotes lethargy, drowsiness, and dizziness.

ETHAMBUTOL HYDROCHLORIDE MYAMBUTOL

Classification Primary antitubercular agent.

General Statement Tuberculostatic. Arrests multiplication of tubercle bacilli but does not affect those microorganisms during their resting state. Probably interferes with RNA synthesis. Readily absorbed after oral administration.

Uses Primary drug for pulmonary tuberculosis. Always use in combination with other tuberculostatic drugs. Now preferred to PAS for primary use in antituberculosis drug combinations.

Contraindications Hypersensitivity to ethambutol, preexisting optic neuritis, and children under 13 years of age. Should be used with caution and in reduced dosage in patients with gout, impaired renal function, and in pregnant patients.

Untoward Reactions Ocular toxicity: optic neuritis, decreased visual acuity, loss of color (green) discrimination, temporary loss of vision or blurred vision.

Renal damage. Also anaphylactic shock, peripheral neuritis (rare), hyperuricemia, and decreased liver function.

Adverse symptoms usually appear during the early months of therapy and disappear thereafter. Periodic renal and hepatic function tests as well as uric acid determinations are recommended.

Dosage **PO, for initial treatment:** 15 mg/kg per day given once daily for 10 to 12 days; **for retreatment:** 25 mg/kg daily as a single dose with at least one other tuberculostatic drug; **after 60 days:** 15 mg/kg administered once daily.

Additional Nursing Implications See also *Nursing Implications* under *Antibiotics* (p. 56) and those at the beginning of this section.

1. Ascertain that patient has had visual acuity test before ethambutol therapy and that patient does not have preexisting visual problems. Also check that patient has vision test every 2 to 4 weeks while on therapy.
2. Reassure patient that effects on eyes generally disappear within several weeks to several months after therapy has been discontinued.
3. Tell female patient that, should she become pregnant, she should discontinue her use of the drug and report to her physician.

ETHIONAMIDE TRECATOR-SC

Classification Secondary antitubercular agent.

Remark This secondary antituberculostatic agent is readily absorbed after oral administration.

Use Pulmonary tuberculosis. Should be given only with other antituberculosis drugs.

Contraindication Children under 12 years of age.

Untoward Reactions Gastric irritation: anorexia, nausea and vomiting, upper abdominal discomfort, and diarrhea. Neurological effects: metallic taste, sialorrhea, mental depression, drowsiness, and asthenia. Also severe postural hypotension, headache, acne and drug rash, jaundice, hepatotoxicity, and peripheral neuropathy.

Periodic hepatic and renal function tests and urine examinations are indicated, as is a blood cell count.

Drug Interactions

Interactant	Interaction
Alcohol, ethyl	↑ CNS toxicity of ethionamide
Cycloserine	Ethionamide potentiates CNS toxicity of cycloserine with possibility of convulsions

Dosage Because of the possible emergence of resistant strains, aim for maximum tolerated dose. This is usually between 0.5 and 1.0 gm daily, given in divided doses concomitantly with pyridoxine. **Children:** 12–15 mg/kg daily (maximum 750 mg) in single or divided doses.

Administration
1. Do not administer to children under 12 years of age unless primary therapy has failed.
2. Administer after meals to minimize gastric irritation.

Additional Nursing Implications
1. Observe for toxic effects, particularly severe nausea, which can be treated with antiemetics.
2. Observe patient for potentiation of toxic effects of cycloserine (congestive heart failure) if given concomitantly.
3. Check urine of diabetic patients more frequently and observe for untoward symptoms related to diabetes. The latter condition is more difficult to control in patients with tuberculosis.

ISONIAZID INH, ISONICOTINIC ACID HYDRAZIDE, HYZYD, LANIAZID, NICONYL, NYDRAZID, ROLAZID, TEEBACONIN

Classification Primary antitubercular agent.

General Statement Isoniazid is the most effective tuberculostatic agent. It is effective against rapidly growing tubercle bacilli. It is well absorbed from its injection site as well as from the GI tract and is well distributed throughout most tissues.

Patients on isoniazid fall into two groups depending on the manner in which they metabolize isoniazid:

1. Slow inactivators—show earlier, favorable response but have more toxic reactions.

2. Rapid inactivators—possibly have poor clinical response due to rapid inactivation. This group requires an increased daily dose of the drug.

Uses
Tuberculosis caused by human, bovine and BCG strains of *Mycobacterium tuberculosis*. The drug should not be used as the sole tuberculostatic agent.

Contraindications
Severe hypersensitivity to isoniazid. Extreme caution should be exercised in patients with convulsive disorders in which case the drug should be administered only when the patient is adequately controlled by anticonvulsant medication. Also, use with caution for the treatment of renal tuberculosis and, in the lowest dose possible, in patients with impaired renal function.

Untoward Reactions
Excess CNS stimulation. Convulsions may occur at higher dosage levels. Peripheral neuritis, optic neuritis, optic atrophy, toxic psychosis, hyperreflexia, parasthesia, ataxia, drowsiness, excitement, euphoria, delay in micturition, dryness of the mouth, and hematological changes.

Neurotoxic reactions are more marked in malnourished individuals.

Excessive dosages of the drug can result in altered thyroid function, elevated blood sugar, acidosis, and hyperkalemia. The drug may cause liver damage that may not be distinguishable from viral hepatitis.

Periodic ophthalmoscopic examinations are indicated.

Patients should be seen monthly, and liver function should be evaluated during each visit.

Drug Interactions

Interactant	Interaction
Aminosalicylic acid	↑ Effect of isoniazid by ↑ blood levels
Atropine	↑ Side effects of isoniazid
Ethanol	↑ Chance of isoniazid-induced hepatitis
Disulfiram (Antabuse)	↑ Side effects of isoniazid (esp. CNS)
Meperidine (Demerol)	↑ Side effects of isoniazid
Phenytoin (Dilantin)	↑ Effect of phenytoin due to ↓ breakdown in liver
Rifampin	Additive liver toxicity

Laboratory Test Interference
Altered liver function tests. False + or ↑ K, SGOT, SGPT, urine glucose (Benedict's, Clinitest).

Dosage
Active Tuberculosis: 5 mg/kg daily (up to 300 mg total) as a single or divided dose; **children and infants:** 10–30 mg/kg/day (up to 300–500 mg total) in single or divided doses. *Prophylaxis:* 300 mg/day in single or divided doses; **children and infants,** 10 mg/kg/day (up to 300 mg total) in single or divided doses.

Administration/ Storage
1. Store in dark, tightly closed containers.
2. Solutions for IM injection may crystallize at low temperature and should be allowed to warm to room temperature if precipitation is evident.

Additional Nursing Implications

See also *Nursing Implications* under *Antibiotics* chapter 1, section 1 (p. 56).

1. Have on hand parenteral sodium phenobarbital for the control of isoniazid-induced neurotoxic symptoms, particularly convulsions.
2. Anticipate that adrenergic drugs, atropine, and certain narcotics (meperidine) may aggravate side reactions.
3. Withhold drug and consult with physician in case of marked CNS stimulation.
4. Explain to patient that pyridoxine is given to prevent neurotoxic effects of isoniazid.
5. Assess diabetic patients closely because diabetes is more difficult to control when isoniazid is administered. Alert patients to this fact.
6. Anticipate that lower doses of the drug are to be given to patients with renal problems and check intake and output of fluids to ascertain that renal output is adequate to prevent systemic accumulation of the drug.
7. Provide patient with only a 1 month supply of the drug as he/she should be examined and evaluated monthly while on isoniazid.
8. Anticipate slight local irritation at site of injection.

PYRAZINAMIDE

Classification

Secondary antitubercular agent.

Remarks

Suitable for short-term use in selected patients. Not suitable for either initial therapy or long-term use. This drug should only be used in conjunction with other antituberculosis agents.

Use

Seriously ill patients hospitalized for tuberculosis who are resistant to other drugs.

Contraindication

Preexistent liver malfunction.

Untoward Reactions

Hepatic damage, especially at doses above 35 mg/kg. Liver damage occurs in 10% to 15% of all patients, and a number of fatal cases are on record. Also: gout, fatal hemoptysis, blood dyscrasias, arthralgia, anorexia, nausea, vomiting, malaise, and fever. **Note:** Frequent liver function tests are required.

Drug Interactions

Interactant	Interaction
Aminosalicylic acid	↓ Pharmacological effect of pyrazinamide
Probenecid (Benemid)	↓ Pharmacological effect of pyrazinamide
Salicylates	↓ Pharmacological effect of pyrazinamide

Dosage

PO: 20–35 mg/kg daily in 3 to 4 divided doses. Maximum daily dose is 3.0 gm. When used in conjunction with surgical treatment, drug therapy for tuberculosis should be initiated 2 weeks before surgery and continued 4 to 6 weeks postoperatively.

Additional Nursing Implications

See also *Nursing Implications* under *Antibiotics* (p. 56) and those at the beginning of this section.

1. Question doses that exceed 35 mg/kg as higher doses tend to promote hepatic damage.
2. Administer only under close medical supervision.
3. Observe for jaundice.
4. Observe diabetic patients closely for hypo- or hyperglycemia because drug affects sugar metabolism.
5. Observe for fatigue, poor appetite, weakness, irritability and signs of anemia.
6. Schedule for frequent liver function tests.

RIFAMPIN RIFADIN, RIMACTANE

Classification

Primary antitubercular agent.

General Statement

Semisynthetic antibiotic derived from *Streptomyces mediterranei*. Bacteriostatic and bactericidal activity that interferes with metabolism of bacteria. Well absorbed from GI tract and distributed throughout all body tissues and fluids.

Uses

Pulmonary tuberculosis. Must be used in conjunction with at least one other tuberculostatic drug (such as isoniazid, ethambutol) but is the drug of choice for retreatment. Also for meningococcal carriers.

Contraindications

Hypersensitivity to rifampin. Safe use in pregnancy has not been established. Use wth extreme caution in patients with hepatic dysfunction.

Untoward Reactions

GI disturbances: heartburn, epigastric distress, anorexia, nausea, vomiting, flatulence, cramps, and diarrhea. Also headaches, drowsiness, fatigue, ataxia, dizziness, mental confusion, visual disturbances, muscular weakness, pruritus, urticaria, purpura, skin rashes, edema, sore mouth, oral monoliasis, transient low frequency hearing loss, transient leukopenia, eosinophilia, decreased hemoglobin, hematuria, casts in urine, and hemoptysis. Thrombocytopenia is rare.

Rifampin may produce liver dysfunction. Such patients should be monitored closely. Drug may interfere with hepatic uptake of bilirubin. This may result in an excess of unconjugated bilirubin in blood, causing jaundice. This is not due to liver necrosis.

Drug Interactions

Interactant	Interaction
Aminosalicylic acid	↓ Effect of rifampin due to ↓ absorption from GI tract
Anticoagulants, oral	Effect ↓ by rifampin
Isoniazid	Additive liver toxicity
Oral contraceptives	↓ Reliability of oral contraceptives

Laboratory Test Interference ↑ in SGOT, SGPT, alkaline phosphatase, BUN, bilirubin, uric acid, BSP retention values. False + Coombs test.

Dosage *Pulmonary tuberculosis*, **PO:** single dose of 600 mg daily; **pediatric over 5 years of age:** 10–20 mg/kg daily, not to exceed 600 mg/day. *Meningococcal carriers:* 600 mg daily for 4 days; **children over 5 years:** 10–20 mg/kg daily for 4 days, not to exceed 600 mg/day.

Administration
1. Administer once daily 1 to 2 hours after meals to assure maximum absorption.
2. Check to be sure there is a desiccant in the bottle containing capsules of rifampin as these are relatively moisture-sensitive.
3. If administered concomitantly with **PAS**, drugs should be given 8 to 12 hours apart as the acid interfers with the absorption of rifampin.

Additional Nursing Implications See *Nursing Implications* under *Antibiotics* (p. 56) and those at the beginning of this section.

1. Observe for jaundice due to liver dysfunction.
2. Check for GI disturbance, impaired renal function, auditory nerve impairment, and blood dyscrasias.
3. Inform the patient that rifampin colors urine, feces, saliva, sputum, and tears orange.

STREPTOMYCIN SULFATE

See *Aminoglycoside Antibiotics,* p. 93.

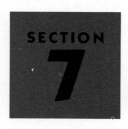

SECTION
7

antimalarials

4-Aminoquinolines   Amodiaquine Hydrochloride   Chloroquine Phosphate
Chloroquine Hydrochloride   Hydroxychloroquine Sulfate

8-Aminoquinoline   Primaquine Phosphate

Miscellaneous Antimalarials   Pyrimethamine   Quinine Sulfate
Quinacrine Hydrochloride

General Statement A knowledge of the life cycle of the causative agent is helpful in understanding the mode of action of the antimalarial drugs.

Malaria is transmitted by the anopheles mosquito. The causative organism is a parasite known as *Plasmodium,* of which there are several species infective to humans: *P. falciparum, P. vivax, P. malariae,* and *P. ovale.*

Plasmodia pass through a complex life cycle, part of which takes place in the gut of the mosquito and part in humans. In the sporozoite stage of development, the organism is transmitted to humans by a mosquito bite. The sporozoite migrates to the human liver where it grows and divides (exoerythrocytic, fixed-tissue stage), emerging as a merozoite. The merozoite enters various tissues, including the red blood cells (asexual erythrocytic stage), causing them to burst. This results in a rise in body temperature. Some merozoites develop into male parasites and others into females. At this stage they are known as gametocytes, which infect the mosquito again when it bites a human carrier. It then reproduces in the gut of the mosquito and develops to the sporozoite stage to complete the cycle.

Clinical manifestations of malaria are not evident during all stages of the life cycle, and no single drug can eradicate the parasite at all stages. Treatment is divided into six categories, according to the end result obtained and the stage at which the malaria is being treated. The categories of treatment are as follows.

1. Causal prophylaxis: eradication of the parasite during the primary exoerythrocytic state (killing of sporozoites). This prevents the disease from spreading.
2. Suppressive prophylaxis: prevents parasites from developing into erythrocytic state (inhibition of erythrocytic stage). This form of treatment prevents clinical manifestations of malaria. Suitable drugs: chloroquine, chloroguanide, pyrimethamine. Symptoms reappear if drug therapy is stopped. When antimalarials are used prophylactically, the drug is administered up to 2 weeks before entering the malarious area and is continued for varying periods of time (depending on the drug) after the person leaves the area.
3. Clinical cure: halts further development of erythrocytic stage and terminates a clinical attack. Suitable drugs: chloroquine, amodiaquine, quinine.
4. Suppressive cure: complete elimination of malarial parasite from affected individual. Suitable drug: pyrimethamine.
5. Radical cure: eradication of erythrocytic and exoerythrocytic forms of the parasite and relief of symptoms. Suitable drug: primaquine.
6. Gametocytocidal therapy: destruction of sexual form of malarial parasite. Suitable drug: primaquine.

4-AMINOQUINOLINES

General Statement   Three 4-aminoquinolines—amodiaquine (Camoquin), chloroquine (Aralen), and hydroxychloroquine (Plaquenil)—are widely used for the treatment of malaria. They are all synthetic agents that resemble quinine. They also are used as amebicides and in the treatment of rheumatic diseases.

The 4-aminoquinolines are rapidly and almost completely absorbed from the GI tract. They are metabolized and excreted extremely slowly and the presence of some members of the group has been demonstrated in the bloodstream weeks and months after the drug has been discontinued.

Urinary excretion is increased by acidifying the urine and slowed by alkalinization.

Uses   Acute attacks of vivax and falciparum malaria. Suppressive prophylaxis and clinical cure of ovale, malariae, vivax, and falciparum malaria. Does not prevent relapses of vivax infection. The drugs are only effective against the erythrocytic stages and therefore will not prevent infections. They are used only against established infections. Other uses include extraintestinal amebiasis, usually together with an intestinal amebicide, giardiasis, discoid lupus erythematosus, systemic lupus erythematosus, and occasionally, rheumatoid arthritis.

Contraindications   To be used with extreme caution in the presence of hepatic, severe GI, neurological, and blood disorders.

Unless deemed essential, the drugs should not be used in the presence of psoriasis, porphyria, and pregnancy. Not to be used concomitantly with gold or phenylbutazone or in patients receiving drugs that depress blood-forming elements of bone marrow.

Untoward Reactions   Gastrointestinal disturbances, pruritus, and other dermatological manifestations. Retinopathy, most often after prolonged administration, visual disturbances, dryness of mouth, headaches, fatigue, lassitude, nervousness, irritability, emotional changes including real psychosis, neurological effects, neuromyopathy manifested as muscle weakness, bleaching of hair, reversible cytotoxicity, and blood dyscrasias. Acute toxicity may develop within 30 minutes after administration and is characterized by respiratory collapse, convulsions, and the like.

Drug Interactions   (amodiaquine hydrochloride, chloroquine, hydroxychloroquine)

Interactant	*Interaction*
Acidifying agents—urinary (Ammonium chloride, etc.)	↑ Urinary excretion of antimalarial and thus ↓ its effectiveness
Alkalinizing agents— urinary (Bicarbonate, etc.)	↓ Excretion of antimalarial and thus ↑ amount of drug in system
Antipsoriatics (Anthralin, Resorcinol)	4-Aminoquinolines inhibit antipsoriatic drugs
MAO inhibitors (isocarboxazid, nialamide, tranylcypromine, pargyline, phenelzine)	↑ Toxicity of 4-aminoquinolines due to ↓ breakdown in liver

Laboratory Test Interference   Colors urine brown.

Dosage   See individual drug entries.

Nursing Implications

1. Assess patients receiving chloroquine therapy in high dosage for a long period of time for *GI disturbances, dermatological manifestations,* such as pruritis, pigmentary changes, dryness, and desquamation; *neuromyopathy,* manifested by muscle weakness; *CNS disturbances,* such as headache, fatigue, nervousness, irritability, emotional changes, psychoses, ototoxicity, and other neurological effects; and *blood dyscrasias.* Reactions are not always reversible.

2. Observe all patients for retinopathy manifested by visual disturbances. Retinal changes are not reversible. Regular ophthalmological examinations are mandatory during prolonged therapy.

3. *Acute toxicity*—observe patients for acute toxicity, which may occur in accidental overdosage in children or in suicidal patients. Symptoms of acute toxicity develop within 30 minutes of ingestion. Death may occur within 2 hours.

   a. *Symptoms of acute toxicity* are headache, drowsiness, visual disturbances, cardiovascular collapse, convulsions, and cardiac arrest.

   b. Have on hand emergency equipment, including setup for gastric lavage, barbiturates, vasopressors, and oxygen. Observe for 6 hours after acute toxicity has been treated.

   c. Check TPR and BP as well as intake and output and state of consciousness at frequent intervals.

   d. Anticipate that fluids will have to be forced and ammonium chloride administered for weeks to months to acidify urine and promote renal excretion of the drug.

   e. Warn patients to keep drug out of reach of children.

4. Check toxic effects of other drugs being used as the combination with chloroquine may reinforce toxic effects.

5. Explain to patients that the drug may turn urine yellow or brown.

6. For suppressive therapy, give drug on same day each week. Give immediately before or after meal so as to minimize gastric irritation. For discoid lupus erythematosus, give with evening meal.

7. Store in amber-colored containers.

8. When the drug is given for rheumatoid arthritis:

   a. Reassure patient and indicate that benefits usually do not occur until 6 to 12 months after therapy has been initiated.

   b. Anticipate that side effects may necessitate a reduction of therapy. After 5 to 10 days of reduced dosage, it may gradually again be increased to the desired level.

   c. Anticipate that dosage will be reduced when the desired response is attained. Drug again will be effective in case of flareup.

   d. To reduce GI irritation, administer drug with meal or glass of milk.

AMODIAQUINE HYDROCHLORIDE CAMOQUIN HYDROCHLORIDE

Classification   4-Aminoquinoline.

Remarks   See *Malaria,* page 140 and 4-*Aminoquinolines,* page 141.

Additional Untoward Reactions   Occasionally, blood dyscrasias at high dosage. Abnormal grayish-green pigmentation on nail beds, palate, and lips. Also, rarely, CNS disturbances such as spasticity and convulsions.

Dosage   *Malaria suppressive therapy, suppressive prophylaxis,* **PO:** 300–600 mg weekly; **pediatric:** 5 mg/kg weekly; give dose on same day of week. *Acute attacks: initial,* 600 mg, followed by 300 mg 6 hr later and 300 mg at 24 and 48 hr, **pediatric:** 10 mg/kg in 3 doses at 12-hour intervals. Do not exceed adult dose.

CHLOROQUINE HYDROCHLORIDE ARALEN HCL

CHLOROQUINE PHOSPHATE ARALEN PHOSPHATE

Classification   4-Aminoquinoline.

Remarks   See *Malaria,* page 140 and 4-*Aminoquinolines,* page 141.

Dosage   *Hydrochloride,* **IM;** 200–250 mg initially and repeated in 6 hr if necessary. Dose should not exceed 800 mg of base in first 24 hr. **PO** treatment should be started as soon as possible; **children and infants:** 5 mg/kg initially; may be repeated in six hrs. Dose should not exceed 10 mg/kg in any 24 hr period. *Phosphate; Suppression:* 5 mg (base)/kg up to maximum of 300 mg/week. *Acute attack: initial,* 600 mg; **then,** 300 mg after 6 hr and 300 mg/day for next 2 days. **children:** *initial,* 10 mg/kg; **then,** 5 mg/kg after 6 hr and 5 mg/kg for next 2 days. Children's dose should not exceed 600 mg for initial dose or 300 mg for subsequent doses.

HYDROXYCHLOROQUINE SULFATE PLAQUENIL SULFATE

Classification   4-Aminoquinoline.

Remarks   See *Malaria,* page 140 and 4-*Aminoquinolines,* page 141.

Additional Untoward Reactions   The appearances of skin eruptions or of misty vision and visual halos are indications for withdrawal.

Dosage   *Malaria, suppressive prophylaxis,* **PO:** to 310 mg weekly. *Acute attacks: initial,* 620 mg; **then,** 310 mg after 6 to 8 hr; 310 mg on days 2 and 3; **pediatric:** *initial,* 10 mg/kg; **then,** 5 mg/kg after 6 hr; 5 mg/kg on days 2 and 3. Should not exceed adult dose. *Giardiasis:* 200 mg t.i.d. for 5 days. *Lupus and polymorphic light eruptions: initial,* 400 mg 1 to 2 times/day for several weeks or months; **maintenance:** 200–400 mg daily. *Rheumatoid arthritis:* 400–600 mg daily; **maximum:** 1 gm daily.

8-AMINOQUINOLINE

PRIMAQUINE PHOSPHATE

Classification	8-Aminoquinoline.
General Statement	See also *General Statement* at beginning of section. This drug is readily absorbed from the GI tract. It is active against primary exoerythrocytic forms of vivax and falciparum malaria. It produces radical cure of vivax malaria by eliminating both exoerythrocytic and erythrocytic forms. It cures suppressed infections after the patient leaves endemic areas and prevents relapse. For this reason, the drug is administered concurrently with quinine or chloroquine.
Uses	Exoerythrocytic and erythrocytic forms of vivax and falciparum malaria.
Contraindications	Very active forms of vivax and falciparum malaria.
Untoward Reactions	Abdominal cramps, epigastric distress, mild hemolytic anemia, methemoglobinemia (cyanosis), leukocytosis, and leukopenia. Blacks and members of certain Mediterranean ethnic groups (Sardinians, Sephardic Jews, Greeks, Iranians), all of whom have a high incidence of glucose-6-phosphate dehydrogenase deficiency, and therefore a low tolerance for primaquine, may manifest marked intravascular hemolysis (hemolytic anemia) after administration of this drug.

Drug Interactions

Interactant	*Interaction*
Bone marrow depressants Hemolytic drugs	Additive untoward reactions
Quinacrine (Atabrine)	Quinacrine interferes with metabolic degradation of primaquine and thus enhances its toxic side reactions. **Do not give primaquine** to patients who are receiving or have received quinacrine within the past 3 months.

Dosage	**PO:** 26.3–52.6 mg daily for 14 days.
Administration/ Storage	1. Administer drug with meals or antacids, as ordered. This reduces or prevents GI distress. 2. Store in tightly closed containers.
Nursing Implications	1. Observe for dark urine indicating hemolysis, a marked fall in hemoglobin, or erythrocyte count as these are indications for withdrawal of drug. Monitor intake and output. 2. Closely observe dark-skinned patients. Because of a possible inborn deficiency of glucose-6-phosphate dehydrogenase, these patients are particularly susceptible to hemolytic anemia while on primaquine.

MISCELLANEOUS ANTIMALARIALS

PYRIMETHAMINE DARAPRIM

Classification Antimalarial, antitoxoplasmotic, folic acid antagonist.

General Statement See also *General Statement* on malaria at beginning of this section.

It has a slow onset of action; a faster acting antimalarial, such as chloroquine or amodiaquine, should be used during acute attacks. Pyrimethamine has some antitoxoplasmotic activity. For treatment of toxoplasmosis, drug is given together with a sulfonamide. The drug is completely absorbed from the GI tract.

Uses Falciparum malaria: causal prophylaxis, suppressive prophylaxis, radical cure, primary attacks, and relapses.

Vivax malaria: suppressive cure and possibly some causal prophylaxis. Toxoplasmosis (a sulfonamide is usually given concomitantly).

Contraindication Not recommended for treatment of resistant parasites.

Untoward Reactions Few toxic effects at usual dosage. Occasional dermatoses. Large doses may cause anorexia, vomiting, megaloblastic anemia, leukopenia, thrombocytopenia, pancytopenia, and atrophic glossitis. Very large doses and overdosage may cause convulsions.

Drug Interactions

Interactant	Interaction
Folic acid	↓ Effect of pyramethamine
Para-aminobenzoic acid (PABA)	↓ Effect of pyramethamine
Quinine	↑ Effect of quinine due to ↓ in plasma protein binding

Dosage *Malaria, suppressive prophylaxis, suppressive cure;* **PO, adults and children over 10 years of age:** 50 mg taken before entering an endemic area followed by 25 mg 1 time a week and continued for 10 weeks; **pediatric: 4 to 10 years:** 12.5 mg 1 time a week; **infants and children under 4 years:** 6.25 mg/week. *Toxoplasmosis,* **individualized:** usually 50–75 mg/day with 1–4 gm of sulfapyrimidine, continue for 1–3 weeks; **pediatric:** 1 mg/kg/day in 2 divided doses; reduce after 2 to 4 days to one-half.

Nursing Implications
1. Anticipate slow onset of action. A faster acting drug is usually used for an acute malarial attack.
2. Administer for suppressive prophylaxis during the seasons of malarial transmission.
3. Administer at weekly intervals in recommended dosages to avoid interference with blood cell formation and the development of resistance, both of which necessitate changes in therapy.
4. Anticipate that with high doses, as given to patients with toxoplasmosis, signs of folic acid deficiency, such as megaloblastic anemia,

thrombocytopenia, leukopenia, or GI side effects, may develop. The drug should be discontinued or reduced, and folic acid (Leucovorin) administered.

5. Have available barbiturates and folic acid for emergency treatment for convulsions resulting from ingestion of large overdoses.
6. Observe patients for symptoms of malaria as resistance to the drug can develop.
7. Administer with meals to reduce gastric irritation.

QUINACRINE HYDROCHLORIDE ATABRINE HYDROCHLORIDE

See *Anthelmintics*, page 129.

QUININE SULFATE COCO-QUININE

Classification   Antimalarial.

General Statement
See also *General Statement* on malaria at beginning of this section.

This drug is a natural alkaloid obtained from the bark of the cinchona tree. In addition to its antimalarial properties, it has antipyretic and analgesic properties similar to those of the salicylates. It relieves muscle spasms and is used as a diagnostic agent for myasthenia gravis. Quinine has been used increasingly in the last several years since resistant forms of vivax and falciparum were observed in Southeast Asia. No resistant forms of the parasite have been found for quinine.

Uses
In combination with synthetic antimalarials for the radical cure of relapsing vivax malaria and for resistant forms of *P. falciparum*. Diagnosis of myasthenia gravis.

Contraindications
Patients with tinnitus and optic neuritis. To be used with caution in patients with optic neuritis.

Untoward Reactions
Quinine causes a typical group of symptoms referred to as cinchonism. Mild cinchonism is characterized by ringing of the ears, headaches, nausea, slightly disturbed vision. A single large dose, however, may also cause severe toxicity including acute hemolytic anemia, renal damage, GI disturbances (nausea, vomiting, diarrhea), CNS disturbances (particularly headaches, fever, and vomiting), and respiratory stimulation, as well as cyanosis of the skin, and severe impairment of hearing and vision.

Drug Interactions

Interactant	Interaction
Anticoagulants, oral	Additive hypoprothrombinemia
Heparin	Effect ↓ by quinine
Pyramethamine	↑ Effect of quinine due to ↓ in plasma protein binding

Skeletal muscle relaxants (surgical)
  Succinylcholine
  d-Tubocurarine
	↑ Respiratory depression and apnea

Dosage: **PO:** 325 mg q.i.d. for 7 consecutive days; **children:** 15 mg/kg t.i.d. for 10 days.

Nursing Implications
1. Observe for cinchonism (ringing of ears, blurring of vision, and headache, which may be followed by digestive disturbances, impairment of hearing and sight, confusion, and delirium), indicating overdosage. Quinine overdosage should be treated by thorough gastric lavage or induced emesis.
2. Observe for tremor and palpitation, tinnitus, impaired hearing, dizziness, which may appear with therapeutic doses.

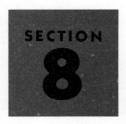

SECTION 8
amebicides and trichomonacides

Carbarsone	Metronidazole
Chloroquine	Paromomycin Sulfate
Diiodohydroxyquin	Povidone-Iodine
Emetine Hydrochloride	Tetracyclines
Erythromycin	

General Statement   Amebiasis is a widely distributed disease caused by the protozoan *Entamoeba histolytica*. The disease has a high incidence in areas with low standards of hygiene. In the United States, the average rate of infestation is generally from 1% to 10%; however, in certain southern localities the incidence is as high as 40%.

Entamoeba histolytica has two forms: (1) an active motile form known as the trophozoite form, and (2) a cystic form that is very resistant to destruction and responsible for the transmission of the disease.

The overt manifestations of amebiasis vary. Some patients manifest violent acute dysentery (sudden development of severe diarrhea, cramps, and passage of bloody, mucoid stools), while others have few overt symptoms or are even completely asymptomatic.

Diagnosis is based on microscopic examination of fresh, or at least moist, stools by a trained examiner. More than one sample of stool must be negative before amebiasis can be ruled out.

Amebae often migrate from the GI tract to other parts of the body (extraintestinal amebiasis). The spleen, lungs, or liver are frequently affected. The amebae colonize in these organs and form abscesses that may rupture and thereby serve as infectious foci.

Drugs used for the treatment of this disease fall into two main categories; some are more suitable for the treatment of intestinal forms of the disease, while others are required for extraintestinal infestations. At present, no one drug can cure all types of amebic infestations, and many physicians prefer to use a combination of several therapeutic agents. Often the more effective, but very toxic agents, are used initially for a short period of time, while long-term eradication or prophylaxis is carried out with less toxic agents.

Since many of the agents used in the treatment of amebiasis are also used for trichomoniasis, nursing implications and dosages for the treatment of *Entamoeba histolytica* will be given in this section.

Infestation with the parasite *Trichomonas vaginalis* causes vaginitis characterized by an irritating, profuse, creamy or frothy vaginal discharge associated with severe itching and burning. Diagnosis is based on demonstrating the presence of the trichomonad microscopically in the vaginal secretion.

Vaginitis caused by *Trichomonas vaginalis* is treated by various locally applied antitrichomonal agents—often effective amebicides—and also by the oral administration of metronidazole (Flagyl). This drug is usually prescribed for both sexual partners so as to prevent reinfection.

Acid douches (vinegar or lactic acid) are a helpful adjunct to treatment.

Eradication of the infectious agent—which frequently becomes resistant—should be ascertained for 3 months after treatment has ceased. The examination usually is made after menstruation, since trichomonas infections often flare up during menstruation.

Nursing Implications

Amebicides

1. Observe patients on therapy for acute dysentery or extraintestinal amebiasis closely because the agents of choice are highly toxic.
2. Anticipate that the patient frequently will be on a combination of drug therapy for amebiasis and must be observed for toxic reactions to all drugs.
3. Be prepared to give intensive supportive nursing care to patients having acute dysentery, assist in the effort to control diarrhea, maintain electrolyte balance, and prevent complications caused by malnutrition. The patient's activity may have to be curtailed during the acute phase of the disease.
4. Administer drugs only for the period of time ordered and allow for rest periods between courses of therapy. Advise patients against self-medication.
5. Encourage carriers to continue with drug therapy, stressing the benefit to themselves, their families, and co-workers.
6. Teach others the necessity for thorough handwashing, especially in industry, schools, and other institutions where disease is likely to be spread.
7. Emphasize the need for food handlers to be particularly conscientious about handwashing after toileting. Emphasize the need for the availability of soap, water, and towels.

8. Encourage patients and carriers to have regular stool examinations to check for recurrence.

Trichomonacides

1. Instruct the patient in the proper method of douching and good feminine hygiene.
2. Instruct the patient in methods of insufflation or insertion of vaginal suppository, depending on drug regimen.
3. Explain that sexual partner may be an asymptomatic carrier and also may require therapy to prevent reinfection of female.
4. Advise the patient to wear a pad to prevent clothing or bed linen from becoming stained by the medication in vaginal suppositories, especially if they contain iodine, which has a tendency to stain. Stress that the pad must be changed frequently and must not be worn moist for any length of time because it may serve as a growth medium for the infecting organism.

CARBARSONE

Classification Amebicide.

Remarks Carbarsone is an organic arsenical, effective against both the motile and cystic forms of amebae. It is readily absorbed from the GI tract.

Uses Acute and chronic amebiasis. Particularly suitable for the treatment of carriers.

Contraindications Renal and hepatic disease, including amebic hepatitis or amebic abscesses of the liver. Also, patients with arsenic intolerance or previous loss of vision.

Untoward Reactions Toxic effects are relatively rare and include vomiting, increased diarrhea, cutaneous rash, weight loss, and abdominal distress. Arsenic intoxication is marked by exfoliative dermatitis, encephalitis, and damage to the optic nerve.

Dosage *Amebiasis,* **PO:** 250 mg 2 to 3 times/day for 10 days. Dosage can be repeated after a rest period of 14 days; **children 2 to 4 years:** 2 gm, total over a 10-day period (66 mg t.i.d.); **5 to 8 years:** 3 gm total over a 10-day period; **9–12 years:** 4 gm total over a 10-day period; **12 years and older:** 5 gm total over a 10-day period.

Additional Nursing Implications **Amebiasis**
1. Observe for dermatitis, CNS inflammation, and visual disturbances, which are all signs of arsenic intoxication.
2. Have dimercaprol (BAL) on hand as an antidote to arsenic poisoning.
3. Maintain patient on light diet and allow only moderate activity.

CHLOROQUINE ARALEN
See *Antimalarials*, page 144.

DIIODOHYDROXYQUIN YODOXIN

Classification	Amebicide, trichomonacide, and local anti-infective.
Remarks	Effective against *Trichomonas vaginalis* and against various fungi and bacteria. Mostly unabsorbed from the GI tract.
Uses	Acute and chronic intestinal amebiasis. Effective in the treatment of mild cases and asymptomatic carriers. Suitable for mass therapy and for prophylaxis. *Trichomonas vaginalis* and bacterial and fungal infections of the skin, including seborrheic dermatitis.
Contraindications	Hepatic or renal damage or iodine intolerance. Severe thyroid conditions.
Untoward Reactions	Diarrhea, constipation, transitory abdominal distress, anal irritation and pruritis, lethargy, an increased sense of warmth occurs occasionally as do symptoms of iodism, such as furunculosis, dermatitis, sore throat, rhinitis, headache, chills, and fever.
Laboratory Test Interference	Certain thyroid function tests ($\downarrow$ uptake of I^{131}) for up to 6 months after discontinuation of therapy.
Dosage	*Amebiasis,* **adults and children over 12 years:** 650 mg t.i.d. after meals for 20 days; **children:** 30–40 mg/kg/day in 2 to 3 divided doses (maximum of 1.95 gm/day) for up to 3 weeks. Course may be repeated after a rest period of 2 to 3 weeks. *Trichomonas vaginalis,* **vaginal tablets:** 2 tablets, 1 or more times daily. *Dermatitis:* Use as cream or shampoo as indicated.
Additional Nursing Implications	**Amebiasis** Observe for symptoms of iodism, such as furunculosis, dermatitis, sore throat, chills, and fever.

Trichomoniasis
1. Anticipate that treatment initially may cause an increase in vaginal discharge.
2. During latter months of pregnancy, suppositories should be inserted by physician.
3. Moisten suppositories before insertion into vagina.
4. Cream should be inserted morning and night.
5. To counteract favorable growth conditions of trichomonas during and immediately after menstruation, treatment should be intensified during these periods. Vaginal tablets should be inserted 2 to 3 times daily.

6. Treatment should be continued until smears are negative for 3 consecutive months.
7. Treatment can be supplemented by lukewarm acid douches (2 tablespoons of vinegar in 1 quart of water).

Dermatologic Use

In seborrheic dermatitis, diiodohydroxyquin is applied as a shampoo usually after hair and scalp have been washed with a nonmedicated shampoo. After the medication has been on the scalp for 5 minutes, it is rinsed off and hair and scalp washed with nonmedicated shampoo so as to remove medication completely.

EMETINE HYDROCHLORIDE

Classification

Amebicide.

Remark

Emetine is an alkaloid that kills the motile (trophozoite) form of ameba but not amebic cysts.

Uses

Acute amebic dysentery, amebic hepatitis, and extraintestinal amebiasis.

Contraindications

Emetine is potentially a very toxic compound, not to be used for minor cases, for prophylaxis, or for carriers. Its main toxic effect is on the cardiovascular system. It is contraindicated for patients with cardiac or renal disease; aged, debilitated persons; children; or during pregnancy, unless the condition does not respond to other therapy.

Untoward Reactions

Side effects range from transitory nausea, vomiting, vertigo, and increased diarrhea to tachycardia and cardiac failure. Cellular degeneration of the heart, GI tract, kidneys, and skeletal muscle.

Dosage

Amebiasis, **adults:** 65 mg daily in 2 divided doses; usually given for 3 to 5 days by deep **SC** or **IM** injection until acute symptoms subside. Some recommend a dose of 1 mg/kg. Period of treatment should not exceed 10 days, and a rest period of 6 weeks should be observed before treatment is repeated. The dose should be halved in underweight or debilitated patients. **Children 8 years or older:** no more than 20 mg/day; **8 years and younger:** no more than 10 mg/day. *Amebic hepatitis:* 65 mg/day for 10 days followed by a 1-week rest period and 6 more days of therapy. Treatment with emetine usually is followed by treatment with a milder amebicide.

Administration

1. Injection may cause local irritation, induration and swelling. Keep record of injection site and rotate.
2. Apply heat to relieve pain and hasten absorption of drug.
3. Aspirate syringe before injecting because accidental IV administration of emetine is dangerous.
4. Oral administration causes gastrointestinal irritation.

Additional Nursing Implications

1. Maintain patient at bedrest during the course of treatment and for several days after therapy has been completed.
2. Advise patient of physician's specific recommendations for limited activity after a course of therapy so that patient can plan his activities.
3. Warn patient to report promptly any unusual symptoms he/she experiences during the post-treatment period.
4. Monitor blood pressure and pulse rate several times daily during the course of therapy. Report a rise in pulse rate above 110, tachycardia, and a fall in blood pressure because such symptoms require that the drug be discontinued.

ERYTHROMYCIN

See Chapter 1, Section 1, page 71.

METRONIDAZOLE FLAGYL

Classification Systemic trichomonacide, amebicide.

Remark Metronidazole is readily absorbed from the GI tract.

Uses Trichomoniasis, amebiasis.

Contraindications Blood dyscrasias, active organic disease of the CNS, pregnancy, especially during the first trimester and near term.

Untoward Reactions GI disturbances, including anorexia, nausea, vomiting, abdominal cramps, diarrhea, and constipation. Also a metallic taste, sharp bitter taste, dry mouth, blurred vision, headache, joint pain, numbness, paresthesia of the extremities, flushing, edema, confusion, irritability, depression, insomnia, drowsiness, superinfections with oral fungus, furry tongue, glossitis, stomatitis, and other side effects. Ataxia, tremor, or other signs of CNS toxicity necessitate drug withdrawal.

Drug Interactions

Interactant	Interaction
Alcohol, ethyl	"Antabuselike" reaction possible
Disulfiram (Antabuse)	Additive effects

Dosage *Trichomoniasis, Female,* **PO:** 250 mg b.i.d. to t.i.d. for 7 days. An interval of 4 to 6 weeks should elapse between courses of therapy. *Male,* **PO:** 250 mg t.i.d. for 7 days. *Amebiasis,* **PO:** 750 mg t.i.d. for 5 to 10 days; **pediatric:** 35–50 mg/kg/day in 3 equal doses for 10 days.

Additional Nursing Implications

1. Warn patients that consumption of alcohol when on drug therapy with metronidazole may result in abdominal cramps, vomiting, flushing, and headache.

2. Explain to patient the necessity for male partner to have therapy since organisms may also be located in the urogenital tract of the male.
3. Warn patient that the drug may turn urine brown.
4. Observe for symptoms of CNS toxicity, such as ataxia or tremor which necessitate withdrawal of the drug.

PAROMOMYCIN SULFATE

See *Miscellaneous Antibiotics*, page 102.

POVIDONE-IODINE BETADINE, PHARMADINE

Classification Antiseptic/germicide.

General Statement This product is a nonstinging, nonstaining iodine complex with all the antiseptic properties of iodine. Bactericidal for gram-positive and gram-negative bacteria, antibiotic resistant organisms, fungi, viruses, protozoa and yeasts. It is only used topically. After product application the coloration of skin is an indication of area of antimicrobial activity. Povidone-Iodine is available in various forms (gauze pads, solutions, aerosol spray, for surgical scrub, douche or as skin cleaner and ointment).

Uses Topical disinfectant (surgery, skin, wounds), vaginitis, vaginal moniliasis, *Trichomonas vaginalis*, vaginitis, common skin infections, stasis ulcers.

Contraindications Rare cases of skin sensitivity.

Dosage The following products are used as indicated on the package or are suitable as topical dressing, degerming of skin, as disinfectant for wounds, burns, or abrasions, or preoperatively. All solutions and ointments are used full strength, and all pads, swabs, and so forth are used only once. Treated area can be bandaged.
Aerosol, Antiseptic Gauze Pad, Gargle, Helafoam Solution, Ointment, Perineal Wash, Skin Cleanser, Solution, Shampoo, Surgical Scrub, Spray, Vaginal Gel.

Additional Nursing Implication Inform patient that Betadine stains wash off easily.

TETRACYCLINES

See Chapter 1, Section 1, page 75.

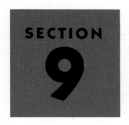

SECTION 9

urinary germicides

Ethoxazene Hydrochloride
Furazolidone
Methenamine
Methenamine Hippurate
Methenamine Mandelate

Methenamine Sulfosalicylate
Nalidixic Acid
Nitrofurantoin
Nitrofurazone
Oxolinic Acid

Urinary tract infections are commonly treated by several of the antimicrobial agents considered in other sections (*Miscellaneous Antibiotics, Sulfonamides*). Agents used specifically for urinary tract infections are listed in this section.

ETHOXAZENE HYDROCHLORIDE SERENIUM HYDROCHLORIDE

Remark Ethoxazene hydrochloride is an azo dye with local anesthetic action.

Uses Pain relief in chronic urinary tract infections, including cystitis, urethritis, and pyelitis. As an adjunct to sulfonamide and antibiotic therapy of acute urinary tract infections.

Contraindications Uremia, severe hepatitis, and chronic glomerular nephritis. Use with caution and at reduced dosage in patients who are pregnant or who have pyelonephritis or GI conditions.

Dosage PO: 300 mg daily in divided doses; **pediatric under 8 years:** 200 mg in equally divided doses.

Nursing Implications 1. Warn patient that drug colors urine orange-red.
2. Administer drug before meals.

FURAZOLIDONE FUROXONE

Classification Trichomonacide, antibacterial.

Remarks Kills *Trichomonas vaginalis*. Bactericidal against many pathogens of the GI tract. Available preparations also contain nifuroxine, a substance active against *Candida*.

Uses Trichomonas vaginitis; bacterial or protozoal diarrhea; enteritis caused by *Salmonella, Shigella, Staphylococcus, Aerobacter,* and *Escherichia;* urinary tract infections.

Contraindications Nursing mothers and infants under 1 month of age.

Untoward Reactions Hypersensitivity to drug, nausea, vomiting, headaches, hypotension, hypoglycemia, hemolysis. Topical: vulvar edema, pruritus, irritation, burning, erythema.

Drug Interactions

Interactant	Interaction
Alcohol, ethyl	"Antabuselike" reaction possible
Antidepressants, tricyclic Amitriptyline Nortriptyline	Toxic psychoses possible
Guanethidine (Ismelin)	Hypotensive effect ↑ by furazolidone
Methyldopa (Aldomet)	Hypotensive effect ↑ by furazolidone
Monoamine oxidase inhibitors	↑ Effect due to monoamine oxidase inhibitor activity of furazolidone
Reserpine	Hypotensive effect ↑ by furazolidone

Laboratory Test Interference False + urine glucose values.

Dosage *Intestinal and urinary tract infections;* **PO:** 400 mg daily in 4 equally divided doses; **pediatric:** 5 mg/kg daily in four equally divided doses.

Nursing Implications

1. Observe for hypersensitivity reactions demonstrated by a drop in blood pressure, arthralgia, fever, and urticaria. Withhold drug if any of these symptoms is observed.
2. Observe for GI symptoms, malaise, or headache that subside when dosage is reduced or drug is withdrawn.
3. Advise patient not to eat food containing tyramine (such as broad beans, strong unpasteurized cheeses, yeast extracts, beer, pickled herring, chicken livers, bananas, avocados, or fermented food) because furazolidone is a monoamine oxidase inhibitor. These reactions are more likely to occur in patients receiving doses larger than those usually recommended or who receive the drug for more than 5 days.
4. Advise the patient to use sedatives, antihistamines, tranquilizers, and narcotic drugs concurrently with therapy only with the knowledge of the physician.
5. Instruct the patient not to drink alcohol during therapy or for 4 days after because an antabuselike reaction, characterized by flushing, palpitation, dyspnea, hyperventilation, tachycardia, nausea, vomiting, drop in blood pressure, and even profound collapse, may occur.
6. Warn patient that drug may color urine brownish.
7. Anticipate withdrawal of drug if clinical response does not occur within 7 days.

8. Store drug in amber-colored bottles.
9. In the treatment of trichomoniasis, instruct the patient to discontinue treatment, administer a cleansing douche, and report to physician if irritation, pruritus, burning, edema, or erythema occur.

METHENAMINE

METHENAMINE HIPPURATE HIPREX, UREX

METHENAMINE MANDELATE MANDALAY, MANDELAMINE, MANDELETS, METHENDELATE, PROV-U-SEP, RENELATE

METHENAMINE SULFOSALICYLATE HEXALET

Remarks This drug decomposes in an acid medium with the formation of formaldehyde, which is the active principle. The drug is thus only effective when urine is very acid (pH 5.5 or less).

Uses Acute, chronic, and recurrent urinary tract infections by susceptible organisms, especially gram-negative organisms including *E. coli*. As a prophylactic before urinary tract instrumentation.

Contraindications Renal insufficiency, severe liver damage, or severe dehydration. Methenamine sulfosalicylate is contraindicated for patients with salicylate sensitivity.

Untoward Reactions GI disturbances including nausea and vomiting. Skin reactions. Withdraw the drug if a skin rash appears. Large doses may cause bladder irritation, painful and frequent micturition, albuminuria and hematuria, tinnitus and muscle cramps.

Drug Interactions

Interactant	Interaction
Acetazolamide (Diamox)	↓ Effect of methenamine due to ↑ alkalinity of urine by acetazolamide
Sodium bicarbonate	↓ Effect of methenamine due to ↑ alkalinity of urine by sodium bicarbonate
Sulfonamides	↑ Chance of sulfonamide crystalluria due to acid urine produced by methenamine
Thiazide diuretics	↓ Effect of methenamine due to ↑ alkalinity of urine produced by thiazides

Laboratory Test Interference False positive urinary glucose with Benedict's solution. Drug interferes with determination of urinary catecholamines and estriol levels by acid hydrolysis technique (enzymatic techniques not affected.)

Dosage   *Methenamine,* **PO, adults:** 1 gm q.i.d.; **children 6 to 12 years:** 500 mg q.i.d; **under 6 years:** 50 mg/kg/day in 3 divided doses. *Mandelate,* **PO, adults:** 1 gm q.i.d.; **children 6 to 12 years:** 500 mg q.i.d.; **5 years and under:** 18.3 mg/kg q.i.d. *Hippurate:* 1 gm b.i.d.; **children 6 to 12 years:** 0.5–1 gm b.i.d. *Sulfosalicylate,* **adults:** 1 gm q.i.d.; **children 6 to 12 years:** 500 mg q.i.d.

Administration   Administer with one-half glass of water after meals and at bedtime.

Nursing Implications
1. Observe patient for skin rash, which is an indication for drug withdrawal.
2. Clearly indicate on chart that patient is receiving drug because drug will interfere with urinary estriol, catecholamines, and HIAA tests.
3. Maintain an adequate fluid intake (between 1500 and 2000 ml daily).
4. Monitor intake and output.
5. Use Labstix or Nitrazine paper daily to test that pH of urine is 5.5 or lower.
6. Observe patients on high dosage for bladder irritation, painful and frequent micturition, albuminuria, and hematuria.
7. Observe for idiosyncratic effect characterized by nausea, vomiting, dermatologic reaction, tinnitus, and muscle cramps.
8. Dysuria may be relieved by reducing dosage and/or reducing acidity.
9. Anticipate possible restriction of alkalinizing medication or alkalizing foods such as fruits, vegetables, milk, peanuts, walnuts, and brazil nuts.
10. Warn patient that urine may become turbid and full of sediment when mandelamine is administered concomitantly with sulfamethizole.

NALIDIXIC ACID NEGGRAM

General Statement   Depending on the organism, nalidixic acid is either bacteriostatic or bactericidal. It is rapidly absorbed from the GI tract. Sensitivity determinations are recommended before and periodically during prolonged administration. Renal and liver function tests are advisable if course of therapy exceeds 2 weeks.

Uses   Acute and chronic urinary tract infections caused by susceptible gram-negative organisms, including *E. coli, Proteus, Aerobacter, Klebsiella,* and *Shigella.*

Contraindications   To be used with caution in patients with liver disease, severely impaired kidney function, epilepsy, and severe cerebral arteriosclerosis. Safety in pregnancy has not been established.

Untoward Reactions GI disturbances: nausea, vomiting. Also drowsiness, headache, dizziness, weakness, and some visual effects. High doses may affect the CNS, producing convulsions.

Drug Interactions

Interactant	Interaction
Antacids, oral	↓ Effect of nalidixic acid due to ↓ absorption from GI tract
Anticoagulants, oral	↑ Effect of anticoagulants due to ↓ in plasma protein binding.
Nitrofurantoin	↓ Effect of nalidixic acid

Laboratory Test Interference False + for urinary glucose with Benedict's solution, Fehling's solution or Clinitest Reagent tablets. Falsely elevated 17-ketosteroids.

Dosage Administer 4 gm daily in divided doses for 1 to 2 weeks, then 2 gm daily; **pediatric:** 50 mg/kg body weight daily in 2 to 4 divided doses. Not for use in infants younger than 3 months.

Nursing Implications Use Clinistix Reagent Strips or Tes-Tape for urinary tests, as other methods may result in a false positive reaction.

NITROFURANTOIN CYANTIN, FURADANTIN, FURALAN, FURATOIN, J-DANTIN, MACRODANTIN, NITREX, SARODANT

General Statement Nitrofurantoin interferes with bacterial enzyme systems. It is bacteriostatic at low concentrations and bactericidal at high concentrations. Tablets are readily absorbed from the GI tract. Nitrofurantoin macrocrystals (Macrodantin) are available; this preparation maintains effectiveness while decreasing GI distress.

Uses Severe urinary tract infections refractory to other agents. Useful in the treatment of pyelonephritis, pyelitis, or cystitis caused by susceptible organisms, including *E. coli*, *Staphylococcus aureus*, and *Streptococcus faecalis*.

Contraindications Anuria, oliguria, and patients with impaired renal function (creatinine clearance below 40 ml/min); pregnant women, especially near term; infants below 3 months of age; and nursing mothers. To be used with extreme caution in patients with anemia, diabetes, electrolyte imbalance, avitaminosis B, or a debilitating disease.

Untoward Reactions Nitrofurantoin is a potentially toxic drug with many side effects, including GI disturbances (vomiting, nausea), headache, dizziness, malaise, nystagmus, neuropathy, skin rash, generalized myalgia, and arthralgia. Allergic reactions have been noted in long-term users and subacute or chronic pulmonary hypersensitivity reactions may lead to pulmonary fibrosis. Transitory hemolytic anemia may occur in patients with glucose-6-phosphate deficiency. Pain at site of injection. Superinfection of the genitourinary tract.

Drug Interactions

Interactant	Interaction
Acetazolamide (Diamox)	↓ Effect of nitrofurantoin due to ↑ alkalinity of urine produced by acetazolamide
Antacids, oral	↓ Effect of nitrofurantoin due to ↓ absorption from GI tract
Nalidixic acid	Nitrofurantoin ↓ effect
Sodium bicarbonate	↓ Effect of nitrofurantoin due to ↑ alkalinity of urine produced by sodium bicarbonate

Dosage

Adults: 50–100 mg q.i.d; **children up to 7 kg:** 1.5 mg/kg q.i.d.; **7 to 11 kg:** 12.5 mg q.i.d.; **12 to 21 kg:** 25 mg q.i.d.; **22 to 31 kg:** 37.5 mg q.i.d.; **32 to 40 kg:** 50 mg q.i.d.

Administration/ Storage

1. To reduce gastric irritation administer drug with meals or milk.
2. Store oral medications in amber-colored bottles.
3. Mix, store, and administer parenteral preparations as ordered on vial.

Nursing Implications

1. Observe patient for acute or delayed anaphylactic reaction and have emergency equipment available.
2. Observe for peripheral neuropathy manifested by numbness and tingling in the extremities. These are indications for drug withdrawal since the condition may become worse and irreversible.
3. Observe for superinfection of the GI tract.
4. Warn patient that drug may turn urine brown.
5. Label chart showing patient is on drug because it may alter certain laboratory determinations.
6. Anticipate severe pain at site of injection. This may require that the drug be discontinued. The IM route should not be used for more than 5 days.
7. Nausea and vomiting may be relieved by reducing the dosage or slowing IV administration.
8. Preferably administer capsules containing crystals instead of tablets because crystals cause less GI intolerance.
9. Maintain input and output.
10. Withhold drug if urinary output is scant.
11. Observe blacks and ethnic groups of Mediterranean and Near-Eastern origin for symptoms of anemia.

NITROFURAZONE FURACIN, FURAZYME, NISEPT, NITROFURASTAN

General Statement

The drug is a broad-spectrum, mostly bactericidal agent for both gram-positive and gram-negative organisms. Mechanism of action unknown. Used topically for infections of the skin and mucous membranes.

Nitrofurazone is available as a solution, soluble powder, cream, soluble dressing, and urethral inserts. The latter is also available containing hydrocortisone.

Uses Adjunctive therapy for patients with second- and third-degree burns or skin grafts. Intravaginally and intraurethrally for nonspecific bacterial infections. To prevent complications after urethral instrumentation (diagnosis and surgery).

Untoward Reactions Overgrowth by nonsusceptible microorganisms including fungi. Very low incidence of contact dermatitis.

Dosage **Creams, sprays,** and so forth, once daily or as indicated. **Urethral inserts:** once or twice daily for 1 to 2 weeks until symptoms disappear.

Administration/ Storage
1. Store in light-resistant containers and prevent exposure to light, heat, and/or alkaline materials.
2. Discard cloudy solutions because they suggest microbial contamination of the drug.
3. Discoloration does not indicate a loss in strength of the material.
4. Reautoclaving may be done at 121° C for 30 minutes at 15–20 pounds of pressure but discoloration usually occurs and the consistency of the base (particularly an ointment) is changed.

Nursing Implications
1. Protect skin adjacent to chronic stasis ulcers by covering the skin with zinc oxide ointment and using Furacin only on the lesion.
2. Observe and report rash, pruritis, and/or irritation which are indications for termination of treatment with Furacin.
3. Minimize adverse effects by removing medication by irrigation at the first sign of irritation.
4. Flush dressing with sterile saline at time of removal to prevent dressing adhering to wound.
5. Use sterile technique to remove Furacin pad and roll from sterile container.

Furacin Roll
1. After removing roll from jar, free both ends of the gauze to prevent twisting or unraveling as it is unrolled.
2. Resterilization of the roll in its original container may be done by autoclave, but the original cap must be replaced by aluminum foil.

Furacin Soluble Dressing
1. Either apply directly with a tongue blade or place first on gauze.
2. To prepare sterile impregnated gauze:
   a. Place sterile gauze strips in a tray and cover with Furacin soluble dressing.
   b. Repeat above adding several layers of gauze for each layer of soluble dressing.
   c. To minimize discoloration caused by autoclaving, sprinkle sterile water on each layer of dressing.

    d. Cover the tray loosely and autoclave at 121° C for 30 minutes at 15–20 pounds of pressure.
3. Impregnate bandage rolls by putting some soluble dressing in the bottom of the glass jar. Stand rolls on end and place more dressing on top. Then autoclave as above.

Furacin Soluble Powder
Apply directly from shaker top of a non-metallic powder insufflator.

Furacin Stretch Gauze Roll
1. To maintain continuous wet dressings, moisten with Furacin solution diluted 1:1 with sterile water.
2. Cover dressings with a layer of dry gauze or a blanket to minimize loss of heat through evaporation.

OXOLINIC ACID UTIBID

Classification   Urinary germicide.

General Statement   Oxolinic acid is believed to interfere with the nucleic acid synthesis of the bacteria and thus prevent their reproduction. Its spectrum, which is almost identical with that of nalidixic acid, includes most gram-negative bacteria. Sensitivity determinations are indicated before and during therapy. The drug is well absorbed from the GI tract. Therapeutic levels are attained after 2 to 4 hours and persist for 12 hours. The drug causes more CNS manifestations than nalidixic acid, and the latter may thus be preferred for the treatment of elderly patients.

Uses   Primary and recurrent non-obstructive urinary tract infections caused by gram-negative organisms.

Contraindications   Hypersensitivity to oxolinic acid. Convulsive disorders. Nursing mothers and infants. Use only for 4 weeks. Use with caution in patients with impaired renal function. Not recommended for children under 12 years of age.

Untoward Reactions   CNS manifestations: insomnia, dizziness, nervousness, and headache. Less frequently GI disturbances: abdominal pain, nausea, cramps, anorexia, vomiting, diarrhea, weakness, constipation. Also elevation of liver function tests, blood dyscrasias, swelling of extremities, photophobia, urticaria, rash, soreness of mouth and gums, and metallic taste.

Drug Interactions   ↑ Effect of anticoagulants due to ↓ plasma protein binding.

Dosage   **PO:** 750 mg b.i.d. for 2 weeks; **pediatric (investigational), 7 to 12 years:** 400–600 mg b.i.d.; **6 years:** 300 mg b.i.d.; **4 to 5 years:** 200 mg b.i.d.; **1 to 3 years:** 100 mg b.i.d. Administer for minimum of 5 weeks.

Nursing Implications

1. Report untoward reactions because these may necessitate that drug be withdrawn.
2. Provide safety measures for patients with excessive CNS stimulation.
3. Advise patients to use caution in driving or operating dangerous machinery because drug may cause dizziness.
4. Observe patients with renal impairment for crystalluria, oliguria, and increased BUN or creatinine levels.

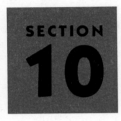

SECTION 10 antiviral drugs

Amantadine Hydrochloride
Idoxuridine

Vidarabine

General Statement

Viruses, sometimes called naked genes, are the most elementary of the infectious agents. They consist of a core of nucleic acid and a coat of protein. To replicate, viruses must penetrate suitable cells whose machinery they take over to make copies of themselves. Viruses do not have cell walls, whose synthesis is usually interfered with by antibiotics like penicillin. This is why most antibiotics are ineffective against viruses.

Many virus infections (measles, small pox, polio) are prevented by means of immunization. Others, like influenza, just run their natural course. Recently several drugs have been developed that are moderately effective against certain viruses.

AMANTADINE HYDROCHLORIDE

Classification

Antiviral agent.

General Statement

This agent has been used for a number of years for the prophylaxis of influenza. The drug apparently prevents the virus from penetrating the host cell.

Use

Influenza A virus infections (prophylaxis and treatment of high risk patients). Parkinsonism (see appropriate section).

Contraindications

Hypersensitivity to drug. Use with caution in the presence of epilepsy or history of congestive heart disease.

Untoward Reactions

CNS: depression, psychosis, convulsions, hallucinations, confusion, ataxia, irritability, anorexia, dizziness. Cardiovascular: congestive heart failure, orthostatic hypotension, peripheral edema. Other: urinary retention, constipation, nausea, leukopenia, neutropenia, mottling of skin of the extremities due to poor peripheral circulation (livedo reticularis).

Drug Interaction

When used concomitantly with anticholinergic drugs, may ↑ incidence of atropine-like side effects.

Dosage

PO: 200 mg daily as a single or divided dose; **children 1 to 9 years:** 4–8 mg/kg/day up to maximum of 150 mg/day in 2 to 3 divided doses; **9 to 12 years:** 100 mg b.i.d. Prophylactic treatment should be instituted prior to or immediately after exposure: for 10 to 21 days if used concurrently with vaccine or for 90 days without vaccine. *Symptomatic management:* initiate as soon as possible and continue for 24 to 48 hr after disappearance of symptoms.

Overdosage

Gastric lavage or induction of emesis followed by supportive measures. Ensure that patient is well hydrated; give fluids by IV if necessary.

Administration/ Storage

Protect capsules from moisture.

Nursing Implications

1. Advise patient not to drive a car or work in a situation where alertness is important because medication can affect vision, concentration, and coordination.
2. Advise the patient to rise slowly from a prone position because orthostatic hypotension may occur.
3. Advise patient to lie down if he/she feel dizzy or weak to relieve the orthostatic hypotension.
4. Observe patient with history of epilepsy or other seizures for an increase in seizure activity and take appropriate precautions.
5. Observe patient with a history of congestive heart failure or peripheral edema for increased edema and/or respiratory distress and report promptly.
6. Observe patient with renal impairment for crystalluria, oliguria, and increased BUN or creatinine levels and report promptly.
7. Alert the patient to report any exposure to rubella because drug may increase susceptibility to disease.

IDOXURIDINE DENDRID, HERPLEX LIQUIFILM, STOXIL

Classification

Antiviral agent.

General Statement

Idoxuridine ressembles thymidine. It interferes with the replication of certain DNA viruses in the cell.

Uses

Herpes simplex keratitis, especially for initial epithelial infections characterized by the presence of threadlike extensions. *Note:* Idoxuridine will control infection but will not prevent scarring, loss of vision, or vascularization. Alternate form of therapy must be instituted if no improvement is noted after 7 days, or if complete re-epithelialization fails to occur after 21 days of therapy. Corticosteroids can be used concurrently.

Contraindications   Hypersensitivity; deep ulcerations involving stromal layers of cornea. Safe use in pregnancy not established.

Untoward Reactions   Localized to eye: Temporary visual haze, irritation, pain, pruritus, inflammation, folicular conjunctivitis with pre-auricular adenopathy, mild edema of eyelids and cornea, allergic reactions (rare), photosensitivity, corneal clouding and stippling, small punctuate defects.

Dosage   **Ophthalmic 0.1% soln: initial,** 1 drop q hr during waking hr, q 2 hr during sleeping hr; or 1 drop 5 times at 1 minute intervals q 4 hr around the clock. **Following improvement:** 1 drop q 2 hr during day and q 4 hr at night. Continue for 3 to 5 days after healing is complete. **Ointment (0.5%):** 5 times/day q 4 hr with last dose at bedtime; usual course is 21 days.

Administration/ Storage
1. Store idoxuridine solution at 2°–8°C and protect from light.
2. Do not mix with other medications.
3. Store idoxuridine ointment 2°–15°C.
4. Administer ophthalmic medication as scheduled even during the night.
5. Do not use drug that was improperly stored because of loss of activity and increased toxic effects.

Nursing Implications
1. Reassure patients that hazy vision which follows instillation of medication will be of short duration.
2. *Do not* apply boric acid to the eye when patient is on idoxuridine therapy because it may cause irritation.
3. Encourage patients to wear dark glasses if they suffer from photophobia.
4. Observe patients for symptoms of vision loss.
5. Anticipate that if idoxuridine has been used concurrently with corticosteroids, the idoxuridine will be continued longer than the steroid to prevent reinfection.

VIDARABINE VIRA-A

Classification   Antiviral agent.

General Statement   Vidarabine specifically interferes with the propagation of a number of viruses within the cell. It is effective against herpes simplex, probably by inhibiting viral DNA synthesis. Vidarabine is more effective than idoxuridine for deep or recurrent infections.

Uses   Herpes simplex epithelial keratitis, acute keratoconjunctivitis, herpes.

Contraindications   Hypersensitivity to drug. Safe use in pregnancy not established. Systemic: use with caution in patients susceptible to fluid overload, cerebral edema, or with impaired renal or hepatic function. Topical: hypersensitivity to drug or any component of mixture.

Untoward Reactions   Systemic: mild to moderate GI disturbances seldom requiring discontinuation of drug. CNS: tremor, dizziness, hallucinations, confusion, psychosis, and ataxia. Hematological: decrease in hemoglobin and hematocrit. Also weight loss, malaise, pruritus, rash, hematemesis, and pain at injection site. Topical: temporal visual haze, burning, itching, mild irritation. Also lacrimation, foreign body sensation, conjunctival injection, superficial punctate keratitis, pain, photophobia, punctal occlusion and sensitivity.

Dosage   **Systemic, IV infusion:** 15 mg/kg/day for 10 days. **Ophthalmic:** ½ inch of 3% ointment applied into lower conjunctival sac 5 times daily at 3-hr intervals. Continue therapy for 7 days after complete re-epithelialization.

Administration
1. Systemic: slowly infuse total daily dose at constant rate over 12 to 24 hours.
2. 2.2 ml of IV solution are required to dissolve 1 mg of medication. A maximum of 450 mg may be dissolved in 1 liter.
3. Any carbohydrate or electrolyte solution is suitable as diluent. Do not use biological or colloidal fluids.
4. Shake vidarabine vial well before withdrawing dosage. Add to prewarmed (35°–40°C) infusion solution. Shake mixture until completely clear.
5. For final filtration use an in-line filter (0.45 micron pore size).
6. Dilute just prior to administration and use within 48 hours.

Nursing Implications
1. Assess patient on systemic therapy for fluid overload.
2. Assess patient for renal, liver, and hematologic dysfunction, precipitated by vidarabine.
3. Inform patient that he/she are to continue under close supervision of an ophthalmologist while receiving therapy for optic problem.
4. Advise patient that ophthalmic ointment will cause a haze after application.

CHAPTER 2

ANTINEOPLASTIC AGENTS

Asparaginase
Bleomycin Sulfate
Busulfan
Calusterone
Carmustine
Chlorambucil
Cisplatin
Cyclophosphamide
Cytarabine
Dacarbazine
Dactinomycin
Doxorubicin Hydrochloride
Dromostanolone Propionate
Floxuridine
Fluorouracil
Gold Au 198 injection
Hydroxyurea
Lomustine
Mechlorethamine Hydrochloride

Melphalan
Mercaptopurine
Methotrexate
Methotrexate Sodium
Mithramycin
Mitomycin
Mitotane
Pipobroman
Procarbazine Hydrochloride
Sodium Iodide I^{131}
Sodium Phosphate P 32
Tamoxifen
Testolactone
Thioguanine
Triethylenethiophosphoramide
  (Thiotepa)
Uracil Mustard
Vinblastine Sulfate
Vincristine Sulfate

General Statement

With rare exceptions, neoplastic disease cannot yet be cured by drugs. However, there are many compounds that slow down the disease process or induce a remission.

All antineoplastic agents are cytotoxic (i.e., cell poisons) and therefore interfere with normal cells as well as with neoplastic cells. However, neoplastic cells are much more active and multiply more rapidly than normal cells and are thus more affected by the antineoplastic agents.

Normal tissue cells, such as those of the bone marrow and the GI mucosal epithelium, are naturally very active and particularly susceptible to antineoplastic agents. The margin between the dose of antineoplastic drug needed to destroy the neoplastic cells and that needed to cause bone marrow damage is very narrow. Thus, patients who receive antineoplastic agents are closely watched for signs of bone marrow depression, which is characterized by low blood counts (leukocytes, erythrocytes, platelets). Since white blood cells (WBC) or platelets show the effect of an overdose more rapidly than do erythrocytes, the platelet and WBC count is often used as a guide to dosage. If a blood or marrow test indicates a precipitous fall in the WBC or platelet count, the antineoplastic agent may have to be discontinued. Sometimes the effect of the antineoplastic drugs on the bone marrow is cumulative, with the depression of WBCs and platelets occurring weeks or months after initiation. Thus patients must be followed carefully.

Drugs are usually withheld when the WBC count falls below 2,000/mm³ and the platelet count falls below 100,000/mm³.

Antineoplastic agents should only be administered by people knowledgeable in their management. Facilities must be available for frequent laboratory evaluations, especially total blood counts and bone marrows. Intravenous medications must be administered by the physician.

The toxicity of the antineoplastic agents is also manifested in the lining of the GI tract. Oral ulcers, intestinal bleeding, or diarrhea are warning signs of excess toxicity.

Antineoplastic agents fall into several broad categories.

1. **Alkylating Agents.** These drugs are believed to attach themselves to the nucleic acid inside the nucleus of the cell, thus interfering with mitosis (cell division). The nitrogen mustards, cyclophosphamide, and thiotepa are examples of alkylating agents.

2. **Antimetabolites.** These drugs interfere with important processes in cell metabolism. Some of these drugs resemble a necessary cell metabolite so closely that the cell absorbs it by mistake, but since it cannot use it, the entire machinery of cell division comes to a halt. The antimetabolite group includes the folic acid analogs, such as methotrexate; the purine analogs, including 6-mercaptopurine; and the pyrimidine analogs, such as 5-fluorouracil.

3. **Natural Products.** Certain natural substances (alkaloids and antibiotics) have proven useful; these drugs also probably interfere with cell division. Vinblastine, an alkaloid, and dactinomycin, an antibiotic, belong to this group.

4. **Hormones.** Hormones, especially sex hormones, are used for palliative treatment of neoplasms, especially those of the reproductive organs. (These drugs are discussed in chapter 7.)

5. **Radioactive Isotopes.** Radioactive phosphorus, iodine, and gold are effective against some specific forms of cancer. These drugs destroy the tumor cells by irradiation.

A combination of several antineoplastic agents usually increases the chance of remission. Combination therapy often includes a corticosteroid.

Hodgkin's disease and other lymphomas often respond well to a combination containing mechlorethamine, vincristine (Oncovin), procarbazine, and prednisone. This combination is commonly referred to as MOPP therapy. During a typical course of MOPP therapy the patient receives drugs daily for 14 days. The course is repeated six times during a 6-month period.

Uses   Most of the drugs discussed in this section are used exclusively for neoplastic disease. A few are used for patients experimentally for some of the rheumatic diseases.

Contraindications   Hypersensitivity to drug. Most antineoplastic agents are contraindicated for a period of 4 weeks after radiation therapy or chemotherapy with similar drugs. Use with caution, and at reduced dosages, in patients with preexisting bone marrow depression, malignant infiltration of bone marrow or kidney, or liver dysfunction.

The safe use of these drugs during pregnancy has not been established, and they are contraindicated during the first trimester.

Untoward Reactions

Bone marrow depression (leukopenia, thrombocytopenia, agranulocytosis, anemia) *is the major danger of antineoplastic therapy. Bone marrow depression can sometimes be irreversible. It is mandatory that the patient have frequent total blood counts and bone marrow examinations. Precipitous falls must be reported to a physician.*

Other untoward reactions include GI distress ranging from mild anorexia or nausea to severe vomiting, hemorrhagic diarrhea, and death. Ulcerations of the oral and intestinal mucosa (cheilitis, stomatitis) are also common. Various dermatological manifestations, such as dermatitis, erythema, and macupapular rash, increased susceptibility to infections, hyperuricemia, acute renal failure, alopecia (reversible), temporary amenorrhea, serum sickness, lassitude, malaise, and fatigue may also occur.

Nursing Implications

1. Utilize a team approach involving the nurse, doctor, social worker, and other staff personnel to develop a therapeutic plan for the patient's physical, social, and spiritual problems.
2. Protect the patient from exposure to communicable diseases.
3. Use strict medical asepsis at all times and reverse isolation when WBC is below 2,000–3,000/mm^3.
4. Report sudden sharp drop in WBC or platelet count since this may indicate a need for reduction of dosage or withdrawal of the drug.
5. Be prepared to explain to and reassure the patient about a bone marrow aspiration and to assist the physician in the procedure.
6. Report signs of anemia or bleeding in any part of the body.
7. Observe for signs of a developing stomatitis, including dryness, erythema, and a white patchy area of the oral mucous membrane.
8. Teach patient not to use a toothbrush or rub his gums because this may cause bleeding and ulceration.
9. Provide mouthwashes and a soft, bland diet to help prevent oral ulceration.
10. Observe for signs of liver involvement, such as abdominal pain, high fever, nausea, and diarrhea, which may be followed by yellowing of skin, sclera, and mucous membranes. Ascertain if liver function tests have been performed.
11. Wait for nausea and vomiting to pass before serving food.
12. Ask the physician if the patient may be administered an antiemetic to prevent or treat nausea and vomiting.
13. Provide nourishing foods liked by the patient to counteract anorexia.
14. Weigh the patient at least twice a week. If patient is edematous, corrected weight should be used to compute dosage.
15. Teach the patient about the toxic effects of the drugs, and stress the importance of medical supervision and the need for reporting untoward symptoms.
16. Tell the patient that loss of hair and amenorrhea are usually reversible and will be corrected with reduction in dosage or completion of therapy.

17. Check the site of IV infusion of vesicant drugs to detect extravasation. Should this occur, discontinue IV, report, and provide care for local tissue as ordered by doctor, because infiltration by vesicant drugs requires an individualized approach.

18. To evaluate response of patient, ascertain that hematological studies are done, before initiation of therapy and at regular intervals thereafter.

19. Share the patient's pleasure at remission but avoid contributing to the development of unrealistic attitudes.

20. For Intra-arterial Infusion see Part I Division D, p. 21.

ASPARAGINASE ELSPAR

Remarks Therapy with the enzyme asparaginase is based on the presumed inability of certain malignant cells to synthesize the amino acid asparagine. Asparaginase, which degrades asparagine, thus interferes with the growth of malignant cells that cannot replace the crucial amino acid. Asparaginase is more toxic in adults than in children.

Use Acute lymphocytic leukemia, in combination with other drugs.

Contraindications Anaphylactic reactions to asparaginase, acute hemorrhagic pancreatitis. Institute retreatment with great care. Also use with caution in presence of liver dysfunction.

Untoward Reactions Allergic reactions: skin rash, urticaria, arthralgia, respiratory disease, acute anaphylaxis. (Acute reactions can occur in patients with negative skin tests). Sharp decrease in lymphocytes, increase in uric acid levels. Also hyperglycemia, bleeding, CNS effects, azotemia and renal malfunction, liver function abnormalities, transient bone marrow depression, fatal hyperthermia.

Dosage *Individualized, in combination with other agents (i.e. prednisone and vincristine sulfate)* **IV**: 1000/IU kg/day for 10 days. **IM**: 6000 IU/M² on every third day of a 28-day treatment plan. *When used as sole agent (rare),* **IV**: 200 IU/kg/day for 28 days.

Administration 1. An intradermal skin test (0.1 ml of a 20 IU/ml solution) is to be done at least 1 hour prior to initial administration of drug and when 1 week or more has elasped between treatments.

2. A desensitization procedure, with increasing amounts of asparaginase is sometimes carried out in patients hypersensitive to drug.

3. Treatment should be initiated only in hospitalized patients.

Additional Nursing Implications 1. Have emergency equipment ready to counteract anaphylactic shock (oxygen, epinephrine, and corticosteroids) at each administration of asparaginase because a severe reaction may occur.

2. Ascertain that serum amylase determinations are done as a baseline and periodically during therapy to detect pancreatitis.

3. Monitor patient for hyperglycemia, glycosuria, and polyuria, which may be precipitated by asparaginase.
4. Have available IV fluids and regular insulin should hyperglycemia occur. Anticipate discontinuance of asparaginase.
5. Monitor intake and output, assessing patient for renal failure.
6. Assess patient for peripheral edema due to hypoalbuminemia triggered by asparaginase.

BLEOMYCIN SULFATE BLENOXANE

General Statement Antineoplastic antibiotic, derived from *Streptomyces verticillus*, with relatively low bone marrow depressant activity. Agent is suitable for patients whose hematopoietic function has been adversely affected by radiation or other chemotherapy.

Uses Palliative treatment of certain solid tumors, lymphomas, Hodgkin's disease, and squamous cell carcinomas. Some effectiveness in testicular carcinomas.

Additional Contraindications Renal or pulmonary diseases.

Additional Untoward Reactions Pulmonary toxicity, especially in older patients. Mucocutaneous toxicity and hypersensitivity reactions.

Dosage **SC, IM, IV: initial** 0.25–0.50 units/kg 1 to 2 times/week; **maintenance (after a 50% response):** 1–5 units IV/week. Lymphoma patients should be given a test dose of 2 units or less prior to initiating regular dosage schedule.

Administration/ Storage
1. Reconstituted bleomycin is stable for 2 weeks when stored at room temperature and for 4 weeks when stored at 2° to 8° C.
2. Administer IV slowly over period of 10 minutes.
3. Intra-arterial perfusion: administer over period of 12 to 24 hours.

BUSULFAN MYLERAN

General Statement Alkylating agent. Bone marrow depressant. Adequately absorbed from the GI tract.
  An increased appetite and sense of well-being may occur a few days after therapy is started. WBC drops in second or third week. Issue no more than 3 or 4 days' supply to a patient at one time since constant medical supervision, including lab tests, is mandatory.

Uses Chronic myelocytic (granulocytic) leukemia (drug of choice) and polycythemia vera.

Dosage   **PO:** Individualized according to WBC count. *Initial, usual dose:* 4–8 mg daily until leukocyte count falls below 10,000 mm³; **maintenance:** 1–3 mg daily if remission is shorter than 3 months. Discontinue therapy if there is a precipitous fall in WBC count.

CALUSTERONE METHOSARB

Remarks   Synthetic steroid related to testosterone.

Uses   Palliative treatment of inoperable, disseminated mammary cancer in postmenopausal or ovariectomized women.

Additional Contraindications   Breast cancer in men or premenopausal women.

Additional Untoward Reactions   Mild virilization, hypercalcemia, and edema. (Also see *Androgens*.)

Additional Drug Interaction

Interactant	Interaction
Anticoagulants	↑ Sensitivity to oral anticoagulants

Dosage   **PO:** *usual*, 50 mg q.i.d. **Range:** 150–300 mg/day. Therapy should be for a minimum of 3 months unless disease progresses.

Additional Nursing Implications
1. Ascertain that plasma calcium levels are routinely determined because hypercalcemia may occur during remissions.
2. Encourage fluid intake to prevent formation of renal calculi.
3. Observe for drug-related edema by assessing feet and ankles, weighing patient at least twice weekly, and monitoring intake and output.
4. Anticipate that diuretics will be used if drug related edema occurs.
5. Ascertain that liver function tests are performed to evaluate whether changes are drug related or progressive disease is occurring with liver involvement. Increases in serum bilirubin and alkaline phosphatase suggest drug related dysfunction.
6. Provide appropriate supportive care and analgesia for patients experiencing osseous flares.
7. Reassure female patients that acne and growth of facial hair are reversible once the drug is withdrawn.
8. Be alert to and report onset of permanent signs of virilization, such as deepening of voice and clitoral enlargement.

CARMUSTINE (BCNU) BiCNU

Remarks   Alkylating agent, nitrosourea type. Bone marrow depressant. Passes blood brain barrier producing high concentrations in cerebrospinal fluid (15%–70% greater than plasma concentration). The drug is very similar to lomustine.

Uses Palliative treatment of primary and metastatic brain tumors. Multiple myeloma (in combination with prednisone). Advanced Hodgkin's disease and non-Hodgkin's lymphomas (in combination with other agents).

Additional Untoward Reactions Nausea and vomiting within 2 hours after administration, lasting 4 to 6 hours. Rapid IV administration may produce transitory intense flushing of skin and conjunctiva (onset after 2 hours; duration 4 hours).

Dosage **IV:** 200 mg/m² q 6 weeks as a single or divided dose (on consecutive days). Subsequent dosage based on blood count of patient.

Administration/ Storage
1. Discard vials in which powder has become an oily liquid.
2. Store unopened vials at 2°–8° C and protect from light. Store diluted solutions at 4° C and protect from light.
3. Reconstitute powder with absolute ethanol (provided); then add sterile water. For injection, these dilutions are stable for 24 hours when stored as noted above.
4. Stock solutions diluted to 500 ml with 0.9% sodium chloride for injection or 5% dextrose for injection are stable for 48 hours when stored as noted above.
5. Administer by IV over 1- to 2-hour period, as faster injection may produce intense pain and burning at site of injection.
6. *Do not use vial for multiple doses*, since there is no preservative in vial.

Additional Nursing Implications
1. Assess for extravasation, if patient complains of burning or pain at site of injection.
2. If there is no extravasation, reduce rate of flow if patient complains of burning at site of injection.
3. Slow IV rate if patient demonstrates intense flushing of skin and/or redness of conjunctiva.

CHLORAMBUCIL LEUKERAN

Remarks Alkylating agent; bone marrow depressant. Relatively nontoxic agent. Absorbed from the GI tract.

Uses Chronic lymphocytic leukemia, malignant lymphomas, giant follicular lymphomas, and Hodgkin's disease.

Dosage **PO:** *Individualized* according to response of patient; *initial usual dose:* 0.1–0.2 mg/kg body weight (or 4–10 mg) daily for 3 to 6 weeks. The drug should be taken 1 hr before breakfast or 2 hr after the evening meal; **maintenance:** 0.03–0.1 mg/kg daily.

CISPLATIN PLATINOL

Remarks   Alkylating agent containing platinum. The drug concentrates in the liver, kidneys, large and small intestines, with little penetrating the central nervous system.

Uses   Palliative treatment of metastatic testicular and ovarian tumors in combination with other drugs, surgery, and/or radiotherapeutic procedures.

Additional Contraindications   Preexisting renal impairment, bone marrow suppression, hearing impairment, and allergic reactions to platinum.

Additional Untoward Reactions   Severe cumulative renal toxicity. Ototoxicity characterized by tinnitus, especially in children, anaphylactic reactions.

Dosage   *Metastatic testicular tumors: Cisplatin* is usually administered together with *bleomycin sulfate* and *vinblastine sulfate; usual dosage, Cisplatin,* **IV:** 20 mg/m² daily for 5 days q 3 weeks for 3 courses. *Bleomycin sulfate,* **IV:** 30 units **(rapid infusion)** weekly (on day 2 of each week) for 12 consecutive weeks. *Vinblastine sulfate,* **IV:** 0.15–0.2 mg/kg q 3 weeks (2 times week on days 1 and 2) for 4 courses (i.e., 8 doses total). *Metastatic ovarian tumor, as single agent,* **IV:** 100 mg/m² once q 4 weeks. *In combination with doxorubicin hydrochloride, Cisplatin,* **IV:** 50 mg/m² once q 3 weeks (on day 1); *doxorubicin hydrochloride:* 50 mg/m² once q 3 weeks (on day 1). The drugs are given sequentially. **Note:** Repeat courses should not be administered until *a)* Serum creatinine is below 1.5 mg/100 ml and/or the BUN is below 25 mg/100 ml, *b)* Platelets are equal to or greater than 100,000/mm³ and white blood cells are equal to or greater than 4,000/mm³, and *c)* auditory activity is within the normal range.

Administration/ Storage

1. Hydrate patient prior to dose with 1 to 2 liters of fluid infused only by IV over period of 8 to 12 hours.
2. Dilute drugs as directed by manufacturer to 2 liters of 5% dextrose or 0.3% or 0.45% saline (containing 37.5 gm mannitol). Infuse over period of 6 to 8 hours.
3. Store vials in refrigerator at 2°–8° C. Reconstituted solutions are stable for 20 hours at room temperature. Do not refrigerate reconstituted solution, as this will cause precipitation.

Additional Nursing Implications

1. Monitor intake and output of patient for adequate hydration and urinary output for 24 hours following treatment.
2. Ascertain that baseline renal tests are performed for BUN and creatinine levels before therapy is instituted.
3. Anticipate that additional doses will not be administered until the patient's renal function has returned to normal values.
4. Schedule patient for audiometry prior to initiation of therapy and before administering subsequent doses.

5. Anticipate that allopurinol may be ordered to reduce uric acid levels.
6. Report untoward neurological symptoms when they are first noted, as peripheral neuropathy may be irreversible in some patients and drug may have to be discontinued.

CYCLOPHOSPHAMIDE CYTOXAN

Remarks   Alkylating agent. Cyclophosphamide is related to the nitrogen mustards.

Uses   Lymphomas, including lymphosarcoma, Hodgkin's disease, reticulum cell sarcoma, multiple myeloma, chronic lymphatic leukemia, acute leukemia, and mycosis fungoides. Also, palliative treatment of cancer of the ovaries, breasts, uterus, neuroblastoma, bronchus. Used experimentally for rheumatoid arthritis.

Drug Interactions

Interactant	Interaction
Insulin	Insulin ↑ hypoglycemia
Phenobarbital	↑ Rate of metabolism in liver of cyclophosphamide
Succinylcholine	↑ Succinylcholine-induced apnea due to ↓ breakdown in liver

Additional Untoward Reactions   Hemorrhagic cystitis. Bone marrow depression appears frequently during ninth to fourteenth day of therapy. WBC and platelet counts should be made weekly until maintenance dosage is determined. Alopecia occurs more frequently than with other drugs.

Dosage   **Loading dose: IV:** 40–50 mg/kg in divided doses over 2 to 5 days. **PO:** 1–5 mg/kg depending on patient tolerance. **Maintenance;** various schedules. **PO:** 1–5 mg/kg/day; **IV:** 10–15 mg/kg q 7 to 10 days or **IV:** 3–5 mg/kg 2 times a week. Attempt to maintain leukocyte count between 3000–4000/mm^3.

Administration/ Storage

1. IV: Dissolve 100 mg cyclophosphamide in 5 ml sterile water. Let solution stand until it clears but use within 3 to 4 hours after preparation.
2. PO: Administer preferably on empty stomach. Give with meals in case of GI disturbance.
3. Store in tightly closed containers, preferably in refrigerator.

Additional Nursing Implications

1. Keep patient well hydrated to help prevent hemorrhagic cystitis due to excessive concentration of drug in urine.
2. Encourage frequent voiding.
3. Observe for dysuria and hematuria.
4. Reassure patient with alopecia that hair will grow back when drug is stopped or a maintenance dosage alone is given.

CYTARABINE ARA-C, CYTOSAR, CYTOSINE ARABINOSIDE

Remark Synthetic antineoplastic acting as antimetabolite.

Uses Acute myelocytic (granulocytic) leukemia in adults *and* other acute leukemia in adults and children. In combination with thioguanine, it is the treatment of choice for acute myeloblastic leukemia in adults. Blood counts continue to fall for 5 to 7 days after therapy is discontinued, but therapy should be reinstituted before counts are completely normal; otherwise patient may again be out of control. Therapy should be initiated in the hospital. Therapy should be stopped or adjusted when platelet count drops below 50,000/mm^3 or polymorphs under 1,000/mm^3.

Additional Untoward Reactions Fever, rash, cellulitis, and pain at injection site. Renal dysfunction, sepsis, pneumonia, sore throat, conjunctivitis, hepatitis, freckling, chest pain, joint pain, urinary retention, and various CNS manifestations.

The incidence of side effects is higher in those receiving rapid IV injection than in those receiving drug by IV infusion.

Dosage **IV injection or infusion, highly individualized,** determine by clinical and hematological response. **IV injection: initial,** 2 mg/kg daily for 10 days; in the absence of toxicity or beneficial effect, increase to 4 mg/kg daily. **IV infusion: initial,** 0.5–1 mg/kg daily. In absence of toxicity or therapeutic response, increase to 2 mg/kg daily after 10 days. **Maintenance (SC):** 1 mg/kg weekly or semiweekly.

Administration/ Storage 1. Until reconstituted, cytarabine must be stored in refrigerator.
2. Reconstituted solution should be stored at room temperature and used within 48 hours.
3. Discard hazy solution.
4. Use water containing 0.9% benzyl alcohol for reconstitution of drug.

DACARBAZINE DTIC-DOME

Remarks Synthetic compound related to purines, which probably acts as an alkylating agent. The drug has little immunosuppressive activity. Limited amounts of the agent (14% of plasma level) cross the blood-brain barrier into the cerebrospinal fluid.

Uses Metastatic malignant melanoma. Investigational: refractory Hodgkin's disease, soft tissue sarcoma, and neuroblastoma.

Additional Untoward Reactions Especially serious (fatal) hematological toxicity. Over 90% of patients develop nausea, vomiting, and anorexia 1 hour after initial administration, persisting for 12 to 48 hours. Rarely, diarrhea, stomatitis, and intractable nausea. Also, flu-like syndrome, severe pain along injected vein, facial flushing, alopecia. Elevation of SGOT, SGPT and other enzymes, CNS symptoms.

Dosage   **IV and IV infusion,** *preferred:* 2–4.5 mg/kg daily for 10 days, may be repeated at 4-week intervals; or 250 mg/m²/day for 5 days, may be repeated at 3-week intervals.

Administration/ Storage

1. In order to minimize GI effects, antiemetics, fasting (4 to 6 hours preceding treatment), and good hydration (1 hour prior to treatment) have been suggested.
2. Extreme care should be taken to avoid extravasation.
3. Drug can be given by IV push over 1-minute period or further diluted and administered by IV infusion (preferred) over 15 to 30 minute period.
4. Protect dry vials from light and store at 2°– 8° C.
5. Reconstituted solutions are stable for up to 72 hours at 4° C or 8 hours at 20° C. More dilute solutions for IV infusion are stable for 24 hours when stored at 2°– 8° C.

Additional Nursing Implications

1. Ascertain whether doctor wishes patient to fast 4 to 6 hours before treatment to reduce emesis or to maintain good hydration by allowing fluids up to 1 hour prior to administration to minimize dehydration following treatment.
2. Alert patient to the possibility of a flu-like syndrome with fever, myalgia, and malaise which may occur after treatment.
3. Advise patient to report to medical supervision if he/she experiences flu-like syndrome.
4. Report nausea and vomiting that may last from 1 to 12 hours after injection.
5. Have available phenobarbital and/or prochlorperazine (Compazine) for palliation of vomiting following administration of dacarbazine.
6. Advise patient that after the first 1 to 2 days of administration of dacarbazine, vomiting ceases because tolerance develops to the drug.

DACTINOMYCIN ACTINOMYCIN D, COSMEGEN

General Statement   Antineoplastic antibiotic produced by *Streptomyces parvullus.* The drug reacts with DNA and inhibits rapid cell proliferation. Initiate therapy in hospitalized patients. During therapy, leukocyte counts should be performed daily and platelet counts every 3 days. Frequent liver and kidney function tests are recommended. All toxic manifestations may be delayed by several weeks. Irreversible bone marrow depression may occur in patients with preexisting renal, hepatic, or bone marrow impairment.

Uses   In combination with surgery and/or irradiation for treatment of Wilms' tumor (nephroblastoma) and its metastases; metastatic tumor of the testes. Osteogenic sarcoma. Has some effect in rhabdomyosarcoma in children.

Drug Interaction   Penicillin is inhibited by dactinomycin.

Dosage   **IV:** *individualized, usual,* 0.5 mg for maximum of 5 days; **pediatric:** 15 μg/kg daily for 5 days. Dosage course may be repeated after 3 weeks unless contraindicated because of toxicity. **Isolation-Perfusion:** 0.05 mg/kg for pelvis and lower extremities; 0.035 mg/kg for upper extremities.

Administration   1. For IV use, dactinomycin is available in a lyophilized dactinomycin-mannitol mixture that turns gold upon reconstitution with sterile water. Use only sterile water without a preservative to reconstitute the drug for IV use as it will precipitate. Solutions should not be exposed to direct sunlight.
2. The drug is extremely corrosive. It is most safely administered through the tubing of a running IV. It may be given directly into the vein, but the needle used to draw up the solution should be discarded and another sterile needle attached, before injection, to prevent subcutaneous reaction and thrombophlebitis.
3. Any portion of the solution not used for the injection should be discarded.

Additional Nursing Implications   1. Report erythema of the skin that may lead to desquamation sloughing, particularly in areas previously affected by radiation.
2. Warn patient of the possibility of delayed toxic reactions and stress importance of returning for blood tests.

DOXORUBICIN HYDROCHLORIDE ADRIAMYCIN

General Statement   Antineoplastic antibiotic isolated from *Streptomyces peucetius* var. *caesius*. Believed to interfere with nucleic acid synthesis. Because of cardiotoxicity of drug, baseline and monthly ECGs are indicated during therapy and for several months thereafter.

Uses   Acute lymphoblastic leukemia, acute myeloblastic leukemia, Wilms' tumor, soft tissue and osteogenic sarcoma, neuroblastoma, cancer of the breast, ovaries, lungs, and thyroid, lymphomas.

Additional Contraindications   Depressed bone marrow or cardiac disease.

Additional Untoward Reactions   Leukopenia. Cardiotoxicity, acute left ventricular failure (usually several weeks after initiation of therapy). Alopecia (almost universal). GI symptoms: severe stomatitis and esophagitis (week 2 of therapy) progressing to ulceration of oral mucosa (symptoms usually do not require cessation of therapy). Nausea, vomiting, and diarrhea. Extravasation may cause severe cellulitis and tissue necrosis. Hyperpigmentation of nailbeds. Drug may reactivate previous tissue radiation damage.

Dosage   **IV;** *highly individualized:* 60–75 mg/m² of body surface q 21 days; or 30 mg/m² of body surface for 3 successive days q 4 weeks. Total dose by either regimen 550 mg/m² of body surface. Use reduced dosage in patients with hepatic dysfunction (based on BSP retention or serum bilirubin levels).

Administration

1. Initiate therapy only in hospitalized patients.
2. In order to minimize danger of extravasation, inject into tubing of freely flowing IV infusion.
3. If stinging or burning occurs during IV administration, stop and restart infusion at another site.
4. Should not be mixed with heparin, since a precipitate may form.

Additional Nursing Implications

1. Inform patient that urine will turn red for 1 to 2 days after initiation of therapy.
2. Advise patient that alopecia will occur, and reassure him/her that hair will grow back 2 to 3 months after discontinuation of therapy.
3. Observe patient for cardiac arrhythmias and/or respiratory difficulties that may be indicative of cardiac toxicity.
4. Monitor IV administration carefully. Stinging, burning, or edema at injection site are indicative of extravasation. Administration should be stopped, and injection site moved so as to avoid tissue necrosis.
5. If medication reactivates previous radiotherapy damage, such as erythema, edema, and desquamation, reassure patient that these symptoms will disappear after 7 days.

DROMOSTANOLONE PROPIONATE DROLBAN

Remarks

Synthetic variant of testosterone with fewer side effects than parent compound.

Uses

Palliative treatment of inoperable, advanced, or disseminated mammary cancer in postmenopausal or ovariectomized women.

Additional Contraindications

Breast cancer in men, premenopausal women.

Additional Untoward Reactions

Mild virilization, hypercalcemia, edema, increased libido. Local irritation at injection site. (Also see *Androgens*.)

Dosage

IM: 100 mg 3 times/week. Other treatment should be instituted if the disease *progresses* during the first 6 to 8 weeks of therapy.

Administration, Additional

Do not refrigerate.

Additional Nursing Implications

1. Ascertain that calcium levels are determined in patients with bone metastasis.
2. Anticipate that patients with edema may require diuretics before or during therapy.

FLOXURIDINE FUDR

Remarks   Floxuridine is an antimetabolite, which is rapidly degraded in the body to fluorouracil (see Fluorouracil, below). It basically has the same indications and side effects as this agent.

Uses   Palliative management of certain cancers in selected patients believed to profit from intra-arterial therapy, including carcinomas of the neck, head, brain, liver, gallbladder, and bile ducts. Used in patients with disease limited to an area capable of infusion by a single artery.

Additional Untoward Reactions   Complications of intra-arterial administration are arterial aneurism, arterial ischemia, arterial thrombosis, bleeding at catheter site, occluded, displaced or leaking catheters, embolism, fibromyositis, infection at catheter site, thrombophlebitis.

Dosage   **Intra-arterial infusion:** 0.1–0.6 mg/kg/day.

Administration   Higher doses (0.4–0.6 mg) are best given by hepatic artery infusion because the liver metabolizes the drug and reduces the possibility of systemic toxicity.

Nursing Implications   See *Nursing Implications* for administration by intra-arterial infusion, page 21.

FLUOROURACIL EFUDEX, 5-FLUOROURACIL, 5-FU, FLUOROPLEX

General Statement   Antimetabolite. Pyrimidine antagonist. Well distributed into tumor and other tissues. Highly toxic. Interferes with synthesis of DNA and RNA. Therapy should be initiated in hospitalized patients. Initially, the topical cream causes a local inflammatory reaction and eventually will produce ulceration. Complete healing of the lesion may not occur for 1 or 2 months following cessation of topical fluorouracil therapy.

Uses   Systemic: palliative management of certain cancers of the GI tract, rectum, liver, ovaries, colon, pancreas, and breast. Relieves pain and reduces size of tumor. Topical (as solution or cream): actinic or solar keratosis, superficial basal cell carcinoma.

Additional Contraindications   Systemic: patients in poor nutritional state, with severe bone marrow depression, severe infection, or recent (4-week-old) surgical intervention. To be used with caution for patients with hepatic or liver dysfunction. Pregnancy.

Additional Untoward Reactions   Bone marrow depression, anorexia, nausea, acute cerebellar syndrome, photophobia, ataxia, euphoria, stomatitis, or alopecia.

Dosage IV: *initial*, 12 mg/kg/day for 4 days not to exceed 800 mg/day. If no toxicity seen, administer 6 mg/kg on days 6, 8, 10, 12. Discontinue therapy on day 12. **Maintenance:** repeat dose of first course every 30 days or when toxicity from initial course of therapy is gone; or, give 10–15 mg/kg/week as a single dose. Do not exceed 1 gm/week. **Topical:** Apply 1–5% cream or solution b.i.d. to cover lesion.

Administration/
Storage **IV**
1. Store in a cool place (50°–80° F, 10°–27° C). Do not freeze. Excessively low temperature causes precipitation.
2. Do not expose the solution to light.
3. Solution may discolor slightly during storage but potency and safety are not affected.
4. If precipitate forms, resolubilize by heating to 140° F with vigorous shaking. Allow to return to room temperature and allow air to settle out before withdrawing and administering medication.
5. Further dilution is not needed, and solution may be injected directly into the vein with a 25-gauge needle.
6. Drug can be administered by IV infusion for periods of ½ hour to 8 hours. This method has been reported to produce less systemic toxicity than rapid injection.

Topical
1. Apply with fingertips, nonmetallic applicator, or rubber gloves. Wash hands immediately thereafter.
2. Avoid contact with eyes, nose, and mouth.
3. Limit occlusive dressings to lesions since they cause an increased incidence of inflammatory reaction in normal skin.

Additional
Nursing
Implications
1. Observe for intractable vomiting, stomatitis, and diarrhea, all of which are early signs of toxicity and cause for immediate discontinuation of drug. Drug should also be discontinued if WBC and platelet counts are depressed below 3,500/mm³ and 100,000 mm³, respectively.
2. Practice reverse isolation when WBC is below 2,000/mm³.
3. Prevent exposure to strong sunlight and other ultraviolet rays because they intensify skin reaction to the drug.

GOLD AU 198 INJECTION AUREOTOPE-198

Classification Radioactive agent, antineoplastic.

Remarks This sterile, colloidal solution of radioactive gold, gelatin, and suitable reducing agents is rapidly absorbed and excreted.

Uses Diagnostic agent for liver scanning. Palliative treatment of pleural and peritoneal effusions associated with metastatic malignancies. Prevention of metastases.

Contraindications   Therapeutic: dying patients, ulcerative tumors. Therapeutic and diagnostic: pregnancy, nursing mothers, or children under 18 years of age.

Untoward Reactions   Radiation sickness, nausea, vomiting, diarrhea, low-grade fever (after 1 to 6 days), bone marrow depression (very rare), or skin rash. Pain and allergic reaction at injection site.

Dosage   **Diagnostic IV:** 50–500 *micro*curies. **Therapeutic, intraperitoneal, intrapleural:** 25–100 *milli*curies. Dosage may be repeated after 4 or more weeks. *Ascites:* 35–100 *milli*curies.

Administration
1. For diagnosis, give drug while patient is in supine position.
2. Great care should be taken to prevent subcutaneous infiltration of gold Au 198 or bowel injury during administration.
3. Drug may be administered through polyethylene catheter.
4. Do not remove lead shield during administration.
5. Note expiration date of drug. It is only stable for 8 days after standardization.
6. Store in container that provides adequate radiation protection.
7. Protect from heat or freezing.
8. Do not use solutions that are not cherry-red.
9. Avoid contact with aluminum, which may precipitate gold Au 198.
10. For radiation protection, follow procedure of the hospital in which the gold Au 198 is administered.

Nursing Implication   In order to ensure proper distribution of radiopharmaceutical within cavity, change the position of the patient frequently, especially during the first hour.

HYDROXYUREA HYDREA

Remark   This miscellaneous antineoplastic probably functions as an antimetabolite.

Uses   Melanoma, resistant chronic myelocytic (granulocytic) leukemia, inoperable ovarian carcinoma, and carcinomas of head and neck.

Additional Contraindication   Give with caution to patients with marked renal dysfunction.

Additional Untoward Reactions   Renal tubular function, hyperuricemia, or uric acid stone development.

Dosage   **PO: Individualized,** *solid tumors, intermittent therapy,* 80 mg/kg as a single dose q third day; **continuous therapy:** 20–30 mg/kg daily as a single dose. Intermittent dosage offers advantage of reduced toxicity. If effective, maintain patient on drug indefinitely unless toxic effects preclude such a regimen. Therapy should be discontinued if WBC drops below 2,500/mm^3 or platelet count below 100,000/mm^3.

Administration   If the patient cannot swallow a capsule, contents may be given in glass of water that should be drunk immediately, even though some material may not dissolve and may float on top of glass.

Additional
Nursing
Implications
1. Check for exacerbation of postirradiation erythema.
2. Anticipate that the dosage for the elderly will be smaller.

LOMUSTINE CeeNU

Remarks   Alkylating agent, nitrosourea type. Bone marrow depressant. Lomustine is rapidly absorbed from GI tract. It crosses the blood-brain barrier. Levels in cerebrospinal fluid are 50% of those attained in plasma. The compound is very similar to carmustine.

Uses   Primary and metastatic brain tumors. Disseminated Hodgkin's disease (in combination with other antineoplastics).

Additional
Untoward
Reactions
High incidence of nausea and vomiting 3 to 6 hours after administration and lasting for 24 hours.

Dosage   **PO: adults and children:** *initial*, 130 mg/m^2 as a single dose q 6 weeks. Subsequent dosage based on blood counts of patient.

Administration/
Storage,
Additional
1. Reduce GI distress by the administration of antiemetics prior to drug, or by giving drug to fasting patient.
2. Teach patient that medication comes in capsules of 3 strengths and that a combination of capsules will make up the correct dose, and that this combination is to be taken at one time.
3. Store below 40°C.

Additional
Nursing
Implications
1. Anticipate that patient may have nausea and vomiting up to 36 hours after treatment and that this may be followed by 2 to 3 days of anorexia. Administer antiemetic as ordered.
2. Emphasize to patient the benefit to be derived from lomustine as he/she is often depressed by prolonged nausea and vomiting.
3. Encourage liquids and small amounts of food as tolerated when antiemetics are effective.
4. Explain to patient that intervals of 6 weeks are necessary between doses for optimum effect with minimal toxicity.

MECHLORETHAMINE HYDROCHLORIDE MUSTARGEN HYDROCHLORIDE, NITROGEN MUSTARD

Remarks   Alkylating agent; nitrogen mustard.

Uses   Malignant lymphomas, including Hodgkin's disease, lymphosarcomas, chronic lymphocytic leukemia, mycosis fungoides, generalized neoplastic disease and inoperable, localized tumors, and bronchogenic carcinoma.

One of the drugs used in MOPP therapy (see p. 168).

Additional Untoward Reactions High incidence of nausea and vomiting. Petechiae, subcutaneous hemorrhages, tinnitus, deafness, Herpes zoster, or temporary amenorrhea.

Drug Interaction Amphoterecin B: combination increases possibility of blood dyscrasias.

Dosage IV, *total dose:* 0.4/mg/kg/course of therapy. This is usually given in 1 to 4 days. Drug can also be given by the intracavitary route. A minimum of 6 weeks must elapse before course is repeated.

Administration
1. Since drug is highly irritating, and contact with skin should be avoided, plastic or rubber gloves should be worn during preparation.
2. Drug is best administered through tubing of a rapidly flowing IV saline infusion.
3. Prepare solution immediately prior to administration.
4. Medication is available in a rubber-stoppered vial to which 10 ml of distilled water should be added.
5. Insert the needle and keep it inserted until the medication is dissolved and the required dose withdrawn. Carefully discard the vial with the remaining solution so that no one will come in contact with it.
6. For intracavitary administration turn patient every 60 seconds for 5 minutes to the following positions: prone, supine, right side, left side, and knee-chest. Lack of effect often results from failure to move the patient often enough.

Additional Nursing Implications
1. Administer phenothiazine and/or sedative as ordered prior to medication and as needed to control severe nausea and vomiting which usually occur 1 to 3 hours after administration of nitrogen mustard.
2. Administer in late afternoon, and follow with sedation (sleeping pill) at an appropriate time so as to control untoward symptoms and induce sleep.
3. After treatment, encourage increased fluid intake to prevent hyperuricemia.
4. Anticipate that extravasation may cause swelling, erythema, induration, and sloughing.
5. In case of extravasation, remove IV and assist in infusion of area with isotonic sodium thiosulfate (4.14% solution of U.S.P. salt) and apply cold compresses. If sodium thiosulfate is not available, use isotonic sodium chloride solution.

MELPHALAN ALKERAN, L-PAM, L-PHENYLALANINE MUSTARD, PAM

General Statement Alkylating agent. Well absorbed from the GI tract. Highly toxic. The drug, in an infusion solution at room temperature, has a half-life of about 13 hours and of slightly less than 2 hours in an infusion solution or blood maintained at body temperature. Response of patients to drug varies from several weeks to several months.

Uses   Multiple myeloma (about one-third of patients have shown some favorable response), malignant melanoma, reticulum cell sarcoma, lymphoma, chronic lymphocytic leukemia, and ovarian carcinoma.

Dosage   **PO:** *Initial,* 6 mg daily. Adjust as required based on frequent (2 to 3 a week) blood counts. Discontinue after 2 to 3 weeks for up to 4 weeks. When WBC increases, reinstitute maintenance therapy. **Usual maintenance:** 2 mg/day. Discontinue if leukocyte count falls below 3,000/mm^3 or if the platelet count falls below 100,000/mm^3.

MERCAPTOPURINE 6-MERCAPTOPURINE, 6-MP, PURINETHOL

Remarks   Antimetabolite; purine antagonist. Readily absorbed from the GI tract. Maintenance dosage usually is given during remissions.

Uses   Drug of choice for acute lymphocytic leukemia, especially in children. Also chronic granulocytic leukemia. Complete or partial remissions noted in 50% of children with acute leukemia. Less effective with adults.

Additional Contraindication   Use with caution in patients with impaired renal function.

Additional Untoward Reactions   Since the maximum effect of mercaptopurine on the blood count may be delayed and blood counts may drop for several days after drug has been discontinued, therapy should be discontinued at first sign of abnormally large drop in leukocyte count.

Produces less GI toxicity than folic acid antagonists, and side effects are less frequent in children than in adults.

Drug Interaction   Allopurinol potentiates mercaptopurine by (↓) breakdown. Requires reduction of antineoplastic agent by 25%.

Dosage   **PO,** *highly individualized:* 2.5 mg/kg daily. *Usual,* **adults:** 100–200 mg; **children:** 50 mg. Dosage may be increased to 5 mg/kg daily after 4 weeks, if beneficial effects are not noted. Dosage is increased until symptoms of toxicity appear. **Maintenance after remission:** 2.5 mg/kg daily.

Administration   Administer drug in one dose daily at any convenient time.

Additional Nursing Implications
1. Encourage increased fluid intake in patients with impaired renal function to aid in excretion of drug and to prevent hyperuricemia.
2. Monitor intake and output.
3. Observe for oliguria and report.
4. Observe for early signs of liver damage, such as upper abdominal pain, nausea, diarrhea, or rash, which may be followed by yellowing of the skin, sclera, or mucous membranes.

METHOTREXATE, METHOTREXATE SODIUM

Remarks   Folic acid antagonist. Interferes with formation of DNA.

Uses   Uterine choriocarcinoma (curative), lymphoma, acute lymphoblastic leukemia, lymphosarcoma, and other disseminated neoplasms in children; meningeal leukemia, some beneficial effect in regional chemotherapy of head and neck tumors, psoriasis. Immunosuppressive agent in kidney transplantation and as an investigational drug in systemic lupus erythematosus and rheumatoid arthritis. Renal function tests are recommended prior to initiation of therapy, and daily leukocyte counts should be taken during therapy.

Additional Untoward Reactions   Methotrexate has a narrow boundary between the desired therapeutic effects and toxic reactions. The most serious side effects are folic acid deficiency and bone marrow depression. Also, hepatoxicity, increased pigmentation, chronic nutritional deficiency, hemorrhagic enteritis, or intestinal perforations. Drug may precipitate diabetes. High intrathecal dosage may cause convulsions.

Dosage   *Methotrexate is administered* **PO;** *methotrexate sodium is administered* **IM, IV, Intra-arterially,** or **intrathecally.** *Dose individualized. Choriocarcinoma,* **PO, IM:** 15–30 mg/day for 5 days. May be repeated 3 to 5 times with 1 week rest period between courses. *Leukemia, initial:* 3.3 mg/m² (with prednisone 60 mg/m² daily); **maintenance:** 30 mg/m² 2 times weekly or 2–5 mg/kg q 14 days. *Meningeal leukemia,* **Intrathecal:** 0.2–0.5 mg/kg q 2 to 5 days, or 12 mg/m² 1 time a week for 2 weeks; **then,** 1 time a month. *Lymphomas,* **PO:** 10–25 mg/day for 4 to 8 days for several courses of treatment with 7 to 10 day rest periods between courses.

Drug Interactions

Interactant	Interaction
Alcohol, ethyl	Additive hepatotoxicity. Combination can result in coma
Anticoagulants, oral	Additive hypoprothrombinemia
Para-aminobenzoic acid	↑ Effect of methotrexate by ↓ plasma protein binding
Phenytoin (Dilantin)	↑ Effect of methotrexate by ↓ plasma protein binding
Salicylates Aspirin	↑ Effect of methotrexate by ↓ plasma protein binding. Also, salicylates block renal excretion
Smallpox vaccination	Methotrexate impairs immunologic response to smallpox vaccine
Sulfonamides	↑ Effect of methotrexate by ↓ plasma protein binding

Administration   1. Use only sterile water, without preservatives, to reconstitute powder for parenteral administration.
2. Prevent the inhalation of particles of medication or skin exposure.

Additional Nursing Implications

1. Monitor intake and output, and encourage fluid intake to facilitate excretion of drug.
2. Report oliguria since this may require discontinuing drug.
3. Observe for oral ulcerations since this is one of the first signs of toxicity.
4. Calcium leucovorin—a potent antidote for folic acid antagonists—should be on hand in case of overdosage. If necessary, 3–6 mg are usually injected intramuscularly. Antidotes are ineffective if not administered within 4 hours of overdosage. Corticosteroids are sometimes given concomitantly with initial dose of methotrexate.

MITHRAMYCIN MITHRACIN

General Statement

This agent is derived from *Streptomyces plicatus*. It affects calcium metabolism leading to a decrease in blood calcium levels. Should be used only for hospitalized patients. Therapy should be interrupted if WBC count goes below 3,000/mm³ or if prothrombin time is more than 4 seconds higher than the control. Daily platelet count should be performed on patients who had x-rays of abdomen and mediastinum.

Uses

Malignant testicular tumors usually associated with metastases. Hyperglycemia and hypercalciuria associated with advanced malignancy.

Additional Contraindications

Thrombocytopenia, coagulation disorders, and increased tendency to hemorrhage. Not to be used for children under 15 years of age.

Additional Untoward Reactions

Hepatotoxicity or hemorrhagic diathesis. Mithramycin toxicity is characterized by facial flushing, thrombocytopenia, and prolongation of prothrombin time.

Dosage

Individualized according to hematopoietic and clinical response. **IV infusion,** *testicular tumor:* 25–30 (maximum) μg/kg daily for 10 (maximum) days. A second approach is 50 μg/kg on alternate days for an average of 6 doses. *Hypercalcemia, hypercalciuria:* 25 μg/kg daily for 3 to 4 days. Additional courses of therapy may be warranted at monthly intervals if initial course is unsuccessful.

Administration/ Storage

1. *Store vials of medication in refrigerator at temperature below 10° C (36–46° F). Discard unused portion of drug.*
2. Reconstitute fresh for each day of therapy.
3. Drug is unstable in acid solution (pH 5 and below) and in reconstituted solutions (pH 7) and thus deteriorates rapidly.
4. Add sterile water to the vial as recommended on the package insert and shake the vial to dissolve the drug.
5. Add the calculated dosage of the drug to the IV solution ordered (recommended 1 liter of 5% D/W) and adjust the rate of flow as ordered (recommended time is 4 to 6 hours for 1 liter).

Additional Nursing Implications

1. Observe patients for any sign of hemorrhage, such as epistaxis, hemoptysis, hematemesis, purpura, or ecchymoses.
2. If antiemetic drugs are ordered, administer prior to or during therapy with mithramycin.
3. Check IV closely for extravasation which may cause local irritation and cellulitis. This may necessitate interrupting infusion and restarting it at another site.
4. Check flow of injection frequently because rapid IV infusions of the drug tend to cause more severe GI side effects.

MITOMYCIN MUTAMYCIN

Remarks   Antineoplastic antibiotic isolated from *Streptomyces caespitosus*. This compound inhibits synthesis of DNA in the cell.

Uses   Palliative treatment and adjunct to surgical or radiological treatment of adenocarcinoma of the stomach, pancreas, colon, and rectum. Squamous cell carcinoma of the head, neck, lungs, and cervix; adenocarcinoma and duct cell carcinoma of the breast; hepatic cell carcinoma; and malignant neoplasms.

Additional Contraindications   Hypersensitivity to drug. Patients with depressed platelet and/or WBC counts, coagulation disorders, increased bleeding tendencies, or serious infections. Use with extreme caution in presence of impaired renal function.

Additional Untoward Reactions   Bone marrow depression: thrombocytopenia, leukopenia, anemia (these symptoms may develop from 2 to 8 weeks after initiation).

GI symptoms: nausea and vomiting (transitory) or anorexia. Fever, malaise, weakness, weight loss, alopecia (rare), oral ulcerations, pain at injection site, induration, or thrombophlebitis. Extravasation causes severe necrosis of surrounding tissue. Renal toxicity.

Dosage   **IV only:** 20 mg/m^2 as a single dose via infusion or 2 mg/m^2/day for 5 days. After 2-day rest period, 2 mg/m^2/day for 5 more days.

Administration   Drug is very toxic, and extravasation is to be avoided.

MITOTANE LYSODREN

Remarks   Mitotane is an antineoplastic agent related to the insecticide DDT. Its mode of action is unknown. The drug seems to suppress the function of the adrenal cortex. Steroid replacement therapy may have to be instituted (increased) to correct adrenal insufficiency.

Use   Inoperable cancer of the adrenal cortex (functional and nonfunctional).

Contraindications Hypersensitivity to drug. Discontinue temporarily after shock or severe trauma. Use with caution in the presence of liver disease other than metastatic lesions. Long-term usage may cause brain damage and functional impairment.

Untoward Reactions Adrenal insufficiency. GI disturbances (80%): anorexia, nausea, vomiting, and diarrhea. CNS reactions (40%): depression, lethargy, somnolence, dizziness and vertigo. Skin reactions (15%). Also, infrequently, ocular manifestations, hematuria, hemorrhagic cystitis, albuminuria, hypertension, orthostatic hypotension, flushing, generalized aching, hyperpyrexia.

Dosage **PO:** *initial,* 9–10 gm/day in 3 to 4 equally divided doses. Adjust dosage upward or downward according to severity of side effects or lack thereof. **Usual maintenance:** 8–10 gm/day. **Range:** 2–19 gm/day.

Administration 1. Institute treatment in hospital until stable dosage schedule is achieved.
2. Continue drug as long as it seems effective. Beneficial effect may only become manifest after 3 months.

Additional Nursing Implications 1. Assess for symptoms of adrenal insufficiency, such as weakness, increased fatigue, lethargy, and GI symptomatology.
2. Assess for brain damage by participating in behavioral and neurological assessments of patient.
3. Withhold medication and report to doctor if shock or severe trauma occurs because of drug-induced suppression of adrenal function.
4. To counteract shock or trauma, be prepared to administer steroid medications in high doses because depressed adrenals may not produce sufficient steroids.
5. Stress importance of wearing Medic Alert identification to patients on mitotane in case of trauma or shock.

PIPOBROMAN VERCYTE

Remarks Alkylating agent. Well absorbed from the GI tract.

Uses Polycythemia vera; chronic granulocytic leukemia.

Additional Contraindication Children under 15 years of age.

Dosage **PO,** *polycythemia vera:* 1 mg/kg daily. When hematocrit has been reduced to 50% to 55%, **maintenance dosage** of 100–200 μg/kg is instituted. *Chronic granulocytic leukemia;* **initial,** 1.5–2.5 mg/kg daily; **maintenance:** 25–175 mg daily to be instituted when leukocyte count approaches 10,000/mm^3.

Administration Administer in divided doses.

Additional Nursing Implication Be alert to the persistence of adverse reactions because they may necessitate withdrawal of the drug.

PROCARBAZINE HYDROCHLORIDE MATULANE, N-METHYLHYDRAZINE, MIH

Remarks Synthetic agent belonging to a new class of antineoplastic drugs. Seems to interfere with cell metabolism. Procarbazine is part of MOPP therapy and is usually given in this combination.

Use Hodgkin's disease

Additional Contraindications Hypersensitivity to drug. Depressed bone marrow. Low white and red blood cell or platelet count.

Additional Untoward Reactions Leukopenia, anemia, or thrombocytopenia (frequent). Bone marrow depression often occurs 2 to 8 weeks after initiation of therapy. Hemorrhages, petechiae, and purpura. GI effects: nausea and vomiting (frequent), anorexia, stomatitis, dysphagia, diarrhea, and constipation. Various CNS effects: fatigue, depression, drowsiness, psychosis, manic reactions, dizziness, headache, nervousness, insomnia, nightmares, falling, unsteadiness, disorientation, foot drop, decreased reflexes, tremors, coma, delirium, convulsions. Dermatological effects: dermatitis, pruritus, hyperpigmentation. Genitourinary effects: depression of spermatogenesis and atrophy of the testes. Miscellaneous: alopecia, myalgia, arthralgia, chills, and fever.

Drug Interactions

Interactant	Interaction
Alcohol	"Antabuse-like" reaction
CNS Depressants	↑ CNS Depression
Sympathomimetics	↑ Chance of hypertension
Tricyclic Antidepressants	↑ Chance of hypertension

Dosage **PO:** 100–200 mg daily, as single or divided doses, during first week; 300 mg daily thereafter until WBC count falls below 4,000/mm^3, platelets below 100,000/mm^3, or until maximum estimated response is attained. Drug should be discontinued if paresthesia, neuropathies, or confusion occur. **Maintenance:** 50–100 mg daily. **Pediatric:** *highly individualized;* often initiated with 50 mg daily. Increase and regulate according to hematopoietic response.

Additional Nursing Implications

1. Observe patient closely and alert family to observe and report untoward CNS reactions which may necessitate withdrawal of the drug.
2. Instruct patients on procarbazine therapy not to drink alcohol as a disulfiram (Antabuse)-type reaction may occur.
3. Advise the patient not to take any other medication before consulting

with physician as procarbazine has monoamine oxidase inhibitory activity. This would contraindicate the use of sympathomimetic drugs and foods that have a high tyramine content.

SODIUM IODIDE I131 IODOTOPE I-131, ORIODIDE-131, SODIUM-RADIO-IODIDE, THERIODIDE-131

See *Thyroid* and *Antithyroid Drugs.*

SODIUM PHOSPHATE P 32 PHOSPHOTOPE

Remarks   Sodium phosphate containing radioactive phosphorus.

Uses   Diagnostic: ocular tumors, especially when other agents are unsuitable. Therapeutic: palliative treatment of polycythemia vera (remissions of 2 or more years are reported in 85% to 90% of patients treated). Chronic myelocytic leukemia and chronic lymphocytic leukemia.

Additional Contraindications   Pregnancy, nursing mothers, children younger than 18 years of age, or acute episodes of leukemia. Polycythemia vera in patients with leukocyte count less than 5,000/mm^3, platelet count less than 150,000/mm^3, or reticulocyte count less than 0.2%. Chronic myelocytic leukemia with a leukocyte count less than 20,000/mm^3.

Additional Untoward Reactions   Bone marrow depression (leukopenia, thrombocytopenia), leukemia, or radiation sickness (rare).

Dosage   *Diagnostic* **IV:** 250–1,000 *micro*curies. *For brain tumor localization,* give 12 to 24 hours prior to surgery. *Therapeutic,* **PO:** *usual, polycythemia vera, 6 milli*curies. **IV:** 3–5 *milli*curies (75% of PO dose). In severe cases, phlebotomy is done in conjunction with radiation. Treatment may be repeated after 2 to 3 months. Older patients usually receive a smaller dosage. *Chronic myelocytic leukemia, individualized: initial, usual dosage,* 40 *micro*curies/kg. **Maximum weekly dose:** 5 *milli*curies.

Administration/ Storage
1. Store in containers suitable for absorption of radiation.
2. Solution and container may darken, but this does not affect efficacy.
3. Note expiration date—should be 2 months after date of standardization.
4. Have patient fast for 2 hours before and 6 hours after administration of drug to minimize the amount of unabsorbed radioactive material.
5. Avoid using milk and milk products, iron, bismuth, and soft drinks for patients on sodium phosphate P 32.

Additional Nursing Implication   For radiation protection, observe the procedure of the hospital in which medication is administered.

TAMOXIFEN NOLVADEX

Remarks A synthetic, non-steroidal agent with marked antiestrogen properties. Believed to compete with estrogen for estrogen binding sites in target tissue, such as the breast.

Uses Palliative treatment of advanced breast cancer in postmenopausal women.

Contraindications The drug is probably not effective in patients with recent negative estrogen receptor assay. Use with caution in patients with leukopenia and thrombocytopenia.

Untoward Reactions Hot flashes, nausea, vomiting (25%). Also, vaginal bleeding and discharge, menstrual irregularities, skin rash. Rarely, hypercalcemia, peripheral edema, distaste for food, pruritus vulvae, depression, dizziness, lightheadedness, headaches, increased bone and tumor pain.

Dosage **PO:** 10–20 mg b.i.d. (A.M. and P.M.).

Additional Nursing Implications
1. Advise patient to report side effects to doctor, because reduction in dosage may be indicated.
2. Explain to patient experiencing increased bone and lumbar pain and local disease flares that these symptoms may be associated with a good response to medication.
3. Be certain that patient with increased pain has adequate orders for analgesics and provide them as needed.

TESTOLACTONE TESLAC

Remarks Synthetic antineoplastic structurally related to androgens. Does not cause virilization.

Uses Palliative treatment of inoperable disseminated mammary cancer in postmenopausal women.

Additional Contraindication Breast cancer in men.

Additional Untoward Reactions Inflammation and irritation at injection site; increases BP during parenteral administration. Hypercalcemia. Also see *Androgens*.

Dosage **PO:** 250 mg q.i.d. **IM:** 100 mg 3 times weekly. Therapy should be continued for 3 months.

Administration
1. Shake vial vigorously before injection.
2. Inject immediately before testolactone settles in syringe.

3. Inject deeply into upper outer quadrant of gluteal region using 1½ in. needle.

Additional Nursing Implications   To minimize local irritation, alternate injection sites and prevent extravasation into subcutaneous tissue.

THIOGUANINE TG, 6-THIOGUANINE

General Statement   Antimetabolite (purine analog). More effective in children than in adults. Platelet counts must be performed at least weekly. Effect of drug is cumulative. Discontinue at first sign of abnormal bone marrow depression.

Uses   Acute and chronic myelocytic leukemia. To be used in patients resistant to busulfan.

Additional Untoward Reactions   Jaundice, loss of vibration sense, unsteadiness of gait, hyperuricemia, or hyperuricosuria. Adults tend to show a more rapid WBC fall than do children.

Dosage   **PO:** *Individualized* and determined by hematopoietic response; **adult and pediatric:** *initial*, 2 mg/kg daily. From 2 to 4 weeks may elapse before beneficial results become apparent. Compute dose to nearest multiple of 20 mg. If no response, dosage may be increased to 3 mg/kg daily. **Usual maintenance** (even during remissions): 2 mg/kg daily.

Additional Nursing Implications
1. Provide assistance to ambulatory patients who may experience loss of vibration sense and thus have unsteady gait (may be unable to rely on canes).
2. Encourage increased fluid intake to minimize hyperuricemia and hyperuricosuria.

TRIETHYLENETHIOPHOSPHORAMIDE THIOTEPA

General Statement   Alkylating agent. The effect of Thiotepa is cumulative and delayed, especially if excretion is delayed. Report when WBC count falls below 4,000/mm^3 or platelet level below 150,000/mm^3. This usually requires reduction in dosage or withdrawal of drug. Prophylactic antibiotics are sometimes ordered when WBC count falls below 3,000/mm^3.

Uses   Advanced metastatic cancer of breast or ovary. Control of serious effusions of pleural, pericardial, and peritoneal cavities. Urinary bladder tumors. Cerebral metastases, chronic granulocytic and lymphocytic leukemia, malignant lymphomas including Hodgkin's disease, and bronchogenic cancer.

Additional Contraindication   Acute leukemia.

Additional Untoward Reactions   Anorexia or decreased spermatogenesis.

Drug Interaction   Thiotepa increases the pharmacologic and toxic effect of succinylcholine due to a decrease in breakdown by the liver.

Dosage   Administered **IV directly into tumor, IP, Intrapleural, Intrapericardial, Intrabladder.** Dose individualized. **Initial:** 60 mg; in cases of *debilitation, surgical shock, cardiovascular,* or *renal disease:* 45 mg, **maintenance:** adjusted weekly on basis of blood counts. **IV:** one-half dose used when drug administered locally. *Carcinoma of bladder:* 60 mg in 30–60 ml distilled water instilled into bladder and retained for 2 hr. Give one time a week for 4 weeks.

Administration/ Storage
1. Minimize pain on injection and retard rate of absorption by simultaneous administration of local anesthetics. Drug may be mixed with procaine HCl 2% or epinephrine HCl 1:1,000 or both, upon order of the physician.
2. Store vials in the refrigerator. Reconstituted solutions may be stored for 5 days in the refrigerator without substantial loss of potency.
3. Since Thiotepa is not a vesicant, it may be injected quickly and directly into the vein with the desired volume of sterile water. Usual amount of diluent is 1.5 ml.
4. Do not use normal saline as a diluent.
5. Discard solutions grossly opaque or with precipitate.

Additional Nursing Implications
1. Encourage patients who recieve drug as bladder instillations to retain fluid for 2 hours.
2. Reposition patient with a bladder instillation every 15 minutes for maximum contact.

URACIL MUSTARD

General Statement   Alkylating agent. Effect of drug is cumulative and delayed for 2 to 4 weeks. Complete blood counts are desirable once or twice weekly during therapy and 1 month thereafter. Effect of drug sometimes takes 3 months to become apparent, and drug should be given that long unless precluded by toxicity reaction.

Uses   Chronic lymphocytic leukemia, lymphomas including Hodgkin's disease, lymphosarcoma, lymphoblastoma, giant follicular lymphomas, and reticulum cell sarcoma. Cancer of ovary, polycythemia vera, and mycosis fungoides.

Dosage   **PO** *individualized* using clinical response and hematologic toxicity as guide. **Typical:** 1–2 mg daily, if possible, until remission obtained; or, 3–5 mg/day for 7 days, the total dose not to exceed 0.5 mg/kg. This is followed by a **maintenance** dose of 1 mg daily.

Administration   Give at bedtime to minimize GI effects.

VINBLASTINE SULFATE VELBAN, VLB

Remarks   Antineoplastic alkaloid isolated from periwinkle; compound probably acts as an antimetabolite.

Uses   Generalized Hodgkin's disease. Cancer resistant to other chemotherapeutic agents.

Additional Untoward Reactions   Toxicity is dose-related and more pronounced in patients over 65 or those suffering from cachexia (profound general ill health) or skin ulceration. The drug can induce leukopenia, thrombocytopenia, anemia, stomatitis, mental depression, neurotoxicity, paresthesias, loss of deep tendon reflexes, nausea, vomiting, diarrhea, or constipation. Overdosage may cause permanent CNS damage.

Drug Interactions

Interactant	Interaction
Glutamic acid	Inhibits effect of vinblastine
Tryptophan	Inhibits effect of vinblastine

Dosage   **IV** *individualized* using WBC as guide. *Initial, usual dose,* 0.1 mg/kg as a single dose once weekly. Take daily WBC count. After 7 days and according to response of patient graded doses of 0.15, 0.2, 0.25, and 0.3 mg/kg (not to exceed 0.5 mg/kg) at intervals of 7 days are given; **maintenance:** single injection every 7 to 14 days of maximum tolerated dose (WBC count above 3,000/mm^3).

Administration/ Storage
1. Dilute vinblastine with 10 ml sterile water or sodium chloride injection.
2. Inject into flowing infusion of 5% dextrose.
3. If extravasation occurs, move infusion to other vein. Treat affected area with injection of hyaluronidase and application of moderate heat so as to decrease local reaction.
4. Remainder of solution may be stored in refrigerator for 30 days.

VINCRISTINE SULFATE ONCOVIN, VCR

Remarks   Antineoplastic alkaloid isolated from periwinkle. Interferes with cell division. Time at which remission occurs varies. Complete remissions have occurred as late as 100 days after initiation of therapy.

Uses   Acute leukemia in children, acute lymphocytic or undifferentiated stem cell leukemia, Hodgkin's disease, and Wilms' tumor

Additional Untoward Reactions   Neurological and neuromuscular manifestations including paresthesia, constipation, depression of tendon reflexes, difficulties in gait, ocular changes, mental depression, and headaches. Also abdominal pain, reversible hair loss, weight loss, and hypertension. Vincristine induces cellular changes or phlebitis at injection site. Care should be taken to avoid extravasation.

Drug Interactions

Interactant	Interaction
Glutamic acid	Inhibits effect of vincristine
Methotrexate	Combination may cause hypotension

Dosage   **IV** *individualized with extreme care as overdose can be fatal.* **Adults:** *usual, initial,* 1.4 mg/m² 1 time a week; **children:** 2 mg/m² 1 time a week.

Administration/ Storage
1. Dissolve powder in sterile water or isotonic saline injection to a concentration ranging from 0.01 mg to 1 mg/ml. Medication is injected either directly into a vein or into the tubing of a flowing IV infusion over a period of one minute.
2. Store in refrigerator. Dry powder is stable for 6 months. Solutions are stable for 2 weeks under refrigeration. Protect drug from exposure to light.

DRUGS AFFECTING BLOOD FORMATION AND COAGULATION

antianemic agents

Ferrocholinate
Ferroglycine Sulfate Complex
Ferrous Fumarate
Ferrous Gluconate
Ferrous Sulfate and Dried Ferrous Sulfate

Iron Dextran Injection
Liver Injection
Polysaccharide-Iron Complex
Soy Protein-Iron Complex

General Statement

Anemia refers to the many clinical conditions in which there is a deficiency in the number of red blood cells (RBCs) or in the hemoglobin level within these cells. Hemoglobin is a complex substance consisting of a large protein (globin) and an iron-containing chemical referred to as "heme." The hemoglobin is contained inside the red cells. Its function is to combine with oxygen in the lungs and transport it to all tissues of the body where it is exchanged for carbon dioxide (which is transported back to the lungs).

A lack of either RBCs or hemoglobin may result in an inadequate supply of oxygen to various tissues. The average life span of a RBC is 120 days; thus, new ones have to be constantly formed. They are produced in the bone marrow, with both vitamin B_{12} and folic acid playing an important role in their formation. In addition, a sufficient amount of iron is necessary for the formation and maturation of RBCs. This iron is supplied in a normal diet and also is salvaged from old RBCs.

There are many types of anemia. However, the two main categories are (1) iron deficiency anemias—resulting from greater than normal loss or destruction of blood cells, and (2) megaloblastic anemias— resulting from deficient production of blood cells. Iron deficiency anemia can result from hemorrhage or blood loss; the bone marrow is unable to replace the quantity of red cells lost even when working at maximum capacity (due to iron-deficient diet or failure to absorb iron from the GI tract). The RBCs in iron deficiency anemias (also called microcytic or hypochromic anemias) contain too little hemoglobin. When examined under the microscope, they are paler and sometimes smaller than normal. The cause of the iron deficiency must be determined before therapy is started.

Therapy consists of administering compounds containing iron so as to increase the body's supplies. Such drugs are discussed in this chapter (Table 7).

Megaloblastic anemias may result from insufficient supplies of the necessary vitamins and minerals needed by the bone marrow to manufacture blood cells. Pernicious anemia, for example, results from inadequate vitamin B_{12}. The RBCs characteristic of the megaloblastic anemias are enlarged and particularly rich in hemoglobin. However, the blood contains fewer mature RBCs than normal and usually contains a relatively higher number of immature red cells (megaloblasts) that have been prematurely released from the bone marrow.

Iron Preparations

These agents are usually a complex of iron and another substance and are normally taken by mouth. The amount absorbed from the GI tract depends on the dose administered; therefore the largest dose that can be tolerated without causing side effects is given. Under certain conditions, iron compounds must be given parenterally particularly when (1) there is some disorder limiting the amount of drug absorbed from the intestine, or (2) when the patient is unable to tolerate oral iron.

Iron preparations are only effective in the treatment of anemias specifically resulting from iron deficiency. Blood loss is almost always the only cause of iron deficiency in adult males and postmenopausal females. The daily iron requirement is increased by growth and pregnancy, and iron deficiency, therefore, is particularly common in infants and young children on diets low in iron. Pregnant women and women with heavy menstrual blood loss may also be deficient in iron.

Iron is available for therapy in two forms: bivalent and trivalent. Bivalent (ferrous) iron salts are administered more often than trivalent (ferric) salts because they are less astringent and less irritating than ferric salts and are better absorbed.

Iron preparations are particularly suitable for the treatment of anemias in infancy, in children, in blood donors, during pregnancy, and in patients with chronic blood loss. Optimum therapeutic responses are usually noted in 2 to 4 weeks of treatment.

The RDA for iron is 90–300 mg daily.

Contraindications Patients with hemosiderosis, hemachromatosis, peptic ulcer, regional enteritis, and ulcerative colitis. Hemolytic anemia, pyridoxine responsive anemia, and cirrhosis of the liver.

Drug Interactions

Interactant	Interaction
Allopurinol	May ↑ hepatic iron levels
Antacids, oral	↓ Effect of iron preparations due to ↓ absorption from GI tract
Chloramphenicol (Chloromycetin)	Chloramphenicol ↓ response to iron toxicity
Cholestyramine (Questran)	↓ Effect of iron preparations due to ↓ absorption from GI tract
Pancreatic extracts	↓ Effect of iron preparations due to ↓ absorption from GI tract
Tetracyclines	↓ Effect of tetracyclines due to ↓ absorption from GI tract
Vitamin E	Vitamin E ↓ response to iron therapy

Untoward Reactions

GI effects: constipation, gastric irritation, mild nausea, abdominal cramps, and diarrhea. These effects may be minimized by administering preparations as a coated tablet. Soluble iron preparations may stain teeth.

Toxic reactions are more likely to occur after parenteral administration and include nausea and vomiting, fever, peripheral vascular collapse, and fatal anaphylactoid reactions. These symptoms may occur within 60 seconds of a toxic dose. Symptoms may then disappear for 6 to 24 hours, followed by a second crisis. Symptoms including nausea and diarrhea or constipation may occur after use of oral preparations.

Treatment of Iron Toxicity

The treatment of iron intoxication is symptomatic. It concentrates on removing iron from the body and combating shock and acidosis. Vomiting should be induced immediately, followed by the administration of eggs and milk. Other measures include gastric lavage with aqueous solutions of sodium bicarbonate or sodium phosphate, followed by oral bismuth subcarbonate as a protectant and IV dextrose and sodium chloride injection to correct dehydration. Plasma, whole blood, calcium disodium edetate, deferoxamine, methionine, oxygen, and antibiotics may be ordered.

Some patients may report late manifestations 1 to 2 months after toxic overdosage. These late manifestations include GI distress caused by necrotic alterations of the gastric or intestinal mucosa. Residual effects may also include pyloric stenosis, fibrosis of the liver, and dilatation of the right side of the heart with pulmonary congestion and hemorrhage.

Laboratory Test Interference

Iron containing drugs may affect electrolyte balance determinations.

Nursing Implications

1. Inform patients of possible untoward effects, such as constipation, gastric irritation with abdominal cramps, and diarrhea. Encourage patient to report these symptoms since they can be relieved by a change in medication, dosage, or time of administration.
2. Administer iron preparations with meals to reduce gastric irritation.
3. Administer with citrus juice to enhance absorption of iron.
4. Do not administer the drug with milk or an antacid as these will interfere with the absorption of iron (except for ferrous lactate, which may be given with milk).
5. Administer liquid preparations well diluted with water or fruit juice through a straw to prevent staining the teeth. To infants and young children, administer liquid preparation with a dropper. Deposit liquid well back against the cheek.
6. Encourage the patient to eat a nutritious diet. Stress the intake of foods high in iron, such as liver, raisins, apricots, and green vegetables.
7. Warn parents to keep iron preparations out of the reach of children.

8. Be prepared to assist with treatment of poisoning, as discussed under Untoward Reactions.
9. Monitor vital signs of patients suffering from iron poisoning for at least 48 hours, particularly since a second crisis may occur within 12 to 48 hours.
10. Encourage an individual with symptoms of anemia to seek medical supervision rather than medicate themselves with iron.

IRON DEXTRAN INJECTION FEOSTAT, FERRODEX, HEMATRAN, HYDEXTRAN, I.D.-50, IMFERON, K-FERON, NORFERAN

Classification Iron preparation, parenteral.

General Statement Parenteral iron is indicated only when the patient cannot tolerate oral iron or is suffering from very severe anemia (hemoglobin less than 7.5 gm/100 ml).

Iron dextran is absorbed slowly from the injection site, that is, 1% to 15% is absorbed within 2 hours; 60% to 68% within several days; and the remainder over a period of up to 6 months.

Iron dextran usually is given IM but can be given IV (this route is not recommended). Also, iron dextran injection can cause fatal anaphylactoid reactions; therefore, a small test dose is recommended. Iron dextran should not be given concurrently with oral iron and should be discontinued unless the hemoglobin level increases by at least 2 gm/100 ml in 3 weeks.

Additional Contraindications Pernicious anemia, acute leukemia in the absence of iron depletion by blood loss, anemia associated with chronic leukemia or bone marrow depression, and other anemias not resulting from iron deficiency. Hypersensitivity to drug. Siderosis, hemochromatosis or severe renal or hepatic failure.

Additional Untoward Reactions Headache, fever, malaise, nausea, vomiting, aching of lower limbs, arthralgia, transient loss of taste, lymphadenopathy, local pain, persistent staining of skin at site of injection, mild urticaria, severe anaphylactic reactions, or transient leukocytosis.

Side Effects After IV Injection
Local phlebitis, dyspnea, shock, cyanosis, urticaria, edema of the face, photophobia, joint pain, and thrombosis in veins remote from the site of infusion.

Dosage See Table 7, page 203.

Administration 1. Prevent staining skin by using a separate needle to withdraw medication from the container and by using the Z-track method of injection.
2. Insert the solution deeply with at least a 2-inch needle, 19–20 gauge, into the upper outer quadrant of the gluteus maximus muscle.

TABLE 7 ANTIANEMICS

Drug	Dosage	Remarks
Ferrocholinate (Chel-iron, Ferrolip, Firon, Kelex)	*Liquid, syrup and tablets*, **PO:** 330 mg (equivalent to 40 mg elemental iron) t.i.d.; **infants and children less than 6 years:** 104 mg daily.	Better tolerated than ferrous gluconate or ferrous sulfate; 12% elemental iron.
Ferroglycine Sulfate Complex (Ferronord)	*Tablets,* **PO:** 250 mg b.i.d.	Each 250 mg tablet contains 40 mg iron.
Ferrous fumarate (Eldofe, Feostat, Ferranol, Fumasorb, Fumerin, Ircon, Laud-Iron, Palmiron, Toleron)	*Tablets, chewable tablets, extended release,* **PO, adults:** 600–800 mg (equivalent to 200–260 mg elemental iron) daily in 3 to 4 divided doses; **children under 5 years and infants:** 100–300 mg (equivalent to 33–99 mg elemental iron) daily in 3 to 4 divided doses.	Better tolerated than ferrous gluconate or sulfate; 33% elemental iron.
Ferrous gluconate (Entron, Fergon, Ferralet)	*Capsules, Elixir, Tablets,* **PO:** 320–640 mg (equivalent to 40–80 mg elemental iron) t.i.d.; **infants and children less than 6 years:** 120–300 mg daily; **children 6–12 years:** 100–300 mg t.i.d.	Particularly indicated for patients who cannot tolerate ferrous sulfate because of gastric irritation; 11.6% elemental iron.
Ferrous sulfate (Fero-Gradumet, Ferospace, Mol-Iron) Dried ferrous sulfate (Arne Modified	**PO:** 300–1200 mg (equivalent to 60–240 mg elemental iron) daily in divided doses; **children less than 6 years:** 1–3 ml (equivalent to 25–75 mg elemental iron) of the pediatric	Least expensive, most effective iron salt for oral therapy; 20% elemental iron.

Drug	Dosage	Comments
Timsules, Feosol, Fer-In-Sol, Festotyme, Sterasol)	preparation; **children 6–12 years:** 120–600 mg (equivalent to 24–120 mg elemental iron) daily in divided doses. Prophylaxis for premature or poorly developed infants: 3–6 mg/kg daily. **Pregnancy:** 300–600 mg daily (equivalent to 60–120 mg elemental iron).	Used mainly for patients intolerant to oral iron. (See drug entry.)
Iron dextran injection (Imferon) (See also special drug entry in text, p. 203)	Dosage formula, **IM, adults over 50 kg:** 50 mg first day and up to 250 mg every other day or twice weekly until the total calculated dose is given; **adults and children 9–50 kg:** no more than 100 mg daily; **infants 3.5–9 kg:** no more than 50 mg daily; **infants under 3.5 kg:** no more than 25 mg daily. **IV, adults:** 15–30 mg to start, increase by 10 mg daily until hemoglobin levels return to normal (maximal daily dose, 100 mg).	
Polysaccharide-Iron Complex (Ferrocol, Hytinic, Niferex, Nu-Iron)	*Tablets, capsules, elixir*, **PO:** 100–300 mg; **children 6–12 years:** 100 mg/day; **2–6 years:** 50 mg/day; **under 2 years:** 25 mg.	Easily absorbable iron-polysaccharide complex with relatively low toxicity and little GI disturbance. Does not stain teeth. Tablets contain 50–150 mg elemental iron, elixir 100 mg elemental iron/5 cc.
Soy Protein-Iron Complex (Fe-Plus)	**PO:** 50 mg t.i.d.	Easily absorbable iron-soy protein complex. Take with meals. Swallow with water.

3. Withdraw with syringe to check that the needle is not in a blood vessel before injecting medication.
4. Injection sites should be alternated. Chart the site of injection to facilitate alternating sites.
5. Instruct the patient standing for the injection to bear weight on the leg opposite the injection site. If he is in bed, position so that patient is in a lateral position with the injection site uppermost.

Additional Nursing Implications

1. Discontinue medication and investigate illness further if 500 mg of iron does not cause hemoglobin to rise at least 2 gm/100 ml in 3 weeks.
2. Check that a small test dose is ordered prior to initiating therapy.
3. Do not administer iron products and tetracyclines within 2 hours of each other because iron reduces absorption of tetracycline.
4. Do not administer antacids together with iron compounds because former decreases absorption of iron.

LIVER INJECTION LIVER INJECTION CRUDE, LIVER INJECTION REFINED, PERNAEMON

Classification Liver preparations.

General Statement These preparations contain the soluble, heat-resistant fraction of mammalian liver. Liver injection refined has vitamin B_{12} activity equivalent to 20 μg of cyanocobalamin per milliliter. Liver injection crude is a less purified preparation and has vitamin B_{12} activity equivalent to 1 or 2 μg cyanocobalamin/ml. The potency of both preparations is 100% to 150% of the labeled quantity.

The liver injection labeled 20 μg of vitamin B_{12} is considered therapeutically equivalent to preparations formerly labeled 15 U.S.P. units/ml.

Uses Pernicious anemia and other macrocytic anemias.

Additional Untoward Reactions Three percent of all patients develop allergic manifestations.

Dosage **Initial,** 20 μg of cyanocobalamin (1 ml of liver injection refined or 10–20 ml of liver injection crude) 3 times weekly for 2 weeks until RBC count is approximately 5,000,000/mm³; **then** reduce to 20 μg q 2 weeks until blood count is normal; **maintenance:** 20 μg q 2 weeks. Double the dose temporarily if RBCs fall below normal or patient develops an infection.

Administration See *Administration* under *Iron Dextran Injection.*

Additional Nursing Implication Read label carefully so that liver injection refined (10–20 μg cyanocobalamin/ml) and liver injection crude (1–2 μg cyanocobalamin/ml) are not confused.

anticoagulants and hemostatics

Anticoagulants	Acenocoumarol Anisindione Bishydroxycoumarin Diphenadione Heparin (and Protamine Sulfate)	Phenindione Phenprocoumon Warfarin Potassium Warfarin Sodium
Hemostatics: Topical Agents	Cellulose, Oxidized Gelatin, Absorbable Gelatin Film, Absorbable	Microfibrillar Collagen Hemostat Negatol Thrombin, Topical
Hemostatics: Systemic Agents	Aminocaproic Acid Antihemophilic Factor (Human) Carbazochrome Salicylate	Factor IX Complex (Human)

General Statement

Blood coagulation is a precise mechanism that can be broken down as follows:

1. It is initiated when an inactive precursor escapes from the damaged platelets and activates *thromboplastin*.
2. The activated thromboplastin helps convert the protein *prothrombin* to *thrombin*.
3. *Thrombin* mediates the formation of the threadlike *fibrin*—an insoluble protein—from the soluble *fibrinogen*. The latter forms a clot, trapping blood cells and platelets. Vitamin K, calcium, and various accessory factors manufactured in the liver are essential for blood coagulation.

Once formed the blood clot is dissolved by another enzymatic chain reaction involving a substance called fibrinolysin.

Blood coagulation can be affected by a number of diseases. An excessive tendency to form blood clots is one of the main factors involved in cardiovascular disorders, and a defect in the clotting mechanism is the cause of hemophilia and related diseases.

Since several of the factors that participate in blood clotting are manufactured by the liver, severe liver disease can also affect blood clotting, as does vitamin K deficiency.

Drugs that influence blood coagulation can be divided into three classes: (1) *anticoagulants*, or drugs that prevent or slow blood coagulation; (2) *thrombolytic agents*, which increase the rate at which an existing blood clot dissolves; and (3) *hemostatics*, which prevent or stop internal bleeding. Protamine sulfate, whose sole use is to correct heparin overdosage, is listed at the end of the anticoagulant section.

The dosage of all agents discussed in this chapter must be very carefully adjusted since overdosage can have serious consequences.

ANTICOAGULANTS

General Statement

There are three major types of anticoagulants: (1) coumarin or coumarin-type drugs (bishydroxycoumarin, warfarin); (2) indandione derivatives (diphenadione, phenindione); and (3) heparin. The following considerations are pertinent to all types.

Anticoagulant drugs are used mainly in the management of patients with thromboembolic disease; they do not dissolve previously formed clots, but they do forestall their enlargement and prevent new clots from forming.

Some physicians also prescribe anticoagulants prophylactically. However, there is still considerable controversy about the long-term use of these agents.

Uses

Venous thrombosis, pulmonary embolism, acute coronary occlusions with myocardial infarctions, and strokes caused by emboli or cerebral thrombi.

Prophylactically for rheumatic heart disease, atrial fibrillation, traumatic injuries of blood vessels, vascular surgery, major abdominal, thoracic, and pelvic surgery, prevention of strokes in patients with transient attacks of cerebral ischemia, or other signs of impending stroke.

Contraindications

Patients with possible defects in the clotting mechanism (hemophilia) or with frail or weakened blood vessels, peptic ulcer, chronic ulcerations of the GI tract, hepatic and renal dysfunction, subacute bacterial endocarditis, or severe hypertension. Also after neurosurgery or recent surgery of the eye, spinal cord, or brain, or in the presence of drainage tubes in any orifice. Alcoholism.

Coumarin and Indandione-type Anticoagulants

General Statement

These drugs interfere with the synthesis of prothrombin and related clotting factors by the liver. Their onset of action is slow (12 to 72 hours). They can be taken orally.

The drugs increase prothrombin time by decreasing the concentration of prothrombin in circulating blood. Their therapeutic effect persists for 24 to 96 hours after the drug is withdrawn. Indandiones have a faster onset and shorter duration than coumarins; prothrombin time returns to normal within 24 to 48 hours.

The aim of therapy is to keep prothrombin time at 10% to 30% of normal, as determined before and after therapy is started.

Uses

Prophylaxis and treatment of intravascular clotting, postoperative thrombophlebitis, pulmonary embolism, acute embolic and thrombotic occlusions of the peripheral arteries, acute coronary thrombosis, and recurrent idiopathic thrombophlebitis.

Heparin is often used concurrently during the therapeutic initiation period.

Contraindications Hemorrhagic tendencies, blood dyscrasias, ulcerative lesions of the GI tract, diverticulitis, colitis, subacute bacterial endocarditis, threatened abortion, recent operations on the eye, brain, or spinal cord, regional anesthesia and lumbar block, vitamin K deficiency, leukemia with bleeding tendencies, thrombocytopenic purpura, open wounds or ulcerations, acute nephritis, impaired hepatic or renal function, or severe hypertension.

The drugs should be used with caution in menstruating women, in pregnant women (because they may cause hypoprothrombinemia in the infant), in nursing mothers, during postpartum, and following cerebrovascular accidents.

Untoward Reactions Hemorrhagic accidents are the chief danger of anticoagulant therapy. Frequent prothrombin time determinations should be performed for patients on long-term therapy to ascertain that values remain within safe levels.

Blood in urine may be a first warning of impending hemorrhage.

Antidotes

Coumarin-type drugs can be counteracted by oral (100–200 mg) or IV administration (50–100 mg) of vitamin K (phytonadione).

Fresh whole blood or plasma transfusions may be required in emergencies.

Dosage PO: *individualized.* See Table 8, page 211.

Drug Interactions These drugs are responsible for more adverse drug interactions than any other group. Patients on anticoagulant therapy must be monitored very carefully each time a drug is added or withdrawn.

Monitoring usually involves determination of prothrombin time. In general, a lengthened prothrombin time means potentiation of the anticoagulant. Since potentiation may mean hemorrhages, a lengthened prothrombin time warrants **reduction of the dosage of the anticoagulant.** However, the anticoagulant dosage must again be increased when the second drug is discontinued.

A shortened prothrombin time means inhibition of the anticoagulant and may require an increase in dosage.

Interactant	Interaction
Acetaminophen	Slight ↑ in hypoprothrombinemia
Alcohol, ethyl	↑ Effect of oral anticoagulants

Aminoglycoside antibiotics
  Gentamicin
  Kanamycin
  Neomycin
  Streptomycin
	Potentiate pharmacologic effect of anticoagulants

Drug Interactions (*Continued*)

Interactant	Interaction
Aminosalicylic acid	Potentiates pharmacologic effect of anticoagulants
Anabolic steroids	Potentiate pharmacologic effect of anticoagulants
Antacids, oral	↓ Effect of anticoagulants due to ↓ absorption from GI tract

Antidepressants, tricyclic
  Amitriptyline
  Nortriptyline
	↑ Effect of anticoagulants due to ↓ in breakdown by liver

Barbiturates	↓ Effect of anticoagulants due to ↓ absorption from GI tract and ↑ breakdown by liver
Carbamazepine (Tegratol)	↓ Effect of anticoagulants due to ↑ breakdown by liver
Cephaloridine (Loridine)	↑ Effect of anticoagulants due to ↑ prothrombin time
Chloral hydrate (Noctec, Somnos)	↑ Effect of anticoagulants by ↓ plasma protein binding
Chloramphenicol (Chloromycetin)	Potentiates pharmacologic effect of anticoagulants
Chlorthalidone (Hygroton)	↓ Response to oral anticoagulants
Cholestyramine (Cuemid, Questran)	↑ Hypoprothrombinemia
Clofibrate (Atromid S)	↑ Effect of anticoagulants by ↓ plasma protein binding
Contraceptives, oral	↓ Anticoagulants' response by ↑ activity of certain clotting factors
Contrast media containing iodine	↑ Effect of anticoagulants by ↑ prothrombin time
Corticosteroids, corticosterone	↓ Effect of anticoagulants by ↓ hypoprothrombinemia; also risk of hemorrhages due to vascular effects of the corticosteroids
Dextrothyroxine	↑ Effect of anticoagulants by ↓ hypoprothrombinemia
Diazoxide (Hyperstat)	↑ Effect of anticoagulants by ↓ plasma protein binding
Disulfiram (Antabuse)	↑ Effect of anticoagulants by ↑ hypoprothrombinemia
Estrogens	↓ Anticoagulant response by ↑ activity of certain clotting factors
Ethacrynic acid (Edecrin)	↑ Effect of anticoagulants by ↓ plasma protein binding
Ethchlorvynol (Placidyl)	↓ Effect of anticoagulants due to ↑ breakdown by liver
Glucagon	↑ Effect of anticoagulants by ↑ hypoprothrombinemia
Glutethimide (Doriden)	↑ Effect of anticoagulants due to ↑ breakdown by liver
Griseofulvin	↓ Effect of anticoagulants due to ↑ breakdown by liver

Haloperidol (Haldol)	↓ Effect of anticoagulants due to ↑ breakdown by liver
Heparin	↑ Effect by ↑ prothrombin time
Indomethacin (Indocin)	↑ Effect of anticoagulants by ↓ plasma protein binding; also indomethacin is ulcerogenic and may inhibit platelet function leading to hemorrhage
Kanamycin (Kantrex)	Potentiates pharmacologic effect of anticoagulants
Mefenamic acid (Ponstel)	↑ Effect of anticoagulants by ↓ plasma protein binding
Methotrexate	Additive hypoprothrombinemia
Methylphenidate (Ritalin)	↑ Effect of anticoagulants due to ↓ in breakdown by liver
Mineral oil	↑ Hypoprothrombinemia by ↓ absorption of vitamin K from GI tract; also mineral oil could ↓ absorption of anticoagulants from GI tract
Methylthiouracil	Additive hypoprothrombinemia
Nalidixic acid (NegGram)	↑ Effect of anticoagulants by ↓ in plasma protein binding
Neomycin	Potentiates pharmacologic effect of anticoagulants
Oxyphenbutazone (Tandearil)	↑ Effect of anticoagulants by ↓ plasma protein binding; oxyphenbutazone may also produce GI ulceration and therefore ↑ chance of bleeding
Penicillin	Penicillin may potentiate the pharmacologic effect of anticoagulants
Phenformin (DBI)	Phenformin-induced ↑ in fibrinolytic activity can lead to ↑ chance of hemorrhage
Phenylbutazone (Butazolidin)	↑ Effect of anticoagulants by ↓ plasma protein binding; phenylbutazone may also produce GI ulceration and therefore ↑ chance of bleeding
Phenyramidol (Analexin)	↑ Effect of anticoagulants by ↓ breakdown by liver
Phenytoin (Dilantin)	↑ Effect of phenytoin due to ↓ in breakdown by liver; also possible ↑ in anticoagulant effect by ↓ plasma protein binding
Propylthiouracil	Additive hypoprothrombinemia
Quinidine	Additive hypoprothrombinemia
Rifampin	Anticoagulant effect ↓ by rifampin
Salicylates	↑ Effect of anticoagulants by ↓ plasma protein binding, ↓ plasma prothrombin, and ↓ platelet aggregation
Streptomycin	Potentiates pharmacologic effect of anticoagulants
Sulfonamides	↑ Effect of sulfonamides by ↑ blood levels; also ↑ anticoagulant effect by long-acting sulfonamides by ↓ plasma protein binding

**Drug
Interactions
(Continued)**

Interactant	Interaction
Tetracyclines	IV tetracyclines ↑ hypoprothrombinemia
Thiazide diuretics	↓ Effect of anticoagulants by concentrating circulating clotting factors and ↑ clotting factor synthesis in liver
Tolbutamide	Initial ↑ effect of anticoagulants by ↓ plasma protein binding followed by ↓ effect of anticoagulants due to ↑ breakdown in liver; also ↑ effect of tolbutamide by ↓ breakdown in liver
Xanthines	↓ Effect of anticoagulants by ↑ plasma pro-thrombin and factor V

**Nursing
Implications**

1. Assist the health team in evaluating the patient's reliability, which is essential in coumarin therapy. The aged, psychotics, and alcoholics cannot be relied on to take medication without supervison.

2. Ask a reliable relative or friend of the patient to report any untoward effects and to make sure that the patient takes medication and comes in for blood tests.

3. Alert the patient to the possibility of bleeding and the signs to look for, but avoid unduly frightening him/her.

4. Advise patient that should there be any bleeding (e.g., from the gums), black and blue areas on the skin, or blood in urine, to stop taking medication and call physician for further instructions.

5. Advise the patient on indandione-type anticoagulants that medication turns alkaline urine red-orange. Discoloration resulting from the drug can be differentiated from hematuria by acidifying urine.

6. Advise patients on coumarin-type therapy to carry a card stating that they are on anticoagulant therapy in order to alert medical or paramedical personnel should an accident or excessive bleeding occur or surgery be required.

7. Emphasize the necessity for remaining under medical supervision for blood tests and adjustment of dosage to the patient.

8. Check that prothrombin times are done at prescribed intervals.

9. Warn the patient that other medications, changes in diet, and physical state may affect the action of the anticoagulant. Illness should be promptly reported to the physician.

10. Warn the patient not to take nonprescription drugs, particularly aspirin, alcohol, or vitamin preparations high in vitamin K, without checking with the physician responsible for coumarin therapy.

11. Advise the patient to use an electric razor rather than a razor blade for shaving.

12. Observe the patient closely for evidence of hemorrhage during initial therapy (bleeding gums, hematuria, tarry stools, hematemesis, ecchymosis, petechiae).

13. Report the sudden appearance of lumbar pain in patients receiving anticoagulant therapy since this may indicate retroperitoneal hemorrhage.

14. Report abdominal symptoms in a patient on anticoagulant therapy since these may indicate intestinal hemorrhage.
15. Anticipate that a patient with a history of ulcers of the GI tract or who recently underwent surgery should have frequent lab tests for blood in urine or feces to assess for GI bleeding.
16. Have vitamin K available for parenteral emergency use.

TABLE 8   ANTICOAGULANTS

Drug	Dosage	Remarks
Acenocoumarol (Sintrom)	**PO:** Day 1: 16–28 mg. Day 2: 8–16 mg. **Maintenance:** 2–10 mg daily.	Coumarin type. Intermediate action; peak effect in 24 to 48 hr; effect persists for 48 to 72 hr after drug is discontinued.
Anisindione (Miradon)	**PO:** Day 1: 300 mg. Day 2: 200 mg. Day 3: 100 mg. **Maintenance:** *Usual:* 75–150 mg daily. *Extreme:* 25–250 mg daily.	Indandione type. Long-acting; peak effect in 48 to 72 hr; effect persists for 24 to 72 hr.
Bishydroxycoumarin (Dicumarol)	**PO:** Day 1: 300 mg. Day 2: 200 mg. Day 3: 100 mg. **Maintenance:** 25–150 mg daily.	Coumarin type. Activity appears only 24 to 72 hr after therapy is started and persists 24 to 96 hr after withdrawal. *Additional Nursing Implications* Explain to patient prothrombin times since effect of drug is cumulative and persistent.
Diphenadione (Dipaxin)	**PO:** Day 1: 20–30 mg. Day 2: 10–15 mg. **Maintenance:** 3–5 mg daily.	Indandione type. Peak effect in 48 to 72 hr; effect may persist for 20 days.
Phenindione (Hedulin)	**PO, initial, patients up to 70 kg:** 200 mg; **over 70 kg:** 300 mg in 2 equally divided doses in morning and at bedtime **Maintenance:** 50–100 mg daily in divided doses.	Indandione type. Peak effect in 48 to 72 hr; effect persists 24 to 48 hr after withdrawal. *Additional Contraindications* Open wounds and ulcerations.

(*Continued*)

TABLE 8 ANTICOAGULANTS (*Continued*)

Drug	Dosage	Remarks
		Additional Nursing Implications Explain need for daily prothrombin time determinations for first 3 days and every 7 to 14 days thereafter.
Phenprocoumon (Liquamar)	**PO:** Day 1: 21–30 mg. Day 2: 2–12 mg. Day 3: 1–4 mg. **Maintenance:** 0.75–6 mg daily.	Peak effect in 48 to 72 hr; cumulative effect noticeable up to 14 days after withdrawal. Dosage should be adjusted carefully (difficult; check prothrombin time frequently) in patients with uncontrolled congestive heart failure or those receiving large doses of salicylates, barbiturates, phenothiazines, antibiotics, corticosteroids, or corticotropin. *Additional Untoward Reaction* Diarrhea. Recovery may take up to 7 days.
Warfarin potassium (Anthrombin-K) Warfarin sodium (Coumadin sodium, Panwarfin)	**PO,** *potassium salt,* **PO, IM, IV,** *sodium salt.* Doses are identical regardless of salt or route. **Initial loading dose:** 40–60 mg daily. *Debilitated patient:* 20–40 mg daily. **Maintenance:** 2–10 mg daily regulated according to prothrombin time. If no loading dose, give 10–15 mg daily until desired prothrombin time achieved.	Response to drug more uniform than with other anticoagulants. Only coumarin-type drug for parenteral administration. Onset in 12 hr; peak in 36 hr; duration 2 to 5 days or more. Daily prothrombin time recommended during start of therapy and weekly thereafter. *Additional Contraindications* Liver or kidney disease *Administration* After reconstitution, sodium warfarin injection may be stored for several days at 4° C. Discard solution if precipitate becomes noticeable. Store in light-resistant containers.

Heparin and Protamine Sulfate

HEPARIN SODIUM HEPATHROM, HEPRINAR, LIPO-HEPIN, LIQUAEMIN SODIUM, PANHEPRIN

Classification   Anticoagulant, natural.

General Statement   Heparin is a naturally occurring substance isolated from porcine intestinal mucosa or bovine lung tissue. Its main advantage is the rapidity of its anticoagulant effect. Its main drawback is that it must be given parenterally. Maximal effects occur within minutes, and the clotting time of blood returns to normal within 2 to 6 hours.

It has not yet been determined precisely how heparin works, although it is known to interfere with several steps of the coagulation process. Heparin does not interfere with wound healing and has anti-inflammatory and diuretic effects. Diuresis usually starts 36 to 48 hours after the first dose is administered and lasts for about 36 hours after the drug is withdrawn.

Uses   As an anticoagulant, heparin is used to prevent the extension of clots or to prevent thrombi and emboli from recurring. It is also used prophylactically in the management of thromboembolic disease and to prevent complications after cardiac and vascular surgery. Heparin has also been used for the treatment of hyperlipemia and in renal dialysis to prevent clotting.

Contraindications   Active bleeding, blood dyscrasias (or other disorders characterized by bleeding tendencies such as hemophilia), purpura, thrombocytopenia, liver disease with hypoprothrombinemia, suspected intracranial hemorrhage, suppurative thrombophlebitis, inaccessible ulcerative lesions (especially of the GI tract), open wounds, extensive denudation of the skin, and increased capillary permeability (as in ascorbic acid deficiency).

The drug should not be administered during surgery of the eye, brain, or spinal cord or during continuous tube drainage of the stomach or small intestine. Use is also contraindicated in subacute endocarditis, shock, advanced kidney disease, threatened abortion, severe hypertension, or hypersensitivity to drug.

Use with caution during menstruation, pregnancy, and postpartum, as well as in patients with a history of asthma, allergies, mild liver or kidney disease, or in alcoholics.

Untoward Reactions   Hemorrhage ranging from minor local ecchymoses to major hemorrhagic complications. Such reactions are more likely to occur in prophylactic administration during surgery than in the treatment of thromboembolic disease.

Rare allergic reactions characterized by chills, fever, pruritus, urticaria, burning feet, rhinitis, conjunctivitis, lacrimation, asthmalike reactions, hyperemia, arthralgia, or anaphylactoid reactions have been noted. Use a test dose of 1,000 units in patients with a history of asthma or allergic disease. Transient alopecia. Long-term therapy may cause osteoporosis and/or spontaneous fractures and hypoaldosteronism.

Heparin resistance has been observed in some elderly patients. In these cases, large doses may be required.

IM or SC injections of heparin may produce local irritation, hematoma, and tissue sloughing.

Overdosage
Drug withdrawal is usually sufficient to correct heparin over-dosage. In some cases, blood transfusion or the administration of a heparin antagonist (protamine sulfate) may be necessary.

Drug Interactions

Interactant	Interaction
Anticoagulants, oral	↑ Effect by ↑ prothrombin time
Aspirin	Inhibition of platelet adhesiveness by aspirin; this may result in bleeding tendencies
Dipyridamole (Persantin)	Inhibition of platelet adhesiveness by dipyridamole; this may result in bleeding tendencies
Guaifenesin	Inhibition of platelet adhesiveness by guaifenesin; this may result in bleeding tendencies
Quinine	Additive hypoprothrombinemia

Dosage   Adjusted individually based on laboratory tests. **SC: initial loading dose,** 10,000–20,000 units (preceded by 5,000 units IV); **maintenance:** 8,000–10,000 units q 8 hr or 15,000–20,000 units q 12 hr. **Intermittent IV: initially,** 10,000 units; **then,** 5,000–10,000 units q 4 to 6 hr. **IV infusion:** 20,000–40,000 units/day.

Prophylaxis of postoperative thromboembolism: **SC:** 5,000 units 2 hr before surgery and 5,000 units q 8 to 12 hr thereafter for 7 days or until patient is ambulatory. *Open heart surgery:* 150–400 units/kg. *Renal dialysis:* See instructions on equipment.

Administration/ Storage
1. Patient must be in hospital for heparin therapy.
2. Protect solutions from freezing.
3. Heparin should not be administered IM.
4. Administer by deep SC injection to minimize local irritation, hematoma, and tissue sloughing and to prolong action of drug.
   a. Z-track method: Use any fat roll, but abdominal fat rolls are preferred. Use a ½ in- or ⅝ in-needle. Grasp the skin layer of the fat roll and lift it upward. Insert the needle at about a 45° angle to the skin surface and then administer the medication. With this medication it is not necessary to check whether or not the needle is in a blood vessel. Rapidly withdraw the needle while releasing the skin.
   b. "Bunch technique" method: Grasp the tissue around the injection site creating a tissue roll of about ½ inch in diameter. Insert the needle into the tissue roll at a 90° angle to the skin surface and

inject the medication. It is not necessary to check whether or not the needle is in a blood vessel. Remove the needle rapidly when the skin is released.

5. Do not massage before or after injection.
6. Change sites of administration.
7. Caution should be used to prevent negative pressure (with a roller pump), which would increase the rate at which heparin is injected into the system.

Nursing Implications

1. Check to be sure prothrombin times are performed as ordered and that the results are reported to the physician promptly.
2. Anticipate that each dose of heparin will be ordered on an individual basis after prothrombin time is evaluated by the physician, except when small doses are administered for prophylaxis.
3. Check for signs of hemorrhage, such as ecchymosis or hematemesis, or bleeding of mucous membranes.
4. Instruct the patient to report any sign of active bleeding.
5. Advise the patient that he may shave with a razor blade since drug does not affect bleeding time.
6. Explain to the patient that the drug may have a diuretic effect and encourage patient to include orange juice or bananas for potassium in diet.
7. Reassure patients with alopecia that the condition is only temporary.
8. Advise women of menstrual age to report any excessive menstrual flow, since this may be due to the drug and would necessitate a reduction in dosage.
9. Have protamine sulfate available for emergency use.

PROTAMINE SULFATE

Classification   Antiheparin agent.

General Statement   This polypeptide acts as an antiheparin agent by forming a physiologically inactive complex with heparin.

The drug also has a very weak anticoagulant effect and a very rapid onset of action.

Use   Treatment of heparin overdose only. Not suitable for treating spontaneous hemorrhage, postpartum hemorrhage, menorrhagia, or uterine bleeding. Heparin rebound may occur during or after transfusion, extracorporeal dialysis, or cardiopulmonary bypass procedures. This may be corrected by administering more protamine sulfate.

Contraindication   Patients previously shown to have intolerance.

Untoward Reactions   Sudden fall in blood pressure, bradycardia, dyspnea, transitory flushing, and feeling of warmth. Slow administration (1 to 3 minutes) of drug may minimize these side effects; also nausea, vomiting, and lassitude. As a result of its weak anticoagulant effect, overdoses may cause hemorrhage.

Dosage **Slow IV.** Dosage is determined by venous coagulation studies. No more than 50 mg of *protamine sulfate* should be given in any 10-minute interval.

It is estimated that 1 mg of *protamine sulfate* will neutralize 78–95 U.S.P. units of heparin derived from lung tissue, or approximately 115 U.S.P. units of heparin derived from intestinal mucosa.

Administration/ 1. Note expiration date, which is 2 years after manufacture.
Storage 2. Store at 2°–15° C.
3. After reconstitution, store at 2°–15° C and discard if not used within 1 week of preparation.

Nursing 1. Monitor blood pressure before and closely after administration of
Implications drug until pressure is stable. Then check hourly or as indicated by medical supervision.
2. Observe patient closely and report signs of "heparin rebound," which is characterized by increased bleeding, lowered blood pressure, or shock.
3. Anticipate need for repeated doses of protamine sulfate if heparin has been administered in a repository form.
4. Anticipate that the patient may show a sudden fall in blood pressure, bradycardia, dyspnea, transitory flushing, and a feeling of warmth if the drug is administered too rapidly. Reassure the patient that these will pass.

HEMOSTATICS

General These drugs are used to control excessive bleeding in persons who have
Statement an inborn clotting defect, who suffer from a disease that affects the clotting mechanism, or who exhibit continuous leakage from a capillary which cannot be controlled by other (physical, surgical) means.

The mechanism of blood coagulation was detailed at the beginning of this section. Defects in clotting are difficult to treat because excessive, drug-induced blood coagulation is far more dangerous than the hemorrhage itself.

Hemostatic agents are divided into: (1) topically active agents and (2) systemic agents.

Topical Agents

CELLULOSE, OXIDIZED OXYCEL, SURGICEL

Classification Hemostatic, topical.

General This specially treated form of surgical gauze does not participate in the
Statement clotting mechanism of the blood. However, when exposed to blood, it forms a dark, gelatinous mass that acts as an artificial clot. Oxidized

cellulose is systemically absorbed within 2 to 7 days. However, when it has been soaked with blood, reabsorption may take 6 weeks or longer.

The material should not be used on open, external wounds because it interferes with new skin formation. It also should not be used for permanent packing because it interferes with bone regeneration.

Uses Surgery, to control moderate bleeding when suturing or ligation is impractical (such as biliary tract surgery), partial hepatectomy, resections or injuries of the pancreas, spleen, or kidneys, and bowel resections.

Dosage Minimum amount necessary.

Administration
1. Apply minimal amount necessary to control hemorrhage.
2. Apply in dry form.
3. Never pull oxidized cellulose from wound without irrigating material. Otherwise, fresh bleeding may be initiated.

GELATIN, ABSORBABLE GELFOAM POWDER, GELFOAM SPONGE

Classification Hemostatic, topical.

General Statement The sponge is a specially prepared form of gelatin that absorbs approximately 50% of its weight in blood or water. The substance is absorbed systemically within 4 to 6 weeks. It is particularly effective when moistened with thrombin solution.

Uses During surgery to control capillary bleeding. The powder is used in the management of massive gastroduodenal hemorrhage, decubitus ulcers, and chronic leg ulcers.

Dosage Enough thin strips of sponge moistened with *thrombin* or *sterile isotonic saline* to cover bleeding surface.

Administration Moisten sponge with thrombin (1,000–2,000 units/ml) or sterile isotonic sodium chloride solution before applying to bleeding surface.

GELATIN FILM, ABSORBABLE GELFILM, GELFILM OPHTHALMIC

Classification Hemostatic, topical.

Remarks This is a thin, absorbable gelatin film that takes up to 50 times its weight of blood and water. Like absorbable gelatin sponge (see above), it can be left in place and is absorbed within 8 days to 6 months.

Uses Neurosurgery, thoracic surgery, and ocular surgery.

Dosage **Topical:** film 25 × 50 mm (ophthalmic) or as required.

Nursing Implication Have sterile isotonic solution available to moisten gelatin before it is applied to bleeding surface.

MICROFIBRILLAR COLLAGEN HEMOSTAT AVITENE

Classification Hemostatic, topical.

General Statement Absorbable agent derived from bovine collagen. The material attracts platelets, which then release clotting factors and initiate the formation of a fibrinous mass.

Uses During surgery to control capillary bleeding and as an adjunct to hemostasis when conventional procedures are ineffectual or insufficient.

Contraindication Closure of skin incisions because preparation may interfere with healing.

Untoward Reactions Potentiation of infections, abscess formation, hematomas, wound dehiscence, mediastinitis.

Dosage *Individualized:* depending on severity of bleeding. *Usual for capillary bleeding:* 1 gm for 50 cm area. More for heavier flow.

Administration
1. Prior to application of dry product, compress surface to be treated with dry sponge. Use dry smooth forceps to handle.
2. Apply hemostat directly to source of bleeding.
3. After hemostat is in place, apply pressure with a dry sponge and not a gloved hand.
4. When controlling oozing from porous (cancellous) bone, pack hemostat tightly into affected area.
5. Tease off excess material after 5–10 minutes.
6. Apply more hemostat in case of breakthrough bleeding.
7. Avoid spillage on nonbleeding surfaces, especially in the abdomen or thorax.
8. Remove excess material after a few minutes.
9. Do not reautoclave. Discard unused portion.
10. Avoid contacting non-bleeding surfaces with microfibrillar collagen hemostat.

Nursing Implications Assess for shock while monitoring BP and pulse because hemostat may mask a deeper hemorrhage by sealing off its exit site.

NEGATOL NEGATAN

Classification Hemostatic and astringent, topical.

General Statement   This substance has a powerful coagulant effect on proteins. It also exerts a germicidal action. Negatol imparts a transitory greyish area to treated mucous membranes.

Use   Suppuration, bleeding, ulceration, and oozing of skin and mucous membranes including those of the mouth, vagina, and cervix.

Contraindication   Hypersensitivity to drug.

Untoward Reaction   Rarely: local irritation of the skin surrounding the vaginal orifice.

Dosage   Paint surface with full strength product or dilute (1:10).

Administration
1. Cleanse and dry affected area.
2. Paint area with negatol.
3. For oral ulceration dry affected area, apply topical anesthetic as ordered, apply negatol with applicator. Hold latter in place for 1 minute. Rinse with copious amounts of water to neutralize.
4. For cervical use: use 1:10 dilution of product to establish tolerance of patient to negatol. Insert a 1-inch gauze pack, dipped into dilute or full strength negatol into cervical canal. For vaginal involvement: pack vagina with gauze soaked in 1:10 dilution of negatol. Remove all packing within 24 hours and follow with a 2-quart douche of dilute negatol or vinegar.

Nursing Implication   Advise patient to wear a perineal pad to prevent soiling of clothing by the highly acid substance.

THROMBIN, TOPICAL

Classification   Hemostatic, topical.

Dosage   **Topical:** Applied as dry powder, or as a solution, containing 1,000–2,000 units/ml. Thrombin can also be applied as a spray using a syringe or it can be soaked into an absorbable gelatin sponge. **PO:** 10,000 units of thrombin dissolved in 50 ml phosphate buffer solution pH 7.6 (this prevents destruction by gastric juice).

Contraindications   Thrombin should never be injected, particularly IV. IV injections may be fatal.

Administration/ Storage
1. Dry powder may be stored indefinitely.
2. Use aqueous solutions within 24 to 48 hours because thrombin solution only retains its stability for 1 to 2 days at room temperature.
3. Use a fine needle and syringe when administering medication in spray form.

Systemic Agents

AMINOCAPROIC ACID AMICAR

Classification   Hemostatic, systemic.

Remarks   Aminocaproic acid prevents fibrinolysis (clot dissolution). It is only indicated in life-threatening situations.

Uses   Excessive bleeding associated with systemic hyperfibrinolysis and urinary fibrinolysis. Surgical complications following heart surgery and portacaval shunt in cancer of the lung, prostate, cervix, stomach, and other types of surgery associated with heavy, postoperative bleeding. Aplastic anemia.

Contraindications   Patients with active, intravascular clotting possibly associated with fibrinolysis and bleeding. Use with caution, or not at all, in patients with uremia or cardiac, renal, or hepatic disease. First and second trimester of pregnancy.

Untoward Reactions   Nausea, cramping, diarrhea, dizziness, tinnitus, malaise, conjunctival suffusion, nasal stuffiness, headache, or skin rash.

    Side effects usually disappear after withdrawal of drug. Bradycardia, arrhythmias, and hypotension have been noted after rapid IV administration.

Drug Interactions

Interactant	Interaction
Anticoagulants, oral	↓ Anticoagulant effects
Contraceptives, oral (Estrogen)	Combination with aminocaproic acid may lead to hypercoagulable condition

Dosage   **PO and IV.** *Acute bleeding caused by increased fibrinolytic activity:* therapy is aimed at reaching a plasma level of 130 μg/ml necessary for inhibition of systemic hyperfibrinolysis. **Initial priming dose,** 4–5 gm during first hour; **then** 1.0–1.25 gm q hr until plasma level of 130 μg/ml is reached; **maximum daily dose:** 30 gm. *Chronic bleeding tendency:* 5–30 gm daily in divided doses at 3 to 6 hour intervals. Aim for minimum effective dosage.

Administration   Dilute drug as directed.

Nursing Implications

1. Check patient frequently for hypotension, bradycardia, and arrhythmias which indicate that the IV administration is too fast. Slow IV and report if such symptoms occur.
2. With all systemic hemostatics, observe carefully for signs and symptoms of thrombosis, such as leg pain, chest pain, or respiratory distress.
3. Have vitamin K or protamine sulfate available for emergency use.

ANTIHEMOPHILIC FACTOR (HUMAN) FACTORATE, FACTOR VIII, HEMOFIL, HUMAFAC, KOATE, PROFILATE

Classification   Hemostatic, systemic.

General Statement   Antihemophilic factor (AHF) is essential to blood coagulation. The factor can now be isolated and prepared from normal human blood plasma. Several processes are used, and various preparations are on the market. The preparations differ with respect to concentration and impurities. There is considerable variation among preparations produced by the same method and each lot is standardized individually. Carefully note instructions on vial for dilution, storage, concentration, and so forth. The antihemophilic factor assists in the conversion of prothrombin to thrombin.

Use   Control of bleeding in patients suffering from hemophilia A (factor VIII deficiency and acquired factor VIII inhibitors).

Untoward Reactions   Headaches, flushing, tachycardia, paresthesia, nausea, vomiting, back pains, hypotension, clouding or loss of consciousness, disturbance of vision, constriction of the chest, or rigor. Jaundice and viral hepatitis.

Antihemophilic factor contains traces of blood group A and B isohemagglutins. These may cause intravascular hemolysis in individuals with types A, B, or AB blood.

Dosage   **IV:** *overt bleeding,* **initial,** 20 units/kg followed by 10 units/kg q 6–8 hr for 24 hr; **then,** q 12 hr for 3 to 4 days. *Joint and muscle hemorrhage:* 25 units/kg/day; can repeat daily dose if no response. *Surgery:* requires levels of 40% AHF or more; 30–40 units/kg prior to surgery and 20 units/kg q 8 hr after surgery. Post infusion level should be 60% AHF and maintained at 13–30% AHF for at least 10 days postoperatively.

Administration/ Storage
1. Antihemophilic factor is very labile and is inactivated rapidly: within 10 minutes at 56° C and within 3 hours at 49° C. Store vials at 2°–8° C. Check expiration date.
2. Warm the concentrate and diluent to room temperature prior to reconstitution.
3. Place one needle in the concentrate to act as an airway and then aseptically with a syringe and needle add the diluent to the concentrate.
4. Gently agitate or roll the vial containing diluent and concentrate to dissolve the drug. **Do not shake vigorously.**
5. Administer drug within 3 hours of reconstitution to avoid incubation if contamination occurred during mixing.
6. Do not refrigerate drug after reconstitution because the active ingredient may precipitate out.
7. Keep reconstituted drug at room temperature during infusion because, at a lower temperature, precipitation of active ingredients may occur.

Nursing Implications
1. Observe and report cyanosis of lips, nailbeds, or mucous membranes.
2. Report hematuria.
3. Take pulse before administration of drug is started. Monitor pulse during administration and report if it becomes more rapid than base pulse.

CARBAZOCHROME SALICYLATE ANDRENOSEM SALICYLATE

Classification Hemostatic, systemic

Remarks The manner in which this drug acts is unclear; it is not suitable for treatment of massive hemorrhage or arterial bleeding. Drug should not be administered IV.

Uses Prophylactic and therapeutic systemic control of capillary bleeding and oozing.

Contraindications Hypersensitivity to salicylates. Early pregnancy.

Untoward Reactions Repeated use may cause salicylate sensitivity. Pain at site of IM injection.

Dosage *Preoperatively:* 10 mg **IM** night before surgery and 10 mg **IM** with on-call medication. **Children under 12 years:** ½ adult dose. *Postoperatively:* if drug used preoperatively, 5 mg q 2 hr **IM** or **PO.** If not used preoperatively, 10 mg q 2 hr as needed. **Children under 12 years:** 5 mg q 2 hr **IM** or **PO** as needed.

Administration Administer IM injection slowly to minimize pain.

Nursing Implication Observe patient for untoward signs of salicylate sensitivity, such as ringing in ears, mental confusion, profuse sweating, and GI disturbances.

FACTOR IX COMPLEX (HUMAN) KONYNE, PROPLEX

Classification Hemostatic, systemic.

Remarks This is a concentrate of several human coagulation factors (II, VII, IX, and X) prepared from normal human plasma. The factors are essential to the clotting mechanism. Factor II is prothrombin.

Uses For patients with coagulation factor deficiency (II, VII, IX, or X), especially hemophilia. Halting or prevention of dangerous bleeding episodes in hemorrhagic disease of newborn (only in life-threatening situations).

Contraindications Liver disease with suspected intravascular coagulation or fibrinolysis.

Untoward Reactions Transient fever, chills, headaches, flushing, and tingling. Most of these side effects disappear when rate of administration is slowed. Viral hepatitis. The preparation also contains trace amounts of blood groups A and B and isohemagglutins that may cause intravascular hemolysis when administered in large amounts to patients with blood groups A, B, and AB.

Dosage **IV:** each lot is standardized individually. Dosage for patients is also individualized. It depends on weight of patient, degree of deficiency, and severity of bleeding.

It is recommended that the level in persons deficient in factors VII and IX be raised prophylactically to 60% of normal level when patient is undergoing extensive surgery or dental procedure. This level should be maintained for 8 days.

Administration/ Storage
1. Store at 2°–8° C.
2. Avoid freezing the diluent provided with drug.
3. Discard 2 years after date of manufacture.
4. Prior to reconstitution, warm diluent to room temperature but not over 40° C.
5. Agitate the solution gently until the powder is dissolved.
6. Administer drug within 3 hours of reconstitution to avoid incubation in case contamination occurred during preparation.
7. Do not refrigerate after reconstitution because the active ingredient may precipitate out.
8. Administer at the rate of flow ordered.

Nursing Implication Reduce rate of injection if patient reports a tingling sensation, chills, fever and headache, and report to physician.

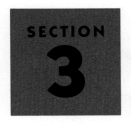

SECTION
3

blood, blood components, and blood substitutes

Albumin, Normal Human Serum
Blood, Whole
Dextran 40
Dextran 70
Dextran 75

Hetastarch
Plasma, Normal Human
Plasma, Protein Fraction
Red Cells, Packed

General Statement

Blood, blood fractions, and blood extenders are not drugs in the ordinary sense. However, since they are often administered and monitored by nurses, they are discussed here briefly.

Blood transfusions have become a reality since it was discovered that blood coagulation can be prevented through the addition of anticoagulants (citrate, heparin) and that blood falls into certain well-defined groups that can be exchanged relatively freely between members of the same group. Nevertheless, the transfusion of whole blood is associated with a certain risk (hypersensitivity, hepatitis), and the recent advent of blood components represents a major advance in therapy because the patient can now receive only the components necessary for treatment. The type of blood or blood substitute to be administered is determined by the need of the patient and the availability of the most suitable preparation.

Uses

Replacement of blood loss resulting from trauma, surgery, or disease. Plasma volume expansion, severe clotting defects, and hemostasis (disease or drug-induced), and agranulocytosis.

Untoward Reactions

These depend on the blood or blood fraction being administered.

Viral Hepatitis
(Onset 4 weeks to 6 months after transfusion.) Characterized by anorexia, nausea, fever, malaise, tenderness and enlargement of liver, jaundice, and GI and skin reactions.

Hypersensitivity Reactions
Mild: urticaria, pruritus. Severe: bronchospasms.

Febrile Reactions
Characterized by fever (103°– 104° F, 39.4°– 40.0° C), tremors, chills, and headaches. Onset: during initial 15 minutes of transfusion.

Hemolysis
Potentially fatal complication caused by mismatching or mislabeling of blood or other human errors. Characterized by flushing, tachycardia, restlessness, dyspnea, chills, fever, headache, sharp pain in lumbar region, pressure feeling in chest, feeling of head fullness, nausea, and vomiting. Also hemoglobinuria and hemoglobinemia, and oliguria and acute renal failure. Usual onset: after administration of 100–200 ml incompatible blood. Shock and/or death may occasionally occur within minutes after initiation of transfusion.

Jaundice
Caused by larger than normal number of hemolyzed RBCs that may be present in blood approaching its expiration date. Occurs more frequently in patients with inadequate liver function.

Hypervolemia (overexpanded blood volume)
Characterized by labored breathing, cough, dyspnea, cyanosis, and pulmonary edema. Occurs more frequently in the very young, the elderly, or patients with cardiac or pulmonary disease.

Pyrogenic Febrile Reaction from Contamination Products (especially bacteria)
Characterized by chills, fever, profound shock, coma, convulsions, and often death. Onset: after transfusion of 50–100 ml.

Administration

1. Use normal saline as part of the Y setup (parallel setup) for blood transfusion. Do not use dextrose injection since this will cause clumping of RBC's. **Never use distilled water as this will cause hemolysis.**
2. Never add medication to blood or plasma.
3. Whenever possible, use plastic bags for transfusion to reduce danger of air embolism.

Nursing Implications for Blood, Blood Expanders, Fractions, and Substitutes

1. Regulate IV to 20 drops/min for the first 10 minutes and remain with the patient to observe for untoward reactions. **Stop the IV at once and notify medical supervision should any of the following untoward reactions occur:**
   a. *Anaphylactic reaction:* urticaria, tightness of chest, wheezing, hypotension, nausea, and vomiting. Have epinephrine, antihistamines, and resuscitative equipment available.
   b. *Circulatory embarrassment:* dyspnea, cyanosis, persistent cough (early sign), frothy sputum (late sign). Position the patient upright with lower extremities dependent. Obtain rotating tourniquets to be used as ordered.
   c. *Febrile (pyrogenic) reaction:* sudden chilling, fever, headache, nausea, and vomiting. Take temperature every half hour after chill and repeat until it is in the normal range.
   d. *Bacterial contamination:* severe chills, high fever, hypotension and shocklike state. Take temperture every half hour after chill and repeat until it is in normal range.
   e. *Hemolytic reaction:* chills, feeling of fullness in head, pressure feeling in the chest, flushing of face, sharp pain in lumbar region, distention of neck veins, hypotension, and circulatory collapse. Have mannitol available. Encourage oral fluids for next few hours. Measure and save all urine voided. Monitor intake and output. Have citrated blood tube available for bloods to be drawn to check for free hemoglobin in plasma.
2. Send the remainder of the material being infused and the equipment used for the infusion to the laboratory for analysis if an untoward reaction has occurred.
3. Increase to rate of flow ordered if no reaction is evident after the first 10 minutes.
4. Anticipate that the rate of flow for elderly and cardiac patients will be slower.

5. Check blood pressure and pulse every half hour during the infusion and report lack of response to therapy or significant deviations from patient's baseline whether elevated or depressed.

ALBUMIN, NORMAL HUMAN SERUM ALBUMINAR-5 AND -25, ALBUSINOL 5% AND 25%, ALBUSPAN 5% and 25%, ALBUTEIN 5% and 25%, BUMINATE 5% and 25%

Classification   Blood volume expander.

Remarks   Is prepared from whole blood and thus eliminates the danger of hepatitis infection. It is supplied as a 5% (isotonic and iso-osmotic with normal human plasma) and 25% (salt-poor solution of which each 50 ml is osmotically equivalent to 250 ml of citrated plasma) strength. It contains sodium, 130–160 mEq/liter.

Uses   Increases serum protein levels in hypoproteinemia; edema nonresponsive to diuretics; blood volume expanders for treatment of shock and burns; hyperbilirubinemia; and erythroblastosis fetalis.

Contraindications   Severe anemia or cardiac failure.

Untoward Reactions   Pulmonary edema, circulatory overload, dehydration, or heart failure.

Dosage   **IV infusion, individualized, 5%,** *Hypoproteinemia:* rate not to exceed 5–10 ml/minute. *Burns:* 500 ml initially; supplement as necessary. *Shock,* **adults and children:** 250–500 ml initially; repeat q 15–30 minutes, if necessary. **25%,** *Hypoproteinemia:* with or without edema; 1 ml/lb/day; rate should not exceed 2–3 ml/minute. *Hepatic Cirrhosis:* 25–50 gm/day or every other day to a total of 250–600 gm. *Nephrosis:* 100–200 ml q 1 to 2 days. *Burns:* determined by extent. *Shock:* Dose determined by condition of patient. *Hyperbilirubinemia* and *Erythroblastosis fetalis:* 1 gm/kg 1 to 2 hr before transfusion of blood.

Administration/ Storage   1. Do not use turbid or sedimented solution.
2. Preparation does not contain preservatives. Use each opened bottle at once.
3. Administer slowly to avoid circulatory overload. Give 5% solution, at rate of 2–4 ml/minute or more; 25% solution at rate of 1 ml/min or more.

Additional Nursing Implications   1. Administer slowly as ordered to prevent circulatory overload, which may result in pulmonary edema.
2. Observe patient for pulmonary edema demonstrated by cough, dyspnea, cyanosis, and rales. Stop administration of albumin immediately should any of these symptoms appear.
3. Monitor intake and output.
4. Observe for diuresis and reduction of edema if present.

5. Observe for dehydration necessitating further administration of IV fluids.
6. Closely monitor blood pressure and pulse.
7. Observe for hemorrhage or shock that may occur because of rapid increase in blood pressure causing bleeding in severed blood vessels that had not been previously noted.
8. Anticipate that after administration of albumin for treatment or prevention of cerebral edema, fluids should be withheld completely during the next 8 hours. Provide the patient with adequate mouth care.

BLOOD, WHOLE

Classification   Blood replacement.

Remarks   Because of the danger of hepatitis, mismatching errors, and allergic reactions, whole blood is only given when absolutely necessary.

Uses   Anemia, severe blood loss, and hypovolemia.

Untoward Reactions   Serum hepatitis and hemolytic (chills, fever, flushing, restlessness, headache, nausea, vomiting) and allergic (bronchospasms) reactions.

Dosage   IV: 500 ml; repeat as necessary.

Administration/ Storage
1. Store between 1°– 10° C.
2. Note expiration date on bottle (21 days for citrated and 40 days for heparinized blood).
3. Check label and ascertain typing and cross-matching of blood and patient.

DEXTRAN 40 GENTRAN-40, L.M.D. 10%, RHEOMACRODEX

DEXTRAN 70 MACRODEX

DEXTRAN 75 GENTRAN 75

Classification   Blood volume expander.

General Statement   Dextran is a biosynthesized, water-soluble, large molecule (polymer). It comes in various molecular weights (sizes). Dextran 40 has a lower molecular weight than Dextran 70 or 75. The lower molecular weight products cause fewer allergic reactions. The preparation is a blood volume expander but is not a substitute for whole blood or its fractions.

Uses   Shock, severe hemorrhage, and cardiovascular surgery.

Contraindications Severe congestive heart failure, renal failure, severe bleeding disorders, and known hypersensitivity. Use with caution in presence of renal, hepatic, or myocardial disease.

Untoward Reactions Anaphylactic reaction, pulmonary edema (chest tightness, angioedema), circulatory overload, increased clotting time, hypotension, tubular stasis, or blockage of kidney.

Dosage *Dextran 40,* **adults and children, IV:** 10–20 ml of 10% solution per kilogram daily. Total daily dose should not exceed 20 ml/kg.
  Dextran 70 and Dextran 75, **adults and children:** 500–1,000 ml of 6% solution up to maximum of 20 ml/kg during first 24 hours; **pediatric:** total dose should not exceed 20 ml.

Administration/ Storage
1. Do not administer unless solution is clear.
2. Dissolve flakes in solution by heating the solution in a water bath at 100° C for 15 minutes or by autoclaving at 110° C for 15 minutes.
3. Store at constant temperature, preferably 25° C, to prevent flake formation.
4. Discard partially used bottles since they do not contain preservatives.

Additional Nursing Implications
1. Complete blood tests should be done prior to administration because values are affected by dextran.
2. Observe for dehydration before initiation of therapy. Additional fluids may be necessary if dehydration develops.
3. Check specific gravity of urine (normal 1.005–1.025) because low values may indicate that dextran is not being eliminated. This may require discontinuation of drug.
4. Monitor output for oliguria or anuria, which may necessitate withdrawal of drug.
5. Report any sudden increase in central venous pressure which is indicative of circulatory overload.
6. Observe salt-restricted patients closely for edema, elevated BP, cough, cyanosis and moist rales. Dextran solutions contain sodium, which may precipitate pulmonary edema.
7. Observe for signs of bleeding (especially 3 to 9 hours after administration) from orifice, site of trauma, or purpura.
8. Check hematocrit after completion of administration.
9. Observe anesthesized patients on dextran 70 or 75 for vomiting or involuntary defecation.
10. Inform patients that administration of dextran may make subsequent crossmatching of blood difficult; patients should report receiving dextran if they require blood transfusions in the future.

HETASTARCH VOLEX

Classification Plasma expander.

General Statement This synthetic water-soluble large molecule (polymer) resembles glycogen. Its action is similar to dextran, but it produces fewer allergic reactions and does not interfere with blood crossmatching. Hetastarch is not a substitute for whole blood or its fractions.

Use Shock (burns, hemorrhages, sepsis, and surgery). Adjunct in removal of white blood cells (leukapheresis).

Contraindications Severe bleeding disorders, severe congestive heart failure, or renal failure with oliguria or anuria.

Untoward Reactions Circulatory overload. Rarely vomiting, mild temperature elevation, chills, itching, mild influenza-like symptoms, peripheral edema, and anaphylactoid reaction.

Dosage **IV infusion only: individualized, usual,** plasma expansion 500–1000 ml of 6% solution up to maximum of 1500 ml/day. *Leukapheresis:* 250–700 ml infused at a constant ratio, usually 8:1 to venous whole blood. *For acute hemorrhage;* rapid rate up to 20 ml/kg/hour. Slower rates for burns and septic shock.

Administration Discard partially used bottles.

Nursing Implications
1. Monitor output for oliguria or anuria necessitating withdrawal of hetastarch.
2. Monitor specific gravity of urine (normal 1.005–1.025). Low values indicate that hetastarch is not being excreted and mandate discontinuation of plasma expander.
3. Monitor hematocrit after administration of 500 ml of hetastarch. Values lower than 30% by volume should be avoided.
4. Report any sudden rise in central venous pressure indicating a circulatory overload.
5. Observe salt-restricted patient closely for edema, elevated BP, cough, cyanosis, and moist rales because sodium in hetastarch may precipitate pulmonary edema in patients with cardiac or kidney dysfunction.
6. Observe for purpura or other signs of bleeding from orifices or wounds, especially 3 to 9 hours after administration, because hetastarch may temporarily prolong bleeding time.

PLASMA, NORMAL HUMAN; PLASMA PROTEIN FRACTION PLASMANATE, PLASMA-PLEX, PLASMATEIN, PROTENATE

Classification Blood volume expander.

General Statement The cell-free portion of the blood, or a 5% solution of human plasma proteins in sodium chloride injection, are used when whole blood is unnecessary or unavailable. Preparations contain albumin, globulins, and electrolytes. Contains sodium 130–160 mEq/liter.

Uses   Hypovolemic shock, burn patients, hypoproteinemia, hemorrhages when whole blood is unavailable, and dehydration in infants and small children.

Plasma, normal human, which is available in fresh, frozen, and dried form, contains clotting factor; plasma protein fraction does not.

Untoward Reactions   Rarely, nausea, vomiting, and increased salivation. Hepatitis (plasma, normal human, only).

Dosage   **Individualized.** Plasma, normal human, **IV:** 250–500 ml. Plasma protein fraction, 1–1.5 liters of 5% solution (50–75 gm of plasma protein); **pediatric:** 33 ml/kg of 5% solution.

Administration/ Storage
1. Note expiration date. Preparations are stable for a long time when refrigerated.
2. Check administration rate with physician. Usual rate of administration: adult and infants, 5–10 ml/minute.

RED CELLS, PACKED

Classification   Blood replacement.

General Statement   Packed red blood cells or concentrates are prepared by removing plasma from whole blood. The preparation sometimes goes through a freeze-thaw process that yields a purer product. Administration of packed red cells reduces the risk of circulatory overload and the amount of transfused blood antibodies and electrolytes (sodium, potassium, citrate). Other dangers associated with blood transfusions (hepatitis, allergic reactions, mismatching) are not reduced.

Uses   Aplastic anemia, hemorrhages, and when it is desirable to replace red cells without expanding blood volume. Especially suitable for the elderly, infants, and patients with cardiopulmonary or renal disease.

Untoward Reactions   See *Blood, Whole,* page 227.

Dosage   Equivalent of indicated amount of whole blood.

Administration/ Storage
1. Store between 1°–6° C.
2. Check label for expiration date and to ascertain typing and cross-matching of blood and patient.

thrombolytic agents

Fibrinolysin, Human   Urokinase
Streptokinase

General Statement Several enzymes are currently used to promote the dissolution (lysis) of intravascular emboli and thrombi. These contain a large amount of insoluble fibrin. By activating the patient's own fibrinolytic system, the thrombolytic enzymes increase the degradation of the fibrin clots in the blood vessels. Since the enzymes interfere with the clotting mechanism of the body, the most serious complication of thrombolytic therapy is hemorrhage. Anticoagulant therapy is contraindicated during treatment with thrombolytic enzymes. Heparin therapy usually follows treatment with these agents.

Uses Acute, massive pulmonary embolism, pulmonary emboli accompanied by unstable hemodynamics, deep vein thrombosis, cleaning of occluded arteriovenous cannulae.

Contraindications Any condition presenting a risk of hemorrhage, such as recent surgery or biopsies, delivery within 10 days, pregnancy, ulcerative disease. Also hepatic or renal insufficiency, TB, recent cerebral embolism, thrombosis, hemorrhage, subacute bacterial endocarditis, rheumatic valvular disease, thrombocytopenia. The use of the drugs in septic thrombophlebitis may be hazardous. Safe use in children has not been established.

Untoward Reactions Hemorrhage, decreased hematocrit, fever, allergic reactions, phlebitis near site of IV infusion, increased tendency to bruise.

Drug Interaction Concomitant use of aspirin, indomethacin or phenylbutazone may ↑ chance of bleeding.

Dosage When administering thrombolytic agents monitor thrombin time q 4–12 hour. It should lie between 2 and 5 times normal control value. Dosage of thrombolytic enzyme should be decreased when values are lower than 2 times normal, increased when they exceed 5 times normal.

Nursing Implications
1. Avoid unnecessary handling of patient to prevent bruising.
2. Avoid intramuscular, intra-arterial, and intravenous injections to prevent bleeding at site of these invasive procedures.
3. Should IM injection be necessary, apply pressure after withdrawing needle to prevent a hematoma and bleeding from puncture.

4. Should intra-arterial injection be necessary, do not use femoral artery but rather use either the radial or brachial artery.
5. Apply manual pressure and a pressure dressing for 15 minutes after intra-arterial or intravenous injection. Retain pressure dressing in place for the next hour, and check frequently for bleeding.
6. Check that patient has had blood typed and crossmatched when receiving thrombolytic therapy.
7. Discontinue therapy if bleeding from an invasive procedure is serious, and call for packed red cells and plasma expanders (other than dextran). Have corticosteroids and aminocaproic acid (Amicar) on hand.
8. Check that thrombin time is less than 2 times normal control value (10 to 15 seconds) before starting an infusion. After therapy with thrombolytic agents, heparin should not be started until the thrombin time again is less than 2 times the normal control value. Take blood for thrombin time to lab in ice bath.
9. Anticipate the use of IV heparin and oral anticoagulants after thrombolytic therapy is concluded to prevent rethrombosis.
10. Observe sites of injection and postoperative wounds for bleeding during thrombolytic therapy.
11. Observe for allergic reactions ranging from anaphylaxis to moderate and mild reactions, which can usually be controlled with antihistamines and corticosteroids.
12. Provide symptomatic treatment for fever reaction. Acetaminophen rather than aspirin is recommended when thrombolytic agents are being administered.
13. Observe for redness and pain at site of IV infusion. If necessary, dilute solution further to prevent phlebitis.
14. Do not administer drugs such as indomethacin, phenylbutazone, or aspirin, which alter platelet function, without consulting medical supervision.

FIBRINOLYSIN, HUMAN THROMBOLYSIN

Classification Thrombolytic agent.

Remarks Fibrinolysin is a modified component of normal blood which promotes the dissolution (lysis) of thrombi. Anticoagulant therapy is usually used concurrently.

Uses Thrombophlebitis, phlebothrombosis, pulmonary embolism, and thrombosis of arteries (except thrombosis of cerebral or coronary arteries). Prophylactically, when indicated.

Contraindications Hemorrhagic diathesis, major liver dysfunction, hypofibrinogenemia. Use with caution after major hemorrhage, anesthesia, surgery, or myocardial disease.

Untoward Reactions   Acute allergic reactions, fever (3 to 4 hours after initiation of therapy), chills, nausea, vomiting, dizziness, headaches, hypotension, tachycardia, flushing, hypertension, urticaria, proteinuria, and angioneurotic edema.

Dosage   **IV infusion:** 50,000–100,000 units/hour for 1 to 6 hours daily. Treatment can be repeated for 3 to 4 consecutive days. *Acute, uncomplicated thrombophlebitis* may respond to a single dose of 100,000 units. *Excessive venous thrombi* present for 5 days or longer; 250,000–500,000 units/day for 1 to 3 days. *Arterial thrombi,* 250,000–500,000 units/day for 1 to 3 days.

Administration/ Storage

1. Dissolve in sterile water or 5% dextrose for injection. Do not reconstitute with solutions containing NaCl.
2. Reconstitute gently, by adding diluent slowly and rolling vial without shaking. Since preparation contains no preservative, its administration should be completed within 2 hours after reconstitution.
3. The reconstituted solution can be kept at 4° C for 8 hours (loss of activity < 10%).
4. Store dry powder at 2°–8° C.

Nursing Implications   Be prepared to assist in the treatment of acute allergic reactions, especially in patients receiving second course of therapy. Have oxygen, epinephrine, and corticosteroids available.

STREPTOKINASE STREPTASE

Classification   Thrombolytic agent.

Remarks   Most patients have a natural resistance to streptokinase that must be overcome with the loading dose before the drug becomes effective. Thrombin time and streptokinase resistance should be determined before initiation of the therapy.

Additional Contraindication   Streptokinase resistance in excess of one million as determined by immune assay.

Dosage   **IV:** 250,000 IU or more over period of 30 minutes; **maintenance:** 100,000 IU/hr for 24 to 72 hours.

Administration/ Storage (Additional)

1. Sodium chloride injection USP is preferred diluent.
2. Reconstitute gently as directed by manufacturer without shaking vial.
3. Use within 24 hours after reconstitution.

UROKINASE ABBOKINASE

Classification   Thrombolytic agent.

Dosage **IV: loading dose,** 4,400 IU/kg administered over 10 minutes; **maintenance, IV:** 4,400 IU/kg administered continuously over 12 hours.

Administration/ Storage (Additional)

1. Reconstitute only with sterile water for injection USP without preservatives. Do not use bacteriostatic water.
2. Reconstitute immediately prior to use.
3. Discard any unused portion.
4. Dilute reconstituted urokinase prior to IV administration in 0.9% normal saline.
5. Total volume of fluid administered not to exceed 200 ml.

CARDIOVASCULAR DRUGS

CHAPTER
4

cardiac glycosides

Acetyldigitoxin　　　　　　　　　　　Digoxin
Deslanoside　　　　　　　　　　　　　Gitalin
Digitalis, glycosides mixture　　　　　Lanatoside C
Digitalis Leaf, powdered　　　　　　　Ouabain
Digitoxin

General Statement

Cardiac glycosides, such as digitalis, are alkaloids obtained from plants. Their exact mode of action is unknown. They are used to (1) strengthen the myocardial contraction and thus improve the efficiency of the heart, and (2) improve disorders of the heartbeat known as arrhythmias. In many cardiac diseases, myocardial contraction is too weak to completely empty the ventricles of blood; therefore, not enough blood is pumped to organs of the body to sustain their normal function. In an attempt to satisfy the oxygen and nutrient requirements of the body, the myocardium contracts more rapidly, which enlarges (hypertrophies) the cardiac muscle, but normal cardiac output usually is not attained.

The cardiac glycosides stimulate the heart muscle to contract more forcefully and thus pump more blood to the body to maintain organ functions. The pulse rate then drops to normal levels. By increasing blood circulation to the kidney, cardiac glycosides also cause diuresis and correct the edema often associated with cardiac insufficiency.

Cardiac glycosides alter the transport of electrolytes across the myocardial membrane. In particular, the drugs cause an efflux of potassium and an influx of sodium and calcium. These changes are believed to affect the contractility of the myocardium, resulting in an increased force of contraction.

When digitalis compounds are used to treat certain disorders of the heartbeat (cardiac arrhythmias), they often slow conduction of the cardiac impulse through the atrioventricular node.

The cardiac glycosides are cumulative in action, and this effect is partially responsible for the difficulties associated with their use.

Uses

Prophylactic management and treatment of congestive heart failure, resulting from many causes; control of the ventricular contraction rate in patients with atrial fibrillation or flutter; and termination of paroxysmal supraventricular tachycardia (rapid atrial beating). Cardiac glycosides are often used in combination with other cardiac agents.

Contraindications

Coronary occlusion or angina pectoris in the absence of congestive heart failure or hypersensitivity to cardiogenic glycosides. Use with caution in patients with ischemic heart disease, acute myocarditis, ventricular tachycardia, hypertrophic subaortic stenosis, hypoxic or myxedemic states, Adams-Stokes or carotid sinus syndromes, cardiac amyloidosis, or cyanotic heart and lung disease, including emphysema and partial heart block.

Electric pacemakers may sensitize the myocardium to cardiac glycosides.

The cardiac glycosides should also be given cautiously and at reduced dosage to elderly debilitated patients, pregnant women and nursing mothers, and to newborn, term, or premature infants with immature renal and hepatic function. Similar precautions also should be observed for patients with reduced renal and/or hepatic function since such impairment retards excretion of cardiac glycosides.

Untoward Reactions Cardiac glycosides are extremely toxic and have caused death even in patients who have received the drugs for long periods of time. There is a very narrow margin of safety between an effective therapeutic dose and a toxic dose. Overdosage caused by the cumulative effects of the drug is a constant danger in therapy with cardiac glycosides.

Overdosage is characterized by a wide variety of symptoms, which are hard to differentiate from the cardiac disease itself. They include: changes in the rate, rhythm, and irritability of the heart and the mechanism of the heartbeat. Extrasystoles, bigeminal pulse, coupled rhythm, ectopic beat, and other forms of arrhythmias have been noted. Death most often results from ventricular fibrillation. Cardiac glycosides should be discontinued in adults when pulse rate falls below 60 beats per minute (70 in children). All cardiac changes are best detected by an ECG, which is also most useful in patients suffering from intoxication. Other, often early, signs of intoxication include anorexia, nausea, vomiting, excessive salivation, epigastric distress, abdominal pain and diarrhea, acute hemorrhage, and bowel necrosis; also headaches, fatigue, lassitude, irritability, malaise, muscle weakness, insomnia, stupor, neurological pain involving the lower third of the face and lumbar areas, paresthesia, chest pain, coldness of the extremities, and psychotomimetic effects (especially in elderly or arteriosclerotic patients) including disorientation, confusion, depression, aphasia, delirium, hallucinations, and rarely, convulsions. Visual disturbances, including blurred vision, flickering dots, white halos, borders around dark objects, diplopia, amblyopia, and disturbances in color perception, have also been observed.

Patients on digitalis therapy may experience two vomiting stages: The first is an early sign of toxicity and is a direct effect of digitalis on the GI tract. Late vomiting indicates stimulation of the vomiting center of the brain, which occurs after the heart muscle has been saturated with digitalis.

Instances of hypersensitivity reactions 5 to 7 days after initiation of therapy, including skin reactions (urticaria, fever, pruritus, facial and angioneurotic edema), have also been reported.

Patients suffering from digitalis intoxication should be admitted to the intensive care area for continuous monitoring of ECG. Administration of digitalis should be halted. If serum potassium is below normal, potassium salts should be administered. Antiarrhythmic drugs, such as phenytoin or lidocaine can be given if ordered by the physician.

Drug Interactions

One of the most serious side effects of digitalis-type drugs is hypokalemia (lowering of serum potassium levels). This may lead to cardiac arrhythmias, muscle weakness, hypotension, and respiratory distress. Other agents causing hypokalemia reinforce this effect and increase the chance of digitalis toxicity. Such reactions may occur in patients who have been on digitalis maintenance for a very long time.

Interactant	Interaction
Amphotericin B	↑ K depletion caused by digitalis: ↑ incidence of digitalis toxicity
Barbiturates	↓ Effect of digitalis glycosides due to ↑ breakdown by liver
Calcium preparations	Cardiac arrhythmias if parenteral calcium given with digitalis
Chlorthalidone (Hygroton)	Produces ↑ K and Mg loss with ↑ chance of digitalis toxicity
Cholestyramine	Cholestyramine binds digitoxin in the intestine and ↓ its half-life
Ethacrynic acid (Edecrin)	Produces ↑ K and Mg loss with ↑ chance of digitalis toxicity
Furosemide (Lasix)	Produces ↑ K and Mg loss with ↑ chance of digitalis toxicity
Glucose infusions	Large infusions of glucose may cause ↓ in serum K and ↑ chance of digitalis toxicity
Phenylbutazone (Butazolidin)	↓ Effect of digitalis glycosides by ↑ breakdown by liver
Phenytoin (Dilantin)	↓ Effect of digitalis glycosides by ↑ breakdown by liver
Propranolol (Inderal)	Propranolol potentiates digitalis-induced bradycardia
Reserpine	↑ Chance of cardiac arrhythmias
Succinylcholine	↑ Chance of cardiac arrhythmias
Sympathomimetics	↑ Chance of cardiac arrhythmias
Thiazides	Produce ↑ K and Mg loss with ↑ chance of digitalis toxicity

Laboratory Test Interferences

May ↓ prothrombin time. Alters tests for 17-ketosteroids and 17-hydroxycorticosteroids.

Dosage

PO, IM, or IV. *Highly individualized.* (See Table 9, p. 239, for usual dosages.)

Initially the drugs are usually given at higher ("digitalizing" or loading) doses. These are reduced as soon as the desired therapeutic effect is achieved or undesirable toxic reactions develop. The response

TABLE 9   CARDIAC GLYCOSIDES

Drug	Digitalizing Dose (DD) and Maintenance (MD)	Onset (ON) and Duration (DR)	Remarks	Additional Nursing Implications
Acetyldigitoxin (Acylanid)	**DD: PO, rapid:** 1.6–2.2 mg in 1 to 4 doses for 24 hr; **slow:** 1.8–3.2 mg for 2 to 6 days. **MD:** 0.1–0.2 mg daily.	**ON: (PO):** 1 to 2 hours. **DR:** 1 to 3 days.	More rapid onset and more quickly eliminated from the body than digitoxin. It is not completely absorbed from the GI tract	
Deslanoside (Cedilanid-D, Desacetyllanatoside-C)	**DD: IM** or **IV,** 1.2–1.6 mg in 1 to 2 equal doses. **Pediatric, IM** or **IV:** 22 μg/kg body weight. **MD:** Switch to **PO** preparation.	**ON:** 10 to 30 minutes. **DR:** 3 to 6 days.	Used for rapid digitalization in emergency situations (acute cardiac failure with pulmonary edema, atrial arrhythmias). Injection vehicle contains ethyl alcohol and glycerin. Protect from light.	
Digitalis, glycosides mixture (Digiglusin)	**DD: PO,** 10–15 U.S.P. units; **IV** 4 U.S.P. units. **MD:** 0.8–1.6 units **PO** daily.	**ON:** 25 minutes to 2 hours. Maximum effect: 4 to 12 hours. **DR:** 2 to 3 weeks.		
Digitalis leaf, powdered (Digifortis, Pil-Digis)	**DD: PO:** 50–150 mg 3 to 4 times daily for 3 to 4 days to a maximum of 1 gm. **MD:** 100–200 mg daily	**ON:** 25 minutes to 2 hr. Maximum effect: 4 to 12 hours. **DR:** 2 to 3 weeks.	This preparation contains standardized amounts of dried leaves of *Digitalis purpurea* plant for PO use.	

(Continued)

TABLE 9   CARDIAC GLYCOSIDES (*Continued*)

Drug	Digitalizing Dose (DD) and Maintenance (MD)	Onset (ON) and Duration (DR)	Remarks	Additional Nursing Implications
Digitoxin (Crystodigin, Detone, Digitaline Nativelle, Purodigin)	**DD: PO, IV, rapid:** 0.6 mg followed by 0.4 mg; **then** 0.2 mg q 4 to 6 hours; **slow:** 0.2 mg b.i.d. for 4 days; **pediatric:** 33 μg/kg. **MD:** 0.05–0.3 mg daily, **PO.**	**ON:** 25 min to 2 hours. Maximum effect: 4 to 12 hours. **DR:** 2 to 3 weeks	Most potent of digitalis glycosides. Its slow onset of action makes it unsuitable for emergency use. Drug of choice for maintenance. 1 mg digitoxin is therapeutically equivalent to 1 gm digitalis leaf. Is almost completely absorbed from GI tract Therapeutic plasma level 10–25 ng/ml	Withhold drug and check with doctor if plasma level exceeds 35 ng/ml indicating toxicity *Administration:* Inject deeply into gluteal muscle *Storage:* Incompatible with acids and alkali. Protect from light.
Digoxin (Lanoxin, SK-Digoxin)	**DD: PO, IM:** 2.0–3.0 mg over a 24-hr period. Give ¼–½ of total dose initially, and the remainder in ¼ doses at 6-hour intervals. **IV** 1–1.5 mg. Give 0.5–1.0 mg every 2 to 4 hr as required. **Pediatric:** 40–80 μg/kg **PO.** **MD:** 0.125–0.5 mg per day.	**ON:** 5 to 30 minutes. Maximum effect: 2 to 5 hours. **DR:** 2 to 6 days.	Action more prompt and shorter than digitoxin. Injection vehicle contains propylene glycol, sodium phosphate, and citric acid. May be drug of choice for congestive heart failure because of (a) rapid onset, (b) relatively short duration, (c) can be administered PO, IM, IV. Therapeutic plasma levels range from 0.5–2.0 ng/ml.	Give full DD only if patient has not received digoxin during previous week; if patient has received an even more slowly excreted cardiac glycoside, full DD should be withheld for 2 weeks. Withhold drug and check with doctor if plasma level exceeds 2.0 ng/ml indicating toxicity. *Administration:* Inject deeply into muscle and follow by vigorous massage. Rotate IM injection site. *Storage:* Incompatible with acids and alkali. Protect from light

				Storage
Gitalin (Gitaligin)	**DD: PO, rapid:** 2.5 mg **initially,** 0.75 mg q 6 hr thereafter for 24 hr; **slow,** 1.5 mg for 4 to 6 days. **MD:** 0.25– 1 mg daily; **pediatric:** 100 μg/kg in 3 doses.	**ON:** 10 to 20 min **DR:** 10 to 12 days	Oral only. Give only to patients who have not received digitalis therapy during previous 2 weeks.	*Storage:* Protect from light
Lanatoside C (Cedilanid)	**DD: PO:** 8– 10 mg. Give 3.5 mg on day 1, 2.5 mg on day 2, 2.0 mg on day 3, 1.5 mg daily thereafter. **MD:** 0.5– 1.5 mg daily.	**DR:** 16 hr to 3 days.	Oral only. Only give to patients who have not received digitalis during previous 2 weeks. Rarely given due to poor absorption from GI tract	*Storage:* Protect from light
Ouabain (G-Strophanthin)	**DD: IV:** 1 mg. Initiate with 0.25 mg followed by 0.1– 0.25 mg at 30 to 60 minute intervals or until 1 mg total given. Switch to **PO** therapy.	**ON:** 3 to 10 minutes. Peak effect: 30 to 60 minutes. **DR:** 1 to 3 days.	Most potent of the pure cardiac glycosides. IV only. Used only for rapid digitalization for emergency treatment of acute congestive heart failure; paroxysmal, atrial, or nodal tachycardia; or atrial flutter. Only given to patients who have not received digitalis therapy during previous 3 weeks	*Storage:* Protect for light

of the patient to cardiac glycosides is gauged by clinical and ECG observations.

There are considerable differences in the rates at which patients become digitalized. Patients with mild signs of congestion can often be digitalized gradually over a period of several days. Patients suffering from more serious congestion, for example, those showing signs of acute left ventricular failure, dyspnea, or lung edema, can be digitalized more rapidly by parenteral administration of a fast-acting cardiac glycoside.

Once digitalization has been attained (pulse between 68–80 beats/ minute) and symptoms of congestive heart failure have subsided, the patient is put on maintenance dosage. Depending on the drug and the age of the patient, the daily maintenance dose is often approximately 10% of the digitalizing dose.

Administration

1. Check the order, the medical card, and the bottle of medication to be given, since many of the cardiac glycosides have similar names. Their dosage and duration of effect differ markedly.
2. Measure all PO liquid cardiac medication exactly with a calibrated dropper or a syringe.
3. Administer after meals to lessen gastric irritation.

Nursing Implications

1. Take the adult patient's radial pulse for at least 1 minute before administering the drug. If the pulse is 60 or below or an arrhythmia that had not previously occurred is noted, take the apical pulse for 1 minute. If the apical pulse is 60 or below or an arrhythmia that had not previously occurred is noted, withhold the drug and check immediately with the physician. The apical, not the radial, pulse rate should be taken for infants and young children. Consult with the physician at what rates (both high and low) he/she wishes the drug withheld. The baseline rate usually is higher in infants and children than in adults.
2. Observe the cardiac monitor for arrhythmias.
3. Observe the patient for nonspecific symptoms that may precede toxicity, such as anorexia, headache, fatigue, lassitude, irritability, malaise, generalized muscle weakness, insomnia, stupor, facial pain, or visual disturbance.
4. Observe the patient and withhold the drug should anorexia, nausea, vomiting, or arrhythmia occur.
5. Observe elderly patients particularly for psychotomimetic effects (tachycardia, dilatation of the pupils, tightness in the chest and abdomen, and nausea followed by hallucinations, anxiety, and delusions).
6. Weigh the patient daily under standard conditions, preferably before breakfast.
7. Observe extremities of patients for edema and listen for chest rales.
8. Monitor intake and output.
9. Observe carefully for symptoms of hypokalemia, such as weakness, fatigue, ileus, and postural hypotension. Provide the patients with foods that have a high potassium content, such as orange juice and bananas.
10. Use cardiac monitor for newborn to identify early toxicity mani-

fested by excessive slowing of sinus rate, sinoatrial arrest, and prolongation of PR interval.

11. Be alert to cardiac arrythmias in children as they occur more frequently as signs of toxicity.

12. Observe the patient for positive response to digitalization as shown by improvement in rate and rhythm of heartbeat, improvement in breathing, reduction in weight, and diuresis.

13. Refer elderly or debilitated patients without adequate home supervision to a public health agency to ensure proper health supervision at home.

14. Teach the patient and a responsible family member:

a. That regular medical supervision is essential.

b. That medication must be taken exactly as ordered. Help develop a checklist that the patient can mark when taking medication. This is particularly helpful with elderly patients whose memory is sometimes poor.

c. Advise the patient that it is best to take medication after meals.

d. Stress that all previously prescribed cardioglycoside medication should be discarded to avoid mistakes.

e. Demonstrate taking a radial pulse and check that the patient or family member knows how to take it. The pulse should be taken before medication is administered.

f. Teach the patient to recognize toxic symptoms of cardiac glycosides. Stress importance of reporting toxic symptoms if they occur.

g. Encourage the patient to report symptoms of illness to physician.

h. Write out the directions that the physician wishes the patient to follow.

i. Instruct the patient to weigh himself/herself daily and to bring in the written record to the physician on day of appointment.

j. Teach patient and family how to maintain diet which often has low salt or low sodium content and increased potassium. Stress the importance of the diet.

k. Caution the patient to consult with doctor before taking other medications. Drug interactions occur frequently with cardiac glycosides.

SECTION 2

coronary vasodilators

Amyl Nitrite
Erythrityl Tetranitrate
Dipyridamole

Isosorbide Dinitrate
Nitroglycerin
Pentaerythritol Tetranitrate

General Statement   Most coronary vasodilating drugs are either nitrites or nitrates. Their chemical, pharmacologic, and clinical actions are closely related, and they are treated here as a group.

Drugs that improve the peripheral circulation and are specifically used for the treatment of peripheral vascular disease, are discussed under *Peripheral Vasodilators*, page 249.

Organic nitrites and nitrates are the oldest and still the most widely used vasodilating drugs. Their basic pharmacologic action consists of relaxing smooth muscle, particularly vascular muscle, by dilating the blood vessels, which consequently increases blood flow. A reduction in oxygen requirements of the myocardium (as a result of the drug) may also account for the therapeutic action.

Although nitrites dilate blood vessels in various organs, they are particularly useful for their effects on blood vessels of the heart and skeletal muscle. Therefore, they are used in the treatment of angina pectoris and ischemia of skeletal muscle.

The dilation of the major vessels of the body results in a drop in blood pressure and a decrease in the cardiac stroke volume. The dilation of the capacitance vessels (veins) can cause syncope in a subject in the upright position.

The action of the nitrites on the coronary vessels of the heart (dilation, redistribution of blood flow) and the decrease in cardiac work abolish the acute oxygen shortage (hypoxia) of the heart muscle. This relieves the acute pain characteristic of angina pectoris.

The various nitrites have different durations of action. The onset is usually very rapid and the duration is short when the drugs are given sublingually, which is the usual route of administration. Oral administration results in a slower onset and a prolonged activity.

Uses   Acute attacks of angina pectoris and prophylactic therapy aimed at reducing their number and severity. Investigational: reduce work load of heart in acute myocardial infarction and congestive heart failure.

Contraindications   Sensitivity to nitrites, which may result in severe hypotensive reactions, myocardial infarction, or tolerance to nitrites. Use with caution in patients with glaucoma, head trauma, cerebral hemorrhage or in anemic patients.

Untoward Reactions   Headaches (usually disappear with continued use and respond to salicylates), postural hypotension (fainting spells), nausea, vomiting, dizziness, and weakness. Occasionally, there is a drug rash, particularly with pentaerythritol tetranitrate. Chronic administration of nitrites can cause tolerance. Nitrites readily change hemoglobin to methemoglobin, large amounts of which impair the oxygen-carrying capacity of blood, resulting in anemic hypoxia. This interaction is particularly dangerous in patients with pre-existing anemia.

Extensive toxicity is rarely encountered during therapeutic use.

Drug Interactions	*Interactant*	*Interaction*
	Alcohol, ethyl	Hypotension due to vasodilator effect of both agents
	Pentaerythritol tetranitrate (Peritrate)	↓ Effect of nitroglycerin due to production of tolerance after long-term use of pentaerythritol tetranitrate

Laboratory Test Interference   ↑ urinary catecholamines.

Dosage   Most nitrites are administered sublingually and are rapidly absorbed through the buccal mucosa. They are also administered orally and, on occasion, parenterally. Amyl nitrite is administered by inhalation. (See individual drugs for specific dosage.)

Nursing Implications

1. Instruct patients carrying sublingual tablets for use in aborting an attack to observe the expiration date on bottle and to obtain a fresh bottle when needed.
2. Instruct the patient to sit or lie down to take sublingual tablet to prevent postural hypotension.
3. Allow the hospitalized patient to keep the drug at bedside but the nurse must note: (a) how much of the drug the patient requires to relieve angina, (b) how frequently drug is taken, (c) whether the relief is partial or complete, (d) length of time before relief, and (e) whether side effects are occurring. Chart observations.
4. Observe the patient for tolerance, which may begin several days after treatment is started and which is manifested by no response to the usual dose. Nitrites may be discontinued temporarily until such tolerance is lost and then reinstituted. During the interim, other vasodilators may be ordered.
5. Advise patients receiving nitrites not to drink alcohol because nitrite syncope, a severe shocklike state, may occur.
6. For patients taking nitrites that have prolonged effects, observe for nausea, headache, vomiting, drowsiness, and visual disturbances during long-term prophylaxis.
7. Observe patients for sensitivity to the hypotensive effects of nitrites, symptoms of which include nausea, vomiting, pallor, restlessness, and collapse.
8. Observe patients on additional therapy with other drugs that cause hypotension for potentiation of that effect.

AMYL NITRITE

Classification   Coronary vasodilator.

Remarks   This drug is more likely to produce headaches and a fall in blood pressure than other nitrites. The drug is most rapidly effective in treating acute attacks of angina pectoris. Onset of action: 30 seconds. Due to possible abuse, this drug should be kept well secured.

Uses   Angina pectoris; antidote for cyanide poisoning.

Dosage   *Angina pectoris;* **inhalation:** 0.18–0.3 ml (1 container crushed and inhaled). *Cyanide poisoning;* **inhalation:** every 30 to 60 seconds until patient becomes conscious and at increasingly longer intervals for the next 24 hours. Switch to **IV** administration of sodium nitrite as soon as feasible.

Additional Nursing Implications
1. Instruct the patient that fabric-covered ampule is to be enclosed in a handkerchief or piece of cloth and crushed by hand.
2. Advise the patient to sit down while breathing the vapors to avoid possible postural hypotension.
3. Advise the patient that the medication has a strong, pungent odor but that several deep breaths must nevertheless be taken.
4. Amyl nitrite vapors are highly flammable. Do not use near a flame or intense heat that could cause the substance to ignite.

ERYTHRITYL TETRANITRATE CARDILATE

Classification   Coronary vasodilator.

General Statement   Not suitable for control of acute attacks of angina pectoris. Tolerance to the therapeutic effect may develop over the course of long-term therapy. The drug has an onset of action of 5 to 10 minutes after sublingual administration and its effects last for 3 to 4 hours.

Use   Prophylactically to decrease the frequency and severity of attacks of angina pectoris.

Dosage   **Sublingual:** 5–15 mg. **PO: initial,** 10 mg t.i.d. to 30 mg. t.i.d.

Additional Nursing Implications
1. Inform the patient that all restrictions on activity cannot be removed even though the drug may permit more normal activity.
2. Advise the patient that a tingling sensation may occur at the point of contact with the mucous membrane when the drug is taken sublingually. If the patient finds this too objectionable, the tablet may be placed in the buccal pouch.
3. Report vascular headaches, should the patient complain of these during the first few days of therapy, because dosage may have to be reduced temporarily.
4. Administer analgesics if they are ordered to relieve headache.
5. Report GI disturbances. They may be controlled by reducing dosage.

DIPYRIDAMOLE PERSANTINE

Classification Coronary vasodilator.

General Statement This non-nitrate coronary vasodilator increases coronary blood flow primarily by selective dilation of the coronary arteries. This effect seems to be related to dipyridamole's ability to increase tissue concentration of adenosine diphosphate, itself a powerful vasodilator. Dipyridamole also decreases clotting time (platelet aggregation).

Uses Chronic angina pectoris (long-term treatment). Not indicated for acute attacks.

Contraindications Use with caution in patients with hypotension.

Untoward Reactions Minor and transitory: headaches, dizziness, nausea, flushing, weakness or syncope, GI distress, and skin rashes. Rarely aggravation of angina pectoris.

Dosage **PO:** 50 mg t.i.d.

Administration At least 1 hour before meals.

Nursing Implications
1. Observe patients for aggravation of angina pectoris which necessitates discontinuation of therapy.
2. Encourage continued drug compliance because patient may become discouraged by delayed clinical response (1 to 3 months).
3. Report untoward reactions because dosage adjustment may be necessary.
4. Instruct hypotensive patients to report subjective signs of hypotension, such as weakness, dizziness, and faintness, that may have been potentiated by medication and warrant a change in regimen.
5. Assess with patient positive clinical response demonstrated by increased exercise tolerance, reduced nitroglycerin requirement, and reduction or elimination of anginal attacks.

ISOSORBIDE DINITRATE ISDN, ISO-BID, ISORDIL, ISOGARD, ISOTRATE, LASERDIL, ONSET, SORATE, SORBIDE, SORBITRATE, VASOTRATE

Classification Coronary vasodilator.

General Statement Not preferred for relief of acute attacks of angina pectoris or coronary insufficiency. Onset of action is 2 minutes sublingually and 30 minutes orally. Duration of action is 1 to 2 hours after sublingual administration and 4 hours after oral administration.

Use Prophylactically to decrease frequency of attacks.

Additional Untoward Reaction Vascular headaches occur especially frequently.

Dosage **PO:** *prophylaxis*, 5–30 mg q.i.d. **Sublingual:** *acute attack*, 2.5–10 mg as tolerated, or q 2 to 6 hours.

Administration Administer with meals to eliminate or reduce headaches.

NITROGLYCERIN (GLYCERYL TRINITRITE) ANG-O-SPAN, DIALEX, GLY-TRATE, NITRINE-TDC, NITRO, NITRO-BID, NITROBON-TR, NITROCAP, NITROCELS, NITROCOT, NITROGLYN, NITROL, NITROLIN, NITRO-LOR, NITRONG, NITROSPAN, NITROSTAT, NITROSULE, NITRO-T.D., NITROTYM, NITROVAS, NITROZEM, TRATES, VASOGLYN

Classification Coronary vasodilator.

Remarks Tolerance develops rapidly. Onset of action is 1 to 2 minutes; duration is 30 minutes. Is available as sublingual, sustained release, and topical preparations.

Use Drug of choice for angina pectoris (prophylaxis and treatment).

Dosage **Sublingual:** 150–600 μg every 2 to 3 hr, as required. *Acute attacks*, 400 μg every 5 minutes until pain is relieved. Too great an increase in dosage causes headaches. **Sustained release:** 1 capsule or tablet (1.3–6.5 mg), q 8 to 12 hr. **Topical:** 1 to 2 inches q 3 to 4 hr, however, some patients require 4–5 inches. Optimum dosage is determined by starting with ½ inch, and increasing it by ½ inch increments for each successive application until headache occurs. Then decrease to largest dose that does not cause a headache. When terminating treatment, reduce both the dose and the frequency of administration over a period of 4 to 6 weeks to prevent sudden withdrawal reactions.

Additional Nursing Implication
1. Tell patient to store tablets in a tightly closed container and in a cold place; otherwise medication will lose its potency.
2. Ointment should be spread in a uniform thin layer on skin. Do not rub in.
3. To prevent skin inflammation, sites of application of ointment should be rotated.

PENTAERYTHRITOL TETRANITRATE ANGIJEN, ANGITRATE, ANTORA TD, DESATRATE, DIVASO, DUOTRATE, KAYTRATE, NAPTRATE, NEO-CORVAS, PENTETRA, PENTRASPAN, PENTRITOL, PENTRYATE, PENTHLAN, PERIHAB, PERITRATE, P.E.T.N., RATE, RATE-T, REITHRITOL, VASO-80

Classification Coronary vasodilator.

Remarks Not used sublingually. Available in combination with rapid-acting nitrites (Peritrate with nitroglycerin) and in extended release forms. Slow acting.

Uses Prophylaxis to reduce frequency and severity of attacks of angina pectoris.

Drug Interaction After long-term use, the drug may cause a decrease in the effect of nitroglycerin as a result of tolerance buildup.

Dosage PO: 10–30 mg before meals and at bedtime. **Extended release:** 30 or 80 mg b.i.d.

SECTION 3

peripheral vasodilators

Cyclandelate
Dioxyline Phosphate
Ethaverine Hydrochloride
Isoxsuprine Hydrochloride
Nicotinyl Alcohol

Nylidrin Hydrochloride
Papaverine Hydrochloride
Phenoxybenzamine Hydrochloride
Tolazoline Hydrochloride

General Statement Many conditions, including arteriosclerosis, reduce blood flow to the limbs. The resulting peripheral vascular disease may have serious consequences, such as tissue hypoxia and gangrene. Treatment usually involves relaxation of the muscles surrounding the small arteries and capillaries. Many of the drugs that act on various components of the autonomic nervous system (see chapter 6) are used for the treatment of peripheral vascular disease. The drugs that specifically act on the peripheral blood vessels are discussed here.

CYCLANDELATE CYCLANFOR, CYCLOSPASMOL, CYDEL

Classification Peripheral vasodilator, spasmolytic.

General Statement Cyclandelate relaxes the vascular smooth muscles and produces mild peripheral vasodilation. This results in an increase in peripheral circulation and in a slight rise in skin temperature of the extremities.
The drug has little effect on blood pressure and heart rate.

Its onset of action is about 15 minutes, with the peak effect occurring at about 60 to 90 minutes; its duration is about 3 to 4 hours. The beneficial effects of therapy are noticeable gradually.

Uses Symptomatic management of occlusive vascular disease and vasospastic conditions including peripheral arteriosclerosis, intermittent claudication, thromboangiitis obliterans, acute thrombophlebitis, erythrocyanosis, Raynaud's disease, scleroderma, noctural leg cramps, diabetic ulcers of the leg, frostbite, and selected cases of occlusive cerebrovascular disease.

Contraindications Should be used with extreme caution in patients with obliterative coronary artery or cerebrovascular disease. Safe use in pregnancy has not been established. Administer with caution to patients with glaucoma.

Untoward Reactions Flushing, tingling of extremities, sweating, dizziness, headaches, GI distress, and tachycardia. Side effects are dose related and occur more frequently at high dosage.

Dosage **PO:** 200 mg q.i.d. before meals. Dosage can be increased to 400 mg q.i.d. **Usual maintenance dosage:** when improvement has occurred, 100 to 200 mg q.i.d.

Nursing Implications
1. For patients experiencing gastric distress, emphasize the need to take the drug with meals or with antacids. The latter must be ordered by a physician.
2. Encourage the patient to continue taking medication by explaining that cyclandelate improvement usually occurs gradually.
3. Teach the patient to report untoward symptoms but inform him that flushing, headache, weakness, and tachycardia occur frequently during the first few weeks of therapy.

DIOXYLINE PHOSPHATE PAVERIL PHOSPHATE

Classification Peripheral vasodilator.

General Statement This drug resembles papaverine both chemically and pharmacologically. It acts directly on the heart muscle, depressing conduction and prolonging the refractory period. It decreases blood pressure and, at higher doses, increases the cardiac and respiratory rate.

Uses Vascular spasms associated with angina pectoris, acute myocardial infarction, peripheral and pulmonary embolism, and vasospastic vascular disease.

Untoward Reactions Nausea, vomiting, dizziness, sweating, flushing, drowsiness, and abdominal cramps.

Dosage   **PO:** 200 mg 3 to 4 times daily before meals and at bedtime. Single doses of 500 mg and daily doses of 2 gm have been used without ill effects.

Nursing Implication   Advise the patient to take medication at meals and at bedtime to minimize GI discomfort.

ETHAVERINE HYDROCHLORIDE CEBRAL, CIRCUBID, ETHAQUIN, ETHATAB, ETHAVEX-100, ISOVEX-100, LAVERIN, MYOQUIN, NEOPAVRIN-FORTE

Classification   Peripheral vasodilator.

General Statement   Ethaverine closely resembles papaverine. It is a nonspecific relaxing (spasmolytic) agent affecting peripheral blood vessels.

Uses   Various circulatory disorders accompanied by spasms of the blood vessels resulting in circulatory insufficiency. Spastic conditions of the genitourinary and gastrointestinal tracts.

Contraindications   Complete A–V block, serious arrhythmias, severe liver disease. Administer with extreme caution in presence of coronary insufficiency, pulmonary embolism, and glaucoma. Safe use during pregnancy and lactation not established.

Untoward Reactions   Nausea, anorexia, abdominal distress, dryness of throat, hypotension, skin rash, vertigo, respiratory and cardiac depression, arrhythmias, and headache.

Dosage   100 mg t.i.d., up to 200 mg t.i.d. **Time-release capsule:** 150 mg q 12 hr.

Nursing Implications
1. Urge patient to report untoward reactions because they will necessitate reduction of dosage or discontinuation of drug.
2. Very carefully assess patients with coronary insufficiency, pulmonary embolus, or glaucoma who are receiving ethaverine hydrochloride.

ISOXSUPRINE HYDROCHLORIDE ISOLAIT, VASODILAN, VASOPRINE

Classification   Peripheral vasodilator.

Remarks   The drug relaxes the vascular and uterine vasculature. This increases peripheral and cerebrovascular blood flow and relaxes the uterus.

Uses   Symptomatic treatment of cerebrovascular insufficiency, improves peripheral blood circulation in arteriosclerosis, Buerger's disease, dysmenorrhea, and Raynaud's disease. Threatened abortion.

Contraindications   Use with caution in patients with hypotension and tachycardia.

Untoward Reactions Occasional lightheadedness, dizziness, and palpitations.

Dosage **PO:** 10–20 mg t.i.d.–q.i.d. **IM:** 5–10 mg b.i.d. or t.i.d.

Administration Switch to PO as soon as possible.

Nursing Implication Monitor frequency, intensity, and duration of contractions when given during premature labor to counteract threatened abortion.

NICOTINYL ALCOHOL RONIACOL (AS TARTRATE)

Classification Peripheral vasodilator.

Remarks The drug produces direct peripheral vasodilation and increases blood flow to the extremities.

Uses Intermittent claudication associated with peripheral arteriosclerosis and thromboangiitis obliterans, diabetic vascular disease, and ischemic ulcers.

Untoward Reactions Flushing of the face and neck, GI distress, paresthesia. Tolerance to drug may develop after prolonged use.

Dosage **PO:** 50–100 mg t.i.d. before meals. Dosage can be increased to 150–200 mg 3 to 4 times daily. Nicotinyl alcohol (sustained-release): 150–300 mg b.i.d. morning and night.

Nursing Implication Advise patient to continue with good skin care, and refrain from smoking and excessive standing even though the drug offers symptomatic relief.

NYLIDRIN HYDROCHLORIDE ARLIDIN, CIRCLIDRIN, ROLIDRIN

Classification Peripheral vasodilator.

Remarks Produces vasodilation by stimulating *beta*-receptors. At present, drug is not considered very effective.

Uses Peripheral vascular disease, night leg cramps, Raynaud's phenomenon, frost-bite, and circulatory disturbances of inner ear.

Contraindications Acute myocardial infarctions, angina pectoris, tachycardia, or thyrotoxicosis. Use with caution in all patients with cardiac disease.

Untoward Reactions Nervousness, palpitations, nausea, and vomiting.

Dosage **PO:** 3–12 mg t.i.d.–q.i.d.

Nursing Implications

1. Inform patient that palpitations should subside as therapy continues.
2. Advise patient that improvement of symptoms may not be seen for several weeks.

PAPAVERINE HYDROCHLORIDE BLUEPAV, CEREBID, CERESPAN, DELAPAV, DILART, DIPAV, DYLATE, J-PAV, KAVRIN, LAPAV, LEMPAV, MYOBID, ORAPAV, PAPACON, PAVA-2, PAP-KAPS-150, PAVABID, PAVACAP, PAVACELS, PAVACEN, PAVACRON, PAVADEL, PAVADUR, PAVADYL, PAVAKEY, PAVA-MEAD, PAVA-PAR, PAVARINE, PAVASED, PAVASULE, PAVATEST, PAVATRAN, PAVA-WOL, PAVEROLAN, RO-PAPAV, SUSTAVERINE, VASAL, VASOCAP, VASOSPAN

Classification   Peripheral vasodilator.

Remarks   Nonspecific relaxing (spasmolytic) agent affecting peripheral blood vessels.

Uses   Various circulatory disorders accompanied by spasms of the blood vessels, resulting in circulatory insufficiency (myocardial, renal, cerebral, or peripheral). At present, drug is not considered to be very effective.

Contraindications   Complete A-V block; administer with extreme caution in presence of coronary insufficiency and glaucoma.

Untoward Reactions   General discomfort, flushing of face, sweating, dryness of mouth and throat. Pruritus, hypotension, increased blood pressure and depth of respiration. Various GI effects. Thrombosis at injection site. Rapid IV administration may cause arrhythmia or fatal apnea.

Laboratory Test Interference   ↑ SGOT, SGPT, and bilirubin.

Dosage   **PO:** 100 mg or more 3 to 5 times daily, or one 150 mg time-release capsule q 12 hr. **IM, IV:** 30– 120 mg given slowly (over 1 to 2 minutes); may be given q 3 hrs. **Pediatric:** 6 mg/kg.

Administration

1. IV injections must be given by physician or under his immediate supervision.
2. Do not mix with Ringer's Lactate Solution because a precipitate will form.

Nursing Implications

1. Monitor pulse, respiration, and BP closely for at least a half hour after IV injection of papaverine.
2. Report untoward autonomic nervous system and GI symptoms to physician.

PHENOXYBENZAMINE HYDROCHLORIDE DIBENZYLINE

See *Adrenergic Blocking Agents* (Sympatholytic), page 493.

TOLAZOLINE HYDROCHLORIDE PRISCOLINE HCL

See *Adrenergic Blocking Agents* (Sympatholytic), page 496.

SECTION 4

antihypertensive agents

Rauwolfia Alkaloids	Alseroxylon Deserpidine Rauwolfia Serpentina	Rescinnamine Reserpine
Veratrum Alkaloids	Alkavervir Cryptenamine Acetate Cryptenamine Tannate	Veratrum Viride Veratrum Viride Alkaloids
Ganglionic Blocking Agents	Mecamylamine HCl	Trimethaphan Camsylate
Agents That Depress the Activity of the Sympathetic Nervous System	Clonidine Guanethidine Sulfate Methyldopa Methyldopate HCl	Metoprolol Tartrate Phenoxybenzamine Hydrochloride Phentolamine Hydrochloride Phentolamine Mesylate
Monoamine Oxidase Inhibitor	Pargyline Hydrochloride	
Agents That Act Directly on Vascular Smooth Muscle	Diazoxide Hydralazine Hydrochloride	Prazosin Hydrochloride Sodium Nitroprusside

General Statement

Hypertension is a condition in which the mean arterial blood pressure is elevated. It is one of the most widespread chronic conditions for which medication is prescribed and taken on a regular basis. Most cases of hypertension are of unknown etiology and result from a generalized increase in resistance to flow in the peripheral vessels (arterioles). Such cases are known as primary or essential hypertension. The treatment of essential hypertension is aimed at reducing blood pressure to normal or near-normal levels because this is believed to prevent or halt the slow albeit permanent damage caused by constant excess pressure.

Essential hypertension is commonly classified according to its severity into mild, moderate, or severe. Most early cases of hypertension are mild. Patients exhibit only a transient increase in blood pressure when under emotional stress. This stage of the illness is called labile hypertension. Moderate or severe (malignant) hypertension can result in degenerative changes in the brain, heart, and kidneys and can be fatal.

Other types of hypertension (secondary hypertension) have a known etiology and can result from a complication of pregnancy (toxemic hypertension) or certain other diseases impairing kidney function. It can also be caused by a tumor of the adrenal gland (pheochromocytoma) or by blockage of certain arteries leading into the kidney (renal hypertension). The latter two cases can be corrected by surgery.

Most pharmacologic agents used to treat hypertension lower blood pressure by relaxing the constricted arterioles, which decreases the resistance to peripheral blood flow. These drugs exert this effect by decreasing the influence of the sympathetic nervous system on smooth muscle of arterioles, by directly relaxing arteriolar smooth muscle, or by acting on the centers in the brain that control blood pressure.

The drugs used to treat hypertension vary according to the severity of the condition and the patient's individual response. The most important classes of antihypertensive drugs are:

1. **Sedatives and Anti-Anxiety Agents.** These are used for the management of mild hypertension. Some of these agents, like mebutamate, seem to be particularly suitable for these cases. See Chapter 5, Sections 2 and 3.
2. **The rauwolfia alkaloids.** Alone or in combination with a diuretic, these drugs are used to control mild and moderate hypertension.
3. **Diuretic (saluretic) agents.** Very important antihypertensive agents, especially those belonging to the thiazide group. Often used in conjunction with other antihypertensive agents because they potentiate their effects.
4. **The veratrum alkaloids.** Used for essential, renal, and malignant hypertension.
5. **Ganglionic blocking agents.** Used to treat moderate to severe hypertension.
6. **Agents that depress activity of the sympathetic nervous system.**
7. **Monoamine oxidase inhibitors.**
8. **Agents that act directly on vascular smooth muscle.**
9. **Combination therapy** is often used.

RAUWOLFIA ALKALOIDS

General Statement   By depleting the nerve terminals, the rauwolfia alkaloids decrease the amount of certain neurohormones (norepinephrine, serotonin) involved in nerve impulse transmission. This results in a decrease in the effects of the peripheral sympathetic nervous system on blood vessels (the sympathetic nervous system normally constricts arterioles, thus raising blood pressure). The rauwolfia alkaloids decrease blood pressure and have a sedative effect accompanied by bradycardia. Cardiac output is usually reduced, and renal flow remains unaffected. However, they are not potent antihypertensive agents when given alone except in doses that produce unacceptable adverse effects.

When given orally, the drugs are cumulative, and maximum effects are only obtained 2 weeks after therapy is initiated. They do not induce tolerance or habituation.

Uses Primary hypertension of the mild or labile type, especially when associated with anxiety and emotional factors. Neurotic conditions characterized by anxiety and tension, chronic psychoses, psychomotor hyperactivity, or compulsive aggressive behavior.

Contraindications History of mental depression, colitis, or peptic ulcer. Use with caution in the presence of cardiac arrhythmias or asthma. Because the drugs have been reported to cause uterine contractions and pass the placental barrier, they should be administered with caution during pregnancy. In nursing mothers, they may cause nasal congestion in the infant, which can result in serious respiratory problems during feeding.

Untoward Reactions Nasal congestion, bradycardia, fatigue, lethargy, headache, dizziness, weakness, weight gain (appetite stimulation), nausea, GI disturbances, increased gastric secretion (especially at high dosage levels), nightmares, and muscular pain.

High dosages or long-term administration may cause severe depression, including suicide attempts. Alteration of sleep pattern is an early sign of depression.

Rare side effects include nosebleeds, insomnia, paradoxical anxiety, nervousness, dry mouth, sialorrhea, edema, decreased libido, gynecomastia, and Parkinson-like syndrome.

Rauwolfia alkaloids may cause acute cardiovascular collapse in patients under sudden stress, and administration should be discontinued 2 weeks prior to surgery. Complications have been noted during the administration of anesthesia.

Rauwolfia alkaloids must be discontinued 1 week prior to electroshock therapy.

Sodium and water retention may progress to congestive heart failure.

Rauwolfia alkaloids stimulate appetite, causing weight gain.

Overdosage is characterized by CNS depression, hypotension, miosis, and catatonia.

Sudden stress, such as surgery, may cause cardiovascular collapse in patients on chronic reserpine therapy, resulting in death.

Drug Interactions	*Interactant*	*Interaction*
	Anticonvulsant drugs	Reserpine ↓ convulsive threshold and shortens seizure latency. Anticonvulsant drug dose may have to be adjusted.

	Antidepressants, tricyclic
	  Amitriptyline
	  Nortriptyline
		↓ Hypotensive effect of reserpine

	Digitalis glycosides	↑ Chance of cardiac arrhythmias
	Ephedrine	Effects of ephedrine ↓ in reserpine-treated patients
	Furazolidone (Furoxone)	Additive hypotensive effect
	Levodopa	Reserpine inhibits the response to levodopa
	Methotrimeprazine (Levoprome)	Additive hypotensive effect

	Monoamine oxidase inhibitors
	  Pargyline (Eutonyl)
	  Tranylcypromine (Parnate)
		Reserpine-induced release of accumulated norepinephrine caused by monoamine oxidase inhibitors results in excitation and hypertension

	Phenothiazines	Additive hypotensive effect
	Procarbazine (Matulane)	Additive hypotensive effect
	Quinidine	Additive hypotensive effect and ↑ chance of cardiac arrhythmias
	Thiazide diuretics	Additive hypotensive effect
	Thioxanthines	Additive hypotensive effect

	Vasodilator drugs
	  Isoxsuprine (Vasodilan)
	  Nicotinyl alcohol (Roniacol)
	  Nylidrin (Arlidin)
		Additive hypotensive effect

Laboratory Test Interference ↑ serum glucose, urine glucose. ↓ Urine catecholamines, 17-hydroxycorticosteroids, and 17-ketosteroids.

Dosage **Usually PO.** See individual compounds, Table 10, page 258.

Nursing Implications
1. Observe the patient for personality changes, nightmares, or changes in sleep patterns since these are early symptoms of depression that may lead to suicide attempts.
2. Explain to responsible family members the signs that may precede depression, and stress the importance of medical supervision should these occur.
3. Have a sympathomimetic agent (ephedrine) on hand to use in case of overdose.
4. Monitor BP under standard conditions and compare with baseline and other previous BP readings. Report significant changes (obtain significant guidelines for a particular patient from physician).

5. Weigh the patient at least twice weekly under standard conditions to monitor fluid retention and evaluate severity by pitting.
6. Teach the patient and family about possible side effects and how to check for edema. Advise them to report condition should it occur.

Nursing Implications for Parenteral Rauwolfia

1. Observe the patient for respiratory depression.
2. Observe for postural hypotension.
3. Caution the patient not to get out of bed without assistance.
4. Monitor blood pressure before each parenteral dose of reserpine.

TABLE 10   RAUWOLFIA ALKALOIDS

Drug	Dosage	Remarks
Alseroxylon (Rautensin, Rauwiloid)	**PO: initial,** 2–4 mg in single or divided doses; **maintenance:** 2 mg daily.	Reserpine preferred for institutionalized patients.
Deserpidine (Harmonyl)	**PO: initial,** 0.25 mg 3 to 4 times daily for up to 2 weeks; **maintenance:** 0.25 mg daily.	Reserpine preferred for institutionalized patients.
Rauwolfia serpentina (Hiwolfia, Hyper-Rauw, Hywolfia, Raudixin, Rauserpa, Rauserpin, Rauval, Rawfola, Serfolia, Wolfina)	**PO: initial,** 200–400 mg daily in AM and PM; **maintenance:** 50–300 mg/day in one or two doses.	
Rescinnamine (Cinnasil, Moderil)	**PO: initial,** 0.5 mg b.i.d. for 2 weeks; **maintenance:** 0.25–0.5 mg daily.	Causes less bradycardia than reserpine. Reserpine preferred for institutionalized patients
Reserpine (Alkarau, Geneserp, Hiserpia, Lemiserp, Raurine, Rau-Sed, Releserp, Resercen, Reserjen, Reserpoid, Rolserp, Sandril, Serpalan, Serpanray, Serpasil, Sèrpate, SK-Reserpine, Tri-Serp, Vio-Serpine, Zepine)	**PO: initial,** 0.25–0.5 mg daily; **maintenance:** 0.1–0.25 mg daily. **Children:** 0.25–0.5 mg daily. **IM:** *Hypertensive crisis, initially,* 0.5–1 mg; **then,** 2 and 4 mg at 3 hr intervals.	Drug of choice for institutionalized patients. May cause postural hypotension and respiratory depression. Determine BP before each administration. 10 mg or more may cause delayed hypotensive reaction. When used alone, may not provide reliable control of hypertension. Most often used with thiazide diuretics or combined with hydralazine

VERATRUM ALKALOIDS

Classification   Antihypertensive agent.

**General
Statement**   The veratrum alkaloids are obtained chiefly from plants. They reduce both systolic and diastolic blood pressure and produce bradycardia by stimulating pressor receptors in the carotid sinus and heart which results in decreased arterial resistance and increased peripheral vasodilatation.

At usual therapeutic doses, the veratrum alkaloids do not produce orthostatic hypotension or adrenergic or ganglionic blockade; also, they do not affect renal blood flow. Cardiac output remains unchanged except in some cases of congestive heart failure associated with increased pulmonary artery pressure. These drugs are ineffective in the presence of severely impaired renal function.

At higher dosage levels, the veratrum alkaloids depress respiration and cause bronchoconstriction.

Some members of the veratrum family affect skeletal muscle, causing myotonia.

The range between an effective therapeutic dose and a toxic dose of veratrum alkaloids is very narrow. Therefore, the drug must be administered cautiously and blood pressure monitored frequently, especially during parenteral administration.

The onset and duration of the action of veratrum alkaloids depend on the mode of administration: PO: onset is 2 hours; duration, 4 to 6 hours; IM: onset 30 to 90 minutes, duration 3 to 6 hours; IV: onset immediate, duration 1 to 3 hours.

Uses   Essential, renal, and malignant hypertension (alone or in combination with other antihypertensive or diuretic agents). Hypertensive crises, eclampsia, preeclampsia and other toxemias of pregnancy, and hypertensive encephalopathy. These drugs are not in extensive use today.

Contraindications   Hypotension, aortic coarctation, digitalis intoxication, increased intracranial pressure not associated with hypertension, or pheochromocytoma. Use with caution in patients with chronic uremia.

Caution: If given to digitalized patient, it causes cardiac arrhythmias.

**Untoward
Reactions**   Hypotension, bradycardia, nausea, vomiting, excessive salivation, perspiration, hiccups, transient irregular heart rate and rhythm, tingling in fingers and mouth, feeling of warmth, flushing, dizziness, mental confusion, blurred vision, muscular weakness, and epigastric burning. All of these reactions are much more pronounced after parenteral administration.

Drug Interactions

Interactant	*Interaction*
Digitalis	Combination may cause dangerous arrhythmias. Use extreme caution
MAO inhibitors	↑ Effect of veratrum alkaloids
Morphine	Additive bradycardia
Quinidine	Combination may cause cardiac arrhythmias
Spironolactone	↑ Effect of veratrum alkaloids
Thiazide diuretics	↑ Effect of veratrum alkaloids. May require adjustment in dosage
Triamterene	↑ Effect of veratrum alkaloids
Tricyclic antidepressants	Hypotensive effects of veratrum alkaloids

Dosage   See Table 11, below.

1. Usually given after meals and at bedtime to reduce nausea. Morning dose is usually larger than afternoon dose. Patient should not eat or drink for 2 hours after taking the drug.

TABLE 11   VERATRUM ALKALOIDS

Drug	*Dosage*	*Remarks*
Alkavervir (Veriloid)	**PO, adults:** 3–5 mg t.i.d. p.c. Evening dose may be 1–2 mg larger than other doses.	May induce tolerance. Observe minimum interval of 4 hr between doses.
Cryptenamine acetate (Unitensen Aqueous) Cryptenamine tannate (Unitensen)	**PO,** *tannate,* **adult: initial,** 2 mg (equivalent to 260 CSR units); **maximum** 12 mg daily. *Acetate* **IV:** *Hypertensive crisis, convulsive toxemia:* 130 CSR units diluted with 20 ml 5% dextrose. Administer 1.0 ml/min. Repeat if necessary. **IM:** 130 CSR units (0.5 ml) Repeat if necessary.	If necessary, increase dosage weekly in ambulatory patients, daily in hospitalized patients. Solutions incompatible with alkaline solutions. No food for 2–3 hr after parenteral administration. Check blood pressure every minute during IV administration. Adjust dosage. Check blood pressure and switch to IM after it has been stable at desirable level for 1 hr. Switch to oral when feasible.
Veratrum viride (Veralzem)	**PO:** initial, 50 mg t.i.d. after meals.	Careful titration of dose is necessary in each patient due to variable GI absorption.
Veratrum viride alkaloids (Vera-67)	**PO:** 2.67 mg t.i.d.–q.i.d. after meals and at bedtime.	

2. Increase dose every few days and check blood pressure 2 to 3 hours after **PO** administration.

Administration Intravenous

1. Mix medication in a suitable IV fluid and administer slowly by drip infusion.
2. Take patient's BP every minute during the initial administration and adjust the rate of administration accordingly.
3. Discontinue the drug if systolic pressure falls 20 mm Hg or diastolic pressure falls 10 mm Hg or more.
4. Temporarily discontinue the drug if nausea or vomiting occur.

Intramuscular
IM injections should be spaced to allow time for each dose to become effective.

Nursing Implications

1. Observe the patient for hypotension, bradycardia, and respiratory distress which indicate overdosage.
2. Monitor blood pressure at least 2 to 3 hours after each oral dose. Blood pressure must be measured frequently with parenteral administration.
3. Have on hand at least 50 mg of pentobarbital sodium to use if emesis occurs when the patient is receiving IV therapy with a veratrum alkaloid.
4. Have on hand pressor amines (epinephrine) and atropine for emergency use with IV administration.
5. Monitor intake and output.
6. Weigh the patient daily and check for edema.
7. Advise the patient that side effects after oral administration are usually transient and may be relieved by changes in dosage or time schedule. Administer oral dose and instruct the patient not to eat or drink for 2 hours to minimize nausea.
8. Follow instructions very carefully for parenteral administration as patient may suffer cardiovascular collapse characterized by excessive hypotension, tachycardia, cold clammy-skin, and cyanosis.
9. Instruct the patient on IV therapy not to stand or sit up alone after being recumbent. Provide assistance for these patients.

GANGLIONIC BLOCKING AGENTS

General Statement This group of drugs depresses blood pressure by blocking the transmission of nerve impulses at the ganglionic sites in the autonomic nervous system and thus blocking nerve impulses that constrict the vascular walls. This results in a fall in blood pressure.

When the patient is standing, there may be an accumulation of blood in the lower limbs with a resultant decrease in the volume of blood returned to the heart. This causes postural hypotension, which can result in fainting.

Normally a decrease in the volume of blood returned to the heart would trigger an increase in the heart rate. The ganglionic blocking agents, however, also block baroreceptor reflexes. This prevents the increase in heart rate, and the systolic blood pressure thus remains low.

Uses   Moderate to severe hypertension; malignant hypertension; alleviates signs, symptoms, and complications of hypertensive vascular disease such as headaches, angina pectoris, retinopathy; congestive heart failure (dyspnea, cardiac asthma, pulmonary and peripheral edema, hepatomegaly); ECG abnormalities; and decreases cardiac dilatation. These drugs are of limited value in long-term management of chronic hypertension because of severe orthostatic hypotension, adynamic ileus, and urinary retention.

Contraindications   Mild or labile hypertension, uncooperative patients, glaucoma, organic pyloric stenosis, recent myocardial infarctions, uremia, and coronary insufficiency.

Abdominal distention, decreased bowel signs, and other signs of bowel stasis are reasons for discontinuing the drug.

Untoward Reactions   Most untoward reactions are related to the blocking of parasympathetic and sympathetic nervous systems because the drugs block ganglia to all organs of the body—not just to the blood vessels. As with other powerful drugs that cause a major alteration of physiological processes, it is often difficult to decide when an untoward reaction becomes excessive.

Severe reactions to ganglionic blocking agents include marked hypotension, constipation, paralytic ileus, and urinary retention. Milder reactions include dry mouth, blurred vision, diarrhea followed by constipation, anorexia, nausea, vomiting, weakness, fatigue, sedation, interference with sexual function, dizziness, syncope, and paresthesia.

High doses may cause tremors and mental disturbance.

Patients on low sodium diets or those who have had sympathectomy and hypertensive encephalopathy are particularly sensitive to the ganglionic blocking agents.

Drug Interactions

Interactant	Interaction
Alcohol	↑ The hypotensive effect of ganglionic blocking agents
MAO inhibitors	↑ Hypotensive effects of ganglionic blocking agents
Reserpine	↑ Hypotensive effects of ganglionic blocking agents
Thiazide diuretics	↑ Hypotensive effects of ganglionic blocking agents. Concomitant use permits reduction of dosage of ganglionic blocking agents to about one-half

Dosage   Highly individualized. (See individual drug entries.) The required amount of drug depends on the time of day (higher doses are generally required at night), on the season (lower doses are required in warm weather), and on the position of the patient (higher doses are required for an ambulatory patient than for one confined to bed).

It is important always to measure blood pressure in patients taking ganglionic blocking agents in the standing position or as the physician orders.

Nursing Implications

1. Teach patients that orthostatic hypotension is manifested by weakness, dizziness, and fainting and that these symptoms may occur when they rapidly change from a supine to a standing position. To prevent this, patients should slowly rise from the bed to a sitting position, dangle legs for a few minutes until they feel stable enough to stand up. A nurse or family member should assist as necessary.
2. Teach patients that if they feel weak, dizzy, or faint after standing or exercising for a long time, they should lie down if possible or otherwise sit down and lower head between knees.
3. Monitor blood pressure and pulse at the specific times ordered and have the patient in position as ordered for all readings (either standing or sitting). If this is not possible, alterations in time and position should be indicated on the chart.
4. Weigh the patient daily and examine for edema to determine whether weight gain is due to fluid or increased appetite.
5. Monitor intake and output since oliguria may occur due to excessive hypotension.
6. Prevent constipation if possible. Check with the physician regarding orders for laxatives, such as saline or other irritating cathartics, which could be administered if the patient fails to have regular bowel movements. Should constipation occur, the drug must be discontinued. Bulk-producing cathartics are ineffective.

MECAMYLAMINE HCL INVERSINE

Classification   Ganglionic blocking agent, antihypertensive.

General Statement   Also used for peripheral vascular disease.

The response to mecamylamine is gradual rather than abrupt. Mecamylamine HCl does not cause a sudden drop in blood pressure, and its effects last up to 12 hours.

The drug is less prone to induce tolerance than other ganglionic blocking agents. Tolerance to mecamylamine may necessitate an increase in dosage. Withdraw or substitute mecamylamine slowly. Sudden withdrawal or switching to other antihypertensive agents may result in severe hypertensive rebound. Since mecamylamine reduces peristalsis, it is a useful addition to a thiazide-guanethidine regimen in patients who experience persistent diarrhea with guanethidine.

Dosage   **PO: initial,** 2.5 mg b.i.d. Increase by increments of 2.5 mg every 2 or more days; **maintenance:** 25 mg daily in three divided doses.

TRIMETHAPHAN CAMSYLATE ARFONAD

Classification Ganglionic blocking agent, antihypertensive.

Remarks This drug also dilates the blood vessels directly. It acts very rapidly.

Uses During surgery when controlled hypotension is desirable, as in the case of brain tumors, cerebral aneurysms, arteriovenous fistula repair, aortic grafts and transplants, coarctation, anastomosis, and fenestration operations.

Trimethaphan is also indicated in hypertensive crises and in pulmonary edema resulting from hypertension.

Additional Contraindications Shock, severe arteriosclerosis, anemia, hypovolemia, polycythemia, kidney or liver disease, degenerative disease of the central nervous system, severe cardiac disease, asphyxia, or impaired renal function.

Additional Untoward Reactions May cause urinary retention and orthostatic hypotension. Also may precipitate anginal attacks in angina patients.

Dosage **IV infusion:** 1.0 mg/ml in 5% dextrose: 3–4 mg/min. Check blood pressure frequently. Effects appear almost immediately and persist 10 to 20 minutes after administration is discontinued.

Additional Nursing Implications
1. Monitor blood pressure closely. Systolic blood pressure should be maintained above 60 mm or at two thirds the usual value in hypertensive patients.
2. Observe for peripheral vascular collapse as demonstrated by excessive hypotension, rapid pulse, cold clammy skin, and cyanosis.
3. Levarterenol, ephedrine, methoxamine, and phenylephrine should be on hand to correct undesirable low blood pressure.

AGENTS THAT DEPRESS THE ACTIVITY OF THE SYMPATHETIC NERVOUS SYSTEM

CLONIDINE HYDROCHLORIDE CATAPRES

Classification Antihypertensive—depresses activity of sympathetic nervous system by action on the CNS.

General Statement Clonidine reduces the activity of the peripheral sympathetic nervous system (reduction in peripheral resistance) and produces bradycardia and a fall in systolic and diastolic blood pressure. The mechanism of action involves the stimulation of the alpha-adrenergic receptors of the CNS which in turn result in an inhibition of the sympathetic vasomotor centers. The drug also decreases plasma renin. Peripheral venous pressure remains unchanged. The drug has few orthostatic effects. It is well absorbed from the GI tract. A decrease in blood pressure is manifested 30 to 60 minutes after an oral dose. The maximum effect is attained after 3 to 4 hours and lasts up to 8 hours. Clonidine markedly decreases sodium chloride excretion. Potassium elimination remains unaffected. Tolerance to the drug may develop.

Uses Mild to moderate hypertension. A diuretic is often used concurrently. Investigationally for prophylaxis of migraine headaches, dysmenorrhea, and menopausal flushing.

Contraindications Safe use in pregnancy not established. Use with caution in presence of severe coronary insufficiency, recent myocardial infarction, cerebrovascular disease, or chronic renal failure.

Untoward Reactions Dry mouth (40%), drowsiness (35%), sedation (8%); also, sodium retention, edema, weight gain, constipation, dizziness, headache, fatigue, anorexia, malaise, nausea, vomiting, congestive heart failure, Raynaud's phenomenon, nightmares, nervousness, restlessness, anxiety, mental depression, various skin reactions, impotence, urinary retention, dryness of mucous membranes, itching of the eyes.

Drug Interactions

Interactant	Interaction
CNS depressants	↑ Depressant effect
Tolazoline	Blocks antihypertensive effect
Tricyclic antidepressants	Blocks antihypertensive effect

Laboratory Test Interference Transient ↑ of blood glucose and serum creatinine phosphokinase. Weakly + Coombs test. Alteration of electrolyte balance.

Dosage **PO: initial,** 0.1 mg b.i.d. Increase by 0.1–0.2 mg daily until desired response is attained; **maintenance:** 0.2–0.8 mg daily in divided doses. Tolerance necessitates increased dosage or concomitant administration of a diuretic. Gradual increase of dosage after initiation minimizes side effects.

Administration Drug should be discontinued gradually over period of 2 to 4 days. Administer last dose of day at bedtime to insure overnight blood pressure control.

Nursing Implications
1. Monitor BP closely during initiation of therapy, because a decrease occurs within 30 to 60 minutes after administration and may persist for 8 hours. Determine frequency of monitorings with medical supervision.
2. Observe patient closely for 3 to 4 days after initiation of therapy for weight gain (weigh daily in AM) and for edema, caused by sodium retention. Fluid retention should disappear after 3 to 4 days.
3. Report side effects because dosage is based on patient's blood pressure and tolerance. Side effects can be minimized by increasing dosage gradually.

4. Warn patient not to engage in activities that require alertness, such as operating machinery or driving a car, because the drug may cause drowsiness.
5. Observe for fluctuations in BP to determine whether it is preferable to use clonidine alone or concomitantly with a diuretic. A stable BP reduces orthostatic effects of postural changes.
6. Instruct patients that they are not to discontinue medication abruptly but are to consult with medical supervision before initiating any change in medication regimen. Rebound hypertension is prevented by gradual withdrawal of medication.
7. Assess patient with a history of mental depression for further depressive episodes that may be precipitated by the drug.
8. Emphasize the need for regular ophthalmologic examinations to determine retinal degeneration in patients on long-term therapy.
9. Have on hand IV tolazoline (Priscoline) for treatment of acute toxicity caused by clonidine.

GUANETHIDINE SULFATE ISMELIN SULFATE

Classification Antihypertensive—depresses activity of sympathetic nervous system.

General Statement Produces selective blockade of efferent, peripheral sympathetic pathways by depleting norepinephrine and inhibiting release of norepinephrine. The drug is not a ganglionic blocking agent and does not produce central or parasympathetic blockade.

Induces a gradual prolonged drop in systolic and diastolic blood pressure usually associated with bradycardia, decreased pulse pressure, a decrease in peripheral resistance, and small changes in cardiac output.

Full therapeutic effect is attained only after 2 to 7 days. Residual effects of the drug on blood pressure persist for 7 to 10 days after the drug is discontinued.

A slight tolerance to the drug may develop after prolonged use.

Uses Moderate to severe hypertension.

Contraindications Mild, labile hypertension, pheochromocytoma, or congestive heart failure not due to hypertension.

Administer with caution and at a reduced rate to patients with impaired renal function, coronary disease, cardiovascular disease, especially when associated with encephalopathy, or to those having suffered a recent myocardial infarction. During prolonged therapy, cardiac, renal, and blood tests should be performed.

Guanethidine sulfate should be discontinued or dosage decreased at least 2 weeks prior to surgery.

Untoward Reactions Dizziness, weakness, lassitude and exertional hypotension, bradycardia, increased frequency of bowel movements (persistent diarrhea is cause for discontinuing the drug), or edema (progressive edema and

congestive heart failure are also reasons for discontinuing the drug).
Acute cardiovascular collapse during stress.

More rarely, inhibition of ejaculation, dyspnea, fatigue, nausea,
vomiting, nocturia, urinary incontinence, dermatitis, alopecia, xerosto-
mai, increased blood urea nitrogen levels, drooping of upper eyelid,
blurred vision, parotid tenderness, myalgia, muscle tremors, psychic
depression, angina, chest paresthesia, and nasal congestion.

Side effects are usually dose related.

Drug Interactions

Interactant	Interaction
Alcohol, ethyl	Additive orthostatic hypotension
Amphetamines	↓ Effect of guanethidine by displacement from its site of action
Antidepressants, tricyclic Amitriptyline Nortriptyline	↓ Effect of guanethidine by ↓ uptake of the drug to its site of action
Cocaine	↓ Effect of guanethidine by displacement from its site of action
Digitalis	Additive bradycardia
Doxepin (Sinequan)	↓ Effect of guanethidine by displacement from its site of action
Hydroxyamphetamine (Paredrine)	↓ Effect of guanethidine by displacement from its site of action
Levarterenol	See norepinephrine
Levodopa	↑ Hypotensive effect of guanethidine
Methotrimeparzine (Levoprome)	Additive hypotensive effect
Methylphenidate (Ritalin)	↓ Effect of guanethidine by displacement from its site of action
Monoamine oxidase inhibitors Pargyline (Eutonyl) Tranylcypromine (Parnate)	Reverse effect of guanethidine
Norepinephrine	↑ Effect of norepinephrine probably due to ↑ sensitivity of norepinephrine receptor and ↓ uptake of norepinephrine by the neuron
Oral contraceptives	Reduce hypotensive effect of guanethidine
Phenothiazines	↓ Effect of guanethidine by displacement from its site of action
Phenylephrine	↑ Response to phenylephrine in guanethidine-treated patients
Procainamide (Pronestyl)	Additive hypotensive effect
Procarbazine (Matulane)	Additive hypotensive effect
Propranolol (Inderal)	Additive hypotensive effect
Quinidine	Additive hypotensive effect
Reserpine	Excessive bradycardia, postural hypotension, and mental depression
Thiazide diuretics	Additive hypotensive effect

Drug Interactions (*Continued*)

Interactant	Interaction
Thiothixene (Navane)	Reverses hypotensive effect of guanethidine
Vasodilator drugs	Additive hypotensive effect
Isoxsuprine (Vasodilan)	
Nicotinyl alcohol (Roniacol)	
Nylidrin (Arlidin)	
Vasopressor drugs	↑ Effect of vasopressor agents probably due to ↑ sensitivity of norepinephrine receptor and ↓ uptake of vasopressor agent by the neuron

Laboratory Test Interference

↑ BUN, SGOT, and SGPT. ↓ prothrombin time, serum glucose, and urine catecholamines. Alteration of electrolyte balance.

Dosage

PO, *Ambulatory patients:* **initial,** 10 mg. Increase in 10 mg increments every 7 days; **maintenance:** 25–50 mg once daily. *Hospitalized patients:* **initial:** 25–50 mg daily, increase and maintenance, as needed.

Drug given daily or every other day.

Often used concomitantly with thiazide diuretics to reduce severity of sodium and water retention caused by guanethidine.

When control is achieved, dosage should be reduced to the minimal dose required to maintain lowest possible blood pressure.

Nursing Implications

1. Caution the patient to arise slowly from bed by sitting on the edge of the bed for a few minutes with feet dangling before standing. This is especially important in the morning when patient should be assisted after lying flat all night since hypotension may be more severe.
2. Caution patient to lie down or sit down with head bent low should he/she feel weak or dizzy.
3. Caution patient to avoid sudden or prolonged standing or exercise.
4. Take blood pressure of ambulatory patient in both the standing and supine positions when visiting a physician.
5. Take a standing blood pressure on hospitalized patients regularly, if possible.
6. Observe for bradycardia and diarrhea and report. An anticholinergic drug (atropine) may be given.
7. Weigh patient daily and observe for edema.
8. Monitor intake and output, observing for reduced urine volume in particular.
9. Observe patients on therapy for stress, as this may precipitate cardiovascular collapse.

METHYLDOPA ALDOMET

METHYLDOPATE HCL ALDOMET HYDROCHLORIDE

Classification

Antihypertensive—depresses activity of sympathetic nervous system.

General Statement

Believed to reduce blood pressure by formation of α-methyl norepinephrine (which has less activity than norepinephrine). May also decrease plasma renin. Causes little change in cardiac output. The drug has a slow onset of action: 6 to 12 hours after PO administration and 4 to 6 hours after IV administration. Full effects of the drug are attained after 1 to 4 days of continued administration.

Tolerance may develop after prolonged therapy (usually between 2 and 3 months). Drug is less effective than guanethidine or ganglionic blocking agents. It is often administered in conjunction with a thiazide diuretic.

Uses

Moderate to severe hypertension. Particularly useful for patients with impaired renal function, renal hypertension, resistant cases of hypertension complicated by stroke, coronary artery disease or nitrogen retention, and for hypertensive crises.

Contraindications

Sensitivity to drug, labile and mild hypertension, pregnancy, active hepatic disease, or pheochromocytoma. Use with caution in patients with a history of liver disease.

Untoward Reactions

Sedation (tends to disappear with use), vertigo, headache, asthenia and weakness, orthostatic hypotension, syncope, aggravation of angina pectoris, paradoxical pressor response, sodium retention, edema, anemia, or fever (during initial weeks of therapy).

Rare side effects include jaundice, bradycardia, nasal stuffiness, dry mouth, GI symptoms, "black tongue," breast enlargement, lactation, impotence, skin rash, mild arthralgia, myalgia, paresthesias, parkinsonism, and psychic disturbances. Affects Coombs test.

Many of these untoward reactions are dose related and disappear with continued use of the drug.

Drug Interactions

Interactant	Interaction
Amphetamines	↓ Hypotensive effect of methyldopa by ↑ sympathetic activity
Antidepressants, tricyclic Amitriptyline Nortriptyline	Tricyclic antidepressants may block hypotensive effect of methyldopa
Barbiturates	↓ Hypotensive effect of methyldopa by ↑ breakdown by liver
Ephedrine	Action of ephedrine ↓ in methyldopa-treated patients
Furazolidone (Furoxone)	Additive hypotensive effect
Levodopa	Methyldopa inhibits effect of levodopa
Methotrimeprazine (Levoprome)	Additive hypotensive effect
MAO inhibitors Pargyline (Eutonyl) Tranylcypromine (Parnate)	Monoamine oxidase inhibitors may reverse hypotensive effect of methyldopa and cause headache and hallucinations

Drug Interactions (*Continued*)

Interactant	Interaction
Norepinephrine (Levophed)	Magnitude and duration of pressor response to norepinephrine ↑ in patients receiving methyldopa
Phenothiazines	Additive hypotensive effect
Procarbazine (Matulane)	Additive hypotensive effect
Propranolol (Inderal)	Additive hypotensive effect
Quinidine	Additive hypotensive effect
Thiazide diuretics	Additive hypotensive effect
Thioxanthines	Additive hypotensive effect
Vasodilator drugs Isoxsuprine (Vasodilan) Nicotinyl alcohol (Roniacol) Nylidrin (Arlidrin)	Additive hypotensive effect

Laboratory Test Interference

False + or ↑: Alkaline phosphatase, bilirubin, BUN, BSP, cephalin flocculation, creatinine, SGOT, SGPT, uric acid, Coomb's test, prothrombin time as well as others.

Dosage

Methyldopa, **PO: initial:** 250 mg b.i.d.– t.i.d. for 2 days. Adjust dose every 2 days. If increased, start with evening dose. Usual **maintenance:** 0.5– 2.0 gm daily in divided doses; **maximum:** 3 gm daily. Transfer to and from other antihypertensive agents should occur gradually, with initial dose of methyldopa not exceeding 500 mg. *Remarks:* Do not use combination medication to initiate therapy. **Pediatric: initial,** 10 mg/kg daily, adjusting maintenance to a maximum of 65 mg/kg.

Methyldopate HCl: 250– 500 mg q 6 hr; **maximum:** 1 gm q 6 hr by **IV infusion** for *hypertensive crisis.* Switch to oral methyldopa, at same dosage level, when blood pressure is brought under control. **Pediatric:** 20– 40 mg/kg q 6 hr; **maximum:** 65 mg/kg up to maximum of 3 gm daily.

Nursing Implications

1. Caution patients to arise from bed slowly and to dangle feet from edge of bed to prevent dizziness and fainting. Adjusting dosage may prevent morning hypotension.
2. Observe for signs of tolerance which may occur during the second or third month of therapy.
3. Weigh patient daily and observe carefully for edema.
4. Monitor intake and output, observing particularly for reduced urine volume.
5. Sedation may occur when therapy is first started but disappears after the maintenance dose is established.
6. Advise patient that in rare cases methyldopa may darken urine or turn it blue but that this reaction is not harmful.

METOPROLOL TARTRATE LOPRESSOR

Classification Antihypertensive, beta-blocker.

General Statement Metoprolol is a beta-adrenergic receptor blocking agent (beta-blocker) that preferentially acts on the receptors located in the cardiac muscle. It is an effective antihypertensive agent. At higher doses, the drug has broncho- and vasodilating effects. The agent is rapidly absorbed after PO administration.

Uses Hypertension, alone or with other antihypertensive drugs or thiazide diuretics.

Contraindications Sinus bradycardia, heart block, cardiogenic shock and overt cardiac failure. Use with caution in patients with cardiac conditions, diabetes mellitus, thyrotoxicosis, impaired renal and hepatic function and during major surgery. Safe use in children or during lactation not established. Only use during pregnancy when clearly needed.

Untoward Reactions Mostly mild and transitory. CNS: tiredness, drowsiness and dizziness (10%), mental depression (5%). Cardiovascular: shortness of breath and bradycardia (3%), also palpitations, cold extremities, congestive heart failure. GI Tract: diarrhea (5%), nausea, gastric pain, flatulence, heartburn. Allergic pruritus.

Drug Interactions Additive hypotensive effects if administered with reserpine or other drugs that deplete norepinephrine.

Dosage **PO, individualized: usual, initial,** 50 mg b.i.d., alone or with diuretic. **Maintenance:** 100 mg b.i.d. up to 450 mg/day in divided doses. Better control is attained in some patients when drug is administered t.i.d. Abrupt discontinuation may result in angina being precipitated.

Nursing Implications
1. Monitor blood pressure prior to administering dose of metoprolol tartrate to determine whether satisfactory control is being maintained throughout care.
2. Monitor patient for dyspnea, increasing cough, edema, fatigue, and altered voice and facial expression—signs and symptoms of congestive heart failure that may be precipitated by metoprolol tartrate.
3. Warn patient not to interrupt therapy without consulting with doctor because angina pectoris or even myocardial infarction may be precipitated.
4. Warn patient to use caution driving a car or operating hazardous machinery because drug may cause dizziness. Report effect to doctor.
5. Instruct patient to notify doctor if diarrhea occurs because it may be drug related.
6. Teach diabetic patients to be alert for hypoglycemia because metoprolol tartrate masks the characteristic signs of acute hypoglycemia, such as changes in pulse, tachycardia, and onset of sweating.
7. Be alert to symptoms of mental depression, hallucinations, disorientation, and sensory impairment.
8. Monitor patients on catecholamine depleting drugs for hypotension and/or marked bradycardia, which may lead to vertigo, syncope, or postural hypotension.

9. Mark clearly chart of pre-op patient who has been receiving metoprolol tartrate as anesthetist should be aware of therapy, which may cause hypotensive problems during and after surgery.

PHENOXYBENZAMINE HYDROCHLORIDE DIBENZYLINE

Classification   Antihypertensive—depresses activity of sympathetic nervous system. (See page 493.)

PHENTOLAMINE HYDROCHLORIDE REGITINE HCl

PHENTOLAMINE MESYLATE REGITINE MESYLATE

Classification   Antihypertensive—depresses activity of sympathetic nervous system. (See page 494.)

MONOAMINE OXIDASE INHIBITOR

PARGYLINE HYDROCHLORIDE EUTONYL

Classification   Antihypertensive agent, monoamine oxidase inhibitor.

General Statement   See *Monoamine Oxidase Inhibitors*, Chapter 5, Section 9. The full effect of this drug is achieved only after several weeks and residual effects may persist for 3 weeks after the drug is discontinued. Tolerance develops readily. Discontinue the drug at least 2 weeks prior to elective surgery.

Uses   Moderate to severe hypertension.

Contraindications   Labile and mild hypertension, advanced renal failure, pheochromocytoma, paranoid schizophrenia, or hyperthyroidism.

Untoward Reactions   See Chapter 5, Section 9.

Drug Interactions and Laboratory Test Interference   See Chapter 5, Section 9.

Dosage   **PO, adult, initial:** 25–50 mg once daily for 1 to 2 weeks. Increase at weekly intervals by 10–25 mg until desired therapeutic effect is attained. **Initial dose** *for elderly or sympathectomized patients:* 25 mg daily. **Maintenance:** 50–75 mg or higher daily but not to exceed 200 mg. Do not use in children under 12 years of age.

Nursing Implications

1. Warn patients not to take any other medication (particularly decongestants) unless they consult with their physician first.
2. Caution patients not to eat aged or natural cheeses (e.g., Cheddar, Camembert, and Stilton) as well as other foods that require the actions of molds or bacteria for their preparation, such as pickled herring. Alcoholic beverages in any form should not be consumed. Concomitant use of pargyline with such foods may lead to hypertensive crisis.
3. Advise patients that they may feel dizzy or faint particularly when changing position from supine to standing. Patients should rise slowly from bed. If they feel dizzy or faint, they should lie or sit down with head lowered.
4. Instruct patients to report headache or other unusual symptoms.
5. Advise patients, particularly those with angina or coronary heart disease, not to increase their physical activity while on medication, although they may feel better.
6. Weigh the patient daily and check for edema. Observe whether weight gain is due to fluid or increased appetite.
7. Monitor intake and output.
8. Check on the patient's bowel function. Report to physician if a laxative is needed.
9. Provide good mouth care to counteract nausea and dry mouth.

AGENTS THAT ACT DIRECTLY ON VASCULAR SMOOTH MUSCLE

DIAZOXIDE HYPERSTAT IV

Classification Antihypertensive—acts directly on vascular smooth muscle.

General Statement This drug produces direct vasodilation of the peripheral arterioles. Produces immediate fall in blood pressure (1 to 5 minutes), with a 24-hour return to pretreatment levels. Diazoxide is considered, by many authorities, an agent of choice for hypertensive crisis.

A potent diuretic is often administered concomitantly.

Uses Hypertensive crisis (malignant hypertension). Especially suitable for patients with impaired renal function, hypertensive encephalopathy, hypertension complicated by left ventricular failure and in eclampsia.

Contraindications Hypersensitivity to drug or thiazide diuretics.

Untoward Reactions Severe hyperglycemia. Sodium and water retention. Hypotension (rare), transient myocardial and/or cerebral ischemia, transient tachycardia, palpitations, or bradycardia. GI distress: nausea, vomiting, abdominal discomfort, diarrhea, or constipation. Pain at injection site.

Drug Interactions	*Interactant*	*Interaction*
	Anticoagulants, oral	↑ Effect of oral anticoagulants due to ↓ plasma protein binding
	Reserpine	↑ Hypotensive effect
	Thiazide diuretics	↑ Hyperglycemic, hyperuricemic, and antihypertensive effect of diazoxide
	Vasodilators, peripheral	↑ Hypoglycemic effect

Laboratory Test Interference   False positive or ↑ uric acid

Dosage   **IV:** 300 mg or 5 mg/kg; **pediatric:** 5 mg/kg. Do not administer **IM** or **SC.**

Administration/ Storage
1. Protect from light, heat, and freezing.
2. Inject rapidly (30 seconds) undiluted into a peripheral vein to maximize response.

Nursing Implications
1. Have the patient recumbent during and for 30 minutes after injection.
2. Have the patient recumbent for 8 to 10 hours if furosemide (Lasix) is administered as part of therapy.
3. Closely monitor BP after injection until it has stabilized and then every hour thereafter.
4. Check final BP of patients on arising after injection.
5. Monitor urine for glycosuria while the patient is on therapy.

HYDRALAZINE HYDROCHLORIDE APRESOLINE, DRALZINE, NOR-PRESS 25, ROLAZINE

Classification   Antihypertensive—acts directly on vascular smooth muscle.

General Statement   Hydralazine reduces elevated blood pressure (diastolic more than systolic), increases cardiac output, and increases blood flow through the kidneys. It acts both on the central nervous system and directly on arteriolar smooth muscle causing vasodilatation.

When used alone, the dosage required to produce an antihypertensive effect usually causes a high incidence of unwanted side effects. Thus, to minimize side effects, lower dosages of hydralazine are often given in combination with other drugs.

Uses   Various hypertensive states, including those associated with pregnancy and after sympathectomy. Early malignant hypertension.

Contraindications   Coronary artery disease, angina pectoris, advanced renal disease (as in chronic renal hypertension), and chronic glomerulonephritis.

Untoward Reactions   Postural hypotension, tachycardia, generalized severe headache, dizziness, faintness, palpitation, angina, numbness and tingling of the extremities, malaise, depression, disorientation, and anxiety. Myocardial infarction. GI disturbances, severe GI hemorrhages, localized edema, sodium retention, decreased urine volume, influenzalike symptoms including fever and muscle pain, and rheumatoid arthritis syndrome also occur. The drug can also cause disseminated lupus. Most of these effects disappear with continued use. Side effects are less severe when dosage is increased slowly and when corticosteroids are administered if necessary.

Drug Interactions

Interactant	Interaction
Methotrimeprazine (Levoprome)	Additive hypotensive effect
Procainamide	Additive hypotensive effect
Propranolol (Inderal)	Additive hypotensive effect
Quinidine	Additive hypotensive effect
Sympathomimetics	↑ Risk of tachycardia and angina

Dosage

PO, adult: initial, 10–25 mg b.i.d.–t.i.d. Daily dose may be increased by 10–25 mg until desired effect is achieved. **Maximal daily dose:** 400 mg usually in 4 divided doses; **children: initial,** 0.75 mg/kg daily in 4 divided doses. Dosage may be increased gradually up to 7.5 mg/kg daily.

IV, IM, *hypertensive crisis,* **adults:** 10–20 mg, increased to 40 mg if necessary. Oral therapy should be instituted as soon as blood pressure is controlled. **Children:** 1.7–3.5 mg/kg daily in 4–6 divided doses.

Adjust as needed. Administer **PO** and at bedtime to ambulatory patients with moderate to severe hypertension. Reduce dosage in patients with renal damage. Blood pressure may fall within 5 to 10 minutes after parenteral injection.

Food increases the bioavailability of the drug.

Nursing Implications

1. Observe for an influenza-type syndrome early during therapy or a rheumatoid syndrome which may necessitate discontinuing the drug.
2. Advise the patient of possible side effects. After taking first dose of medication, the patient may experience headache, palpitation, and, possibly, mild postural hypotension. These symptoms may persist for 7 to 10 days on continued treatment.
3. **Caution patients** that they may feel weak and dizzy. Should this occur instruct patients to lie down or sit down with head low.
4. Advise patients to change from supine to sitting position slowly.
5. Monitor blood pressure several times a day under standardized conditions, either sitting or standing, as ordered by physician.
6. Monitor blood pressure within 5 minutes after the parenteral injection of the medication.
7. Weigh the patient daily and check for edema.
8. Monitor intake and output, observing particularly for a reduction in output.

PRAZOSIN HYDROCHLORIDE MINIPRESS

Classification Antihypertensive—acts directly on vascular smooth muscle.

General Statement Prazosin seems to produce direct vasodilation of the peripheral arterioles and is associated with decreased total peripheral resistance. Cardiac output, heart rate, and renal blood flow are unaffected by the drug. The drug is well absorbed from GI tract. Blood pressure begins to decrease within 2 hours after PO administration. The effect peaks after 2 to 4 hours and lasts less than 24 hours. The drug can be used to initiate hypotensive therapy and is most effective when used in conjunction with a diuretic. Tolerance has not been observed in long-term therapy. Often used in conjunction with a diuretic or other antihypertensive drug.

Uses Mild to moderate hypertension.

Contraindications Safe use in pregnancy and during childhood has not been established.

Untoward Reactions Syncope 30 to 90 minutes after administration of initial dose (usually 2 or more mg), increase of dosage, or addition of other antihypertensive agent. Symptoms of decreased blood pressure, such as dizziness (10%) and lightheadedness, headaches (8%), drowsiness (7.6%), fatigue, weakness, palpitations, GI disturbances, edema, dyspnea, tachycardia, nervousness, vertigo, depression, rash, pruritus, urinary frequency, impotence, blurred vision, reddened sclera, tinnitus, dry mouth, nasal congestion, and diaphoresis.

Drug Interactions

Interactant	Interaction
Antihypertensives (other)	↑ Antihypertensive effect
Diuretics	↑ Antihypertensive effect
Propranolol	Especially pronounced additive hypotensive effect

Dosage **PO:** *individualized*, always initiate with 1 mg t.i.d.; **maintenance:** if necessary, increase gradually to 20 mg daily in 2 to 3 divided doses. If used with diuretics or other antihypertensives, reduce dose to 1–2 mg t.i.d.

Administration Food may delay absorption and may minimize side-effects of the drug.

Nursing Implications
1. Encourage patient to be drug compliant though full effect of drug may not be evident for 4 to 6 weeks.
2. Report side effects to medical supervisor because reduction in dosage may be indicated.
3. Instruct patients not to discontinue medication unless they are so directed by medical supervision.
4. Caution patients against taking any cold, cough, or allergy medication, unless they check with medical supervision because sym-

pathomimetic component of such medication will interfere with action of prazosin.

5. Warn patient not to engage in activities which require alertness, such as operating machinery or driving a car as the drug may cause dizziness and drowsiness.
6. Instruct patient to avoid rapid postural changes because these may precipitate weakness, dizziness, and syncope.
7. Instruct patients that if they note a very rapid heartbeat, they should lie down or sit down and put their heads below their knees to avoid fainting.
8. Encourage patient to avoid situations in which fainting would be dangerous.
9. In the event of syncope, place patient in a reclining position, and provide needed supportive measures.
10. Place patient in a supine position should overdosage occur, and provide supportive measures. Treat for shock if necessary with plasma volume expanders and vasopressor drugs.

SODIUM NITROPRUSSIDE NIPRIDE

Classification Antihypertensive—acts directly on vascular smooth muscle.

Remarks The drug acts directly on the vascular smooth muscle and produces peripheral vasodilation. The effect is rapid (2 minutes) but transitory, and the drug must be given by IV infusion.

Use Hypertensive crisis.

Contraindication Compensatory hypertension.

Untoward Reactions CNS symptoms (transitory): restlessness, agitation, and muscle twitching. Vomiting or skin rash.

Drug Interaction Concomitant use of other antihypertensives ↑ response to nitroprusside.

Dosage **IV infusion:** average 3 μg/kg/min. **Range:** 0.5–8 μg/kg/min.
Monitor blood pressure and use as guide to regulate rate of administration so as to maintain desired antihypertensive effect. Rate of administration ranges from 20–400 μg/min and should not exceed 800 μg/min. Smaller dose is required for patients receiving other antihypertensives.

Administration/ Storage
1. Protect drug from heat, light, and moisture.
2. Protect dilute solutions during administration by wrapping flask with opaque material, such as aluminum foil.
3. Dilute with 5% D/W injection or with sterile water **without preservative.**
4. Discard all unused dilute solutions after 4 hr.

5. Discard solutions that are any color but very light brown.
6. Do not add any other drug or preservative to solution.

Nursing Implications
1. Monitor BP closely to assist in regulating rate of administration and to check for excessive hypotensive effect.
2. Adjust the infusion pump or microdrip regulator to conform exactly to the rate of administration ordered.

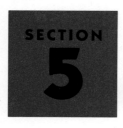

SECTION 5

antiarrhythmic agents

Digitalis Glycosides
Disopyramide
Lidocaine Hydrochloride (XYLOCAINE)
Methoxamine
Phenytoin
Phenytoin Sodium

· Procainamide Hydrochloride (PRONESTYL)
· Propranolol Hydrochloride (INDERAL)
Quinidine Gluconate
Quinidine Polygalacturonate
· Quinidine Sulfate

General Statement
The orderly sequence of contraction of the heart chambers, at an efficient rate, is necessary so that the heart can pump enough blood to the body organs. Normally the atria contract first, then the ventricles.

Altered patterns of contraction, or marked increases or decreases in the rate of the heart, reduce the ability of the heart to pump blood. Such altered patterns are called *cardiac arrhythmias*. Some examples of cardiac arrhythmias are:

1. *Ventricular premature beats* or beats that occasionally originate in the ventricles instead of in the sinus node region of the atrium. This causes the ventricles to contract before the atria and ultimately results in a decrease in the volume of blood pumped into the aorta.
2. *Ventricular tachycardia.* A rapid heartbeat with a succession of beats originating in the ventricles.
3. *Atrial flutter.* Rapid contraction of the atria at a rate too fast to enable it to efficiently force blood into the ventricles.
4. *Atrial fibrillation.* The rate of atrial contraction is even faster than that noted during atrial flutter and more disorganized.
5. *Ventricular fibrillation.* Rapid, irregular, and uncoordinated ventricular contractions that are unable to pump any blood to the body. This condition will cause death if not corrected immediately.
6. *Atrioventricular heart block.* Slowing or failure of the transmission of the cardiac impulse from atria to ventricles, in the atrioventricular

junction. This can result in atrial contraction *not* followed by ventricular contraction.

Antiarrhythmic drugs are used to correct disorders of the heart rate and rhythm. These drugs will either change the rate of the heart to more normal values or restore the origin of the heartbeat to the sinus nodes (pacemaker). The drugs regulate the heartbeat by depressing impulse formation in regions of the heart where the impulse should not arise.

The major antiarrhythmic drugs are:

Disopyramide
Quinidine
Procainamide
Lidocaine
Phenytoin
Propranolol

They are discussed separately under their respective drug entries. However, there are certain general nursing implications that apply to all antiarrhythmic drugs.

Nursing Implications

1. Maintain all patients receiving antiarrhythmic drugs by the IV route on a cardiac monitor.
2. Observe for variations in cardiac rhythm and report changes that may require alteration in drug administration.
3. Observe especially for depression of cardiac activity such as the prolongation of the PR interval, the QRS complex, or aggravation of the arrhythmia.
4. Monitor blood pressure almost continuously during IV therapy because antiarrhythmic patients are particularly susceptible to hypotension and cardiac collapse.
5. Monitor cardiac rate. Bradycardia may be indicative of forthcoming cardiac collapse.
6. Should an adverse reaction occur, be prepared to assist in discontinuing the medication, to administer emergency drugs, and to use emergency resuscitative techniques.

DIGITALIS GLYCOSIDES

See *Cardiac Glycosides*, page 236.

DISOPYRAMIDE NORPACE

Classification Antiarrhythmic.

General Statement Disopyramide depresses the excitability of the cardiac muscle to electric stimulation, and normalizes the time interval during which heart cells cannot be stimulated to contract (refractory period). The drug seems to have fewer side effects than quinidine. The drug has anticholinergic properties. Disopyramide is well absorbed from the intestinal tract. The onset of the therapeutic effects is noted in 30 minutes and lasts

6 hours. The drugs can be used in digitalized and nondigitalized patients. It rarely causes significant alterations in blood pressure.

Uses Prevention, recurrence, and control of unifocal, multifocal, and paired premature ventricular contractions. Arrhythmias in coronary artery disease.

Contraindications Hypersensitivity to drug. Cardiogenic shock, heart failure, heart block, especially preexisting second and third degree A-V block, glaucoma, urinary retention. Safe use during pregnancy, childhood, labor, and delivery has not been established.

Untoward Reactions Anticholinergic: dry mouth (40%), urinary retention (10%–20%), constipation, blurred vision, dry nose, eyes and throat. Genitourinary: urinary frequency and urgency. GI: nausea, pain, flatulence, anorexia, diarrhea, vomiting. General discomforts: dizziness, fatigue, nervousness. Cardiovascular: edema, weight gain, cardiac conduction disturbances, hypotension, shortness of breath, syncope, chest pain. Dermatological: rash/dermatoses.

Dosage **PO:** *individualized,* **loading dose,** 300 mg; **then** 150 mg q 6 hr; **maintenance:** 100–200 mg q 6 hr. *Patients of small stature or those suffering from renal or hepatic insufficiency,* **loading dose:** 200 mg; **maintenance:** 100 mg as determined by creatinine clearance rate.

Administration
1. Administer drug only after electrocardiographic assessment.
2. Administer with caution to individuals receiving (or who have recently received) other antiarrhythmic drugs.

Nursing Implications
1. Do not administer if ECG shows a first-degree heart block. Check with medical supervision for reduced dosage.
2. Monitor patients who are being transferred from another antiarrhythmic to disopyramide very carefully.
3. Monitor BP b.i.d. for hypotensive effect.
4. Observe ECG for QRS widening and QT prolongation, indications for discontinuing disopyramide.
5. Be alert to patients with poor left ventricular function because they are more susceptible to hypotension or worsened CHF manifested by cough, dyspnea, moist rales, and cyanosis.
6. Check that adequate serum potassium levels are present for effective response to disopyramide.
7. Be alert to development of urinary retention, particularly in men with hypertrophy of the prostate.
8. Report untoward reactions because dosage is based on individual's response and tolerance to the medication.

LIDOCAINE HYDROCHLORIDE XYLOCAINE HYDROCHLORIDE, LIDO-PEN AUTO-INJECTOR

Classification Antiarrhythmic.

General Statement Lidocaine does not affect blood pressure, cardiac output, or myocardial contractility in the therapeutic dosage range.

Lidocaine shortens the refractory period and suppresses the automaticity of ectopic foci, but it does not affect conduction of impulses through the cardiac tissue. Since lidocaine does not severely impair conduction in normal antiarrhythmic doses, it should be used acutely instead of procainamide in instances where heart block might occur.

Uses Treatment of acute ventricular arrhythmias such as those following myocardial infarctions or occurring during surgery. The drug is ineffective against atrial arrhythmias.

Contraindications Hypersensitivity to amide-type local anesthetics, Adams-Stokes syndrome, or total or partial heart block. Use with caution in the presence of liver or severe kidney disease, congestive heart failure, marked hypoxia, severe respiratory depression, or shock.

Untoward Reactions CNS effects including dizziness, restlessness, apprehension, euphoria, tinnitus, loss of hearing, visual disturbances, vomiting, difficulties in breathing or swallowing, muscle twitching, tremors, stupor, convulsions, unconsciousness, and respiratory depression. Overdosage may cause hypotension, cardiac conduction disorders (including heart block), cardiovascular collapse, bradycardia, or cardiac and respiratory arrest.

During anesthesia, cardiovascular depression may be the first sign of lidocaine toxicity. During other usage, convulsions are the first sign of lidocaine toxicity.

Drug Interactions

Interactant	Interaction
Procainamide	Additive neurologic side effects
Succinylcholine	↑ Action of succinylcholine by ↓ plasma protein binding

Dosage **IV:** 50–100 mg at rate of 25–50 mg/min. Repeat if necessary after 5-minute interval. Onset of action is 10 seconds. **Maximum dose/hour:** 200–300 mg. **Infusion:** 1–4 mg/min (or 20–50 μg/kg/min for the average 70 kg adult). Onset of action is 10 to 20 minutes. **IM:** 300 mg.

Administration
1. **Do not add lidocaine to blood transfusion assembly.**
2. Lidocaine solutions that contain epinephrine should not be used to treat arrhythmias. Make certain vial states "For Cardiac Arrhythmias."

Additional Nursing Implications
1. Observe for untoward CNS effects, such as twitching and tremors, that may precede convulsions.
2. Observe for respiratory depression by monitoring respiratory rate.
3. Have on hand a short-acting barbiturate such as Seconal for emergency use.

METHOXAMINE VASOXYL

See *Adrenergic Drugs* in Chapter 6, Section 1.

PHENYTOIN (DIPHENYLHYDANTOIN) DILANTIN

PHENYTOIN SODIUM (DIPHENYLHYDLANTOIN SODIUM) DILANTIN SODIUM

Classification	Anticonvulsant, antiarrhythmic.
Remarks	This antiarrhythmic agent is less effective than quinidine, procainamide, or lidocaine.
Uses	PO for certain premature ventricular contractions and IV for premature ventricular contractions and tachycardia. The drug is particularly useful for arrhythmias produced by digitalis overdosage. For all details on this drug, including *Contraindications, Untoward Reactions,* and *Drug Interactions,* see Chapter 5, Section 5, *Anticonvulsants.*
Laboratory Test Interference	False + or ↑ fasting glucose, Coombs test
Dosage	*Arrhythmias;* **PO:** 200–400 mg daily. **IV:** 100 mg q 10 minutes up to maximum of 10 mg/kg.

PROCAINAMIDE HYDROCHLORIDE PROCAMIDE, PRONESTYL, SUB-QUIN

Classification	Antiarrhythmic agent.
General Statement	Procainamide prolongs the refractory period of the heart and depresses the conduction of the cardiac impulse. The drug also has some anticholinergic and local anesthetic effects. Extremely rapid onset of action, ranging from 30 minutes after PO administration to several minutes after IV administration. Effects last approximately 3 hours.
Uses	Ventricular and atrial arrhythmias, resistant paroxysmal atrial tachycardia. Emergency treatment of ventricular tachycardia, digitalis intoxication, prophylactic control of tachycardia for patients at risk during anesthesia or undergoing thoracic surgery.
Contraindications	Sensitivity to drug, complete heart block, or blood dyscrasias. Use with extreme caution in patients for whom a sudden drop in blood pressure

could be detrimental, in patients with liver or kidney dysfunction, and in those with bronchial asthma or other respiratory disorders.

Untoward Reactions Hypotension, especially after parenteral administration, bradycardia, partial or complete heart block, asystole, extrasystole, ventricular tachycardia or fibrillation, and circulatory collapse. Drug-induced systemic lupus erythematosus. For additional *Untoward Reactions*, see *Quinidine*, page 286.

Drug Interactions

Interactant	Interaction
Acetazolamide (Diamox)	↑ Effect of procainamide due to ↓ excretion by kidney
Anticholinergic agents Atropine	Additive anticholinergic effects
Antihypertensive agents	Additive hypotensive effect
Cholinergic agents	Anticholinergic activity of procainamide antagonizes effect of cholinergic drugs
Guanethidine (Ismelin)	Additive hypotensive effects
Kanamycin (Kynex)	Procainamide ↑ muscle relaxation produced by kanamycin
Lidocaine	Additive neurologic side effects
Magnesium salts	Procainamide ↑ muscle relaxation produced by magnesium salts
Methyldopa (Aldomet)	Additive hypotensive effect
Neomycin	Procainamide ↑ muscle relaxation produced by neomycin
Reserpine	Additive hypotensive effects
Skeletal muscle relaxants Succinylcholine	Procainamide ↑ muscle relaxation produced by succinylcholine
Sodium bicarbonate	↑ Effect of procainamide due to ↓ excretion by the kidney

Laboratory Test Interference May affect liver function tests. False + or ↑ serum alkaline phosphatase.

Dosage **Individualized** to achieve plasma levels of 4–8 μg/ml. *Atrial arrhythmias,* **PO: initial,** 1.25 gm. Another 0.75 gm may be given after 1 hr; 0.5 gm q 2 hr until ECG is normal or until toxic symptoms appear; **maintenance:** 50 mg/kg in divided doses. **Pediatric: initial,** 50 mg/kg daily in 4–5 doses. *Ventricular extrasystoles or tachycardia,* **IV:** 0.2–1 gm. *Atrial fibrillation or paroxysmal atrial tachycardia,* **IV:** 0.5–1 m. Monitor with ECG. Switch to **PO** preparation as soon as possible.

Administration/ Storage Discard solutions of drug that are darker than light amber or otherwise colored. Solutions that have turned slightly yellow on standing may be used.

Additional Nursing Implications

1. Monitor IV administration, checking that dose does not exceed 25–50 mg/min.
2. Keep patient in a supine position during IV infusion and monitor blood pressure almost continuously.
3. Report and be prepared to discontinue infusion if diastolic blood pressure falls 15 mm Hg or more during administration.
4. Have on hand phenylephrine hydrochloride injection (Neo-Synephrine) or levarterenol bitartrate (Levopheol) injection to counteract excessive hypotensive response.
5. Observe patients on oral maintenance for symptoms of lupus erythematosus as manifested by polyarthralgia, arthritis, pleuritic pain, fever, myalgia, and skin lesions.

PROPRANOLOL HYDROCHLORIDE INDERAL

Classification   Antiarrhythmic.

General Statement   The antiarrhythmic action of propranolol results from a *beta*-adrenergic blockade and from a direct effect of the drug on the cardiac cell membrane. The drug decreases the rate and force of contraction of the heart. This results in a decrease in cardiac output and in a fall of the systemic arterial pressure.

The onset of action, after PO administration, is 30 minutes. Maximum effect is reached 4 hours after PO and 10 minutes after IV administration.

Uses   Arrhythmias due to hyperactive sympathetic nervous system or to pheochromocytoma; a variety of ventricular arrhythmias; hypertrophic subaortic stenosis; treatment of angina pectoris; slows the ventricular rate during atrial fibrillation.

Contraindications   Patients in whom sudden changes in blood pressure would be detrimental. Patients with sinus bradycardia, partial or total heart block, cardiogenic shock, congestive heart failure, bronchial asthma, or hay fever during season. Administer with caution to patients with acute myocardial infarctions and patients who underwent electric reversion to sinus rhythm. Propranolol should be administered with caution to patients with diabetes, kidney or liver dysfunction. Do not use for arrhythmias resulting from digitalis toxicity.

Untoward Reactions   Can precipitate congestive heart failure or circulatory collapse. Also hypotension, bradycardia, asystole, and A-V block.

The drug also has many untoward effects on the GI tract (nausea, diarrhea) and the CNS (hallucinations, incoordination, vertigo, syncope, dizziness, unsteadiness, insomnia). Skin reactions and urinary retention have also been reported.

Drug Interactions

Interactant	Interaction
Anticholinergics Atropine	Anticholinergics are used to counteract excessive bradycardia produced by propranolol
Antidiabetic agents	Propranolol inhibits the rebound of blood glucose following insulin-induced hypoglycemia
Antihypertensives	Additive hypotensive effects
Digitalis glycosides	Propranolol potentiates digitalis-induced bradycardia
Guanethidine (Ismelin)	Additive hypotensive effect
Isoproterenol	Propranolol blocks the pharmacologic effects of isoproterenol
Methyldopa (Aldomet)	Additive hypotensive effect
Phenothiazines	Additive hypotensive effect
Quinidine	Both produce a negative inotropic effect on the heart
Reserpine	Additive hypotensive effect
Sympathomimetics	Propranolol blocks certain pharmacologic effects of sympathomimetics

Laboratory Test Interference

May ↑ SGOT and SGPT values and ↓ serum glucose values.

Dosage

PO: *Angina: individualized,* **initial,** 10–20 mg t.i.d.–q.i.d. **Average:** 160 mg/day; *Migraine:* 80 mg/day in divided doses initially; **then** 160–240 mg/day. *Arrhythmias:* 10–30 mg t.i.d.–q.i.d. before meals and at bedtime. *Hypertrophic subaortic stenosis:* 20–40 mg t.i.d.–q.i.d. *Hypertension:* **initial,** 80 mg daily in divided doses; **usual range:** 160–480 mg/day. **IV:** 1–3 mg (1 mg/min); a second dose may be administered after 10 to 15 minutes. **IV** use should be reserved for life-threatening arrhythmias. *Pheochromocytoma:* 60 mg/day in divided doses for 3 days before surgery; administer with an alpha-adrenergic blocking agent.

Administration

1. Administer on an empty stomach because food decreases absorption of the drug.
2. Do not administer for a minimum of 2 weeks after patient has received monoamine oxidase inhibitor drugs.
3. Monitor with ECG during IV administration and withhold medication for 4 hours after IV administration.
4. If signs of serious myocardial depression occur following propranolol, isoproterenol (Isuprel) should be slowly infused IV.

Nursing Implications

1. Observe patient for untoward reactions of the GI, CNS, circulatory (bradycardia most common), and integumentary systems.
2. Have on hand atropine (0.25–1 mg) for IV administration to combat hypotension or circulatory collapse after IV administration of propranolol.
3. Observe diabetic patients closely for insulin shock because pro-

pranolol masks the characteristic signs of acute hypoglycemia such as changes in pulse, tachycardia, and onset of sweating.

QUINIDINE GLUCONATE QUINAGLUTE

QUINIDINE POLYGALACTURONATE CARDIOQUIN

QUINIDINE SULFATE CIN-QUIN, QUINIDEX, QUINORA, SK-QUINIDINE SULFATE

Classification Antiarrhythmic.

General Statement Quinidine is an alkaloid isolated from the bark of the cinchona tree. It is marketed as different salts, some of which are suitable for parenteral administration. The rate of absorption of the different salts varies.

The drug depresses the excitability of the cardiac muscle to electrical stimulation and increases the time interval during which the heart cannot be stimulated to contract (refractory period). The drug also slows the rate at which the cardiac impulse is transmitted through the cardiac tissue.

Quinidine decreases cardiac output. The drug has some anticholinergic, antimalarial, antipyretic and oxytocic properties.

The onset of action of quinidine salts varies from 0.5 to 4 hours. Action persists for 6 to 8 hours.

Uses Often the drug of choice for atrial fibrillation and atrial and ventricular arrhythmias. Also used in intractable hiccups (IM administration) and nocturnal cramps. Not indicated for prophylaxis during surgery.

Contraindications Hypersensitivity to drug or other cinchona drugs. Quinidine should be used with extreme caution for patients in whom a sudden change in blood pressure might be detrimental or those suffering from extensive myocardial damage, subacute endocarditis, bradycardia, coronary occlusion, disturbances in impulse conduction, chronic valvular disease, considerable cardiac enlargement, or frank congestive failure.

Cautious use is also recommended in patients with acute infections, hyperthyroidism, myasthenia gravis, muscular weakness, respiratory distress, and bronchial asthma.

Untoward Reactions Severe cardiac manifestations including bradycardia, congestive heart failure, partial or total heart block, changes in heartbeat, precipitation or potentiation of heart failure, syncope, circulatory collapse, and shock.

Effects on respiration: asthmatic attacks, dyspnea, respiratory paralysis, and cyanosis.

Hypersensitivity reactions including skin eruptions, urticaria, exfoliative dermatitis, and maculopapular or scarlitiniform rash.

Thrombocytopenia and thrombocytopenic purpura have also been reported.

GI effects: anorexia, bitter taste, nausea, vomiting, abdominal pain, diarrhea, and increased urge to defecate as well as urinate.

CNS effects: confusion, apprehension, headache, cold sweat, salivation, flushing, periarteritis nodosa, and edema. Signs of cinchonism, including tinnitus, visual disturbances, vertigo, convulsions, and tremors.

Drug Interactions

Interactant	Interaction
Acetazolamide (Diamox)	↑ Effect of quinidine due to ↓ renal excretion
Anticholinergic agents Atropine	Additive effect on blockade of vagus nerve action
Anticoagulants, oral	Additive hypoprothrombinemia
Cholinergic agents	Quinidine antagonizes effect of cholinergic drugs
Digoxin	↑ Symptoms of digoxin toxicity
Guanethidine (Ismelin)	Additive hypotensive effect
Methyldopa (Aldomet)	Additive hypotensive effect
Phenobarbital ⎤ Phenytoin ⎦	↓ Effect of quinidine by ↑ rate of metabolism in liver
Phenothiazines	Additive cardiac depressant effect
Propranolol (Inderal)	Both drugs produce a negative inotropic effect on the heart
Reserpine	Additive hypotensive effect
Skeletal muscle relaxants	↑ Skeletal muscle relaxation

Laboratory Test Interference

False + or ↑ PSP, 17-ketosteroids, prothrombin time.

Dosage

Individualized. ECG monitoring recommended during quinidine therapy. Administration of test doses of approximately 200 mg quinidine sulfate or gluconate is recommended to avoid hypersensitivity reactions.

Quinidine sulfate, **PO: initial,** 400 mg q 2 to 3 hr. Single dose can be increased to 600–800 mg. No more than 5 doses should be administered in 24 hours, **maintenance:** 100–200 mg 1 to 4 times daily.

Quinidine polygalacturonate, **PO:** 275–825 mg q 3 to 4 hr for 4 or more doses; **maintenance:** 275 mg 2 to 3 times daily.

Quinidine gluconate, **PO:** 330–660 mg 2 to 4 times daily; **maintenance:** 330–660 mg 2 to 4 times daily.

Acute tachycardia, **IM: initial,** 600 mg; **maintenance:** 400 mg quinidine gluconate q 2 hr if necessary. *Hiccups:* 800 mg q hr for 3 to 4 hr.

IV infusion (rare): 200–750 mg given slowly as a dilute solution (16 mg/ml) infusion. Check BP and ECG continuously during administration.

Administration/ Storage

1. Use only colorless clear solution for injection because light may cause quinidine to crystallize and this turns solution brownish.
2. Administer with food to minimize GI effects.

Additional Nursing Implications

1. Anticipate that preliminary test dose will be given before instituting quinidine therapy. **Adult:** 200 mg quinidine sulfate or quinidine gluconate administered PO or IM. **Children:** test dose of 2 mg of quinidine sulfate per kilogram of body weight.
2. Observe cardiac monitor and report prolongation of PR intervals, absence of P waves, and cardiac rates above 120 beats/minute, all of which are reasons for discontinuation of drug.
3. Observe patients on oral quinidine for signs of hypotension.
4. Check BP of hospitalized patient on oral quinidine at least once daily.
5. Observe patients for hypersensitivity demonstrated by respiratory and integumentary symptoms.
6. Administer extended release tablets only for maintenance and prophylactic therapy.

SECTION 6
hypocholesterolemic and antilipemic agents

Aluminum Nicotinate
Nicotinic Acid
Cholestyramine Resin
Clofibrate

Colestipol
Dextrothyroxine Sodium
Probucol
Sitosterols

General Statement

It is presently believed that a reduction of the plasma lipids to more normal levels is therapeutically useful in minimizing atherosclerosis. This can often be achieved through diet and, for certain patients, occasionally with the help of specific antilipemic or hypocholesterolemic agents.

Atherosclerosis is characterized by deposits of lipids (fats) within the inner layers of the arteries. This narrowing of the blood vessels increases the likelihood of cardiovascular accidents (strokes).

Atherosclerosis is probably related to a disorder of cholesterol, fat, and/or carbohydrate metabolism. In any case, patients with atherosclerosis often have increased levels of circulating fatty substances. These so-called plasma-lipids consist of triglycerides, phospholipids, free cholesterol, and cholesterol ester all associated with protein (lipoproteins). Plasma also contains free fatty acids.

The exact composition of lipoproteins varies from person to person and with dietary intake of fats and carbohydrates. Persons who have a higher than normal amount of lipoprotein are considered to suffer from hyperlipoproteinemia.

On the basis of their lipoprotein patterns and other physiological characteristics, patients can be separated into five groups:

Lipid Pattern	Characteristic Feature	Treatment
Type I (exogenous or "fat-induced")	High level of triglycerides. Normal levels of cholesterol. This pattern occurs rarely and is related to dietary intake of fat	Low fat diet. Treatment of underlying condition (diabetes, thyroid condition)
Type II (familial hypercholesterolemia)	High plasma cholesterol level, normal or slightly elevated triglycerides	Substitution of unsaturated fats for saturated fats in diet. Nicotinic acid, dextrothyroxine
Type III (endogenous)	Increased low-density lipoproteins, especially beta-lipoproteins. Hypercholesterolemia and hypertriglyceridemia	Weight reduction. Possible drug therapy (clofibrate)
Type IV (endogenous)	Carbohydrate-induced hyperlipoproteinemia, often associated with early onset of atherosclerosis	Weight reduction, reduction in carbohydrate intake. Drug therapy (clofibrate and nicotinic acid)
Type V (mixed exogenous and endogenous)	Mixed I and IV caused both by dietary fat and abnormal carbohydrate metabolism. Hypertriglyceridemia	Weight reduction. Reduced carbohydrate intake. Drug therapy (clofibrate and nicotinic acid)

A number of drugs that lower the blood level of cholesterol and lipids have been introduced. These agents, however, will not remove existing plaques of lipids (atheromas) but it is hoped that they will reduce the rate at which new ones are formed.

The exact mode of action of these agents is not known, although it is likely that some of them interfere with the formation of cholesterol from precursor substances, others speed up the rate at which cholesterol is broken down, and still others interfere with the absorption of cholesterol from the GI tract. Sometimes, despite continuous medication, cholesterol levels return to their pretreatment levels.

At present the hypocholesterolemic agents are only given to poor-risk patients who have already had one or several cardiovascular accidents, to those who are overweight, and/or to those having a family history of atherosclerotic disease.

It is also highly desirable to restrict the dietary intake of cholesterol and saturated fatty acids of patients suffering from atherosclerosis.

Encouragement along these lines by the nurse is very valuable. Serum cholesterol is lowered when foods with unsaturated fatty acids are substituted for foods high in saturated fats. Saturated fatty acids are predominantly of animal origin, whereas unsaturated fatty acids are predominantly of vegetable oil and fish oil origin.

ALUMINUM NICOTINATE NICALEX

NICOTINIC ACID DIACIN, NIAC, NIACELS, NIACIN, NIACINAMIDE, NICALEX, NICL, NICOBID, NICOCAP, NICO-400, NICOLAR, NICO-SPAN, NICOTINAMIDE, NICOTINEX, SK-NIACIN, TEGA-SPAN, VASOTHERM, WAMPOCAP

General Statement

The drug reduces the blood level of cholesterol and, to a lesser extent, that of lipids and free fatty acids.

Nicotinic acid is believed to interfere with the formation of cholesterol.

The drug has been effective in keeping the cholesterol and serum lipid level down for periods up to 5 years. When discontinued the blood levels return to pretreatment levels within 2 to 6 weeks.

The drug stimulates the release of histamine from mast cells and increases gastric secretion.

Uses Hypercholesterolemia, hyperlipidemia.

Contraindications Use with caution in patients with peptic ulcer or a history thereof, gallbladder disease, hepatic conditions, gout, diabetes, tuberculosis (active or arrested), asthma, allergic tendencies, or bronchial disease.

Untoward Reactions

GI: nausea, dyspepsia, flatulence, anorexia, vomiting, epigastric pain, and diarrhea. These reactions can be severe but usually respond to dosage reduction. Concomitant administration of antacids helps.

Other side effects include flushing, pruritus, urticaria, dry skin, dry mouth, panic reactions, nervousness, alteration of sugar metabolism (hyperglycemia, glycosuria, precipitation of diabetes), tingling sensations, ocular effects (blurred vision, amblyopia, ocular edema), reactivation of tuberculosis, activation of peptic ulcer, and acanthosis nigricans (a skin condition characterized by pigmented wartlike growths).

Prolonged therapy has resulted in a slight increase in uric acid levels (precipitation of gouty arthritis) as well as alteration of some blood and liver function tests.

Drug Interactions

Interactant	Interaction
Anticoagulants	Aluminum nicotinate ↑ effect
Antidiabetic agents	Change in sugar metabolism caused by aluminum nicotinate may require change in dosage of antidiabetic drugs
Tetracyclines	Effect ↓ by aluminum nicotinate

Dosage   *Aluminum Nicotinate;* **PO:** *individualized,* 1–2 gm t.i.d. Therapeutic results may not appear until after 2 to 6 weeks.

Niacin; **PO:** 0.5–3 gm daily in 3 to 4 doses. Dosage is initiated slowly to minimize side effects.

Administer preferably with meals, when stomach is full.

Nursing Implications
1. Assist and encourage patients to follow prescribed diet. Administer in divided doses and, if necessary, in reduced doses, with antacids, ordered by a physician.
2. Avoid administering aluminum nicotinate on an empty stomach because, in addition to gastric side effects, the likelihood of flushing is increased. Flushing may be delayed.
3. Reassure the patient that flushing, pruritis, and nausea may subside with continuing therapy.
4. Test the urine of a diabetic patient regularly for sugar because drug tends to cause hyperglycemia and glycosuria, mandating a change in dosage of insulin or oral hyperglycemic agents.
5. Observe patients on anticoagulant therapy for bleeding from any orifice or purpura because drug potentiates anticoagulants.
6. Encourage patients who develop acanthosis nigricans as an untoward reaction that the warts usually disappear two months after discontinuation of the drug.

CHOLESTYRAMINE RESIN QUESTRAN

General Statement   This resin binds large amounts of sodium cholate (bile salt) and is used primarily for the treatment of biliary cirrhosis, cholestatic jaundice, and as an antidiarrheal. By removing the irritating bile salts, it relieves the itching associated with this condition. The symptoms often return after cholestyramine resin is discontinued.

Recently the resin has been used for the treatment of patients with high cholesterol levels. Some patients exhibit a large drop in serum cholesterol levels. Fat-soluble vitamins should be administered IM to patients on long-term therapy.

Uses   Pruritus associated with obstructive jaundice, primary biliary cirrhosis and biliary obstruction, diarrhea for patients with ileac resections, and atherosclerosis.

Contraindications   Complete obstruction or atresia of bile duct.

Untoward Reactions   GI: nausea, vomiting, constipation, diarrhea, abdominal distention. Fecal impaction in elderly patients. Large doses may cause steatorrhea. Osteoporosis, electrolyte imbalance, and CNS and musculoskeletal manifestations.

Prolonged administration may interfere with absorption of fat-soluble vitamins.

Dosage   **PO:** 4 gm of anhydrous resin 3 to 4 times daily before or with meals, for 2 or more weeks. After relief of pruritus, dosage may be reduced.

Drug Interactions

Interactant	Interaction
Anticoagulants, oral	↑ Hypoprothrombinemia
Cephalexin	↓ Absorption of cephalexin from GI tract
Clindamycin	↓ Absorption of clindamycin from GI tract
Digitalis glycosides	Cholestyramine binds digitoxin in the intestine and ↓ its half-life
Iron preparations	↓ Effect of iron preparations due to ↓ absorption from GI tract
Phenobarbital	↓ Absorption of phenobarbital from GI tract
Phenylbutazone (Butazolidin)	Absorption of phenylbutazone delayed by cholestyramine—may ↓ effect
Thiazide diuretics	↓ Effect of thiazides due to ↓ absorption from GI tract
Thyroid hormones	↓ Effect of thyroid hormones due to ↓ absorption from GI tract

Administration

1. Always mix with fluid before administering because resin may cause esophageal irritation or blockage.
2. Disguise unpalatable taste of drug by mixing it with fruit juice, soup, milk, water, applesauce, pureed fruits, or carbonated beverage.
3. After placing contents of one packet of resin on the surface of 4–6 oz. of fluid, allow it to stand without stirring for 2 minutes, occasionally twirling the glass, and then stir slowly (to prevent foaming) to form a suspension.

Nursing Implications

1. Encourage and assist patient to follow prescribed, low-cholesterol diet.
2. Anticipate that vitamins A, D, and K will be administered in a water-miscible form when patient is receiving medication.
3. Observe for bleeding from any orifice or purpura because bleeding tendencies are increased. Such symptoms are usually treated with parenteral administration of vitamin K.
4. Administer other prescribed medications at least 1 hour before or 4 hours after administration of antihyperlipidemic medication to minimize interference with their absorption.
5. Inform patient of constipating effects of medication.
6. Encourage patient to drink extra fluids and to include roughage in diet. Check with physician whether laxatives should be ordered to overcome constipating effect of medication.
7. Check that patient is scheduled for regular clinical laboratory evaluation including serum cholesterol and triglyceride levels.
8. Anticipate that medication will be discontinued if it does not lower cholesterol levels.
9. Inform patient that relief of pruritus may become evident 1 to 3 weeks after initiation but may return after medication is discontinued.

CLOFIBRATE ATROMID-S

General Statement
Clofibrate has several proposed mechanisms of action including (1) interfering with binding of serum-free fatty acids to albumin, (2) inhibiting hepatic release of lipoproteins, (3) increasing excretion of fecal neutral sterols, (4) inhibiting cholesterol biosynthesis, and (5) affecting metabolism of apoprotein. This results in a reduction of serum cholesterol, triglyceride, and phospholipid levels. Free fatty acid levels are usually not affected.

Proportionately, the higher the cholesterol level, the more effective the drug. The drug is more effective in females than males. Clofibrate is ineffective in patients with untreated hypothyroidism.

Liver function tests should be performed during treatment.

Uses
Hypercholesterolemia and/or hypertriglyceridemia. Xanthoma (small lumpy fat deposits in skin). In the latter case, therapy is limited to one year.

Contraindications
Impaired hepatic or renal function, pregnancy or expectation thereof, lactation, children. Use with caution in patients with gout.

Untoward Reactions
GI distress: nausea and dyspepsia occur in 5% to 10% of patients.

Also, less commonly: vomiting, loose stools, flatulence, abdominal distress, headaches, dizziness, fatigue, weakness, skin rash, urticaria, pruritus, stomatitis, dry and brittle hair (in women), and dyspnea. Muscle aches, cramps, and weakness have also been reported.

Potentially severe effects on skeletal and cardiac muscle have been observed. Symptoms include myositis, asthenia, myalgia, and changes in creatine phosphokinase.

Weight gain has been observed in 30% to 55% of patients, although a few report weight loss.

Leukopenia is cause for discontinuation of drug.

Clofibrate may affect blood clotting time and the level of certain enzymes, especially the transaminases.

Drug should be withdrawn if the serum transaminase level keeps increasing after clofibrate has reached its maximum therapeutic response.

Drug Interactions
Clofibrate increases the effect of anticoagulants by decreasing plasma protein binding.

Dosage
PO: 500 mg q.i.d. Therapeutic response may take several weeks to become apparent. Drug must be administered on a continuous basis since lowered levels of cholesterol and other lipids will return to elevated state within several weeks after administration is stopped. Discontinue after 3 months if response is poor.

Nursing Implications
1. Encourage and assist the patient to follow prescribed diet.
2. Observe for symptoms of hyperglycemia and test urine of diabetic patients regularly for sugar as drug tends to cause hyperglycemia and glycosuria.

3. Observe patients on anticoagulant therapy for bleeding from any orifice or for purpura.

COLESTIPOL HYDROCHLORIDE COLESTID

Classification   Antihyperlipidemic.

General Statement   Colestipol is a resin that, like cholestyramine, binds and removes bile acids. This indirectly decreases the concentration of cholesterol levels in the blood by stimulating its oxidation to bile acids. The drug also decreases blood levels of low density lipoproteins (LDL). The effect of colestipol becomes apparent within 24 hours. Since the resin has no effect on triglyceride levels, its effectiveness has been questioned.

Use   Hypercholesterolemia.

Contraindications   Complete obstruction or atresia of bile duct. Use with caution in patients with pre-existing constipation or hemorrhoids. Safe use during pregnancy and childhood not established.

Untoward Reactions   Constipation (10%), usually mild, but can result in fecal impaction, also, abdominal discomfort, GI irritation, muscle pain, headaches, dizziness, and hypersensitivity reactions.

Drug Interactions

Interactant	Interaction
Cephalexin Chlorothiazide Clindamycin Digitalis Phenobarbital Phenylbutazone Tetracycline Trimethoprim Thyroid Preparations Warfarin	Colestipol may delay or ↓ absorption from the GI tract of the drugs listed.

Dosage   **PO:** 15–30 gm daily in 2 to 4 equally divided doses.

Administration
1. Always mix with fluid before administering, because resin may cause esophageal irritation or blockage.
2. Disguise unpalatable taste of drug by mixing it with fruit juice, soup, milk, water, applesauce, pureed fruit, breakfast cereals, carbonated beverages.

Nursing Implication   See *Cholestyramine*.

DEXTROTHYROXINE SODIUM CHOLOXIN

Classification   Antilipemic.

General Statement   This drug is a salt of the dextro isomer of the thyroid hormone. It has only a slight effect on the basal metabolism rate (BMR) but has all the physiological effects of levothyroxine (see chapter 7, section 2).

Sodium dextrothyroxine causes an increase in the rate at which cholesterol is metabolized in the liver. There is an increase in the excretion of cholesterol and its metabolites. The drug causes a decrease in the serum level of cholesterol and total serum lipids including triglycerides.

The drug is most effective in patients with frankly elevated cholesterol levels.

Uses   Hypercholesterolemia in patients with no thyroid or heart disease. Occasionally used for hypothyroidism. Should mainly be used if dietary measures fail.

Contraindications   Euthyroid patients with hypertensive organic heart disease including angina pectoris, history of myocardial infarctions, cardiac arrhythmias or tachycardia, rheumatic disease, and congestive heart failure. The drug is also contraindicated during pregnancy, lactation, and for patients with advanced liver or kidney disease or a history of hypersensitivity to iodine.

Untoward Reactions   The most frequent side effects relate to increased general metabolism. Insomnia, palpitations, tremor, weight loss, nervousness, drooping eyelids, sweating, flushing, fever, hair loss, diuresis, and menstrual irregularities have been reported.

The drug sometimes causes changes in cardiac activity in previously normal subjects.

Many other untoward reactions have been reported. These include a great variety of cardiac conditions, including myocardial infarctions, angina pectoris, arrhythmias, and ischemic myocardial changes. Also, less frequently, headache, changes in libido, bitter taste, hoarseness, tinnitus, dizziness, peripheral edema, malaise, tiredness, visual disturbances, psychic changes, paresthesia, muscle pain, gallstones, cerebrovascular accidents, thrombophlebitis, GI hemorrhages, and increases in blood sugar level of diabetic patients.

Aggravation of existing cardiac disease is cause for discontinuation.

Overdose is characterized by hyperthyroidism, diarrhea, cramps, vomiting, nervousness, twitching, tachycardia, and weight loss.

Drug Interactions

Interactant	Interaction
Anticoagulants, oral	↑ Effect of anticoagulants by ↑ hypoprothrombinemia
Antidiabetics, oral	↓ Diabetic control as dextrothyroxine ↑ blood sugar
Thyroid drugs	↑ Sensitivity in hypothyroid patients

Dosage   **PO:** *individualized,* **initial,** 1–2 mg daily. Daily dosage can be increased every 4 weeks by 1–2 mg; **maintenance:** 4–8 mg daily. **Maximum daily dosage:** 8 mg. It may take 2 to 4 weeks for the therapeutic response to become manifested. **Pediatric: initial,** 0.05 mg/kg daily. Increase by 0.05 mg/kg daily every month up to maximum of 4 mg daily, until satisfactory control is established.

Withdraw drug 2 weeks prior to surgery.

Nursing Implications
1. Assist and encourage patient to follow prescribed diet.
2. Observe patients for attacks of angina.

PROBUCOL LORELCO

Classification   Antihyperlipidemic.

General Statement   The mechanism by which this lipophilic agent reduces cholesterol levels is unknown. Effects on cholesterol levels are usually noted in 2 to 4 weeks. If no effect is observed after 3 months, the drug should be discontinued. Effects on triglyceride levels are variable and uncertain. After prolonged administration, the drug becomes deposited in the adipose tissues, and after discontinuation, persists in the body for up to 6 months. Absorption from the GI tract is variable.

Uses   Hyperlipoproteinemia, especially of type II and IIa. Not indicated when hypertriglyceridemia is the main finding.

Contraindication   Hypersensitivity. Safe use during pregnancy and in childhood has not been established.

Untoward Reactions   Mild and of short duration. Most common are gastrointestinal disturbances, such as diarrhea (10%), flatulence, abdominal pain, nausea, and vomiting; also, hyperhydrosis, fetid sweat, and angioneurotic edema.

Dosage   **Adults only, PO:** 500 mg b.i.d.

Administration/ Storage
1. To be taken with morning and evening meal.
2. Store in dry place, in light-resistant containers away from excessive heat.

Nursing Implications
1. Encourage and assist patient to follow prescribed low cholesterol diet.
2. Advise patient that should diarrhea occur, it is usually transient but to eliminate roughage from diet until diarrhea stops.
3. Advise patient to check with doctor if GI symptoms persist.

SITOSTEROLS CYTELLIN

Classification   Antilipemic.

General Statement Sitosterols are a mixture of sterols obtained from vegetable oils whose chemical structure resembles cholesterol. The compounds seem to interfere with the absorption of dietary cholesterol from the GI tract as well as with the absorption and reabsorption of cholesterol manufactured by the body (endogenous cholesterol). There also is an increase in the excretion of cholesterol and a decrease in the level of total lipids including triglycerides.

The effect of the drug is inconsistent, however.

Uses Hypercholesterolemia and hyperlipidemia. Sitosterols have been used successfully for patients who also suffer from diabetes, hypothyroidism, and idiopathic hypercholesterolemia. The higher the abnormal serum cholesterol level, the more effective the drug.

Contraindication Administer with caution to patients with liver disease.

Untoward Reactions GI effects: anorexia, diarrhea, and abdominal cramps.

Drug Interaction Anticoagulants, oral: potentiated by sitosterols. Anticoagulant dosage must be reduced.

Dosage **PO:** 9–18 gm daily in divided doses before meals, not to exceed 24–36 gm/day. Effect of therapy becomes apparent during first month. Maximum effect usually becomes established during second or third month.

Administration
1. Improve palatability of drug by mixing with milk, coffee, tea, or fruit juice.
2. Suggested dose is 1 tablespoon (15 ml) before each medium-size meal.
3. Increase dose to 1½ or 2 tablespoons when large or high-fat meals are consumed.
4. Precede any additional food taken in between meals with a whole or fractional dose.

Nursing Implications
1. Teach the patient to adjust dosage.
2. Inform the patient that stool will be bulky and light in color because of presence of sitosterols.
3. Restrict roughage in the patient's diet to minimize incidence of diarrhea.

CHAPTER 5

DRUGS AFFECTING THE CENTRAL NERVOUS SYSTEM

barbiturates

Amobarbital	Pentobarbital Sodium
Amobarbital Sodium	Phenobarbital
Aprobarbital	Phenobarbital Sodium
Barbital	Secobarbital
Butabarbital Sodium	Secobarbital Sodium
Hexobarbital	Talbutal
Mephobarbital	Thiamylal Sodium
Metharbital	Thiopental Sodium
Methohexital Sodium	

General Statement

The barbiturates produce all levels of CNS depression. Low doses produce mild depression resulting in sedation, while higher doses result in deeper depression having a sleep-inducing (hypnotic) effect. Still higher doses produce profound depression resulting in coma. Toxic doses of barbiturates also depress the activity of other tissues including the cardiovascular system. By depressing the CNS, certain long-acting barbiturates have anticonvulsant activity.

The barbiturates do not have a specific analgesic action and therefore should not be given to patients suffering pain.

The drugs produce sedation and hypnosis by acting at the level of the reticular activating system and interfering with the transmission of nerve impulses to the cerebral cortex. In some patients, barbiturates have an unusual action inducing an excitatory response.

All barbiturates have the same physiological actions. The main difference between the various types is the rate of absorption and thus the latency until onset and duration of this action. The barbiturates are divided into ultrashort (minutes), short-acting (4 hours), intermediate-acting (4 to 8 hours), and long-acting (6 to 10 hours).

Their principal uses are dictated by their length of action. Ultrashort-acting barbiturates are given only intravenously and are used for anesthesia, alone or in conjunction with other anesthetics. Intermediate- and short-acting barbiturates are used mainly as hypnotics, whereas the long-acting drugs are used for sedative purposes.

The barbiturates, especially their sodium salts, are readily absorbed after oral, rectal, or parenteral administration. They are distributed thoughout all tissues, cross the placental barrier, and appear in breast milk. Except for phenobarbital and barbital, the compounds are totally metabolized in the liver, and the metabolic products are excreted in the urine. Only a small percentage of phenobarbital is metabolized this way. Most of it is excreted unchanged by the kidneys. Barbital is excreted entirely as the nonmetabolized compound.

Uses Anesthesia, sedation, as hypnotics, for the control of acute convulsive conditions as in epilepsy (only phenobarbital, mephobarbital, metharbital), tetanus, eclampsia, and in toxic reactions associated with strychnine. Before the advent of psychotherapeutic agents, the barbiturates were widely used as antianxiety drugs and even today are helpful in the control of manic states. Because of their sedative effects, the barbiturates are often used alone or in conjunction with other drugs, for the treatment of hyperthyroidism, cardiovascular and GI disorders, menopausal syndrome, and pre- and postsurgical anxiety.

Contraindications Hypersensitivity to barbiturates, severe trauma, pulmonary disease, edema, uncontrolled diabetes, history of porphyria, and for patients in whom they produce an excitatory response.

Barbiturates should be used with caution during pregnancy and lactation, and in patients with CNS depression, hypotension, marked asthenia (hypothyroidism), porphyria, fever, anemia, hemorrhagic shock, cardiac, hepatic or renal damage, history of alcoholism, suicidal patients, and the elderly, especially those with senile psychosis.

Untoward Reactions Skin eruptions, blood dyscrasias, photosensitivity, muscle and joint pain, lassitude, vertigo, headache, nausea, diarrhea, and hangover. Also excitement, euphoria, and restlessness. Prolonged administration may produce jaundice and porphyria in susceptible individuals. Elderly patients usually have an increased sensitivity to barbiturates and sometimes respond with excitement.

Barbiturates can induce physical and psychological dependence if high doses are used regularly for long periods of time. Withdrawal symptoms usually begin after 12 to 16 hours of abstinence. Manifestations of withdrawal include anxiety, weakness, nausea, vomiting, muscle cramps, delirium, and even grand mal seizures.

Drug Interactions **General Considerations**

1. Barbiturates stimulate the activity of enzymes responsible for the metabolism of a large number of other drugs by a process known as enzyme induction. As a result, when barbiturates are given to patients receiving such drugs, their therapeutic effectiveness is markedly reduced or even abolished.
2. The CNS depressant effect of the barbiturates is potentiated by many drugs. Concomitant administration may result in coma or fatal CNS depression. Barbiturate dosage should either be reduced or eliminated when other CNS drugs are given.
3. Barbiturates also potentiate the toxic effects of many other agents.

Interactant	Interaction
Alcohol	Potentiation or addition of CNS depressant effects. Concomitant use may lead to drowsiness, lethargy, stupor, respiratory collapse, coma, or death.
Anesthetics, general	See *Alcohol*

Drug Interactions (Continued)

Interactant	Interaction
Antianxiety drugs	See *Alcohol*
Anticoagulants, oral	↓ Effect of anticoagulants due to ↓ absorption from GI tract and ↑ breakdown by liver
Antidepressants, tricyclic	Barbiturates ↑ adverse affects of toxic doses of tricyclic antidepressants—additive respiratory depression
Antidiabetic agents	Prolong the effects of barbiturates

CNS depressants
  anesthetics
  antianxiety drugs
  antihistamines
  narcotics
  phenothiazines
  sedative-hypnotics
	See *Alcohol*

Corticosteroids	↓ Effect of corticosteroids due to ↑ breakdown by liver
Digitalis glycosides	↓ Effect of digitalis glycosides due to ↑ breakdown by liver
Disulfiram	↑ Effect of barbiturates due to ↓ breakdown by liver
Doxycycline	↓ Effect of doxycycline due to ↑ breakdown by liver
Estrogens	↓ Effect of estrogen due to ↑ breakdown by liver
Griseofulvin	↓ Effect of griseofulvin due to ↓ absorption from GI tract
Methotrimeprazine (Levoprome)	Potentiation of CNS depression
Methyldopa	↓ Hypotensive effect of methyldopa by ↑ breakdown by liver

Monoamine oxidase inhibitors
  Pargyline (Eutonyl)
  Tranylcypromine (Parnate)
	↑ Effect of barbiturates due to ↓ breakdown by liver

Narcotic analgesics	See *Alcohol*
Phenytoin (Dilantin)	↓ Effect of phenytoin due to ↑ breakdown by liver
Sedative-hypnotics, nonbarbiturate	See *Alcohol*
Phenothiazines	See *Alcohol.* Also, possible ↓ effect of phenothiazines due to ↑ breakdown by liver
Procarbazine (Matulane)	↑ Effect of barbiturates
Sulfonamides	↑ Effect of barbiturates due to ↓ in plasma protein binding
Tricyclic antidepressants	Additive respiratory depression

Acute Toxicity

Characterized by cortical and respiratory depression; anoxia; peripheral vascular collapse; feeble, rapid pulse; pulmonary edema; decreased body temperature; clammy, cyanotic skin; depressed reflexes; stupor; and coma. After initial constriction the pupils become dilated. Death results from respiratory depression, cardiovascular collapse, or pneumonia.

Chronic Toxicity

Prolonged use of barbiturates at high doses may lead to physical and psychological dependence as well as tolerance. Doses of 600–800 mg daily for 8 weeks may lead to physical dependence. The addict usually ingests 1.5 gm a day. Addicts prefer short-acting barbiturates. Symptoms of dependence are similar to those associated with chronic alcoholism and withdrawal symptoms are as severe. Withdrawal symptoms usually last from 5 to 10 days and are terminated by a long sleep.

Treatment consists of a cautious withdrawal of the hospitalized addict over a 2- to 4-week period. A stabilizing dose of 200–300 mg of a short-acting barbiturate is administered every 6 hours. The dose is then reduced by 100 mg daily until the stabilizing dose is reduced by one half. The patient is then maintained on this dose for 2 to 3 days before further reduction. The same procedure is repeated when the initial stabilizing dose has been reduced by three quarters. If a mixed spike and slow activity appear on the ECG, or if insomnia, anxiety, tremor, or weakness is observed, the dosage is maintained at a constant level or increased slightly until symptoms disappear.

Treatment of Acute Toxicity

This should consist of maintenance of an adequate airway, oxygen intake, and carbon dioxide removal. Absorption following SC or IM administration of the drug may be delayed by the use of ice packs or tourniquets. After oral ingestion, gastric lavage or gastric aspiration may delay absorption. Emesis should not be induced once the symptoms of overdosage are manifested as the patient may aspirate the vomitus into the lungs. Also, if the dose of barbiturate is high enough, the vomiting center in the brain may be depressed. Maintenance of renal function and removal of the drug by peritoneal dialysis or artificial kidney should be carried out. Supportive physiological methods have proven superior to analeptic methods.

Laboratory Test Interference May affect BSP retention; alters prothrombin time and bilirubin values. ↑ SGOT, SGPT. May cause false + lupus erythematosus test.

Dosage Aim for minimum effective dosage. As hypnotics, barbiturates should be administered intermittently because tolerance develops. Elderly patients should receive half dosage, children one-quarter to one-half of adult dose (see Table 12, p. 304).

TABLE 12 BARBITURATES

Drug	Use	Dosage	Remarks
Amobarbital (Amytal) Amobarbital sodium (Amytal sodium)	Sedation, hypnotic, acute convulsive disorders.	Amobarbital is given **PO** only. *Sedation:* 30–50 mg 2 to 3 times daily. *Hypnotic:* 100–200 mg. *Amobarbital sodium,* **IM, IV:** dose highly individualized, essentially the same regardless of route of administration. *Preanesthetic medication:* 200 mg 1 to 2 hr before surgery. *Manic reactions:* 65–500 mg.	Intermediate acting. *Administration:* When dissolving dry-packed ampules with accompanying sterile water for parenteral use, rotate ampule for mixing. Solutions that are not clear after 5 minutes should be discarded. Not more than 30 minutes should elapse between opening of ampule and usage. IM: Inject deeply, in large muscle, no more than 5 ml at 1 site. IV: Inject slowly at rates not exceeding 1 ml/min. Patients requiring IV administration should be closely monitored.
Aprobarbital (Alurate, Alurate Verdum)	Daytime sedation, hypnotic.	**PO,** *Sedation:* 40 mg t.i.d. *Hypnotic:* 80–160 mg. The preparation is supplied as red or green elixir. One teaspoon (5 ml) contains 40 mg.	Intermediate-acting barbiturate.
Barbital Barbital sodium	Mild, prolonged sedation.	**PO,** *Sedation:* 65–130 mg 2 to 3 times daily. *Hypnotic:* 300–600 mg 1 to 2 hr before sleep is desired.	Long-acting barbiturate. Not metabolized by liver.
Butabarbital sodium (Butal, Butazem Butisol Sodium, Buticaps, Sarisol)	Hypnotic, mild sedation for anxiety.	**PO,** *Sedation:* 15–30 mg 3 to 4 times daily. *Hypnotic:* 50–100 mg. **Pediatric,** *Sedation:* 8–30 mg in divided doses daily.	Intermediate-acting barbiturate. Used more as a sedative than as a hypnotic.
Hexobarbital (Sombulex)	Hypnotic, preanesthetic, preoperative or postoperative sedation.	*Hypnotic:* 250–500 mg; **pediatric** dosage has not been established.	Ultra-short-acting barbiturate. May be used preoperatively with atropine if morphine is contraindicated.
Mephobarbital (Mebaral)	Sedation and as anticonvulsant as required in epilepsy (grand mal and focal seizures, not for petit mal or psychomotor), tension, anxiety, neurasthenia, hysteria, mild psychosis, alcoholism, delirium	*Sedation:* 32–100 mg 3 to 4 times daily. *Delirium tremens:* 200 mg 3 times daily. *Epilepsy:* 400–600 mg daily; **pediatric, up to age 5:** 16–32 mg 3 to 4 times daily; **over age 5:** 32–64 mg 3 to 4 times daily. Administer at bedtime	Long-acting barbiturate with anticonvulsant activity. The hypnotic effects are mild and compound causes little drowsiness or lassitude. For epilepsy, mephobarbital is often administered concurrently with phenytoin. Drug has specific antiepileptic

Drug	Uses	Dosage	Remarks
	tremens, and restlessness. As adjunct in cardiovascular disease and allergies.	if seizures are likely to occur at night. Increase dosage gradually until optimum is reached.	action because it is broken down in body to phenobarbital.
Metharbital (Gemonil)	Anticonvulsant, suitable for treatment of petit mal, grand mal, myoclonic epilepsy and mixed types of seizures (not agent of first choice, however)	*Individualized, Usual,* **adult:** 100 mg 1 to 3 times daily, to be increased gradually until control is established; **pediatric:** 5–15 mg/kg daily.	Long-acting barbiturate, anticonvulsant with specific antiepileptic action.
Methohexital sodium (Brevital sodium)	General anesthetic for brief procedures (oral surgery, gynecologic, and genitourinary examinations, reduction of fractures, prior to electroshock therapy).	**Induction:** 50–120 mg; **maintenance:** administer 20–40 mg as required usually q 4 to 7 min (as a 1% solution) or by continuous drip (0.2% solution—1 drop/minute).	Ultrashort acting; duration of anesthesia 5–8 minutes.
Pentobarbital sodium (Nebralin, Nembutal Sodium)	Sedative, hypnotic, adjunct in diagnostic procedures, emergency use in convulsive states.	Drug can be given **PO, IM, rectally,** and even by cautious **IV administration.** *Sedation:* 30 mg 3 to 4 times daily up to maximum of 120 mg daily. *Hypnotic:* 100 mg. **Pediatric** *Sedation:* 8–30 mg; **older children:** 60–120 mg. **IV** *(control of acute convulsions):* 200–500 mg depending on response of patient (see Remarks) **IM, adults:** 150–200 mg; **pediatric:** 25–80 mg. **Rectal, adults:** 120–200 mg; **pediatric 2–12 months:** 30 mg; **1–4 years:** 30–60 mg; **5–12 years:** 60 mg; **12–14 years:** 60–120 mg.	Short-acting barbiturate. *Administration:* Since pentobarbital is a potent CNS depressant that may cause adverse respiratory and circulatory response, the IV dose is given in fractions. Adults receive 100 mg initially; children and debilitated persons 50 mg. Subsequent fractions are administered after 1 minute observation periods. Overdosage or too rapid administration may cause spasms of larynx or pharynx, or both. Pentobarbital solutions are highly alkaline. *Administration:* Administer no more than 5 ml at one site IM because of possible tissue irritation (pain, necrosis, gangrene). *Additional Nursing Implications* (1) Observe closely for respiratory depression, which is the first sign of overdosage. (2) Observe for pain, delayed onset of hypnosis, pallor, cyanosis, and patchy discoloration of skin, signs of intra-arterial injection. (3) Stop IV injection if there is any pain in limb.

(Continued)

TABLE 12 BARBITURATES (*Continued*)

Drug	Use	Dosage	Remarks
Phenobarbital (Eskabarb, Luminal PRB/12, Pheno-Squar, SK-Phenobarbital, Solfoton) Phenobarbital sodium (Luminal sodium)	Sedative, anticonvulsant, antiepileptic (grand mal and focal cortical epilepsy only, can exacerbate psychomotor and petit mal).	Phenobarbital is given **PO**. Phenobarbital sodium is given **PO, IM, IV, SC and rectally**. *Sedation:* 16–32 mg 2 to 4 times daily. *Hypnotic;* **PO:** 100–300 mg. *Anticonvulsant: individualized,* aim at minimum effective dose. **PO:** usual, 120–200 mg daily. **IV, IM:** 200–320 mg. Total adult daily dose should not exceed 650 mg. **IV** dose should not exceed 300 mg. **Pediatric,** *sedative,* **PO:** 2 mg/kg/24 hr in 4 divided doses. **Rectal:** *Anticonvulsant:* 6 mg/kg daily. **Parenteral** (*epilepsy*): 3–5 mg/kg daily.	Long-acting barbiturate. A drug of choice for grand mal epilepsy. Give major fraction of anticonvulsant dosage according to when seizures are likely to occur. On arising for daytime seizures, at bedtime when seizures occur at night. In most cases, when used for epilepsy, drug must be taken regularly to avoid seizures—even when no seizures are imminent. For epilepsy, may be given with amphetamine to overcome sedation. Aqueous solution for injection must be freshly prepared. Some ready-dissolved solutions for injection are available. The vehicle is propylene glycol, water, and alcohol. These solutions are stable. IM administration is preferred. *IV Administration:* Inject very slowly at rate of 50 mg/min

Drug	Use	Dosage	Remarks
Secobarbital (Seconal, Seco-8) Secobarbital sodium (Seconal Sodium)	Mild sedation, hypnotic, acute convulsive disorders, dentistry, minor surgery, obstetrics.	**PO, IM, and rectally:** Same dosage regardless of route. b. *Sedation:* 30–50 mg t.i.d. *Hypnotic:* 100–200 mg. *Preoperative sedation:* 200–300 mg 1 to 2 hr before surgery. **Pediatric,** *sedation:* 6 mg/kg/day in 3 divided doses. *Preoperative sedation:* 50–100 mg 1 to 2 hr before surgery.	Short-acting barbiturate. Not effective for epilepsy. **Adults:** Aqueous solution preferred to polyethylene glycol—which may be irritating to kidneys, especially in patients with signs of renal insufficiency. *Administration:* (1) Aqueous solutions for injection must be freshly prepared from dry-packed ampules. (2) Stable aqueous-polyethylene glycol solutions are available. These should be stored below 10°C.
Talbutal (Lotusate)	Mild sedation, hypnotic	PO, *Hypnotic:* 120 mg.	Intermediate-acting barbiturate.
Thiamylal sodium (Surital Sodium)	Anesthesia	**IV:** 3–4 ml of a freshly prepared 2.5% solution; **maximum dose:** 1 gm (or 40 ml of 2.5% solution). Two-thirds of calculated dose may be sufficient for obstetric cases.	Ultrashort-acting barbiturate. *Administration:* Solution should be administered slowly: 1 ml every 5 seconds. Can also be administered by IV drip as 0.2% or 0.3% solution. *Additional Contraindication* Porphyria
Thiopental sodium (Pentothal Sodium)	Preanesthetic or general anesthesia only	**IV only.** Dosage determined by anesthesiologist to fit needs of situation.	Ultrashort-acting barbiturate. Administer cautiously to avoid severe respiratory depression.

Remarks   Many barbiturates are also supplied as the sodium salt, which is the only suitable form for parenteral administration.

Administration/ Storage

1. Aqueous solutions of sodium salts are unstable and must be used within 30 minutes after preparation.
2. Discard parenteral solutions that contain precipitate.

Nursing Implications

1. Withhold drug and consult with a physician if symptoms of overdosage are observed.
2. Do not awaken a patient to administer a sleeping pill.
3. Note sleeping patterns of patients since these may influence the doctor in deciding what type of barbiturate the patient may need.
4. Anticipate that with some patients sedation is preceded by a period of transient elation, confusion, or euphoria and provide appropriate nursing measures to calm the patient and prevent injury.
5. Use safety measures, such as side rails and assistance when ambulatory, for patients receiving hypnotic doses since they may be unsteady or confused.
6. Do not apply cuffs or other restraints at the first sign of excitement when a patient becomes confused by barbiturates. Attempt to calm the patient and orient him/her by switching on a light and talking quietly and calmly until he/she is calm and relaxed.
7. Utilize supportive nursing measures to enhance the effect of the drug (back rub, warm drink, quiet pleasant atmosphere, and empathetic attitude).
8. Use nursing judgment in deciding whether to administer a second PRN sleeping medication during the night. Try to find out why the patient cannot sleep, utilize comfort measures, and administer analgesics for pain if ordered, or consult with physician. The dazed, dizzy, lethargic hangover effect is sometimes caused by injudicious use of barbiturates during the night.
9. Observe that the patient is actually taking the drug and not hoarding it when medication is given PO.
10. Observe patients for physical and psychological dependence and tolerance.
11. Caution the patient that alcohol potentiates the barbiturates.
12. Warn the patient receiving barbiturates not to drive a car or operate other machinery.
13. Warn patients who take sleeping pills at home not to leave the pill bottle on the bedside table. Patients have been known to forget how many pills they have taken. This may lead to accidental overdosage.
14. Explain to the patient who has been taking large doses of sedative for 8 weeks or more that they should not suddenly discontinue medication because withdrawal symptoms, including weakness, anxiety, delirium, and grand mal seizures, may occur. They should not reduce the dose without checking with their physician.
15. Be alert to the signs of developing porphyria characterized by nausea and vomiting, abdominal pain, and muscle spasm.
16. Teach patients on long-term therapy to report immediately signs of

infection, such as sore throat and fever, or signs of a bleeding tendency, such as bruising easily or nosebleeds, all of which are signs of hematologic toxicity.

17. Anticipate that IV use of barbiturates will be limited to the treatment of acute convulsions and anesthesia.
18. Monitor IV administration of barbiturates closely for correct rate of flow; too rapid an injection may produce respiratory depression, dyspnea, and shock.
19. Monitor the site of the IV injection closely for extravasation which may lead to pain, nerve damage, and necrosis.
20. Monitor the site of the IV injection for thrombophlebitis evidenced by redness and pain along site of vein.
21. Be familiar with the treatment of chronic and acute toxicity associated with barbiturates.

SECTION 2

nonbarbiturate sedatives and hypnotics

Bromisovalum
Chloral Hydrate
Ethchlorvynol
Ethinamate
Flurazepam
Glutethimide

Methaqualone
Methaqualone Hydrochloride
Methyprylon
Paraldehyde
Propiomazine Hydrochloride
Triclofos Sodium

General Statement (See also *Antianxiety Agents*)

This section presents the characteristics of various nonbarbiturate compounds that are used for sedation and as hypnotics. Concomitant use of nonbarbiturate sedative-hypnotics with alcohol, anesthetics, antianxiety drugs, antihistamines, barbiturates, narcotics, or phenothiazines may result in addition or potentiation of CNS depressant effects. Symptoms manifested are drowsiness, lethargy, stupor, respiratory collapse, coma, and possibly death.

BROMISOVALUM BROMURAL

Classification Nonbarbiturate sedative and hypnotic.

Remarks Depresses CNS without causing drowsiness. May be habit forming. Because of its bromide content, this preparation has little advantage over other, potentially less toxic, preparations.

Uses   General hypnotic and sedative.

Contraindications   Hypersensitivity to bromides; marked renal impairment.

Untoward Reactions   Dermatitis and urticaria. Upon metabolism, compound releases free bromide, which can cause bromide intoxication characterized by vomiting, profound stupor, and bromide psychosis.

Dosage   *Sedative:* 324 mg q 3 to 4 hr. *Hypnotic:* 650–975 mg at bedtime. *Overdosage:* discontinue medication, administer 4–8 gm sodium chloride and encourage fluid intake to 4 liters/day.

Nursing Implications
1. Observe the patient for rash or mental disturbances indicating bromism and necessitating discontinuance of medication and treatment of toxicity.
2. Encourage the patient to take a warm bath, drink warm milk, or use other such sedative measures rather than taking bromisovalum because it is habit forming.

CHLORAL HYDRATE AQUACHLORAL, COHIDRATE, FELSULES, NOCTEC, ORADRATE, RECTULES, SK-CHLORAL HYDRATE, SOMNOS

Classification   Nonbarbiturate sedative and hypnotic.

General Statement   CNS depressant. Induces sedation and sleep in therapeutic doses. Drug produces only slight hangover. High dosages produce severe CNS depression and depress respiratory and vasomotor centers (hypotension). Patients can develop tolerance and psychological and physical dependence. Readily absorbed from the GI tract. Well distributed throughout all tissues, passes the placental barrier, and appears in breast milk.

Chloral hydrate is the most popular "chloral" drug. It is rapidly changed in the body to trichloroethanol, which seems to be the active form of the drug. Other chloral derivatives and analogs (chloral betaine, tribromoethanol, and trichloroethanol) have the same characteristics as chloral hydrate.

Uses   General hypnotic and sedative. Treatment of delirium tremens and for patients undergoing narcotic, barbiturate, and alcohol withdrawal. Prior to EEG. Has little analgesic activity and should not be given to patients suffering pain—may cause excitement or delirium.

Contraindications   Marked hepatic or renal impairment, severe cardiac disease, or nursing mothers. Drugs should not be given orally to patients with gastritis or gastric ulcer.

Untoward Reactions   Nausea, vomiting, skin reactions, paradoxical behavior (patient may become somnambulistic and show paranoid reactions), gastritis, renal and hepatic damage, allergic reactions. Drug may increase peristalsis and decrease urine flow and uric acid excretion. Sudden withdrawal of chloral hydrate in dependent patients may lead to "chloral delirium." Also, patients who have tolerated high doses of chloral hydrate for prolonged periods of time may suddenly exhibit intolerance characterized by severe respiratory depression, hypotension, and cardiac effects. These symptoms may result in death. Chronic toxicity is treated by gradual withdrawal and rehabilitative measures as used in treatment of the chronic alcoholic. Poisoning by chloral hydrate resembles acute barbiturate intoxication; the same supportive treatment is indicated.

Drug Interactions

Interactant	Interaction
Anticoagulants, oral	↑ Effects of anticoagulants by ↓ plasma protein binding
Furosemide (IV)	Concomitant use results in diaphoresis, tachycardia, hypertension, flushing

Monoamine oxidase inhibitors
   Pargyline (Eutonyl)
   Tranylcypromine
   (Parnate)
	↑ Effects of chloral hydrate due to ↓ breakdown by liver

Dosage   **PO** (*capsules, elixir, and syrup*) and **rectally.** *Sedative:* 250 mg, t.i.d; **pediatric:** ½ the hypnotic dose. *Hypnotic:* 500–1000 mg; **pediatric:** 55 mg/kg. **Maximum adult dose:** 2 gm daily; **pediatric:** 1 gm daily.

Administration   PO: give after meals with full glass of water. Rectally: Use suppositories or dissolve powder in olive oil and administer as a retention enema.

Nursing Implications

1. Observe for alertness of patient and monitor respiratory, cardiac, and vasomotor depression and dilation of cutaneous blood vessels.
2. Minimize nausea or vomiting by administering the drug in capsules or as a well-diluted syrup. This will disguise the taste and minimize gastritis.
3. Anticipate that a false-positive Benedict's test may occur.
4. Observe for reduced urine output and elevated BUN.
5. Observe patients for tolerance and psychological and physical dependence. Symptoms of dependence resemble those of acute alcoholism but with more severe gastritis.
6. Have equipment ready for physiologic supportive treatment of acute poisoning: suction, respirator, oxygen, IV sets, and sodium bicarbonate and sodium lactate solutions.
7. Warn the patient not to ingest alcohol while on chloral hydrate therapy because the additive effects of these two CNS depressants results in a "Mickey Finn" or "knockout drops" reaction.

ETHCHLORVYNOL PLACIDYL

Classification   Nonbarbiturate sedative and hypnotic.

General Statement Depresses CNS but produces less respiratory depression than barbiturates. Also has some muscle relaxant and anticonvulsive properties. Chronic use can cause psychological and physical dependence.

Uses Mild anxiety and tension. Simple insomnia. Particularly useful for patients who cannot tolerate barbiturates. As adjunct for the treatment of dermatologic disorders and epilepsy. Sedative before EEG. No analgesic effects—not useful in patients suffering pain.

Contraindication Hypersensitivity.

Untoward Reactions Initial excitement, giddiness, vertigo, mental confusion, headache, blurred vision, facial numbness, bad aftertaste, nausea, vomiting, drowsiness, hangover, fatigue, and ataxia. Massive overdose produces symptoms similar to barbiturate intoxication.

Drug Interactions

Interactant	Interaction
Anticoagulants, oral	↓ Effect of anticoagulants due to ↑ breakdown by liver
Antidepressants, tricyclic	Combination may result in transient delirium

Dosage **PO,** *sedative:* 200–600 mg daily in 2 to 3 divided doses. *Hypnotic:* 0.5–1 gm.

Administration With food or milk to reduce or eliminate giddiness and ataxia.

Nursing Implications See *Nursing Implications* under *Barbiturates*, pages 308–309.

ETHINAMATE VALMID

Classification Nonbarbiturate sedative and hypnotic.

General Statement Drug may have some weak anticonvulsant and weak local anesthetic effects. Therapeutic doses produce quiet sleep with little or no hangover. Larger doses produce euphoria. *Overdosage:* respiratory depression. Ethinamate may cause psychological and physical dependence as well as tolerance. Withdrawal symptoms are similar to those of barbiturates.

Uses Simple insomnia, preoperative sedation. Particularly useful for patients with impaired liver or kidney function and for those who cannot tolerate barbiturates. No analgesic effect—not useful in patients suffering pain.

Contraindications Hypersensitivity to drug. Safety in pregnancy, childhood, or during lactation has not been established. *Not recommended* for routine daytime sedation because prolonged use may lead to psychological and physical dependence. **Do not give** to patients receiving other CNS depressant drugs.

Untoward Reactions Few. Thrombocytopenic purpura, mild GI symptoms, skin rashes, and paradoxical excitement in children. Abrupt withdrawal of large doses may be dangerous.

Drug Interactions See *General Statement*, page 309.

Dosage **PO:** 500–1000 mg 20 minutes before bedtime or 1 to 2 hours preoperatively. Elderly or debilitated patients should receive a lower dosage.

Nursing Implications
1. Observe patients receiving large dosages for symptoms of dependence.
2. Caution the patient against abruptly discontinuing drug since withdrawal symptoms may occur.
3. See treatment for acute toxicity under *Barbiturates*.
4. Gastric lavage for acute poisoning must be done immediately to be effective as the drug is rapidly absorbed from the GI tract.

FLURAZEPAM DALMANE

Remarks Although this agent is a benzodiazepine compound like Valium and Librium, it is only used as a hypnotic. For details, see *Antianxiety Agents*, page 326.

Dosage **PO:** 30 mg at bedtime; 15 mg for elderly and/or debilitated patients.

GLUTETHIMIDE DORIDEN, ROLATHIMIDE

Classification Nonbarbiturate sedative and hypnotic.

General Statement Similar to barbiturates in sedative-hypnotic actions. CNS depressant; anticholinergic with some mydriatic (pupil dilating) effect. Also inhibits salivary secretion and is constipating. Small therapeutic doses produce sedation; somewhat larger ones reduce motor activity, leading to sleep. The drug may cause psychological and physical dependence as well as tolerance. At comparable doses, it produces a lesser degree of respiratory depression but a greater degree of hypotension than barbiturates.

Uses Daytime or preoperative sedation, simple insomnia, and first stage of labor. Particularly useful for patients who cannot tolerate barbiturates. No analgesic action.

Contraindications Hypersensitivity to drug. Administer with extreme caution to depressed patients with suicidal tendencies.
     Do not give to patient with glaucoma or to patients with a history of drug dependence, alcoholism, or emotional disorders.

Untoward Reactions

Nausea, vomiting, anorexia, xerostomia, headache, dizziness, confusion, drowsiness, or skin rash. Rarely: acute hypersensitivity, blood dyscrasias, peripheral neuropathy, intermittent porphyria, and jaundice. Skin rashes necessitate discontinuing the drug. Abrupt withdrawal of large doses may be dangerous—withdrawal symptoms are similar to that of barbiturates. Occasionally, symptoms similar to withdrawal occur in patients who have been taking only moderate doses, even when there is no abstention (tremulousness, nausea, tachycardia, fever, tonic muscle spasms, generalized convulsions).

Chronic Toxicity

Characterized by psychosis, confusion, delirium, hallucinations, ataxia, tremor, hyporeflexia, slurred speech, memory loss, irritability, fever, weight loss, mydriasis, xerostomia, nystagmus, headache, and convulsions. Treatment consists of careful, cautious withdrawal of drug over a period of several days or weeks.

Acute Toxicity

Characterized by coma, hypotension, hypothermia, followed by fever, tachycardia, depression or absence of reflexes (including pupiliary response), sudden apnea, cyanosis, tonic muscle spasms, convulsions, and hyperreflexia.

Treatment of acute toxicity is supportive, starting with gastric lavage, CNS stimulants (used with caution), vasopressors, and maintenance of pulmonary ventilation. Parenteral fluids are administered cautiously, and hemodialsis may be necessary. Endotracheal intubation or tracheotomy may be indicated.

Drug Interactions

Interactant	*Interaction*
Anticoagulants, oral	↓ Effect of anticoagulants due to ↑ breakdown by liver
Antidepressants, tricyclic	Additive anticholinergic side effects

Laboratory Test Interference

Alters (↑ or ↓) 17-ketogenic steroids.

Dosage

Daytime sedation: 125–250 mg t.i.d. *Preoperative sedation:* 500 mg the night before surgery; 500–1000 mg 1 hr before anesthesia. *Labor:* 500 mg. This dose may be repeated once, but drug may cause CNS depression in fetus. *Hypnosis:* 500 mg at bedtime, which may be repeated once during the same night. **Maximum daily dose:** 1 gm. **Not recommended for children under 12.**

Administration

After meals.

Nursing Implications

1. Provide special mouth care since the patient may have xerostomia.
2. Check that the patient is having regular bowel movements; glutethimide reduces intestinal motility. Provide extra fluids and roughage in diet. Consult with physician regarding need for a laxative.

3. Observe the patient for tolerance and psychological or physical dependence.
4. Warn patients receiving glutethimide not to drive a car or operate other machinery after taking medication because drug may cause drowsiness.
5. Withhold drug from patients showing signs of depression or suicidal tendencies.

Treatment of Overdosage
6. Be prepared to assist with gastric lavage for treatment of acute toxicity. Monitor vital signs.
7. In addition to providing an adequate airway, oxygen, fluids, electrolyte intake, and parenteral fluids, have on hand CNS stimulants and pressor agents.
8. Have on hand an endotracheal tube and tracheotomy setup.
9. Be prepared to handle request for hemodialysis.

METHAQUALONE QUAALUDE, SOPOR

METHAQUALONE HYDROCHLORIDE PAREST

Classification	Nonbarbiturate sedative and hypnotic.
General Statement	General CNS depressant. Low doses produce sedation. Higher doses induce sleep. Can cause physical and psychological dependence.
Uses	Routine daytime sedation; simple insomnia. Particularly useful for patients who cannot tolerate barbiturates. No analgesic activity.
Contraindications	Hypersensitivity to drug, severe hepatic or renal impairment, pregnancy, children under 14 years of age. Administer with extreme caution to depressed patients or those with suicidal tendencies, renal and hepatic impairment, or cerebral insufficiency.
Untoward Reactions	Neuropsychiatric: headache, hangover, acroparesthesia (tingling and numbness in extremities), fatigue, dizziness, torpor. GI: dry mouth, anorexia, nausea, epigastric distress, diarrhea.
Drug Interactions	*See General Statement*, page 309.
Dosage	*Sedative:* 75 mg t.i.d. or q.i.d. *Hypnotic:* 150–300 mg (200–400 mg methaqualone HCl) at bedtime. Dosage for elderly or debilitated patients should be individualized. **Not recommended for use in children.**
Nursing Implications	1. Prevent patient on methaqualone therapy from engaging in hazardous tasks. 2. Check that hospitalized patient takes his/her dose of methaqualone and does not hoard it.

3. Be alert to flushed appearance, a sign of mild intoxication, and to slightly pale skin, a sign of severe intoxication.
4. Encourage a patient suffering from simple insomnia to try warm baths, warm milk, and so forth to induce sleep rather than becoming dependent on drugs.
5. Advise patient to take prescribed dose as ordered and not to increase dosage though it may take 5 to 7 days before they sleep well.
6. Turn comatose patient on his/her side to prevent aspiration of emesis.
7. Provide safety measures such as padded side rails for the overactive toxic patient.
8. Assist in treatment of toxicity.
   a. Monitor vital signs closely;
   b. Assist in evacuation of stomach contents by lavage;
   c. Provide oxygen and assisted ventilation as necessary;
   d. Monitor IV fluids and electrolytes;
   e. Monitor urinary output;
   f. Have on hand phenothiazines to reduce motor activity.

METHYPRYLON NOLUDAR

Classification   Nonbarbiturate sedative and hypnotic.

Remarks   CNS depressant with activity similar to that of the barbiturates. (See also *Glutethimide*, page 313.)

Uses   Simple insomnia. Especially useful for patients allergic to barbiturates.

Contraindications   Hypersensitivity to drug. Infants under 3 months. Administer with caution in the presence of renal and hepatic disease.

Untoward Reactions   Morning drowsiness, dizziness, mild-to-moderate gastric upset, headache, paradoxical excitement, skin rash. Overdosage is characterized by somnolence, confusion, coma, constricted pupils, respiratory depression, and hypotension.

Drug Interactions   See *General Statement*, page 309.

Dosage   **Administer** 200–400 mg before retiring. **Pediatric** (effectiveness extremely variable), **initial,** 50 mg. If ineffective, may be increased to 200 mg at bedtime.

Nursing Implications
1. Advise patient taking methyprylon not to engage in hazardous activities such as driving because drowsiness may develop.
2. Encourage the patient suffering from simple insomnia to try warm baths, warm milk, and so forth to induce sleep rather than becoming dependent on drugs.
3. Advise the patient not to increase dosage without medical supervision.

4. Assist in treatment of toxicity.
   a. Monitor vital signs closely;
   b. Assist in evacuation of stomach contents by lavage;
   c. Provide oxygen and assist ventilation if necessary; have available caffeine and sodium benzoate or metrazol to be used to stimulate respiration;
   d. Monitor IV fluids and electrolytes; have on hand Levophed or Aramine to be used for hypotension;
   e. Monitor urinary output; hemodialysis may be instituted if urinary output is too scant;
   f. Provide supportive care for the comatose patient; turn patient on side to prevent aspiration of vomitus;
   g. Provide safety measures such as side rails.

PARALDEHYDE PARAL

Classification Nonbarbiturate sedative and hypnotic.

Remarks This CNS depressant resembles chloral hydrate. See page 310 for all general information, including contraindications, untoward reactions, and treatment of toxicity.

Drug Interactions

Interactant	Interaction
Disulfiram (Antabuse)	Combination may produce an Antabuse-like reaction
Sulfonamides	↑ Chance of sulfonamide crystalluria

Dosage **PO, rectal;** *sedative:* 3–8 ml; *hypnotic:* 10–30 ml. **Pediatric;** *sedative:* 0.15 mg/kg; *hypnotic:* 0.3 ml/kg. **IM, IV;** *anticonvulsant:* 3–5 ml. **Use Paraldehyde for Injection.**

Administration/ Storage

1. PO: Drug should be very cold to minimize odor and taste as well as gastric irritation. Mask the taste and odor by mixing drug with syrup, milk, fruit juice, or wine.
2. Rectal: Mix with a thin oil or isotonic sodium chloride solution to minimize irritation—1 part medication to 2 parts diluent.
3. IM: A pure sterile preparation should be used. Prevent extravasation into subcutaneous tissue as drug is very irritating and may cause sterile abscesses.
4. IV: Only in an emergency, dilute with several volumes of physiologic saline and inject slowly with caution; since circulatory collapse or pulmonary edema may occur. Use glass syringe and metal needles because the drug may react with the plastic used in disposable syringes and needles.
5. Store in a tight, light-resistant container, well-filled with a maximum of 120 gm in each container.

Nursing Implications
1. Reassure patients disturbed by the odor that they will become used to it.
2. Observe for dependence and toxicity.
3. See *Nursing Implications* under *Chloral Hydrate* for toxicity and treatment.

PROPIOMAZINE HYDROCHLORIDE LARGON

Classification   Nonbarbiturate sedative and hypnotic phenothiazine.

General Statement   At therapeutic dosages, this phenothiazine drug has sedative, anti-emetic, antihistaminic, and anticholinergic effects. Peak sedation occurs 15 to 30 minutes after IV and 40 to 60 minutes after IM administration. The effect starts to diminish after 3 hours and vanishes after 6 hours.

Uses   Preanesthetic to reduce anxiety and emesis during surgery and labor. Adjunct to narcotic analgesic.

Contraindications   Coma. Use with extreme caution in presence of hypertensive crisis.

Untoward Reactions   Dry mouth, transient decrease in blood pressure during rapid IV administration, tachycardia, GI upset, skin rashes, respiratory depression, altered respiratory pattern. Dizziness and confusion in the elderly. Transient restlessness.
Irritation and thrombophlebitis at injection site.

Dosage   **IM and IV,** *preoperative sedation; usual,* 20 mg up to 40 mg. *Obstetrics:* 20–40 mg. Meperidine—50 mg, *sedation with local anesthesia:* 10–20 mg; **children weighing less than 60 pounds:** 0.55–1.1 mg/kg; or **children 2–4 years:** 10 mg; **4–6 years:** 15 mg; **6–12 years:** 25 mg. All dosages may be repeated after 3 hours.

Administration/ Storage
1. Inject into large, undamaged vein.
2. Avoid extravasation.
3. Never administer subcutaneously or intra-arterially.
4. Do not use solutions that are cloudy or contain precipitate.
5. Aqueous solutions are incompatible with barbiturate salts or alkaline solutions.
6. Store at 15°–30°C and protect from light.

Nursing Implications
1. Anticipate that the dose of other sedatives administered with propiomazine will be reduced by ¼ to ½ in strength.
2. Anticipate that should vasopressor drugs be administered with propiomazine, norepinephrine would be used rather than epinephrine.
3. Warn patients not to drive a car or operate machinery requiring mental alertness for at least 2 weeks after therapy is initiated and then only after consulting with a physician who will evaluate their response to therapy.

4. Provide mouth care to relieve xerostomia except for patients scheduled for surgery for whom a dry mouth is desirable.
5. Monitor BP for 5 hours after IM or IV administration because medication may have a hypotensive effect.
6. Observe patients for untoward reaction remembering that though unlikely, the adverse reactions (blood dyscrasias, hepatotoxicity, extrapyramidal symptoms, reactivation of psychotic processes, cardiac arrest, endocrine disturbances, dermatologic disorders, ocular changes, and hypersensitivity reactions) associated with long-term use of phenothiazines may occur.
7. Provide a safe environment for geriatric patients experiencing dizziness, confusion, or amnesia after administration of the drug.
8. Consider that the antiemetic effect of propiomazine may be masking other pathology, such as toxicity to other drugs, intestinal obstruction, or brain lesions.

TRICLOFOS SODIUM TRICLOS

Classification Nonbarbiturate hypnotic.

General Statement This agent is related to chloral hydrate. At therapeutic doses it produces mild CNS depression and deep sleep. The latter is attained within 20 minutes and lasts 6 to 8 hours.

Uses Hypnotic for simple insomnia, prior to EEG.

Contraindications Hypersensitivity to triclofos or chloral hydrate. Marked renal and hepatic diseases. Children under 12 years of age. Use with caution for patients suffering from cardiac arrhythmia, severe cardiac diseases, mental depression, suicidal tendencies or tendency for drug abuse. Safe use in pregnancy has not been established.

Untoward Reactions Nausea, vomiting, flatulence, "bad taste," hangover, staggering gait, ataxia, lightheadedness, dizziness, vertigo, drowsiness, nightmares, headaches, malaise, ketonuria, urticaria, blood dyscrasias.

Drug Interactions

Interactant	Interaction
Anticoagulants, oral	↑ Effect of anticoagulants by ↓ plasma protein binding
Furosemide (Lasix)	Diaphoresis, flushes, hypotension (only in patients with myocardial infarction and congestive heart failure)
Monoamine oxidase inhibitors	↑ Effect of triclofos due to ↓ breakdown by liver
Warfarin sodium (Coumadin)	↑ Anticoagulant effect during first two weeks of combined therapy as a metabolite of triclofos ↓ plasma protein binding.

Laboratory Test Interference Possibility of false + for urine glucose with Benedict or Fehling's solutions. Fluorometric test for urine catecholamines; Reddy-Jenkins-Thorn procedure for urinary 17-hydroxycorticosteroids.

Dosage **PO:** 1.5 gm, 15 to 30 minutes before retiring. **Pediatric** (*before EEG only*): 22 mg/kg.

Administration/ Storage
1. Store in cool place.
2. Should not be used continuously for more than 6 weeks.
3. After prolonged use discontinue medication gradually to avoid withdrawal symptoms.

Nursing Implications
1. Ascertain that periodic blood and liver function tests are done for patients on long-term use.
2. Warn patient against operating a car or hazardous machinery, because drug may impair alertness and coordination.
3. Observe for signs of sodium retention, such as edema and hypertension, in patients with cardiac and/or renal dysfunction.
4. Report gastric discomfort which may necessitate discontinuation of drug.
5. Anticipate that dosage of other sedatives administered concomitantly will be reduced.
6. Anticipate that the dosage of anticoagulants administered concomitantly will be reduced to prevent bleeding, because triclofos potentiates anticoagulants. After triclofos sodium is discontinued, dosage of anticoagulants may require an increase.
7. Advise diabetic patients to use Tes Tape or Clinitest tablets for testing urine because triclofos causes a false positive with Benedict's or Fehling's solutions.
8. Withdraw drug slowly from physically dependent persons to prevent delirium tremens and hallucinations.
9. Have equipment available for physiologic supportive treatment of acute poisoning: suction, respirator, oxygen, IV sets and sodium bicarbonate and sodium lactate solutions.
10. Observe patients with history of mental depression or suicidal tendencies and report because these patients have a tendency to increase dosage at their own initiative.

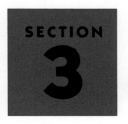

antianxiety agents

Chlordiazepoxide
Chlormezanone
Clorazepate Dipotassium
Clorazepate Monopotassium
Diazepam
Flurazepam Hydrochloride
Hydroxyzine Hydrochloride

Hydroxyzine Pamoate
Lorazepam
Meprobamate
Prazepam
Oxazepam
Tybamate

General Statement

This group of drugs is used for the treatment of mild-to-moderate states of emotional upset, nervous tension, and conditions requiring muscle relaxant activity. The agents are useful in the treatment of neuroses and for normal persons who react adversely to environmental stress.

At higher dosage levels, certain agents are used for acute psychotic agitation in schizophrenics.

They are sometimes prescribed for the management of delirium tremens after alcohol withdrawal.

The pharmacologic actions of this group resemble those of the barbiturates. The drugs are often used for the same purposes. However, they cause less drowsiness and confusion and also have a higher therapeutic/toxic ratio.

Meprobamate and diazepam also have some anticonvulsant activity, relax skeletal muscle spasms, and alleviate tension. This enhances their value as tranquilizers for patients suffering from arthritis and for alcoholic patients suffering from muscle tension and tremors.

All antianxiety agents can cause psychological and physical dependence. Withdrawal symptoms usually start within 12 to 48 hours after stopping the drug and last for 12 to 48 hours. When the patient has received large doses of these drugs for weeks or months, dosage should be reduced gradually over a period 1 to 2 weeks. Alternatively, a short-acting barbiturate may be substituted and then withdrawn gradually. Abrupt withdrawal of high dosage may be accompanied by coma, convulsions, and even death.

The benzodiazepines generally have long half-lives (1 to 8 days). Thus, cumulative effects may occur. Chlordiazepoxide and diazepam are absorbed more rapidly following oral than following IM administration. Diazepam, with a half-life of 1 to 3 days, is metabolized in the liver to active metabolites including N-desmethyl diazepam which can be oxidized to form another active metabolite—oxazepam. Chlordiazepoxide has a half-life of 1 to 2 days and is metabolized to two active compounds. Oxazepam, with a shorter half-life than either chlordiazepoxide or diazepam, is not metabolized to active compounds; therefore, cumulative effects are less likely to occur. Finally, flurazepam has a half-life of 2 to 4 days and is metabolized to the active compound, N-desalkylflurazepam.

Dosage and uses of the benzodiazepines and meprobamate-type drugs are presented in Table 13. The miscellaneous agents are presented individually.

Uses Management of anxiety and tension occurring alone or as a side effect of other conditions including menopausal syndrome, premenstrual tension, asthma, and angina pectoris.

Neurological conditions involving muscle spasms and tetanus. Adjunct in treatment of rheumatoid arthritis, osteoarthritis, trauma, low back pain, torticollis, and selected convulsive disorders including status epilepticus.

Premedication for surgery or electric cardioversion.

Rehabilitation of chronic alcoholics; delirium tremens; nocturnal enuresis in childhood; and to induce sleep.

Contraindications *Absolute:* Hypersensitivity; children under 6 years of age.

Untoward Reactions Lowered tolerance to alcohol. Drowsiness (decreases with usage), allergic reactions, urticaria, blood dyscrasias, dizziness, inability to void and ejaculate, headaches, nausea, vomiting, constipation, hypotension, fainting spells, angioneurotic edema, fever, bronchial spasms, changes in visual accommodation, paradoxical excitement, anaphylactic reactions, weakness, muscle tenderness, slurred speech, talkativeness, emotional instability, confusion, and urinary frequency.

Drug Interactions (Meprobamate, Benzodiazepines)

Interactant	Interaction
Alcohol	Potentiation or addition of CNS depressant effects. Concomitant use may lead to drowsiness, lethargy, stupor, respiratory collapse, coma, or death
Anesthetics, general	See *Alcohol*
Antidepressants, tricyclic	Concomitant use with benzodiazepines (diazepam, chlordiazepoxide, oxazepam) may cause additive sedative effect and/or atropine-like side effects
Antihistamines	See *Alcohol*
Barbiturates	See *Alcohol*
CNS depressants	See *Alcohol*
Narcotics	See *Alcohol*
Phenothiazines	See *Alcohol*
Phenytoin (Dilantin)	Concomitant use with benzodiazepines (chlordiazepoxide, diazepam, oxazepam) may cause ↑ effect of phenytoin due to ↓ breakdown by liver
Sedative-hypnotics, nonbarbiturate	See *Alcohol*

Laboratory Test Interference   Altered liver function tests, including bilirubin values.

Dosage   See Table 13, page 324, and individual agents. Persistent drowsiness, ataxia, or visual disturbances may require dosage adjustment.

Lower dosage is usually indicated for older patients. GI effects are decreased when drugs are given with meals or shortly after.

Withdraw drugs gradually.

Nursing Implications

1. Observe the patient for more frequent requests for the drugs or ingestion of larger than recommended doses. These patients may be developing physical and psychological dependence leading to drug abuse.
2. Observe for ataxia, slurred speech, and vertigo manifestations. Such symptoms are characteristic of chronic intoxication and usually are an indication that the patient is taking more than the recommended dose.
3. Carefully supervise the dose and amount prescribed, especially when prescription is for long-term treatment of alcoholics and other patients with a known predisposition to take excessive quantities of drugs.
4. Stay with patient until drug is swallowed when it is administered on the ward. This prevents omission of the drug or hoarding, which may result in a suicide attempt.
5. Be aware, and inform the patient, that sudden withdrawal of the drug after prolonged and excessive use may cause the recurrence of preexisting symptoms or precipitate a withdrawal syndrome manifested by anxiety, anorexia, insomnia, vomiting, ataxia, tremors, muscle twitching, confusion, hallucinations, and, rarely, convulsive seizures.
6. Warn patients that these drugs may reduce ability required to handle potentially dangerous equipment, such as cars and other machinery.
7. Anticipate that doses to the elderly or debilitated patient will be lowest effective dose.
8. Anticipate that the drug will be prescribed cautiously and in small doses to patients with suicidal tendencies and observe such patients (as indeed all patients) for signs of depression.
9. Warn the patient not to drink alcohol while taking antianxiety agents because the depressant effect of both the alcohol and the antianxiety agents will be potentiated.
10. Provide side rails and assistance for patients affected by ataxia, weakness, or incoordination.
11. Encourage the patient to rise slowly from a supine position and to dangle feet before standing.
12. Advise the patient to lie down immediately if feeling faint.
13. Monitor BP before and after the patient receives an antianxiety agent. Evaluate the presence and degree of hypotensive reaction. Preferably keep the patient in a supine position for 2 to 3 hours after IV administration of drug.

TABLE 13 BENZODIAZEPINES, MEPROBAMATE, AND RELATED DRUGS

Drug	Main Use	Dosage	Remarks
Chlordiazepoxide (Chlordiazachel, J-Liberty, Libritabs, Librium, Sereen, SK-Lygen, Tenax)	Anxiety, acute withdrawal symptoms in chronic alcoholics	**PO, anxiety:** 5–25 mg t.i.d.–q.i.d. *Alcohol withdrawal:* initial, 50–100 mg. May be increased gradually to maximum of 300 mg daily. **Pediatric over 6 years: Initial,** 5 mg b.i.d.–q.i.d. May be increased to 10 mg b.i.d.–t.i.d. *Elderly debilitated patients:* use pediatric dosage. **IM or IV (IV not for children under 12 years);** *acute agitation, severe anxiety:* 50–100 mg initially; **then** 25–50 mg t.i.d.–q.i.d. *Presurgically* 25–100 mg 1 hr prior to surgery. *Alcohol withdrawal:* 50–100 mg. Repeat in 2 to 4 hr if needed. Daily maximum by any route: 300 mg	Benzodiazepine derivative. The drug is excreted slowly. Onset: PO: 30–60 minutes; IM: 15–30 minutes; IV: 3–30 minutes. Action may persist 3 or more hours. The drug has less anticonvulsant activity and is less potent than diazepam. *Additional Untoward Reactions* Jaundice, acute hepatic necrosis, hepatic dysfunction. *Administration* IM: Prepare solution immediately before administration by adding diluent to ampule. Shake until dissolved. Discard any unused solution. Inject slowly into upper, outer quadrant of gluteal muscle. IV: Prepare immediately before administration. Inject directly into vein over 1-min period. Do not add to IV infusion because of instability of drug. Do not use IV solution for IM.
Chlormezanone (Trancopal)	Anxiety, sedative	**PO:** 100–200 mg t.i.d.–q.i.d.; **pediatric 6–10 yr:** 50–100 mg t.i.d.–q.i.d.	Meprobamate-type drug. Exerts effect within 15 to 30 minutes and lasts 4 to 6 hours. Drug is tasteless and can be taken on an empty stomach.
Clorazepate Dipotassium (Tranxene)	Anxiety, tension	**PO:** 15 mg b.i.d. Adjust according to response. **Elderly patients: initial,** 7.5–15 mg daily. Adjust as required. *Alcohol withdrawal,*	Benzodiazepine-type drug. Peak effect attained within 60 minutes. Excreted slowly.

		day 1: 60–90 mg/day; *day 2:* 45–90 mg/day; *day 3:* 22.5–45 mg/day; *day 4:* 15–30 mg/day. Discontinue as soon as possible.	*Additional Contraindications* Depressive patients, nursing mothers. Give cautiously to patients with impaired renal or hepatic function.
Clorazepate Monopotassium (Azene)	Anxiety, psychoneurosis, acute withdrawal symptoms in chronic alcoholism	**PO,** *anxiety:* 13–52 mg in divided doses. Adjust as required. Can be given as single dose at night. *Alcohol withdrawal,* day 1: 26 mg, **then** 13–26 mg b.i.d.; day 2: 19.5–39 mg b.i.d.; day 3: 9.75–19.5 mg b.i.d.; day 4: 6.5–13 mg b.i.d.; **then** reduce gradually to 3.25–6.5 mg b.i.d. and discontinue when patient is stable.	Benzodiazepine derivative. *Additional Contraindications* Narrow angle glaucoma, persons under 18 years. *Additional Untoward Reaction* Decrease in blood pressure.
Diazepam (Valium)	Anxiety, tension (more effective than chlordiazepoxide), alcohol withdrawal, muscle relaxant, anticonvulsive agent. Used prior to gastroscopy and esophagoscopy, preoperatively and prior to cardioversion. Treatment of status epilepticus. Adjunct in cerebral palsy, paraplegia, or tetanus	**PO,** *Anxiety, anticonvulsant, muscle relaxant:* 2–10 mg b.i.d.–q.i.d. *Alcohol withdrawal:* **initial,** 10 mg t.i.d.–q.i.d. Decrease gradually to 5 mg t.i.d.–q.i.d. **Elderly, debilitated patients:** 2.5 mg b.i.d. May be gradually increased to adult level; **pediatric over 6 months: initial,** 1–2.5 mg t.i.d.–b.i.d. **IM, IV:** same as **PO** up to maximum of 30 mg in 8 hr. *Preop or diagnostic use,* **IM:** 5–15 mg 5 to 30 minutes prior to procedure. IV administration should not exceed 5 mg/min. Elderly or debilitated patients should not receive more than 5 mg parenterally at any one time.	Benzodiazepine derivative. Onset: PO: 30 to 60 minutes; IM: 15 to 30 minutes; IV: more rapid; may persist 3 hours. *Additional Contraindications* Narrow angle glaucoma, children under 6 months, and parenterally under 12 years. *Additional Drug Interactions* Potentiates antihypertensive effects of thiazides and other diuretics. Potentiates muscle relaxing effects of curare and gallamine. Administration together with chlordiazepoxide can cause enuresis. *Administration/Storage* Do not mix diazepam with any other injectable. Store protected from light.

(Continued)

TABLE 13 BENZODIAZEPINES, MEPROBAMATE, AND RELATED DRUGS (*Continued*)

Drug	Main Use	Dosage	Remarks
Flurazepam hydrochloride (Dalmane)	Simple insomnia	**PO:** 30 mg at bedtime. **Elderly or debilitated patients:** 15 mg. Do not use for prolonged period.	Benzodiazepine derivative. *Additional Contraindications* Use with caution in patients suffering from depression, renal, or hepatic disease, hypersensitivity to drug, or children under 15 years. *Additional Untoward Reaction* Paradoxical excitement.
Lorazepam (Ativan)	Anxiety, tension, agitation, irritability and insomnia	**PO, range:** 1–10 mg/day in divided doses with a larger dose at bedtime. *Anxiety:* 2–3 mg b.i.d. or t.i.d. *Insomnia:* 2–4 mg at bedtime. Reduce dosage in elderly patients	Benzodiazepine derivative. Absorbed and eliminated faster than other benzodiazepines. Steady state reached after 2 to 3 days, eliminated after 4 days. *Additional Contraindications* Narrow angle glaucoma. Use cautiously in presence of renal and hepatic disease.
Meprobamate (Bamate, Bamo, Canquil-400, Coprobate, Equanil, FM-200 & 400, Mepriam, Meprospan, Miltown, Neuramate, Neurate-400, Promate 400, Robamate, Saronil, Sedabamate, SK-Bamate, Tranmep, Tranqui-Tabs)	Anxiety, simple insomnia, premedication in electroshock therapy, conditions requiring muscle relaxant activity. As adjunct in treatment of chronic alcoholism and selected cases of idiopathic petit mal epilepsy	**PO: initial,** 400 mg t.i.d.–q.i.d. May be increased if necessary, up to maximum of 2.4 gm daily; **pediatric over 6 years:** 100–200 mg b.i.d.–t.i.d.	

Prazepam (Verstran)	Anxiety, psychoneurosis, anxiety associated with various disease states.	**PO: initial,** 30 mg; **maintenance:** 20–60 mg in single (bedtime) or divided doses. **Elderly patients:** 5–7.5 mg b.i.d.	Benzodiazepine derivative
Oxazepam (Serax)	Anxiety, tension. Adjunct in acute withdrawal symptoms in chronic alcoholism	**PO:** 10–30 mg t.i.d.–q.i.d. **Elderly, debilitated patients: initial,** 10 mg t.i.d., can be increased to 15 mg t.i.d.–q.i.d. *Alcohol withdrawal:* 45–120 mg daily in 3 to 4 divided doses	Benzodiazepine derivative. Less effective than diazepam. Drug is reputed to cause less drowsiness than chlordiazepoxide. Paradoxical reactions characterized by sleep disturbances, and hyperexcitement may occur during first weeks of therapy. Hypotension has occurred with parenteral administration.
Tybamate (Tybatran)	Anxiety	**PO:** 250–500 mg t.i.d.–q.i.d.; **maximum:** 3 gm daily; **pediatric 6 years and over:** 20–35 mg/kg daily in 3 to 4 divided doses.	Similar to meprobamate. Onset of action: 30 min–2 hours. Duration: 4–6 hours. *Additional Contraindications* Administer with caution to patients with history of convulsive disorders; grand mal seizures have occurred in a few hospitalized patients who received large doses of drug. *Additional Untoward Reactions* Unsteadiness, confusion, feeling of unreality, lightheadedness, dry mouth, and glossitis. *Additional Nursing Implications* Encourage rinsing mouth with water and increased fluid intake, unless contraindicated, to relieve dryness of mouth and glossitis.

14. Observe and report early symptoms of cholestatic jaundice, such as high fever, upper abdominal pain, nausea, diarrhea, and rash, that would necessitate liver function tests.
15. Withhold the drug and report to the physician should yellowing of skin, sclera, or mucous membranes occur. (These are late signs of cholestatic jaundice indicating biliary tract obstruction.)
16. Observe and report symptoms of blood dyscrasias such as sore throat, fever, and weakness that necessitate withholding the drug and reevaluation of blood tests.
17. Withhold the drug and consult with physician if the patient appears overly sleepy or confused or if comatose.
18. Be prepared to assist in the treatment of overdosage. This may involve respiratory assistance, gastric lavage, and general physiologic supportive measures. During such procedures, BP, respiration, and intake-output should be carefully monitored.
19. Be prepared to assist and have drugs on hand, such as epinephrine, antihistamines, and possibly corticosteroids, for treatment of hypersensitivity reactions.

HYDROXYZINE HYDROCHLORIDE ATARAX, VISTARIL

HYDROXYZINE PAMOATE VISTARIL

Classification Antianxiety agent, miscellaneous.

General Statement Mild CNS depressant closely related to the antihistamines. The drug also has anticholinergic, antiemetic, antispasmotic, local anesthetic, and antihistaminic effects. In addition, the drug has a mild antiarrhythmic activity, produces skeletal muscle relaxation and has antisecretory and mild analgesic effects.

Hydroxyzine hydrochloride is well absorbed from the GI tract. After oral administration, hydroxyzine pamoate is believed to be converted to hydrochloride in the stomach.

After oral administration the drug is effective within 15 to 30 minutes. The drugs have an expiration date of 5 years.

Uses Tranquilizer for psychoneurosis and tension states, anxiety and agitation. Adjunct in the treatment of chronic urticaria. Control of nausea and vomiting accompanying various diseases.

When administered IM for the control of emesis, reduce narcotic requirement during surgery or delivery.

Additional Contraindications Pregnancy; not recommended for the treatment of morning sickness during pregnancy or as sole agent for treatment of psychoses or depression. Hypersensitivity to drug.

Additional Untoward Reactions Low incidence at recommended dosages. Drowsiness, dryness of mouth, involuntary motor activity, dizziness, urticaria, or skin reactions.

Marked discomfort, induration, and even gangrene have been reported at site of IM injection.

Drug Interactions   See *General Drug Interactions*, page 322.

Dosage   **Hydroxyzine hydrochloride** and **hydroxyzine pamoate** (*anti-anxiety*), **PO:** 25–100 mg t.i.d.-q.i.d.; **pediatric under 6 years:** 50 mg daily; **over 6 years:** 50–100 mg daily in divided doses.

Hydroxyzine hydrochloride, IM (*acute anxiety, including alcohol withdrawal*) **initial,** 50–100 mg repeated q 4 to 6 hr as needed. *Nausea, vomiting, pre- and postoperative, pre- and postpartum;* 25–100 mg. Switch to **PO** as soon as possible.

Administration   Inject IM only. Injection should be made into the upper, outer quadrant of the buttock or the midlateral muscles of the thigh.

In children the drug should be injected into the midlateral muscles of the thigh.

Additional Nursing Implication   Encourage rinsing of mouth and increased fluid intake to relieve dryness of mouth.

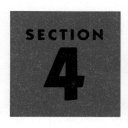

SECTION
4

centrally acting skeletal muscle relaxants

Baclofen	Diazepam
Carisoprodol	Meprobamate
Chlorphenesin Carbamate	Metaxalone
Chlorzoxazone	Methocarbamol
Cyclobenzaprine Hydrochloride	Orphenadrine Citrate
Dantrolene Sodium	Orphenadrine Hydrochloride

General Statement   The centrally acting muscle relaxants decrease muscle tone and involuntary movement and relieve anxiety and tension. They depress the CNS and preferentially act on the spinal polysynaptic reflexes. Chemically, many drugs in this group resemble agents used for the treatment of anxiety.

They are used in musculoskeletal and neurological disorders associated with muscle spasms, hyperreflexia, and hypertonia, including parkinsonism, tetanus, tension headaches, acute muscle spasms caused by trauma, inflammation, and various other conditions in which muscle relaxation is desired.

The centrally acting muscle relaxants affect some of the crucial neurojunctions involved in motor reflex transmission. The beneficial effect may also result from the ability of these drugs to relieve anxiety and tension. However, their mode of action is still poorly understood.

In addition to their muscle-relaxing effects, many of the drugs of this group also have analgesic and tranquilizing properties.

Uses Musculoskeletal conditions involving spasms resulting from peripheral injury and inflammation, including low back syndromes, sprains, and connective tissue disorders (arthritis, bursitis).

Neurological conditions: management of cerebral palsy, multiple sclerosis, parkinsonism.

Contraindications Some agents should not be used for patients with glaucoma, tachycardia, or a tendency toward urinary retention.

Untoward Reactions Hypersensitivity reactions. Drowsiness and dizziness occur most frequently. Blurred vision, flushing, lethargy and lassitude occur rarely after oral and more frequently after parenteral administration. GI distress (nausea, vomiting, heartburn, constipation, diarrhea), respiratory depression, tachycardia, and hypotension occur occasionally after large oral doses.

Drug Interactions Centrally acting muscle relaxants may increase the sedative and respiratory depressant effects of CNS depressants like alcohol, barbiturates, sedatives and hypnotics, and antianxiety agents.

MAO inhibitors potentiate centrally acting muscle relaxants.

Dosage The drugs seem to be more effective when administered parenterally. For dosage, see individual agents.

Nursing Implications Since these drugs cause drowsiness, patients should be instructed not to operate dangerous machinery or drive a car.

BACLOFEN LIORESAL

Classification Centrally acting muscle relaxant.

General Statement Baclofen is believed to work by inhibiting nerve message transmission at the level of the spinal cord. The drug relieves the spasticity associated with multiple sclerosis, and certain diseases and injuries involving the spinal cord. Not effective for the treatment of cerebral palsy, stroke, parkinsonism, or rheumatic disorders.

Uses Multiple sclerosis (flexor spasms, pain, clonus and muscular rigidity) and diseases and injuries of the spinal cord associated with spasticity.

Contraindications Hypersensitivity. Safe use in pregnancy or for children under 12 years of age not established.

Untoward Reactions   CNS: Drowsiness, dizziness, weakness, fatigue, confusion, headaches, insomnia. Cardiovascular: Hypotension. GI: Nausea, constipation. GU; Urinary frequency; also rash, pruritus, ankle edema, increased perspiration, weight gain.

Drug Interaction

Interactant	Interaction
CNS depressants	Additive CNS depression

Dosage   **PO: initial,** 5 mg t.i.d. Increase by 5 mg t.i.d. q 3 days until optimum effective dosage is attained; **maximum:** 20 mg q.i.d.

Nursing Implications
1. Caution patients about operating an automobile or other dangerous machinery because the major side effects of drug are drowsiness, dizziness, weakness, and fatigue.
2. Caution patients against ingestion of alcohol and other CNS depressants because effects may be additive.
3. Report to medical supervision patients who use spasticity to stand upright, maintain balance when walking, or to increase their function. Baclofen may be contraindicated in these instances because it interferes with patients' coping mechanisms.
4. Assess epileptics for clinical signs and symptoms of disease, and arrange for EEG at regular intervals because reduction in seizure control has been associated with baclofen.
5. Assist with lavage and maintain adequate respiratory exchange in treatment of overdosage. Do not use respiratory stimulants.

CARISOPRODOL RELA, SOMA

Classification   Centrally acting muscle relaxant.

General Statement   Drug resembles meprobamate. It has a CNS depressant effect. Onset: 30 minutes; duration: 6 hours. On rare occasions, drug causes idiosyncratic reactions within minutes after administration of first dose, such as extreme weakness, transient quadriplegia, dizziness, temporary loss of or changes in vision, and psychic changes.

Uses   Bursitis, low back disorders, contusions, fibrositism, spondylitis, sprains, muscle strains, and cerebral palsy.

Drug Interactions

Interactant	Interaction
Alcohol	Additive CNS depressant effects
Antidepressants, tricyclic	↑ Effect of carisoprodol
Barbiturates	Possible ↑ effect of carisoprodol, followed by inhibition of carisoprodol
Chlorcyclizine	↓ Effect of carisoprodol
MAO inhibitors	↑ Effect of carisoprodol by ↓ breakdown by liver
Phenobarbital	↓ Effect of carisoprodol by ↑ breakdown by liver
Phenothiazines	Additive depressant effects

Dosage	**PO:** 350 mg q.i.d. **Not recommended for children.**
Administration	For patients unable to swallow tablets, mix with a flavoring agent such as jelly, syrup, or chocolate.

CHLORPHENESIN CARBAMATE MAOLATE

Classification	Centrally acting muscle relaxant.
Remarks	CNS depressant. Peak effect: 1 to 3 hours. Paradoxical effect may occur.
Uses	Muscle spasms and muscle pain secondary to sprains, trauma, or inflammation
Additional Contraindications	Hepatic dysfunction; hypersensitivity to drug.
Dosage	**PO:** 400 mg q.i.d. Treatment can be initiated with 800 mg t.i.d. Therapy should not exceed 21 days.

CHLORZOXAZONE PARAFLEX

Remarks	CNS depressant. Peak effect: 2 to 3 hours. Duration: 6 hours.
Uses	Muscle spasms associated with low back pain, fibrositis, bursitis, myositis, spondylitis, sprains, muscle strain, torticollis, cervical root and disk syndrome.

Drug Interactions

Interactant	*Interaction*
Alcohol Antianxiety drugs Barbiturates Hypnotics Sedatives	Additive CNS depressant effects. Concomitant use may result in severe sedation, respiratory depression, and death

Dosage	**PO:** 250–750 mg t.i.d.–q.i.d. with meals and at bedtime; **pediatric:** 20 mg/kg divided into 3 to 4 doses.
Administration	1. Administer at mealtime to minimize gastric irritation. 2. May be mixed with food or beverages for administration to children.
Additional Nursing Implications	Advise the patient that this drug may cause urine to appear orange or purple-red in color when it is exposed to air.

CYCLOBENZAPRINE HYDROCHLORIDE FLEXERIL

Classification	Centrally acting muscle relaxant.

General Statement Cyclobenzaprine acts primarily within the CNS, producing overall skeletal muscle relaxation that results in decreased muscle spasms, reduction in local pain and tenderness, and increased range of motion. Structurally and pharmacologically, the drug is closely related to the tricyclic antidepressants. Cyclobenzaprine has sedative and anticholinergic effects. It is not indicated for spastic diseases or cerebral palsy. The drug is well absorbed from the GI tract and is slowly excreted.

Uses Adjunct to rest and physical therapy for relief of muscle spasms associated with acute and/or painful musculoskeletal conditions.

Contraindications Hypersensitivity. Arrhythmias, heart block, congestive heart failure, or soon after myocardial infarctions. Safe use in pregnancy has not been established.

Untoward Reactions Drowsiness (40%), dry mouth (28%), dizziness (11%); also tachycardia, weakness, dyspepsia, paresthesia, unpleasant taste, blurred vision, insomnia.

Drug Interactions

Interactant	*Interaction*
Anticholinergics	Additive anticholinergic side-effects
CNS depressants	Additive depressant effects
Guanethidine	Cyclobenzaprine may block effect
MAO inhibitors	Hypertensive crisis, severe convulsions

Dosage **PO:** *usual;* 10 mg t.i.d., up to 60 mg daily in divided doses.

Administration
1. Use cyclobenzaprine for 2 to 3 weeks only.
2. Do not administer for a minimum of 2 weeks after patient has received monoamine oxidase inhibitor drugs.

Nursing Implications Teach patient not to extend course of medication beyond 2 to 3 weeks; longer therapy with this drug is contraindicated. See *Nursing Implications* under *Tricyclic Antidepressants*, page 393.

DANTROLENE SODIUM DANTRIUM

Classification Muscle relaxant, thought to act directly.

General Statement This hydantoin is chemically and pharmacologically unrelated to other skeletal muscle relaxants. It acts directly on the skeletal muscles. Clinically the drug produces general relaxation of the skeletal muscles and decreases the force of reflex muscle contraction, hyperreflexia, spasticity, involuntary movements, and clonus.

 It must be taken for 1 week before beneficial effects become apparent. Since reduction in chronic spasticity is associated with general weakening of muscles, the long-term benefits must be evaluated for each patient.

Uses Muscle spasticity associated with severe chronic disorders, such as multiple sclerosis, cerebral palsy, spinal cord injury, and stroke.

Additional Contraindications Rheumatic diseases, nursing mothers, or children under 5 years of age.

Additional Untoward Reactions These are extensions of beneficial effects: muscle weakness, slurring of speech, drooling, enuresis. Also drowsiness, dizziness, light-headedness, nausea, malaise, and fatigue. Various other GI disturbances including anorexia, cramps, and constipation have been reported.

Untoward reactions are dose related and decrease with usage.

Dosage **Individualized, initial;** 25 mg daily. Increase gradually to 25 mg t.i.d.– q.i.d. Some patients require 200 mg q.i.d. **Pediatric: initial,** 1 mg/kg daily. Can be increased gradually by giving additional 1 mg/kg daily up to 4 times a day.

Administration Can be given in fruit juice or other liquid vehicle.

Additional Nursing Implication Encourage the patient by telling him/her that the effect of drug may become apparent after 1 week and that side effects decrease with usage.

DIAZEPAM

Antianxiety agent and muscle relaxant. For details, see Table 13.

MEPROBAMATE

Antianxiety agent and muscle relaxant. For details, see Table 13.

METAXALONE SKELAXIN

Remarks Muscle relaxant with sedative effects. Drug resembles meprobamate.

Uses Initial phase of acute skeletal muscle spasm associated with sprains, strains, dislocation, and other trauma.

Additional Contraindications Liver disease, epilepsy, impaired renal function, and pregnancy.

Additional Untoward Reactions Drug may cause hepatoxicity and have an adverse effect on hemato-poietic system. Blood and liver tests should be done prior to and during therapy.

Dosage **PO:** 800 mg t.i.d.–q.i.d.; **children over 6 years:** 45 mg/kg daily in divided doses. **Not to be administered for longer than 10 days.**

Additional Nursing Implications

1. Observe for abdominal pain, high fever, nausea and diarrhea (early symptoms of hepatotoxicity).
2. Observe for sore throat, fever, and lassitude (symptoms of blood dyscrasias).
3. Encourage rinsing of mouth and intake of more fluids in diet to relieve dryness of mouth.
4. Observe patients with history of grand mal for accentuation of seizures precipitated by metaxalone.

METHOCARBAMOL DELAXIN, FORBAXIN, METHO-500, ROBAMOL, ROBAXIN, ROMETHOCARB, SPENAXIN

Classification   Centrally acting muscle relaxant.

Remarks   Muscle relaxant of limited usefulness. For acute phase of muscle spasm, drug may be given IM or IV in 50% solution of polyethylene glycol 300. Onset of action is 10 minutes. Substitute PO administration as soon as possible.

Uses   Muscle spasms associated with sprains and/or trauma, acute back pain due to nerve irritation or discogenic disease, postoperative orthopedic procedures, bursitis, and torticollis. Acute phase muscle spasms. Adjunct in tetanus.

Additional Contraindications   Renal disease, preexisting acidosis, pregnancy, or children under 12 years of age.

Additional Untoward Reactions   IV administration may cause blurred vision, flushing, or metallic taste. WBC count should be taken occasionally during long-term administration.

Dosage   **PO: initial and maintenance:** 1–1.5 gm q.i.d.; **pediatric:** 60 (**initial**)– 75 (**maintenance**) mg/kg body weight in 4 divided doses. **IM:** 500 mg maximum in each gluteal region. May be repeated after 8 hr for total of 5 consecutive doses; **pediatric:** 60 mg/kg daily in 4 equally divided doses. **IV:** 1–3 gm daily injected slowly at rate of 3 ml/minute. (Solution for injection contains 100 mg/ml; thus rate of administration is 300 mg/min.) **IV administration should not exceed 3 days.**
   Tetanus: 1–3 gm (1 or 3 10 ml ampules) given into tube of previously inserted indwelling needle. May be given q 6 hr until **PO** administration, via nasogastric tube, is feasible.

Administration

1. Rate of IV not to exceed 3 ml/minute.
2. For IV drip, one ampule may be added to not more than 250 ml of sodium chloride or 5% dextrose injection.
3. Clamp off tubing before removing IV to prevent extravasation of hypertonic solution which may cause thrombophlebitis.
4. For IM use, inject no more than 5 ml into each gluteal region.

Additional Nursing Implications

1. Position the patient in reclining position during IV administration and have him/her maintain this position for 10 to 15 minutes following injection to minimize postural hypotensive side effects.
2. Have the patient rise slowly from a recumbent position and dangle feet before standing up.
3. Advise the patient to lie down immediately if he/she feels faint.
4. Check IV for infiltration frequently because extravasation of fluid may cause thrombophlebitis or sloughing.
5. Have side rails in place unless the patient is attended during IV administration and have padded tongue blade available because convulsions may occur.

ORPHENADRINE CITRATE FLEXON, MYOLIN, NEOCYTEN, NORFLEX, RO-ORPHENA, TEGA-FLEX, X-OTAG

Classification Centrally acting muscle relaxant.

Remarks Antihistamine-type antispasmodic agent. Peak effect: 2 hours; duration of action: 4 to 6 hours.

Uses Possibly effective in acute spasms associated with discogenic disease, tension, and posttrauma.

Additional Contraindications Angle-closure glaucoma or myasthenia gravis. Use with caution in patients with tachycardia or signs of urinary retention.

Additional Untoward Reactions Anticholinergic effects, including blurred vision, dryness of mouth and skin, and mild excitation.

Dosage **PO:** 100 mg b.i.d. **IV or IM:** 60 mg. May be repeated q 12 hr.

Additional Nursing Implications

1. Observe the patient for dryness of mouth, which indicates need for reduction of dosage.
2. Encourage rinsing of mouth and more fluids in diet to relieve dryness of mouth.

ORPHENADRINE HYDROCHLORIDE DISIPAL

Uses Adjunct in all types of parkinsonism.

Additional Contraindications Glaucoma or myasthenia gravis. Use with caution for patients with tachycardia, signs of urinary retention, or in pregnancy.

Dosage **PO:** 50 mg t.i.d. Doses up to 250 mg daily have been used without ill effects.

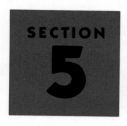

anticonvulsants

Hydantoins	Ethotoin	Phenytoin	
	Mephenytoin	Phenytoin Sodium	
Oxazolidinediones	Paramethadione	Trimethadione	
Succinimides	Ethosuximide	Phensuximide	
	Methsuximide		
Miscellaneous Anticonvulsants	Carbamazepine	Phenacemide	
	Clonazepam	Primidone	
	Diazepam	Valproic Acid	

General Statement

Anticonvulsant agents are used for the control of the chronic seizures and involuntary muscle spasms or movements characteristic of certain neurological diseases. They are most frequently used in the therapy of epilepsy, which results from disorders of nerve impulse transmission in the brain.

Therapeutic agents cannot cure these convulsive disorders, but they attempt to suppress their manifestations without impairing the normal functions of the CNS. This is often accomplished by selective depression of hyperactive areas of the brain responsible for the convulsions. Therefore, these drugs are taken at all times (prophylactically) to prevent the occurrence of the seizures.

There are several different types of epileptic disorders, including grand mal, petit mal, and psychomotor epilepsy. All the drugs listed under this grouping of anticonvulsants are not effective against all types of epilepsy; only certain ones can be used for each type of disorder (see individual drugs). Drugs effective against one type of epilepsy may not be effective against another.

Barbiturates, especially phenobarbital, mephobarbital, and metharbital are effective anticonvulsant drugs. They were discussed in Chapter 5, Section 1.

Anticonvulsant therapy must be individualized. Therapy begins with small doses of the drug, which are continuously increased until either the seizures disappear or drug toxicity occurs. If a certain drug decreases the frequency of seizures but does not completely prevent them, another drug can be added to the dosage regimen and administered concomitantly with the first. Often a drug is ineffective and then another agent must be given. Failure of therapy most often results from the administration of doses too small to have a therapeutic effect and from failure to use two or more drugs together.

If for any reason drug therapy is discontinued, the anticonvulsant drugs must be withdrawn gradually over a period of days or weeks to avoid severe, prolonged convulsions. This rule also applies when one anticonvulsant is substituted for another. The dosage of the second drug is built up at the same time the first drug is being reduced.

With modern drugs, four out of five cases of epilepsy can be controlled adequately, but it may take the physician some time to find the best drug or combination of drugs with which to treat the patient. Anticonvulsants may cause postpartum hemorrhages, birth, and coagulation defects in neonates of patients on these drugs.

Dosage   Dosage is highly individualized. However, trauma or emotional stress may necessitate an increase in drug dosage requirements (e.g., if the patient requires surgery and starts having seizures). For details see individual agents.

Nursing Implications

1. Include the patient and family in all health teaching regarding disease and therapeutic regimen.
2. Warn the patient how to avoid fever, low blood sugar, and low salt since these lower the seizure threshold.
3. Emphasize the need for close medical supervision during anticonvulsant therapy.
4. Check that the patient is taking the prescribed doses of the drug.
5. Emphasize that anticonvulsant drugs are not to be increased, decreased, or discontinued without medical supervision because convulsions may result.
6. Warn the patient that excessive use of alcohol may interfere with the action of anticonvulsants.
7. Caution the patient during initiation of therapy against performing hazardous tasks requiring mental alertness and coordination because the anticonvulsants often cause drowsiness, vertigo, headache, and ataxia. These CNS symptoms are often dose related and may disappear with a change of dosage or continued therapy.
8. Advise the patient that GI distress may be minimized by taking medication with large amounts of fluid or with food.
9. Advise the patient to report rash, fever, severe headache, stomatitis, rhinitis, urethritis, or balanitis (inflammation of the glans penis), which are early signs of hypersensitivity syndromes.
10. Check whether the patient has a history of hypersensitivity to a particular type of anticonvulsant; if so, derivatives of that type should not be administered (e.g., if the patient has shown hypersensitivity to any of the hydantoins, he/she should not be administered any other drug of this type).
11. Advise the patient to report sore throat, easy bruising, petechiae, or nosebleeds, which are signs of hematological toxicity. Hematologic studies should be performed prior to initiation of therapy and at periodic intervals during therapy.
12. Advise the patient to report jaundice, dark urine, anorexia, and abdominal pain, which are signs of hepatotoxicity. Liver function tests should be performed prior to initiation of therapy and at periodic intervals during therapy.

13. Check whether the physician wishes the patient to have folic acid supplementation to avoid megaloblastic anemia.
14. Check whether the physician wishes the patient to have vitamin D supplementation to prevent hypocalcemia (4,000 units of vitamin D/week is the usual dose).
15. Advise women of childbearing age to discuss with doctor the effects of medication on pregnancy prior to becoming pregnant.
16. Anticipate that vitamin K will be administered to pregnant women 1 month prior to parturition to prevent bleeding in the newborn.
17. Observe infants who are being nursed by mothers on anticonvulsant therapy for signs of drug toxicity and report.
18. Advise that the physician should be informed of unusual events in the patient's life since dosage requirements may change when the patient is undergoing trauma or emotional stress.
19. Monitor the patient closely after IV administration of anticonvulsants for respiratory depression and cardiovascular collapse. Be prepared in case of acute toxicity to assist with inducing emesis (provided the patient is not comatose) and with gastric lavage along with other supportive measures such as administration of fluids and oxygen.
20. Anticipate that peritoneal dialysis or hemodialysis may be instituted in the treatment of acute toxicity for barbiturates and hydantoins and hemodialysis for succinimides.

HYDANTOINS

General Statement Three hydantoins are currently used for the treatment of epilepsy and other convulsive manifestations: phenytoin, ethotoin, and mephenytoin. Of these, phenytoin (Dilantin) is used much more frequently than the others. However, patients refractory to phenytoin may respond to one of the other hydantoins. (Phenytoin used to be called diphenylhydantoin).

These hydantoins apparently reduce the spread of electric discharges from the rapidly firing epileptic focus in the brain. This reduces the rate and intensity at which the periodic sudden discharges characteristic of epilepsy spread throughout the nervous system and decreases the severity and frequency of epileptic-type attacks. The drugs have little hypnotic action and are well absorbed from the GI tract.

Uses Chronic epilepsy, especially of the grand mal and psychomotor type. Not effective against petit mal and may even increase the frequency of seizures in this disorder. Also used rarely in Parkinson's syndrome, Meniere's disease, and prophylactically for the control of seizures in neurosurgery. Phenytoin is sometimes used to treat status epilepticus, as well as cardiac arrhythmias, migraine, and trigeminal neuralgia.

Contraindications Hypersensitivity to hydantoins or exfoliative dermatitis. Administer with extreme caution to patients with a history of asthma or other allergies, impaired renal or hepatic function, and heart disease. Should not be administered to nursing mothers.

Untoward Reactions

CNS effects: postural disturbances, incoordination, drowsiness, dizziness, extrapyramidal reactions, paradoxical increase in motor activity, psychotomimetic effects including hallucinations and delusions, fatigue, insomnia, and apathy. Various ocular disturbances.

Skin reactions usually necessitate withdrawal of drug. Gum hyperplasia occurs in 20% of all patients. Hirsutism and blood dyscrasia, including Stevens-Johnson syndrome, occur infrequently. Also, hepatitis, jaundice, and keratosis. May raise blood sugar levels and produce glycosuria.

The hydantoins may interfere with absorption of dietary folic acid. Drug-induced systemic lupus erythematosus and a disorder resembling Hodgkin's disease (enlargement of lymph glands in neck, shoulders, and armpits) have been reported. Rapid parenteral administration may cause serious cardiovascular effects, including hypotension, shock, cardiovascular collapse, and heart block, as well as CNS depression.

Overdosage is characterized by nystagmus, ataxia, dysarthria, coma, unresponsive pupils, hypotension, as well as by some of the CNS effects described above.

Many individuals have a partial deficiency in the ability of the liver to degrade phenytoin, and as a result toxicity may develop after a small oral dose. Liver and kidney function tests and hematopoietic studies are indicated prior to and periodically during drug therapy.

Drug Interactions (Phenytoin)

Interactant	*Interaction*
Alcohol, ethyl	In alcoholics, ↓ effect of phenytoin due to ↑ breakdown by liver
Aminosalicylic acid	↑ Effect of phenytoin
Anticoagulants, oral	↑ Effect of phenytoin due to ↓ breakdown in liver. Also, possible ↑ in anticoagulant effect by ↓ plasma protein binding
Antidepressants, tricyclic	May ↑ incidence of epileptic seizures
Barbiturates	↓ Effect of phenytoin due to ↓ breakdown by liver
Benzodiazepines 　Chlordiazepoxide 　（Librium) 　Diazepam (Valium) 　Oxazepam (Serax)	↑ Effect of phenytoin due to ↓ breakdown by liver
Carbamazepine (Tegretol)	↓ Effect of phenytoin due to ↑ breakdown by liver
Chloramphenicol 　(Chloromycetin)	↑ Effect of phenytoin due to ↓ breakdown by liver
Chlorpromazine 　(Thorazine)	↑ Effect of phenytoin due to ↓ breakdown by liver
Contraceptives, oral	Estrogen-induced fluid retention may precipitate seizures. Also, contraceptive steroids ↑ effect of anticonvulsants by ↓ breakdown in liver and/or ↓ plasma protein binding
Corticosteroids	Effect of corticosteroids ↓ due to ↑ breakdown by liver

Interactant	*Interaction*
Digitalis glycosides	↓ Effect of digitalis glycosides by ↑ breakdown by liver
Disulfiram (Antabuse)	↑ Effect of phenytoin due to ↓ breakdown by liver
Estrogens	See *Contraceptives, Oral*
Folic acid	↓ Phenytoin blood levels due to ↑ breakdown of phenytoin by liver
Isoniazid	↑ Effect of phenytoin due to ↓ breakdown by liver
Methotrexate	↑ Effect of methotrexate by ↓ plasma protein binding
Phenothiazines	↑ Effect of phenytoin due to ↓ breakdown by liver
Phenylbutazone (Butazolidin)	↑ Effect of phenytoin due to ↓ breakdown by liver
Phenyramidol (Analexin)	↑ Effect of phenytoin due to ↓ breakdown by liver
Salicylates	↑ Effect of phenytoin by ↓ plasma protein binding
Sulfonamides	↑ Effect of phenytoin due to ↓ breakdown in liver
Thyroid preparations	↑ Effect of thyroid hormone by ↓ plasma protein binding
Tricyclic antidepressants	↑ Chance of seizures

Laboratory Test Interference

Alters liver function tests, ↑ blood glucose values, and ↓ PBI values.

Dosage

See individual drugs. Full effectiveness of orally administered hydantoins is delayed and may take 6 to 9 days to be fully established. A similar period of time will elapse before effects disappear completely.

When hydantoins are substituted for or added to other anticonvulsant medication, their dosage is gradually increased, while dosage of the other drug is decreased proportionally.

Additional Nursing Implications

1. Advise the patient to practice good oral hygiene and gum massage to minimize bleeding of gums.
2. Instruct the patient to report appearance of excessive hair on face and trunk to physician.
3. Advise the patient on good skin hygiene since the androgenic effect of phenytoin on the hair follicle may cause acne.

ETHOTOIN PEGANONE

Classification

Anticonvulsant of the hydantoin type.

Remarks

Drug is less toxic but also less effective than phenytoin.

Dosage PO: initial, **individualized,** 1 gm daily in 4 to 6 divided doses. Dosage is increased until control has been established. Usual **maintenance:** 2–3 gm daily; **pediatric:** 0.5–1 gm daily in divided doses.

MEPHENYTOIN MESANTOIN

Classification Anticonvulsant of hydantoin type.

General Statement Mephenytoin is a potentially dangerous drug since it is more toxic than the other hydantoins and is to be used only for patients refractory to other anticonvulsants. Blood dyscrasias, skin and mucous membrane manifestations, and central effects are more common than with other hydantoins. Also mephenytoin has a sedative effect which phenytoin does not have. Liver function tests are indicated before initiating therapy.

Dosage **PO, adults and children: initial,** 50–100 mg daily to be increased gradually over a period of 8 to 10 weeks until symptoms are under control. Usual **maintenance, adults:** 200–600 mg in 3 to 4 divided doses; **pediatric maintenance:** 100–400 mg in 3 to 4 divided doses.

Additional Nursing Implications Advise patients against running machinery since drowsiness occurs more frequently with this drug than with other hydantoins.

PHENYTOIN (DIPHENYLHYDANTOIN) DILANTIN

PHENYTOIN SODIUM (DIPHENYLHYDANTOIN SODIUM) DILANTIN SODIUM, DIPHENYLAN SODIUM

Classification Anticonvulsant of the hydantoin type.

Remarks See *General Statement* on *Hydantoins*, page 339 and *Anticonvulsants*, page 337.

Dosage PO: **initial,** 100 mg t.i.d.; increase gradually until seizures are under control. Usual **maintenance:** 300–600 mg daily. **Pediatric:** 3–8 mg/kg; **maintenance:** 4–8 mg/kg. **Children over 6** may require minimum adult dose. **IM** (absorption is erratic): 100–200 mg t.i.d.–q.i.d. **IV:** 150–250 mg (for status epilepticus only).

Administration (Parenteral)
1. Dilute with special diluent supplied by manufacturer. Vials must be shaken until solution is clear. The drug takes about 10 minutes to dissolve. The process can be hastened by warming the vial in warm water after the addition of the diluent. Drug is incompatible with acid solutions. Only a clear solution may be used.
2. Avoid subcutaneous or perivascular injection, as pain, inflammation, and necrosis may be caused by the highly alkaline solution.

3. Administer sodium chloride injection through the same needle or IV catheter after IV administration of the drug to avoid local irritation of the vein due to alkalinity of solution.
4. *Do not* add phenytoin to a running IV solution.
5. Inject IV slowly for treatment of status epilepticus, at a rate not exceeding 50 mg/min. If necessary, dose may be repeated 30 minutes after initial administration.

OXAZOLIDINEDIONES

General Statement
Two oxazolidinediones (paramethadione and trimethadione) are currently used for the treatment of petit mal epilepsy only. The drugs may depress rapid activity of neurons in the epileptogenic focus or depress the spread of seizure from focus by depressing synaptic transmission during rapid activity. The drugs are well absorbed from the GI tract.

Uses
Petit mal epilepsy. Because of its toxicity, it is not the drug of choice; reserved for refractory cases.

Contraindications
Anemia, leukopenia, thrombopenia, renal and hepatic disease, disease of the optic nerve. Pregnancy (may be teratogenic).

Untoward Reactions
May increase frequency of grand mal seizures. Skin rash, exfoliative dermatitis, erythema multiforme, blood dyscrasias (especially leukopenia), aplastic anemia, drowsiness, sedation, nephrotic symptoms (albuminuria), hepatitis, blurred vision (especially in bright light), photosensitivity, pseudolymphomas, lupus erythematosus. Hiccups sometimes occur during early treatment. Alopecia, paresthesias, vaginal bleeding, and changes in blood pressure also may occur. Periodic ophthalmologic examinations are necessary. Blood and urine tests are advisable biweekly; weekly leukocyte counts are indicated.

Drug Interactions

Interactant	Interaction
Aminosalicylic acid (PAS)	PAS ↑ CNS depressant effects of the oxazolidinediones
Anticoagulants, oral	↑ CNS depressant effects of oxazolidinediones
Narcotic analgesics	Concomitant administration may cause severe respiratory depression, coma, and death

Additional Nursing Implications
1. Report increased frequency of grand mal seizures.
2. Alert the patient and family to report signs of renal damage demonstrated by edema, frequency of urination, burning on urination, and albuminuria (cloudy urine). Stress the importance of periodic urine analysis.
3. Explain to the patient and family that drowsiness occurs frequently with these anticonvulsants and that activities should be planned to minimize hazard caused by lack of alertness and coordination.
4. Alert the patient and family that hyperalopia (day blindness) should be reported and that it may be relieved by wearing dark glasses.

5. Check whether there has been a history of visual problems before initiating therapy, and stress need for periodic ophthalmologic exams.
6. Check whether there has been unusual vaginal bleeding.
7. Check whether there has been excessive loss of hair.

PARAMETHADIONE PARADIONE

Classification Anticonvulsant, oxazolidinedione type.

Remarks Less toxic than trimethadione but also less effective.

Dosage **PO; adults and older children:** *highly individualized;* **initial,** 0.9– 2.4 gm daily in divided doses. Adjust dosage after a few days. **Pediatric, infants:** 300– 900 mg daily in divided doses; **2 to 6 years:** 600 mg in divided doses.

Administration Available in capsules and alcoholic solution that must be diluted with milk, juice, or other diluent before administration.

TRIMETHADIONE TRIDIONE

Classification Anticonvulsant, oxazolidinedione type.

Dosage **PO:** *highly individualized;* 0.9– 2.4 gm daily in divided doses. **Pediatric up to 6 years:** *initial,* 150– 300 mg. t.i.d., to be increased if necessary; **maintenance:** 40 mg/kg daily. Do not give in large amounts to children on ketogenic diet.

SUCCINIMIDES

General Statement Three succinimide derivatives are currently used primarily for the treatment of petit mal epilepsy: ethosuximide, methsuximide, and phensuximide. Methsuximide may have some effectiveness against psychomotor epilepsy. Ethosuximide is currently the drug of choice in the treatment of petit mal.

The succinimide derivatives suppress the abnormal brain wave patterns characteristic of petit mal epilepsy. They apparently do so by depressing the motor cortex and raising the threshold of the CNS to convulsive stimuli.

Use Primarily petit mal epilepsy.

Contraindications Hypersensitivity to succinimides. Safe use in pregnancy has not been established. Must be used with caution in patients with abnormal liver and kidney function.

Untoward Reactions   The succinimides may increase the tendency toward grand mal seizures. Blood dyscrasias, including leukopenia and aplastic anemia, may occur.

A great variety of nervous reactions, including drowsiness, apathy, euphoria, depression, dizziness, headaches, ataxia, hiccup, occur. Also various GI disturbances, including nausea, vomiting, diarrhea.

Psychological or psychiatric aberrations and skin eruptions. Various other adverse reactions, including Stevens-Johnson syndrome. Drug induces systemic lupus erythematosus and gum swelling. If ethosuximide is given to patients with both petit mal and grand mal, who are already on therapy for grand mal, it may increase the number of grand mal seizures unless dosage of medication for grand mal is increased simultaneously.

Drug Interactions

Interactant	Interaction
Amphetamines	↓ Effect of succinimides
Anticonvulsant, other	Concomitant administration results in increased libido

Dosage   See individual agents. *Individualized.* As with other anticonvulsants, drug must be withdrawn gradually.

Additional Nursing Implications
1. Report increase in frequency of grand mal seizures.
2. Alert the family to the possibility of transient personality changes, hypochondriacal behavior, and aggressiveness. Stress reporting these psychological abnormalities.

ETHOSUXIMIDE ZARONTIN

Classification   Anticonvulsant, succinimide type.

Remarks   See *General Statement* on *Succinimides,* page 344 and *Anticonvulsants,* page 347.

Dosage   **PO:** *individualized.* **Usual initial; adults and children over 6 years:** 250 mg b.i.d.; **pediatric, children under 6 years:** 250 mg daily.

Dosage may be increased gradually (increments of 250 mg every 4 to 7 days) until control is established. This may require 1–1.5 gm or more daily. Doses exceeding 1 gm daily are seldom more effective than smaller amounts.

METHSUXIMIDE CELONTIN

Classification   Anticonvulsant, succinimide type.

Remarks   See *General Statement* on *Succinimides,* page 344 and *Anticonvulsants,* page 337.

Untoward Reactions   Greater incidence and severity of side effects than other derivatives of succinimide. In addition to those mentioned, these include personality changes, severe mental depression, confused behavior, periorbital edema, albuminuria. Renal and hepatic damage. Periodic blood, liver studies, and kidney function tests are indicated.

Dosage   **PO:** *individualized.* **Initial, adults and children:** 300 mg daily. Can be increased by 300 mg at weekly intervals until control is established. **Maximum daily dose:** 1.2 gm daily in divided doses.

PHENSUXIMIDE MILONTIN

Classification   Anticonvulsant, succinimide type.

Remarks   Less effective than other succinimides but much less toxic. See *General Statement* on *Succinimides*, page 344 and *Anticonvulsants*, page 337.

Uses   Selected cases of petit mal epilepsy that fail to respond to other anticonvulsants.

Untoward Reactions   Alopecia and muscle weakness.

Dosage   **PO:** *highly individualized.* **Adults and children:** 0.5–1.0 gm b.i.d.–t.i.d.

MISCELLANEOUS ANTICONVULSANTS

CARBAMAZEPINE TEGRETOL

Classification   Anticonvulsant.

General Statement   Carbamazepine is related to the tricyclic antidepressants. Its anticonvulsant properties are similar to those of the hydantoins. Its mechanism of action is unknown. The drug also has anticholinergic and sedative effects. The drug has potentially serious effects and a benefit-to-risk evaluation should be done before it is instituted.

Uses   Epilepsy, especially partial seizures with complex symptomatology. Grand mal, psychomotor epilepsy, and disease with mixed seizure patterns. Tic douloureux (trigeminal neuralgia) and glossopharyngeal neuralgia.

Contraindications   History of bone marrow depression. Hypersensitivity to drug or tricyclic antidepressants. Safe use in pregnancy or lactation not established. Do not use when other antiepileptic agents are effective. Use with caution in patients with hepatic, renal, and cardiovascular disease.

Untoward Reactions Blood dyscrasias, including aplastic anemia, agranulocytosis, leukopenia, eosinophilia, leukocytosis, thrombocytopenia, purpura. CNS manifestations (most frequent): dizziness, drowsiness, unsteadiness, nausea, and vomiting. Also abnormal liver function. GU: urinary frequency, retention, oliguria with hypotension, impotence. Ocular manifestations, speech disturbances, depression, agitation, tinnitus, various skin reactions, including Stevens-Johnson syndrome, exfoliative dermatitis, alopecia, erythema multiforme and nodosum. Various GI manifestations: dryness of mucous membranes; various cardiovascular manifestations, including arrhythmias and myocardial infarction. Also, arthralgias, leg cramps, fever, and chills.

Drug Interactions

Interactant	Interaction
MAO Inhibitors	Exaggerated side effects
Troleandomycin	↑ Serum levels of carbamazepine leading to increased risk of toxicity.

Dosage **PO,** *individualized, epilepsy,* **adults and children over 12 years: initial,** 200 mg b.i.d. Increase by 200 mg/day until best response is attained. Divide total dose and administer q 6 to 8 hours. **Maximum dose, children 12 to 15 years:** 1000 mg daily; **adults and children over 15 years:** 1200 mg daily. **Maintenance:** decrease dose gradually to 800–1200 mg daily. *Trigeminal neuralgia:* **initial,** 100 mg b.i.d. on day 1. Increase by no more than 200 mg/day using increments of 100 mg q 12 hr as needed, up to maximum of 1200 mg daily. **Maintenance:** *usual,* 400–800 mg daily. Attempt discontinuation of medicine at least 1 time q 3 months.

Administration/ Storage
1. Do not administer for a minimum of 2 weeks after patient has received MAO inhibitor drugs.
2. Protect tablets from moisture.

Nursing Implications
1. Ascertain that baseline hematological tests, liver function, and renal function tests are completed prior to initiation of therapy. Do not initiate therapy until significant abnormalities have been ruled out.
2. Ascertain that above tests are done periodically (hematological tests are to be done every week during the first 3 months of therapy and monthly thereafter for 2 to 3 years). Withhold drug and report to medical supervision if the test results indicate abnormalities.
3. Use the following guide to assess for bone marrow depression: Erythrocyte count less than 4 million/mm^3; hematocrit less than 32%; hemoglobin less than 11 gram%; leukocytes less than 4000/mm^3; reticulocytes less than 0.3% of erythrocytes (20,000/mm^3); serum iron greater than 150 μg%.
4. Teach patients to withhold drug and check with medical supervision should the following symptoms occur:
   a. Early signs of bone marrow depression: fever, sore throat, mouth ulcer, easy bruising, petechial and purpuric hemorrhages.

     b. Early signs of genito-urinary dysfunction: frequency, acute retention, oliguria, and impotence.
     c. Cardiovascular side effects: symptoms of congestive heart failure, syncope, collapse, edema, thrombophlebitis or cyanosis.
5. Ascertain that baseline and periodic eye examination for opacities and intraocular pressure are completed.
6. Advise patients to report skin eruptions which may necessitate withdrawal of drug.
7. Anticipate that therapy will start gradually with low doses to minimize adverse reactions, such as dizziness, drowsiness, nausea, and vomiting.
8. Advise patients to use caution in operating an automobile or other dangerous machinery because drug interferes with vision and coordination.
9. Assess patients with history of psychosis for activation of symptoms.
10. Assess elderly patients for confusion and agitation and provide protective measures for them.
11. Anticipate that when carbamazepine is added to an antiepilepsy regimen the drug will be gradually added while the other antiepilepsy agents are maintained or gradually decreased.
12. Unless bone marrow depression or other life-threatening side effects occur, the drug should be withdrawn slowly to avoid precipitating status epilepticus.
13. Practice seizure precautions for patients who may have seizures precipitated by abrupt withdrawal of drug.

CLONAZEPAM CLONOPIN

Classification   Anticonvulsant.

General Statement   Clonazepam, like diazepam (Valium) belongs to the benzodiazepine class of drugs. (For details of its pharmacological actions, contraindications, untoward reactions, etc., see page 321.) At present clonazepam is used only as an anticonvulsant.

Uses   Petit mal epilepsy (Lennox-Gastant syndrome), akinetic and myoclonic seizures.

Contraindications   Sensitivity to benzodiazepines. Severe liver disease, acute narrow angle glaucoma. Safe use in pregnancy and childhood not established.

Untoward Reactions   In patients in whom different types of seizure disorders exist, clonazepam may elicit or precipitate grand mal seizures.

Dosage   **PO; adults:** *individualized;* **initial,** 0.5 mg t.i.d. Increase by 0.5–1 mg daily q 3 days until seizures are under control or side effects become excessive; **maximum:** 20 mg/day. **Pediatric up to 10 years or 30 kg:**

0.01–0.03 mg/kg/day in 2 to 3 divided doses to maximum of 0.05 mg/kg/day. Increase by increments of 0.25–0.5 mg q 3 days until seizures are under control or maintenance of 0.1–0.2 mg/kg is attained.

Nursing Implications   See beginning of this section and page 321, under *Benzodiazepines.*

DIAZEPAM VALIUM

See Table 13.

PHENACEMIDE PHENURONE

Classification   Anticonvulsant, miscellaneous.

Remarks   Elevates threshold of psychomotor seizures. The drug is well absorbed from the GI tract.

Uses   Reserved for psychomotor epilepsy, grand mal, petit mal, and mixed seizures refractory to other anticonvulsants. Not the drug of choice for any disorder because of its *severe toxic effects.*

Contraindications   Hypersensitivity to drug or impaired liver function. Use with caution in patients with history of psychoneurosis and allergy.

Untoward Reactions   Phenacemide is more toxic than most other anticonvulsants and its administration requires close supervision of patient. Specific side effects include psychic changes (17% of patients); toxic psychoses with suicidal tendencies; GI symptoms, including anorexia, nausea, and weight loss; dermatologic manifestations; blood dyscrasias, including aplastic anemia and leukopenia, which may be fatal; liver damage; nephritis; and mild sedation.

Liver function tests and complete blood counts are indicated prior to and periodically after therapy has been initiated.

Drug Interactions

Interactant	Interaction
Ethotoin	Concomitant use with phenacemide increases likelihood of paranoid symptoms
Mephenytoin Oxazolidinediones Succinimides	Since these anticonvulsants have similar toxic effects as phenacemide, they should not be used concomitantly

Dosage   **PO:** *highly individualized.* Aim at minimum effective dosage. **Adult Initial,** 250–500 mg t.i.d. Dose may be increased at weekly intervals by 500 mg and up to a maximum of 3 gm daily; **pediatric 5–10 years:** half of adult dose.

Additional Nursing Implications

1. Check if there is any history of allergy and/or personality disorder before administering phenacemide.
2. Observe and report changes in mental attitude, such as loss of interest or depression, since such changes may indicate severe personality change leading to toxic psychoses.
3. Instruct the patient to discontinue drug and check with physician at the first sign of a rash or other allergic manifestation.
4. Alert the patient and family to report signs of renal damage demonstrated by edema, frequency, burning on urination, and albuminuria (cloudy urine). Stress the importance of periodic urine analysis.

PRIMIDONE MYSOLINE, RO-PRIMADONE

Classification   Anticonvulsant, miscellaneous.

General Statement   Primidone is closely related to the barbiturates. The drug has specific antiepileptic actions. It is useful for patients refractory to the barbiturate-hydantoin regimen and produces a greater sedative effect than barbiturates. Side effects usually subside with use.

Uses   Psychomotor seizures, myoclonic epilepsy, or refractory grand mal epilepsy.

Contraindication   Porphyria.

Untoward Reactions   Drowsiness, ataxia, vertigo, irritability, general malaise, headache, skin rash, painful gums, edema of eyelids and legs, megaloblastic anemia, diplopia, nystagmus, alopecia, or impotence. Occasionally has caused hyperexcitability, especially in children. Postpartum hemorrhage and hemorrhagic disease of the newborn.

Drug Interactions   See *Barbiturates*, page 301.

Dosage   **PO, adults and children over 8 years: Initial,** 250 mg daily at bedtime. Increase by 250 mg each week, up to maximum of 2 gm daily until desired effect is attained. **Children under 8 years:** half the adult dose. Transfer from other anticonvulsant in no less than 2 weeks.

Additional Nursing Implications

1. Observe and report hyperexcitability in children.
2. Note excessive loss of hair.
3. Check for edema of eyelids and legs.
4. Ask the patient whether the drug has made him impotent.
5. Check whether the physician wishes a pregnant patient to be administered vitamin K during the last month of pregnancy to prevent postpartum hemorrhage and hemorrhagic disease of the newborn.

VALPROIC ACID DEPAKENE

Classification   Anticonvulsant, miscellaneous.

General Statement   The mechanism of action of this anticonvulsant is unknown. It is rapidly absorbed from GI tract. The drug is supplied as a capsule or syrup; the latter is the sodium salt.

Uses   Alone or in combination with other anticonvulsants for treatment of epilepsy characterized by simple and multiple absence seizures, petit mal.

Contraindications   Safe use in pregnancy and during lactation has not been established. Use with caution in presence of liver disease.

Untoward Reactions   GI (most frequent): nausea, vomiting, indigestion. CNS: sedation. Also transient alopecia, emotional disturbances, changes in behavior, weakness, altered blood coagulation, increase in SGOT, and serum alkaline phosphatase values.

Drug Interactions

Interactant	Interaction
Aspirin	Inhibition of platelet aggregation
Clonazepam	↑ Chance of absence states
CNS depressants	↑ Incidence of CNS depression
Warfarin	Inhibition of platelet aggregation

Laboratory Test Interference   False positives for ketonuria.

Dosage   **PO: initial,** 15 mg/kg/day. Increase at 1-week intervals by 5–10 mg/kg/day; **Maximum:** 30 mg/kg/day.

Administration
1. Divide daily dosage if it exceeds 250 mg/day.
2. Initiate at lower dosage or give with food to patients who suffer from GI irritation.
3. Capsules should be swallowed whole to avoid local irritation.

Nursing Implications
1. Advise diabetic patients on valproic acid therapy that the drug may cause a false + urine test for acetone. Review symptoms of ketoacidosis (dry mouth, thirst, dry flushed skin) so that patients can evaluate whether or not they are acidotic.
2. Do not administer valproic acid syrup to patients whose *sodium* intake must be restricted. Consult doctor if a sodium restricted patient is unable to swallow capsules.
3. Since valproic acid is irritating to mucous membranes of mouth and throat the capsules should not be opened or mixed with food.

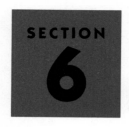

narcotic analgesics

Morphine and Congeners	Butorphanol Tartrate Codeine Codeine Phosphate Codeine Sulfate Fentanyl Citrate Hydrochlorides of Opium Alkaloids Hydromorphone Hydrochloride Levorphanol Tartrate	Methadone Hydrochloride Morphine Sulfate Oxycodone Hydrochloride Oxycodone Terephthalate Oxymorphone Hydrochloride Pentazocine Hydrochloride Pentazocine Lactate
Meperidine and Congeners	Alphaprodine Hydrochloride Anileridine Hydrochloride	Anileridine Phosphate Meperidine Hydrochloride

General Statement

The narcotic analgesics depress the CNS in a rather specific manner. Their most striking and useful effect is the relief of severe pain. They also depress the cough reflex and cause a decrease in propulsive movements of the GI tract. The mode of action of the drugs is unknown.

The narcotic analgesics include opium, morphine, codeine, various opium derivatives, and totally synthetic substances with similar pharmacologic properties. Of these, meperidine (Demerol) is the best known. The relative strength of all narcotic analgesics is measured against morphine.

Opium itself is a mixture of alkaloids obtained since ancient times from the poppy plant. Morphine and codeine are two of the pure chemical substances isolated from opium.

The discussion of the narcotic analgesics is divided into two main parts. The first section includes the drugs closely related to morphine. The second comprises drugs related to meperidine. Although the effect of both groups on various organ systems varies in degree and intensity, their overall actions are similar enough to be considered together.

Dependence and Tolerance

It is important to remember that all drugs of this group are addictive. Psychological and physical dependence and tolerance develop even when using clinical doses. Tolerance is characterized by the fact that the patient requires shorter periods of time between doses or larger doses for relief of pain. Tolerance usually develops faster when the narcotic analgesic is administered regularly and when the dose is large.

Effects of Narcotic Analgesics

The most important effect of the narcotic analgesics is on the CNS. In addition to an alteration of pain perception (analgesia), the drugs, especially at higher doses, induce euphoria, drowsiness, changes in mood, mental clouding, and deep sleep.

The narcotic analgesics also depress respiration. The effect is noticeable at small doses and death, by overdosage, is almost always the result of respiratory arrest.

The narcotic analgesics have a nauseant and emetic effect (direct stimulation of the chemoreceptor trigger zone). They depress the cough reflex, and small doses of narcotic analgesics (codeine) are part of several antitussive preparations.

The narcotic analgesics have little effect on blood pressure when the patient is in a supine position. However, most narcotics decrease the capacity of the patient to respond to stress. Morphine and other narcotic analgesics induce peripheral vasodilation that may result in hypotension.

Narcotic analgesics constrict the pupil. Pupillary constriction is the most obvious sign of dependence.

The narcotic analgesics also decrease peristaltic motility. The constipating effects of these agents ("paregoric") are sometimes used therapeutically in severe diarrhea. The narcotic analgesics also increase the pressure within the biliary tract.

Acute Toxicity

This state is characterized by profound respiratory depression, deep sleep, stupor or coma, and pinpoint pupils. The respiratory rate may be as low as 2–4 breaths/minute. The patient may be cyanotic. The blood pressure falls gradually. Urine output is decreased, the skin feels clammy, and there is a decrease in body temperature. Death almost always results from respiratory depression.

Treatment of Acute Overdosage

Gastric lavage and induced emesis are indicated in case of PO poisoning. Treatment, however, is aimed at combating the progressive respiratory depression (usually artificial respiration). Although respiratory stimulants (caffeine, pentylenetetrazole, nikethamide) have been used, severe depression follows the stimulatory effects. Such depression adds to the depression from the narcotic overdosage.

Narcotic antagonists: levallorphan (Lorfan), 0.5–1.0 mg IV or naloxone (Narcan), 0.4 mg IV are effective in the treatment of acute overdosage. Naloxone is currently the drug of choice.

Chronic Toxicity

The problem of chronic dependence is well known and does not need to be detailed here. Suffice to say, that dependence is not only a problem of "the street" but is often found among those who have easy access to narcotics (physicians, nurses, pharmacists). All the principal narcotic analgesics (morphine, opium, heroin, codeine, and meperidine) are at times used for nontherapeutic purposes.

The nurse must be aware of the problem and be able to recognize signs of chronic dependence. These are constricted pupils, GI effects (constipation), skin infections, needle scars, abscesses, and itching, especially on the anterior surfaces of the body where patient may inject drug.

Withdrawal signs appear after drug is withheld 4 to 12 hours. They are characterized by intense craving for the drug, insomnia, yawning, sneezing, vomiting, diarrhea, tremors, sweating, mental depression, muscular aches and pains, chilliness, and anxiety. Although the symptoms of narcotic withdrawal are uncomfortable, they are rarely life threatening. This is to be contrasted with the withdrawal syndrome from depressants where the life of the individual may be endangered because of the possibility of grand mal seizures.

Uses Severe pain, especially of coronary, pulmonary, or peripheral origin. Hepatic and renal colic. Preanesthetic medication and acute vascular occlusion, especially of coronary, pulmonary, and peripheral origin. Diarrhea and dysentery. Some members of this group are primarily used as antitussives. Methadone is used for heroin withdrawal and maintenance. Details for this use are not discussed in this book.

Contraindications Asthmatic conditions, emphysema, kyphoscoliosis, severe obesity, convulsive states as in epilepsy, delirium tremens, tetanus and strychnine poisoning, diabetic acidosis, myxedema, Addison's disease, hepatic cirrhosis, and children under 6 months. To be used cautiously in patients with head injury or after head surgery because of morphine's capacity to elevate intracranial pressure.

To be used with caution in the elderly, the debilitated, in young children, in cases of increased intracranial pressure, in obstetrics, and with patients in shock or during acute alcoholic intoxication.

Morphine should be used with extreme caution in patients with pulmonary heart disease (cor pulmonale). Deaths following ordinary therapeutic doses have been reported. Use cautiously in patients with prostatic hypertrophy, since it may precipitate acute urinary retention.

To be used cautiously in patients with reduced blood volume such as in hemorrhaging patients who are more susceptible to the hypotensive effects of morphine.

Since the drugs depress the respiratory center, they should be given early in labor, at least 2 hours before delivery, so as to reduce the danger of respiratory depression to the newborn. When given prior to surgery the narcotic analgesics should be given at least 1 to 2 hours preoperatively so that the danger of maximum depression of the respiratory function will have passed before anesthesia is initiated.

These drugs should sometimes be withheld prior to diagnostic procedures so that physician can use pain to locate dysfunction.

Untoward Reactions Respiratory depression, slowed heart beat, nausea, vomiting, constipation, mental clouding, euphoria, increased pressure in the biliary tract, sedation, dizziness, decreased blood pressure (orthostatic), sweating, changes in body temperature, urinary retention, syncope (fainting), or suppression of cough reflex. Idiosyncratic effects such as nausea, vomiting, excitement and restlessness, tremors, delirium, and insomnia also occur. Allergic manifestations (urticaria, skin rash, itching, and sneezing). The drug passes the placental barrier and depresses respiration of newborn.

Drug Interactions

Interactant	Interaction
Alcohol, ethyl	Potentiation or addition of CNS depressant effects. Concomitant use may lead to drowsiness, lethargy, stupor, respiratory collapse, coma, or death.
Anesthetics, general	See *Alcohol*
Antianxiety drug	See *Alcohol*
Antidepressants, tricyclic	↑ Narcotic-induced respiratory depression
Barbiturates	See *Alcohol*
CNS depressants	See *Alcohol*
Methotrimeprazine (Levoprome)	Potentiation of CNS depression

Monoamine oxidase inhibitors
  Pargyline (Eutonyl)
  Tranylcypromine (Parnate)
	Possible potentiation of either monoamine oxidase inhibitor (excitation, hypertension) or narcotic (hypotension, coma) effects. Death has resulted.

Phenothiazines	See *Alcohol*
Sedative-hypnotics, nonbarbiturate	See *Alcohol*

Skeletal muscle relaxants (surgical)
  Succinylcholine
  d-Tubocurarine
	↑ Respiratory depression and ↑ muscle relaxation

Laboratory Test Interference

Alter liver function tests. False + or ↑ urinary glucose test (Benedict's).

Dosage

(See individual drugs.) The dosage of narcotics and the reaction of a patient to the dosage depend on the amount of pain. Two to four times the usual dose may be tolerated for relief of excruciating pain. However, the nurse should be aware that, if for some reason the pain disappears, severe respiratory depression may result. This respiratory depression is not apparent while the pain is still present.

Nursing Implications

1. Account for narcotics (given or wasted) in a written record as required by the provisions of the Controlled Substances Act of 1971 and state law.
2. Request that the physician rewrite order at time intervals required for continued administration.
3. Use discrimination and judgment in evaluating the needs of a patient complaining of pain.
   a. Preferably use supportive nursing care measures, such as repositioning patient and reassurance, to relieve pain.
   b. If there is a choice, preferably administer a nonaddictive type of analgesic.
   c. Do not make the patient wait for resumption of full pain before administering medication, for then effect of drug will be reduced.
   d. Do not withhold medication when it is needed.

4. Observe patients for growing dependence and tolerance.
5. Observe for allergic or idiosyncratic effects.
6. Have naloxone available in case of toxicity.
7. Observe for early signs of toxicity such as depressed respiration (10–12 breaths/minute), deep sleep, and constricted pupils. Withhold drug when any of these symptoms appear and consult physician.
8. Use safety measures (particularly side rails) for the bedridden patient who has been medicated with narcotics.
9. Adequately supervise and assist the ambulatory patient who is more likely to experience dizziness, nausea, and vomiting after medication. Have the patient gradually rise to a sitting position to minimize hypotension.
10. Check on food intake and provide meals that patient can tolerate.
11. Check for abdominal distention, gas, and constipation; report such signs to the physician, who may order laxatives. Encourage more roughage and fluids in diet.
12. Check intake and output and check for bladder distention because drug may inhibit stimulus to void. This may cause urinary retention. Offer fluids and urge the patient to attempt to empty bladder at least every 3 to 4 hours.
13. Be prepared to dry patient and change linens more frequently because the patient perspires when receiving drug.
14. Reassure the patient that flushing and feeling of warmth are sometimes caused by therapeutic doses of narcotics.
15. Nursing care to a dependent patient should be provided in a friendly but firm manner.

MORPHINE AND CONGENERS

BUTORPHANOL TARTRATE STADOL

Classification Narcotic analgesic, synthetic opioid.

General Statement The analgesic effectiveness of butorphanol tartrate approximates that of morphine. Its onset of action is approximately 10 minutes after IV administration and less than 30 minutes following IM administration and lasts for 3 to 4 hours. The compound has both narcotic antagonistic (1/40 of naloxone) and agonistic properties. Overdosage responds to naloxone, however. Two mg butorphanol depresses respiration approximately the same degree as 10 mg morphine.

Uses Moderate to severe pain especially after surgery.

Additional Contraindications Use with extreme caution in patients with acute myocardial infarction, ventricular dysfunction, and coronary insufficiency (morphine or meperidine are preferred). Safe use in pregnancy, during labor or in children under 18 years of age not yet established.

Dosage   **IM: usual;** 2 mg q 3 to 4 hr, as necessary; **range:** 1–4 mg q 3 to 4 hr. **IV: usual:** 1 mg q 3 to 4 hr; **range:** 0.5–2 mg q 3 to 4 hr.

CODEINE

CODEINE PHOSPHATE

CODEINE SULFATE

Classification   Narcotic analgesic, morphine type.

General Statement   Analgesic effect is one sixth that of morphine. Moderately habit-forming and constipating. Produces less respiratory depression, nausea, and vomiting than morphine. Dosages over 60 mg often cause restlessness and excitement and irritate cough center.

It is a potent antitussive and thus is part of many cough syrups. It is often used to supplement the action of nonnarcotic analgesics such as aspirin. Onset of effects is 15 to 30 minutes and duration is 4 to 6 hours.

Uses   Analgesic, antitussive. Analgesia for severe pain and pre- and postoperative medication.

Additional Drug Interaction   Combination with chlordiazepoxide may induce coma.

Dosage   **PO, SC.** Codeine sulfate is given **PO;** codeine phosphate **PO** or **SC.** *Analgesic:* 15–60 mg q 3 to 4 hr. *Antitussive:* 10–20 mg q 4 to 6 hrs up to maximum of 120 mg/day. **Pediatric,** *analgesic:* 3 mg/kg in 6 divided doses. **Pediatric,** *antitussive:* 1–1.5 mg/kg in 6 divided doses. **Do not exceed 60 mg/day.**

FENTANYL CITRATE SUBLIMAZE

Classification   Narcotic analgesic, morphine type.

General Statement   Potent synthetic narcotic analgesic resembling morphine in pharmacologic effect. May be habit-forming. It has short onset of action (almost immediate after IV administration and 7 to 15 minutes after IM) which lasts for 30 to 60 minutes after IV and 1 to 2 hours after IM administration. This makes it faster acting and of shorter duration than morphine and meperidine.

Uses   Analgesia for severe pain, pre- and postoperative medication; especially suitable for minor surgery in outpatients. Tachypnea and postoperative emergence delirium.

Additional Contraindications Myasthenia gravis and other conditions in which muscle relaxants should not be used. Patients particularly sensitive to respiratory depression. Use with caution and at reduced dosage in poor-risk patients, children, the elderly, and when other CNS depressants are used.

Additional Untoward Reaction Skeletal and thoracic muscle rigidity, especially after rapid IV administration.

Dosage *Preoperatively* **IM:** 50–100 μg. *Induction* **IV:** 50–100 μg q 2 to 3 minutes. During *anesthesia* **IV or IM:** 25–50 μg. *Postoperatively:* 50–100 μg IM q 1 to 2 hr as needed. Aim for minimum dose necessary.

Storage Protect from light.

HYDROCHLORIDES OF OPIUM ALKALOIDS PANTOPON

Classification Narcotic analgesic, morphine type.

Remarks This is a mixture of all the alkaloids obtained from opium. It has a low incidence of side effects.

Uses Analgesia for severe pain and pre- and postoperative medication.

Dosage **IM or SC only:** 5–20 mg. Each 20 mg of pantopon is equivalent to 15 mg of morphine.

HYDROMORPHONE HYDROCHLORIDE DILAUDID HYDROCHLORIDE

Classification Narcotic analgesic, morphine type.

General Statement Synthetic compound, 7 to 10 times more analgesic than morphine with shorter duration. Less somnifacient than morphine and thus relieves pain with minimal hypnotic effect. Also causes less vomiting and less nausea. Induces a particularly pronounced respiratory depression. Given rectally for more prolonged activity. Onset is 15 to 30 minutes with effects lasting for 4 to 5 hours.

Uses Analgesia for severe pain; pre- and postoperative medication.

Additional Contraindication Migraine headaches.

Dosage *Analgesic* **PO, IM, IV, SC:** 2–4 mg q 4 to 6 hr as necessary. **Rectally:** 3 mg (suppository).

Additional Nursing Implications
1. Administer slowly by IV to minimize hypotensive effects and respiratory depression.
2. Observe closely for respiratory depression as it is more profound with hydromorphone.

LEVORPHANOL TARTRATE LEVO-DROMORAN

Classification Narcotic analgesic, morphine type.

General Statement Synthetic compound closely resembling morphine. Five times more potent than morphine. Respiratory depression, smooth muscle contraction, and addiction potential are increased proportionally. Long onset (up to 60 minutes) and duration of 4 to 5 hours.

Uses Analgesia for severe pain and pre- and postoperative medication.

Dosage **PO, SC:** 2 mg q 4 to 6 hr. Aim for minimal effective dosage. Use at reduced dosage for poor-risk, elderly, or very young patients.

METHADONE HYDROCHLORIDE DOLOPHINE HYDROCHLORIDE, WESTADONE

Classification Narcotic analgesic, morphine type.

General Statement Although the chemical structure of methadone markedly differs from morphine, its pharmacologic activity closely resembles the morphine-type narcotic analgesic. Methadone produces only mild euphoria, and this is why it is currently used as a heroin withdrawal substitute. Abstinence syndrome develops more slowly when methadone is discontinued. Symptoms are less intense but more prolonged than for morphine. Drug does not produce sedation or narcosis.

Like other narcotic analgesics it is used for the control of moderate and severe pain, but it is not effective for preoperative or obstetrical anesthesia. It is long-acting and less sedating than morphine.

Uses Analgesic, drug withdrawal, and maintenance.

Additional Contraindications IV use, liver disease; give rarely if at all during pregnancy.

Additional Untoward Reactions Marked constipation, excessive sweating, or pulmonary edema.

Additional Drug Interactions
1. It is incompatible with wild cherry syrup, alkaline solution, and the common alkaloid reagents.
2. Rifampin decreases plasma methadone levels by ↑ metabolism of methadone. Thus, symptoms of narcotic withdrawal may develop.

Dosage *Analgesia:* 2.5–10 mg **IM, SC, or PO** q 3 to 4 hr. *Heroin withdrawal (highly individualized):* 20–40 mg/day in divided doses. **Maintenance** *(individualized):* approximately 60–120 mg/day, once stabilized.

Additional Nursing Implications
1. Irritation may be caused by injection. Inspect sites of injection for tissue damage.
2. Anticipate that side effects are more prominent in ambulatory patients and in those who are not suffering acute pain.
3. Relief of nausea and vomiting may be achieved by lowering the dosage and by administering medication only when needed to control pain.
4. Caution patients on withdrawal therapy to store medication out of the reach of children.

MORPHINE SULFATE

Classification Narcotic analgesic.

General Statement Morphine is more effective against dull, continuous pain than against intermittent, sharp pain. Large doses, however, will dull almost any kind of pain.

Morphine should not be used with papaverine for analgesia in biliary spasms but may be used with papaverine in acute vascular occulsion. It is effective in controlling the pain and restlessness that accompany shock, burns, and other trauma. Onset of effects is within 20 minutes and effects last up to 6 hours.

Uses Analgesia for severe pain and pre- and postoperative medication.

Dosage **SC, IM, IV:** 2–20 mg every 4 hr as indicated; **pediatric:** 100–200 μg/kg, up to maximum of 15 mg. Use minimum effective dose. **PO administration (not recommended):** 5–15 mg q 4 hr. For quick relief of acute pain the prescribed dose of morphine sulfate, dissolved in 5 ml of physiological saline, can be injected slowly intravenously.

OXYCODONE HYDROCHLORIDE

OXYCODONE TEREPHTHALATE PERCODAN

Classification Narcotic analgesic, morphine type.

General Statement Produces mild sedation and little or no depression of cough reflex. Most effective for pain of acute nature. Moderate tolerance and dependence potential. Used in combination with aspirin, phenacetin, caffeine.

Uses Moderate acute pain, such as bursitis, injuries, dislocations, simple fractures, pleurisy, and neuralgia. Also for obstetrical, postoperative, postextractional, and postpartum pain.

Additional Drug Interactions Patients with gastric distress, such as colitis or gastric or duodenal ulcer, and patients who have glaucoma should not receive Percodan, which also contains aspirin, phenacetin, and caffeine.

Dosage **PO, adults and older children:** 4.88 mg q 6 hr; **pediatric 6–12 years:** 1.22 mg every 6 hours.

OXYMORPHONE HYDROCHLORIDE NUMORPHAN HYDROCHLORIDE

Classification Narcotic analgesic, morphine type.

General Statement On a weight basis, this synthetic narcotic analgesic is 2 to 10 times as potent as morphine. Potency depends on mode of administration. The drug is fast acting. It produces mild sedation and moderate depression of the cough reflex 5 to 8 minutes after SC injection. The full effect is attained after 10 to 20 minutes and lasts 3 to 6 hours. Effectiveness depends on mode of administration.

Uses Severe pain associated with neoplastic disease, neurological disorders, burns, trauma, biliary spasm, and acute vascular occlusion. Analgesia for severe pain and pre- and postoperative medication.

Dosage **SC, IM, IV, and rectal** suppositories, *initial*, **SC and IM:** 1– 1.5 mg q 4 to 6 hr. **IV:** 0.5 mg; **rectal:** 5 mg q 4 to 6 hr. *During labor:* 0.5– 1 mg. Usually repeated every 4 to 6 hr. Dosage can be cautiously increased if necessary.

PENTAZOCINE HYDROCHLORIDE TALWIN HCl

PENTAZOCINE LACTATE TALWIN LACTATE

Classification Narcotic analgesic, morphine type.

Remarks Pentazocine has analgesic as well as weak narcotic antagonist properties. It is approximately one third as potent as morphine when administered preoperatively for pain.

Uses Obstetrics. Preoperative analgesic and sedative. Moderate to severe pain.

Additional Contraindications Increased intracranial pressure or head injury. Use with caution in impaired renal or hepatic function as well as after myocardial infarction when nausea and vomiting are present. Not recommended for use in children under 12 years of age.
Note: The narcotic antagonist levallorphan is *ineffective* in reversing respiratory depression or overdosage of pentazocine. Naloxone, however, can be used for such purposes.

Additional Untoward Reactions Drowsiness, hyperhidrosis, vertigo, respiratory depression, nausea, and vomiting. Also, tachycardia, palpitations, hypertension, dysphoria, nightmares, and hallucinations. Both psychological and physical dependence are possible, although the addiction liability is thought to be no greater than for codeine.

Dosage *Pentazocine hydrochloride,* **PO:** 50 mg q 3 to 4 hr. Daily dose should not exceed 600 mg. *Pentazocine lactate,* **IM, IV, SC:** 30 mg q 3 to 4 hr. Total daily dose should not exceed 300 mg. For obstetric analgesia, administer a single **IM** dose of 20–30 mg or 20 mg **IV** 2 to 3 times at 2 to 3 hr intervals, if necessary.

Administration A precipitate will occur if soluble barbiturates are mixed in the same syringe with pentazocine.

Additional Nursing Implications
1. Methadone and other narcotics should not be substituted for pentazocine in the treatment of pentazocine withdrawal.
2. Patients should not operate machinery or drive cars because dizziness and sedation may occur.

MEPERIDINE AND CONGENERS

General Statement The chemical structure of these narcotic analgesics is very different from the morphinelike narcotic analgesics. Their physiological action and use is nevertheless very similar. The drugs belonging to this group are more rapidly effective than morphine. They are also shorter acting and are thus more suitable for minor surgery and painful diagnostic procedures (cytoscopy, pyelography, gastroscopy).

However, *these drugs still produce dependence.* They act chiefly on the CNS. The compounds produce analgesia, sedation, and euphoria. They severely depress the respiratory centers (treatment of overdosage is identical to morphine). They also produce moderate spasmogenic effect on smooth muscle.

Uses Any situation that requires a narcotic analgesic: severe pain, hepatic and renal colic, obstetrics, preanesthetic medication, adjunct to anesthesia. These drugs are particularly useful for minor surgery as in orthopedics, ophthalmology, rhinology, laryngology, and dentistry, and for diagnostic procedures such as cystoscopy, retrograde pyelography and gastroscopy.

Additional Contraindications Hypersensitivity to drug, convulsive states as in epilepsy, tetanus and strychnine poisoning, children under 6 months, diabetic acidosis, head injuries, shock, liver disease, respiratory depression, increased cranial pressure, and pregnancy prior to labor. To be used with caution in obstetrics, lactating mothers, and in older or debilitated patients. Use with extreme caution in patients with asthma.

Additional Untoward Reactions   Respiratory depression, dizziness, sweating, dry mouth, constipation, biliary tract spasms, vomiting, weakness, palpitations, dysphoria, drop in blood pressure, or decreased cough reflex. Also euphoria, weakness, headache, agitation, tremor, uncoordinated muscle movements, transient hallucinations, disorientation, visual disturbances, urinary retention, allergic reactions including pruritus, urticaria and other skin rashes, syncope (fainting), or sedation. These reactions are more marked in ambulatory patients. Like morphine, the drug passes the placental barrier and depresses the respiratory rate of the newborn. When used in obstetrics observe same precautions as for morphine. High doses may induce transient hypotension.

Drug Interactions   *Note:* Combination of meperidine and congeners with other drugs that have a CNS depressant effect can lead to serious consequences including severe CNS depression that may result in respiratory depression and coma. Dosage reduction is usually necessary. In addition, meperidine has atropine-like effects which may be adverse in glaucoma, especially when given in combination with another drug that may be hazardous for that condition.

Interactant	*Interaction*
Alcohol	Potentiation or addition of CNS depressant effects. Concomitant use may lead to drowsiness, lethargy, stupor, respiratory collapse, coma, or death
Anesthetics, general	See *Alcohol*
Antianxiety drugs	See *Alcohol*
Antidepressants, tricyclic	Additive anticholinergic side effects
Barbiturates	See *Alcohol*
CNS depressants	See *Alcohol*
Contraceptives, oral	↑ Effect of meperidine due to ↓ breakdown by liver
Estrogens	See *Contraceptives, Oral*
Isoniazid	↑ Side effects of isoniazid

Monoamine oxidase inhibitors
  Pargyline (Eutonyl)
  Tranylcypromine (Parnate)
	Possible potentiation of either monoamine oxidase inhibitor (excitation, hypertension) or narcotic (hypotension, coma) effects. Death has resulted.

Phenothiazines	See *Alcohol*
Sedative-hypnotics, nonbarbiturate	See *Alcohol*

Dosage   See individual agents.

ALPHAPRODINE HYDROCHLORIDE NISENTIL

Classification   Narcotic analgesic, meperidine type.

General Statement Narcotic analgesic of the meperidine type. Drug has a more rapid onset of action, shorter duration than meperidine. Produces analgesia within 5 to 10 minutes for approximately 2 hours. Acts in 1 to 2 minutes and persists 30 to 60 minutes when given IV. More effective than meperidine when given orally. Not for use in children under 12 years of age. IM administration not recommended.

Uses Analgesia for severe pain, pre- and postoperative medication, and diagnostic procedures, especially in urology.

Additional Drug Interaction Chlorpromazine potentiates alphaprodine.

Dosage **SC and IV. SC:** 0.4–1.2 mg/kg every 2 hr as needed up to maximum of 60 mg. **IV:** 0.4 mg/kg repeated every 2 hr as needed up to maximum of 30 mg. **Total maximum daily dose:** 240 mg.

In obstetrics, give initial dose (40–60 mg **SC**) only after cervix has started to dilate. Last dose 2 or more hours prior to expected time of delivery.

ANILERIDINE HYDROCHLORIDE LERITINE HYDROCHLORIDE

ANILERIDINE PHOSPHATE LERITINE PHOSPHATE

Classification Narcotic analgesic, meperidine type.

Remarks More effective orally than meperidine. Narcotic antagonists and equipment for emergency administration of oxygen should be on hand. Onset of effects begins in 15 minutes and lasts 2 to 3 hr. Not for children under 12 years of age.

Uses To relieve moderate-to-severe pain in angina pectoris, biliary colic, dentistry, fractures, and extensive burns. For apprehension in acute congestive heart failure, obstetrics, and pre- and postoperative medication.

Dosage **PO, SC, IM, and IV.**
Anileridine hydrochloride; **PO:** 25–50 mg repeated every 4 to 6 hr if necessary. *Anileridine phosphate;* **IM:** 25–75 mg repeated every 4 to 6 hr if necessary. **Total dose/day should not exceed 200 mg.** *In conjunction with anesthesia:* IV 50–75 mg (in 500 ml 5% dextrose injection). Administer amount corresponding to first 5–10 mg anileridine very slowly. Sudden injection in excess of 10 mg may cause apnea. Administer remainder at rate of 600 μg/min.
Obstetrics; **SC or IM:** 50 mg repeated every 3 to 4 hr up to total of 100–200 mg. **IV (slow):** 5–10 mg initially followed by 0.6 mg/minute until desired amount given.

MEPERIDINE HYDROCHLORIDE DEMEROL HYDROCHLORIDE, PETHADOL

Classification	Narcotic analgesic.
General Statement	Antispasmodic. The compound is one tenth as potent an analgesic as morphine. Its analgesic effect is cut in half when given PO rather than parenterally. The drug has no antitussive properties and does not constrict the pupils. Onset of effects occurs in 10 to 15 minutes and effects last 2 to 4 hours.
Uses	Analgesia for severe pain. Also pain associated with spasm of the lower GI tract, uterus and urinary bladder. Anginal syndrome and distress of congestive failure.
Additional Untoward Reactions	Meperidine occasionally causes tremors and uncoordinated muscular movements. The drug has a slight constipating effect. Respiratory depressions are relatively rare, but dizziness is frequent. The drug may cause postural hypotension in patients out of bed or after rapid IV administration.
Dosage	**PO, IM, IV:** 50–150 mg repeated every 1 to 4 hr as needed. *Obstetrics:* 50–100 mg **IM** or **SC** given 90 minutes or more before expected delivery. **Pediatric:** 1.5 mg/kg q 2 to 4 hr. Maximal dose: 100 mg.

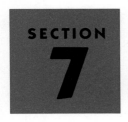

SECTION 7

narcotic antagonists

Levallorphan Tartrate
Naloxone Hydrochloride

General Statement	Narcotic antagonists prevent or promptly abolish many of the actions of the narcotic analgesics of the morphine and meperidine type. They are able to prevent or reverse, within minutes, the respiratory depression induced by narcotic analgesics. The narcotic antagonists also restore blood volume and blood pressure to more normal values.

The mechanism of action by which this is accomplished is unknown; however, it is believed that the drugs displace narcotics from some of the crucial receptor sites.

When used alone, not in conjunction with narcotic analgesics, levallorphan has some of the same effects as the narcotic analgesics themselves; that is, it depresses the respiratory rate. Naloxone does not possess any effects of the narcotic analgesics.

The narcotic antagonists are not effective in reversing the respiratory depression induced by barbiturates, anesthetics, or other nonnarcotic agents.

Narcotic antagonists almost immediately induce withdrawal symptoms in narcotic addicts and are used to unmask dependence.

Nursing Implications

1. Try to obtain a history about cause of respiratory depression from the patient or a friend because narcotic antagonists will not relieve the toxicity of nonnarcotic CNS depressants.
2. Monitor vital signs before and after administration of narcotic antagonist to evaluate response to therapy.
3. Monitor respiration closely when duration of action of narcotic antagonist is over as additional doses may be necessary.
4. Be alert to the appearance of withdrawal symptoms after administration of antagonist. Withdrawal symptoms are characterized by restlessness, lacrimation, rhinorrhea, yawning, perspiration, and pupil dilation.
5. Be prepared to assist in the use of other resuscitative measures for the narcoticized patient such as gastric lavage, maintenance of a patent airway, artificial ventilation, provision of oxygen, cardiac massage, and vasopressor agents.
6. Provide supportive care to the comatose patient by turning him on his side to prevent aspiration and providing side rails etc.
7. When the narcotic antagonists are used to diagnose narcotic use or dependence, the pupil of the eye will dilate initially followed by constriction.

LEVALLORPHAN TARTRATE LORFAN

Classification

Narcotic antagonist.

Remarks

The drug overcomes respiratory depression without abolishing anesthesia. Its onset of action is rapid (1 minute) and its effect lasts for 2 to 5 hours. It increases both the rate and depth of respiration.

Uses

To overcome narcotic-induced respiratory depression. Diagnosis of narcotic dependence.

Contraindications

Mild respiratory depression. Respiratory depression induced by barbiturates and anesthetics (unless levallorphan used in a test dose to determine whether toxicity is due to a narcotic analgesic). Drug may induce severe withdrawal symptoms in narcotic addicts.

Untoward Reactions

Respiratory depression when used alone. Also dysphoria, miosis, lethargy, dizziness, drowsiness, GI upsets and sweating. At high dosages the drug may induce psychotomimetic manifestations.

Dosage *Narcotic overdosage (also in parturient women)*; **IV:** 1 mg. If required give 1 to 2 additional doses of 0.5 mg at 10 to 15 minute intervals up to maximum of 3 mg. **Neonates:** 0.05–0.1 mg injected with 2–3 ml of sodium chloride injection into umbilical vein after delivery. Can also be given **IM or SC.**

NALOXONE HYDROCHLORIDE NARCAN

Classification Narcotic antagonist.

General Statement Naloxone is a narcotic antagonist that resembles oxymorphone. Unlike the narcotic antagonist levallorphan, naloxone does not produce psychotomimetic, circulatory, miotic changes, or respiratory depression when administered alone.

The drug can reverse the respiratory depression induced by narcotic analgesics and that induced by pentazocine (Talwin), propoxyphene (Darvon), and cyclazocine. Since the action of naloxone is shorter than that of the narcotic analgesics, the respiratory depression may return when the narcotic antagonist has worn off.

Uses Respiratory depression induced by natural and synthetic narcotics. Drug of choice when nature of depressant drug is not known. Diagnosis of acute opiate overdosage. Not effective when respiratory depression is induced by hypnotics, sedatives, or anesthetics, and other nonnarcotic CNS depressants.

Contraindications Sensitivity to drug. Narcotic addicts (drug may cause severe withdrawal symtoms). Not recommended for use in neonates. Safe use in children is not established.

Untoward Reactions Nausea and vomiting.

Dosage **IM, IV, or SC. IV** is recommended for emergency situations. **Initial:** 400 µg. May be repeated at 2- to 3-minute intervals until favorable response is achieved: **pediatric:** *narcotic overdose–known or suspected,* 0.01 mg/kg, **IV, IM, SC.**

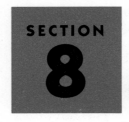
antipsychotic agents

Phenothiazines	Acetophenazine Maleate
	Butaperazine Maleate
	Carphenazine Maleate
	Chlorpromazine
	Chlorpromazine Hydrochloride
	Fluphenazine Decanoate
	Fluphenazine Enanthate
	Fluphenazine Hydrochloride
	Mesoridazine Besylate

Perphenazine
Piperacetazine
Prochlorperazine
Prochlorperazine Edisylate
Prochlorperazine Maleate
Promazine Hydrochloride
Thioridazine Hydrochloride
Trifluoperazine
Triflupromazine Hydrochloride

Thioxanthene Derivatives
Chlorprothixene
Thiothixene

Butyrophenone Derivatives
Droperidol
Haloperidol

Miscellaneous Antipsychotic Agents
Lithium Carbonate
Lithium Citrate
Loxapine Succinate
Molindone

General Statement The advent of antipsychotic drugs was responsible for a major change in the treatment of the mentally ill. Reserpine, an alkaloid derived from *Rauwolfia serpentina*, and chlorpromazine, both of which appeared in the early 1950s, almost singlehandedly revolutionized the care of the mentally ill both inside and outside the hospital. Patients who had not been helped for decades with electroschock, insulin therapy, and/or other forms of treatment could now often be discharged.

Antipsychotic drugs do not cure mental illness, but they calm the intractable patient, relieve the despondency of the severely depressed, activate the immobile and withdrawn, and make some patients more accessible to psychotherapy.

Phenothiazines

General Statement The phenothiazines act on subcortical centers of the brain, which are believed to be involved in the emotional responses of the individual. This is why these agents have a calming effect on aggressive, overactive, disturbed patients. The drugs also depress areas of the brain stem which control vomiting (antiemetic effect).

The agents potentiate the pain-relieving properties of the narcotic analgesics and prolong the action of some CNS depressant drugs. The latter can thus be used at lower dosage levels.

Most phenothiazines induce some sedation, especially during the initial phase of the treatment. Medicated patients can, however, be easily roused. In this manner, the phenothiazines differ markedly from the narcotic analgesics and sedative hypnotics.

The drugs also decrease spontaneous motor activity, as in parkinsonism, and many lower blood pressure.

According to their detailed chemical structure, the phenothiazines belong to three subgroups:

1. The dimethylaminopropyl compounds
2. The piperazine compounds
3. The piperidyl compounds

Drugs belonging to the *dimethylaminopropyl subgroup*, which includes chlorpromazine, are often the first choice for patients in acute excitatory states. Drugs belonging to this subgroup cause more sedation than other phenothiazines and are especially indicated for patients exhausted by lack of sleep.

Members of the *piperazine subgroup* act most selectively on the subcortical sites. This accounts for the fact that they can be administered in relatively small doses. This in turn results in minimal drowsiness and undesirable motor effects. The piperazines also have the greatest antiemetic effects because they specifically depress the chemoreceptor trigger zone (CTZ) of the vomiting center. Members of the *piperidyl subgroup* are less toxic in terms of extrapyramidal effects. Mellaril, a member of this group, has little effectiveness as an antiemetic drug.

Uses
Severe psychoses: schizophrenia, manic phase of manic depressive psychosis, involutional and senile psychoses, confusion, personality disorders.

Neuroses accompanied by anxiety, agitation, tension, and apprehension. Behavior disorders in children.

As an adjunct during alcohol withdrawal; for certain types of nausea, vomiting, intractable hiccups.

Since the drugs enhance and prolong the action of narcotics and hypnotics, they permit and necessitate lower dosage of analgesics and anesthetics during surgery, labor, and delivery. They are also useful in the control of severe pain in cancer when used in conjunction with analgesics.

Contraindications
Hypersensitivity to drugs, comatose states, glaucoma, prostatic hypertrophy, convulsive disorders, and children under 6 months of age.

Use cautiously in patients with cardiovascular and cerebrovascular disease, hypertension, hepatic or renal disease.

Withhold drugs from patients under the influence of barbiturates, alcohol or other CNS depressants.

Untoward Reactions
CNS System Side effects may either manifest themselves as excess depression, including drowsiness, dizziness, lethargy, and fatigue or as excess stimulation (extrapyramidal), such as pseudoparkinsonism

(muscle tremors, rigidity), dyskinesias (spasms), akathisia (extreme restlessness accompanied by increased mental turbulance and motor activity), or dystonia (involuntary movements). Excess extrapyramidal stimulation is particularly marked for the piperazine-type subgroup, which includes most phenothiazines. High dosage may enhance bizarre motor effects.

Convulsive seizures, particularly in patients with a history of epileptic seizures, also occur.

Autonomic Blockage-Type Side Effects *Adrenergic-type blockade:* sharp drop in blood pressure, postural hypotension (most common when drugs are given parenterally), palpitation, faintness.

Cholinergic-type blockade: atropinelike symptoms, dryness of mouth, blurring of vision, stuffy nose, constipation, fever.

Endocrine Effects Menstrual disorders, amenorrhea, false-positive pregnancy tests, abnormal lactation, increased libido in women, decreased libido in men, increased appetite, weight gain, hypoglycemia, delayed ejaculation, peripheral edema.

Hypersensitivity Reactions Cholestatic hepatitis, jaundice, blood dyscrasias including leukopenia and agranulocytosis.

Dermatologic Reactions Purple discoloration of skin, especially after long-term administration, photosensitivity reaction.

Sudden death has also been reported after administration of tranquilizers.

Tardive dyskinesia has been observed with all classes of antipsychotic drugs although the precise cause is not known. The syndrome is most commonly seen in older patients, especially women, and in individuals with organic brain syndrome. It is often aggravated or precipitated by the sudden discontinuance of antipsychotic drugs and may persist indefinitely after the drug is discontinued. Early signs of tardive dyskinesia include fine vermicular movements of the tongue and grimacing or tic-like movements of the head and neck. Although there is no known cure for the syndrome, it may not progress if the dosage of the drug is slowly reduced. Also, a few drug-free days for the patient may unmask the symptoms of tardive dyskinesia and help in early diagnosis.

Drug Interactions	*Interactant*	*Interaction*
	Alcohol, ethyl	Potentiation or addition of CNS depressant effects. Concomitant use may lead to drowsiness, lethargy, stupor, respiratory collapse, coma, or death
	Amphetamine	↓ Effect of amphetamine by ↓ uptake of drug to the site of action.
	Anesthetics, general	See *Alcohol*
	Antacids, oral	↓ Effect of phenothiazines due to ↓ absorption from GI tract

Drug Interactions (*Continued*)	*Interactant*	*Interaction*
	Antianxiety drugs	See *Alcohol*
	Antidepressants, tricyclic	Additive anticholinergic side effects
	Antidiabetic agents	↓ Effect of antidiabetic agents since phenothiazines ↑ blood sugar
	Barbiturates	See *Alcohol*
	CNS depressants	See *Alcohol*
	Guanethidine (Ismelin)	↓ Effect of guanethidine by ↓ uptake of drug at the site of action
	Levodopa	↓ Effect of levodopa in parkinsonism patient
	Lithium carbonate	Additive hyperglycemia
	Methyldopa (Aldomet)	Additive hypotensive effects
	Monoamine oxidase inhibitors Pargyline (Eutonyl) Tranylcypromine (Parnate)	↑ Effect of phenothiazines by ↓ breakdown by liver
	Narcotics	See *Alcohol*
	Phenytoin (Dilantin)	↑ Effect of phenytoin due to ↓ breakdown by liver
	Piperazine (Antepar)	Increase in phenothiazine-induced extrapyramidal effects
	Procarbazine (Matulane)	Additive CNS depression
	Propranolol	Additive hypotensive effects
	Quinidine	Additive cardiac depressant effect
	Reserpine	Additive hypotensive effect
	Sedative-hypnotics, nonbarbiturate	See *Alcohol*
	Succinylcholine	↑ Muscle relaxation

Laboratory Test Interference Alter liver function tests. ↑ Levels of cholesterol, urine catecholamines, estrogens, 17-ketogenic steroids, and 17-ketosteroids.

Dosage The phenothiazines are effective over a wide dosage range. Dosage is usually increased gradually to minimize side effects over a period of 7 days until the minimal effective dose is attained. Dosage is increased more gradually in elderly or debilitated patients, since they are more susceptible to the effects and side effects of drugs. After symptoms are controlled, dosage is gradually reduced to maintenance levels. It is usually desirable to keep chronically ill patients on maintenance levels indefinitely.

Medication, especially in patients on high dosages, should not be discontinued abruptly.

Administration/ Storage
1. When preparing or administering parenteral solutions avoid contact with skin, eyes, and clothing (nurse and patient).
2. Dilution of commercially available injectable solutions in saline or local anesthetic and massaging injection site after administration may reduce pain of administration.

3. Do not mix in syringe with other drug.
4. Discard pink or markedly discolored solutions.
5. Store solutions in a cool place in amber-colored containers.
6. A specific rate of flow should be ordered for parenteral doses. Rate of IV administration and blood pressure should be monitored carefully.
7. Prevent extravasation of IV solution.
8. Inject deeply and slowly IM.

Nursing Implications

1. Stay with patient until medication is swallowed to prevent hoarding or omission of medication.
2. Take a base reading of BP before IV administration.
3. Keep the patient lying flat for at least 1 hour after IV administration and monitor BP closely for hypotensive reaction. After 1 hour, slowly elevate the patient and observe for tachycardia, fainting, or dizziness. Side rails are an advisable precaution.
4. Instruct the patient when dizzy or faint to sit down or preferably to lie down with feet elevated.
5. Prevent exposure of patient to excessive sunlight.
6. Observe and report yellow-brown skin reaction that may turn to grayish purple (usually occurs in patients on long-term therapy).
7. Observe for symptoms of hyperthermic or hypothermic reaction as heat regulating mechanism may be affected by the drug. Warmth for hypothermic reactions should be provided with blankets and *not* hot water bottles or heating appliances since the patient's sensitivity to heat is blocked and burns may occur. Excessive hyperthermia may necessitate cooling baths, but care should be taken that the patient is not chilled.
8. Warn the patient not to drive a car or operate machinery requiring mental alertness for at least 2 weeks after therapy has begun, and then only after consulting physician, who will evaluate response to therapy.
9. Observe and report early symptoms of cholestatic jaundice, such as high fever, upper abdominal pain, nausea, diarrhea, and rash, that would necessitate liver function tests.
10. Withhold drug and report to physician should signs of cholestatic jaundice occur indicating bile-tract obstruction, including yellowing of skin, sclera, or mucous membranes.
11. Observe and report symptoms of blood dyscrasias, such as sore throat, fever, and weakness, that necessitate withholding the drug and practicing reverse isolation until blood tests are reevaluated.
12. Observe and report signs of both physical and emotional depression or excessive stimulation, as well as extrapyramidal symptoms as a change in medication or additional medication may be required.
13. Monitor children with acute infections or dehydration more closely since they are more susceptible to neuromuscular reactions.
14. Encourage rinsing oral cavity with water and increasing fluid intake to relieve excessive dryness of mouth, and to assist in retention of false dentures, if the patient has these.
15. Monitor intake and output and observe for abdominal distention as patient may fail to report urinary retention and constipation.

   a. Report urinary retention as this condition may require reduced dosage, antispasmodics, or change of drug.

   b. Report constipation as this condition may require increased roughage in diet, more fluids, and laxatives.

15. Observe patients for visual difficulties and check that they have periodic ocular examinations.

16. Observe and report changes in carbohydrate metabolism, such as glycosuria, weight loss, polyphagia, increased appetite, or excessive weight gain, that may necessitate dietary or medication changes.

17. Observe and report menstrual irregularities, breast engorgement, lactation, increased libido in women, and decreased libido in men since these symptoms may be very frightening to the patient and a change of medication may be necessitated. Reassurance should be given to the patient that these changes are drug-induced and will be relieved by medication adjustment.

18. Anticipate that barbiturates (to relieve anxiety) will be reduced in dosage when given with phenothiazines but that barbiturates used as anticonvulsants will not be reduced in dosage.

19. Caution patients against abrupt cessation of high doses of phenothiazines since this may cause nausea, vomiting, tremors, feeling of warmth or cold, sweating, tachycardia, headache, and insomnia.

20. Observe and report symptoms of hypersensitivity, such as fever, asthma, laryngeal edema, angioneurotic edema, and anaphylactoid reaction.

21. Encourage patients with respiratory disorders to deep breathe and cough since drug may depress the cough reflex.

22. Consider that the antiemetic effect of phenothiazines may be masking other pathology such as toxicity to other drugs, intestinal obstruction, or brain lesions.

23. Warn patient on phenothiazines that drug may turn urine pink or red brown.

24. Emphasize the need for discharged patients to maintain their medication to avoid the "revolving door syndrome."

25. Inform families and patients of the necessity to continue taking medication after discharge and emphasize need to return for follow-up care.

Note: These nursing implications apply to all antipsychotic agents except lithium.

ACETOPHENAZINE MALEATE TINDAL

Classification Antipsychotic, piperazine-type phenothiazine.

Remarks The drug is much less potent than other phenothiazines with more pronounced sedative effects but fewer extrapyramidal phenomena.

Uses Patients with chronic brain syndrome and severe neurotic conditions; anxiety, tension, agitation, and hyperexcitability in ambulatory patients.

Dosage **PO, adults:** 40–80 mg daily in divided doses for anxiety and tension; 80–120 mg daily in divided doses for hospitalized schizophrenic patients. **Pediatric:** 0.8–1.6 mg/kg daily in 3 doses. **Maximum doses:** 80 mg daily.

Additional Nursing Implication Administer 1 hour before bedtime to those patients who have difficulty sleeping.

BUTAPERAZINE MALEATE REPOISE MALEATE

Classification Antipsychotic, piperazine-type phenothiazine.

Remarks Less of a sedative than chlorpromazine. High incidence of extrapyramidal symptoms.

Uses Chronic schizophrenia, particularly when characterized by paranoid delusions and hallucinations, and for the agitation and confusion associated with chronic brain syndrome.

Dosage **PO; initial** (*hospitalized patients*): 5–10 mg, t.i.d. Increase by 5–10 mg daily q few days up to maximum of 100 mg daily. **Maintenance (after desired response is reached):** ¼–½ of the dose required during the acute phase. **Not recommended for use in children under 12 years of age.**

CARPHENAZINE MALEATE PROKETAZINE MALEATE

Classification Antipsychotic, piperazine-type phenothiazine.

Remarks Full effect may only appear after several months.

Uses Acute and chronic schizophrenia in hospitalized patients.

Dosage **PO; initial** (*hospitalized chronic psychotic patients*): 12.5–50 mg t.i.d. Can be increased q 7 to 14 days by 25–50 mg daily up to maximum of 400 mg/day. *Acute schizophrenia:* 12.5–25 mg t.i.d. Can be increased to 100 mg daily within first 24 hours.

CHLORPROMAZINE

CHLORPROMAZINE HYDROCHLORIDE CHLORAMEAD, ORMAZINE, PROMAPAR, SONAZINE, THORAZINE, OTHERS

Classification Antipsychotic, antiemetic, dimethylamino-type phenothiazine.

Uses Acute and chronic psychoses, including schizophrenia; alcohol withdrawal; antiemetic; control of hiccups; agitation associated with tetanus; and acute intermittent porphyria.

Dosage **Adults;** *psychiatry,* **PO:** 10–25 mg b.i.d.–q.i.d. Up to 200–400 mg/day may be required. **IM:** 25 mg; may be repeated in 1 hr. *Nausea and vomiting;* **PO:** 10–25 mg q 4 to 6 hr; **IM:** 25 mg; **rectal:** 50–100 mg q 6–8 hr. *Hiccups;* **PO, IM:** 25–50 mg t.i.d.–q.i.d. *Surgery;* **PO:** 10–50 mg; **IM:** 12.5–25 mg pre- and/or postoperatively. *Acute intermittent porphyria,* **PO, IM:** 25–50 mg t.i.d.–q.i.d. *Tetanus;* **IV, IM:** 25–50 mg t.i.d.–q.i.d. **Children:** *nausea, vomiting, psychiatry,* **PO, Rectal, IM:** 0.55–1.1 mg/kg q 4 to 8 hr. **Maximum IM dose up to 5 years:** 40 mg/day; **age 5–12 years:** 75 mg/day. Not used in children under 6 months. *Surgery:* **PO, IM:** 0.55 mg/kg. *Tetanus:* **IM, IV:** 0.55 mg/kg q 6 to 8 hr.

FLUPHENAZINE DECANOATE PROLIXIN DECANOATE

FLUPHENAZINE ENANTHATE PROLIXIN ENANTHATE

FLUPHENAZINE HYDROCHLORIDE PERMITIL, PROLIXIN

Classification Antipsychotic, piperazine-type phenothiazine.

General Statement Fluphenazine has a more prolonged action than other phenothiazines. Onset after parenteral administration is slow (24 to 72 hours). When fluphenazine enanthate is injected in fixed oil vehicle (sesame oil), effect lasts up to 3 weeks. This makes it suitable for use by outpatients.

The drug has a high incidence of reversible extrapyramidal side effects. It may also cause polyuria, xerostomia, hypertension, and fluctuating blood pressure.

Fluphenazine hydrochloride can be cautiously administered to patients with known hypersensitivity to other phenothiazines. Fluphenazine enanthate may replace fluphenazine hydrochloride if desired response occurs with hypersensitivity reaction to fluphenazine.

Uses Acute and chronic schizophrenia; manic phase of manic-depressive psychosis; involutional, senile, and toxic psychoses; antiemetic.

Dosage *Individualized.* Fluphenazine hydrochloride is administered **PO and IM.** Fluphenazine enanthate or decanoate are administered **SC and IM.**

Fluphenazine hydrochloride: **initial,** 1.0–10 mg daily to be increased gradually up to maximum of 20 mg daily. **Usual maintenance:** 1–5 mg daily.

Fluphenazine decanoate or enanthate; **initial,** 12.5–25 mg. Subsequent doses determined by patient's response.

Administration Inject with dry syringe.

MESORIDAZINE BESYLATE SERENTIL

Classification	Antipsychotic, piperidine-type phenothiazine.
Remarks	Mesoridazine has pronounced sedative effects, moderate anticholinergic effects, and a low incidence of extrapyramidal symptoms. The drug also causes a moderate degree of orthostatic hypotension. Safe use in children and pregnant women has not been established.
Uses	Schizophrenia, acute and chronic alcoholism, behavior problems in patients with mental deficiency and chronic brain syndrome, psychoneurosis.
Dosage	**PO**, *Schizophrenia:* **initial,** 50 mg t.i.d.; **optimum total dose:** 100–400 mg/day. *Alcoholism:* **initial,** 25 mg b.i.d.; **optimum total dose:** 50–200 mg/day. *Behavior problems:* **initial,** 25 mg t.i.d.; **optimum total dose:** 75–300 mg/day. *Psychoneurosis:* **initial,** 10 mg t.i.d.; **optimum total dose:** 30–150 mg. Total dosage is administered in 2 to 3 divided doses. **IM: initial,** 25 mg. Can be repeated, if necessary, after 30 to 60 minutes. **Optimum IM daily dose** 25–200 mg.
Administration	Maintain patient supine for minimum of 30 minutes after parenteral administration to minimize orthostatic effect.

PERPHENAZINE TRILAFON

Classification	Antipsychotic, antiemetic, piperazine-type phenothiazine.
Uses	Acute and chronic schizophrenia; manic phase of manic-depressive psychosis; involutional, senile, and toxic psychosis; controls nausea and vomiting.
Dosage	**PO, IM, IV:** Administer 16–64 mg daily in divided doses.
Administration/ Storage	Each 5.0 ml oral concentrate should be diluted with 60 ml diluent, such as water, milk, carbonated beverage, or orange juice. Do not mix with tea, coffee, cola, grape juice, or apple juice. Protect from light. Store solutions in amber containers.

PIPERACETAZINE QUIDE

Classification	Antipsychotic, piperidyl-type phenothiazine.
Remarks	Piperacetazine has a low incidence of extrapyramidal reactions. Safety for use in children and pregnant women has not been established.
Uses	Acute and chronic schizophrenia, especially when characterized by hyperactivity, agitation, or anxiety states.

Dosage   **Initial:** 10 mg b.i.d.–q.i.d. Increase gradually over 3 to 5 days; **maintenance:** 100 mg daily, but up to 160 mg daily may be required.

PROCHLORPERAZINE COMPAZINE

PROCHLORPERAZINE EDISYLATE COMPAZINE EDISYLATE

PROCHLORPERAZINE MALEATE COMPAZINE MALEATE

Classification   Antiemetic, antipsychotic, piperazine-type phenothiazine.

Remarks   Compound has greater antiemetic and extrapyramidal effects than other phenothiazines.

Uses   Psychomotor disorders associated with schizophrenia; manic phase of manic-depressive psychosis; involutional, senile, and toxic psychosis; and as antiemetic.

Dosage   **PO, IM, IV, rectal. Range:** 15–150 mg daily. **Usual PO, IM:** 5–10 mg, 2 to 4 times daily. Dosage gradually increased to 75–150 mg daily in divided doses. **Rectal:** 25 mg twice daily. *Preoperative* (not for children): **IM:** 5–10 mg 1 to 2 hours prior to surgery; **IV:** 5–10 mg 30 minutes before anesthesia.

    As an antiemetic after surgery or during labor: 5–10 mg **IM: pediatric above 2 years; PO, rectal:** *antiemetic* 2.5 mg 1–4 times daily depending on body weight. *Antipsychotic,* **PO, rectal:** 2.5 mg b.i.d.–t.i.d. **IM,** *antiemetic, antipsychotic:* 0.13 mg/kg. Usually one dose will suffice.

Administration/ Storage
1. Store all forms of drug in tight closing amber-colored bottles; the suppositories below 37° C.
2. Add the desired dosage of concentrate to 60 ml of beverage (tomato or fruit juice, milk, soup, etc.) or semisolid food just prior to administration to disguise the taste.

Additional Nursing Implications
1. Since children are particularly likely to exhibit extrapyramidal effects, advise parents not to exceed prescribed dose and to withhold drug if child reacts with signs of restlessness and excitement.
2. If the patient received spansule, continue treatment of overdosage until all signs of latter have worn off.
3. In treatment of overdosage, anticipate that saline cathartics may be used to hasten evacuation of pellets that have not already released their medication.

PROMAZINE HYDROCHLORIDE NORAZINE HYDROCHLORIDE, SPARINE HYDROCHLORIDE

Classification   Antipsychotic; dimethylaminopropyl-type phenothiazine.

Remarks   Less potent than chlorpromazine. Most common side effect is drowsiness. Not effective in reducing destructive behavior in acutely agitated psychotic patients.

Uses   Useful for delirium tremens, alcoholic hallucinations, and drug withdrawal symptoms. More effective and less toxic drugs are available for psychoses.

Dosage   **PO, IV, IM:** Oral or IM route preferred. *Severe and moderate agitation:* **initial, IM:** 50–150 mg; **then, PO:** 10–200 mg q 4 to 6 hr. **Total daily dose should not exceed 1000 mg. Children over 12 years:** 10–25 mg q 4 to 6 hr for chronic psychotic disease.

Administration   Dilute concentrate as directed on bottle. Taste can be disguised with citrus fruit juice, milk, or flavored drinks.

THIORIDAZINE HYDROCHLORIDE MELLARIL, MELLARIL-S

Classification   Antipsychotic; piperidyl-type phenothiazine.

General Statement   Thioridazine hydrochloride has a low incidence of extrapyramidal effects. The drug can often be used for patients intolerant to other phenothiazines. Thioridazine has little or no antiemetic effect. Dryness of mouth is especially frequent.

Uses   Acute and chronic schizophrenia. In children: treatment of hyperactivity in the retarded and behavior problems.

Dosage   **PO.** Highly individualized. *Neurosis, anxiety states, alcohol withdrawal, senility,* **range:** 20–200 mg daily; **initial:** 25 mg t.i.d. *Psychotic, severely disturbed hospitalized patients,* **initial:** 50–100 mg t.i.d. If necessary increase to maximum of 200 mg q.i.d. When control is achieved, reduce gradually to minimum effective dosage. **Pediatric above 2 years:** 0.5–3.0 mg/kg daily. *Hospitalized psychotic children,* **initial:** 25 mg 2 to 3 times/day. Increase gradually if necessary.

Administration/ Storage   Dilute each dose just prior to administration with distilled water, acidified tap water, or suitable juices. Preparation and storage of bulk dilutions is not recommended.

TRIFLUOPERAZINE STELAZINE

Classification   Antipsychotic, antiemetic; piperazine-type phenothiazine.

General Statement   Recommended for hospitalized or well-supervised patients only. Drug has antiemetic properties. More potent and with more prolonged activity than chlorpromazine. Drug produces a high incidence of extrapyramidal symptoms. Maximum therapeutic effect is usually attained 2 to 3 weeks after therapy is begun.

Uses Schizophrenia. Suitable for patients with apathy or withdrawal.

Dosage *Hospitalized patients*, **PO: initial**, 2–5 mg b.i.d.–t.i.d.; **maintenance:** 15–20 mg daily in 2 or 3 divided doses. *Outpatients* **PO:** 1–2 mg daily, up to 4 mg daily. **IM:** 1–2 mg q 4 to 6 hr. May be increased to 6–10 mg daily. **Pediatric 6–12 years: PO:** 1–2 mg daily. Increase gradually to maintenance levels, which rarely exceed 15 mg daily.

Administration/ Storage Dilute concentrate with 60 ml of suitable beverage (tomato or fruit juice, milk, etc.) or semisolid food. Dilute just prior to administration. Protect liquid forms from light. Discard strongly discolored solutions.

TRIFLUPROMAZINE HYDROCHLORIDE VESPRIN

Classification Antipsychotic; dimethylaminopropyl-type phenothiazine.

Uses Psychomotor agitation associated with acute and chronic psychoses, alcohol withdrawal, adjunct in obstetrics and surgery. Behavior problems in children. Emesis and nausea of pregnancy.

Dosage **PO**, *neurosis, psychosis:* 10–50 mg b.i.d.–t.i.d. **IM**, *severly agitated patients:* 60–150 mg daily in 2 to 3 doses. **PO**, *antiemesis:* 20–30 mg/day. **IV**, *antiemesis:* 1–3 mg. **Pediatric**, *antipsychotic*, **PO: initial**, 2 mg/kg up to maximum of 150 mg. Reduce gradually to lowest effective level for maintenance. **IM:** 0.25 mg/kg in divided doses up to maximum of 10 mg/day. **PO, IM**, *antiemetic:* 0.2 mg/kg up to maximum of 10 mg/day. The drug should not be used in children under 2½ years of age. **Not recommended for IV use in children.**

Administration/ Storage
1. Triflupromazine is only used in commerically available suspensions.
2. Triflupromazine hydrochloride is available in tablets for injection.
3. Store in amber-colored containers.
4. Do not use discolored (darker than light amber) solutions.

THIOXANTHENE AND BUTYROPHENONE DERIVATIVES

General Statement Drugs belonging to two other chemical families—the thioxanthene derivatives and the butyrophenone derivatives—are used as antipsychotic agents. The thioxanthene derivatives, chlorprothixene and thiothixene, are closely related to the phenothiazines from a chemical, pharmacologic, and clinical point of view.

Although the butyrophenone derivatives (haloperidol and droperidol) differ chemically from the phenothiazines, they are closely related in their pharmacologic actions.

For all general information pertaining to these agents see the *Phenothiazines.*

A totally different pharmacologic agent, lithium carbonate, which recently has been used quite successfully for the treatment of manic-depressive patients, is also presented here.

Thioxanthene Derivatives

CHLORPROTHIXENE TARACTAN

Classification Antipsychotic, thioxanthine derivative.

General Statement This thioxanthene derivative is closely related to chlorpromazine and the other phenothiazines as well as to thiothixene. The drug has CNS depressant, sedative, hypnotic, anticholinergic, and antiemetic properties. It is a more potent inhibitor of postural reflexes and motor coordination than chlorpromazine, but has less pronounced antihistaminic effects. It is effective within 30 minutes after IM administration.

Uses Neurosis, depression, schizophrenia, antiemesis, alcohol withdrawal. Adjunct in electroshock therapy. Drug may be effective in patients resistant to other psychotherapeutic drugs.

Untoward Reactions Drowsiness, lethargy, orthostatic hypotension, tachycardia, dizziness, and dry mouth occur especially frequently.

Drug Interactions

Interactant	Interaction
Methyldopa (Aldomet)	Additive hypotensive effect
Reserpine	Additive hypotensive effect

Dosage **IM, adults and children over 12 years:** 25–50 mg t.i.d.–q.i.d. Doses exceeding 600 mg/day are rarely needed. Switch to oral when feasible. **PO** same as **IM. Pediatric, children 6–12 years:** 10–25 mg t.i.d.–q.i.d.

Administration/ Storage 1. Inject deeply into large muscle mass.
2. Patient should be supine during administration because of postural hypotension.
3. Protect from light.

Nursing Implications See **Nursing Implications** under *Phenothiazines*.

THIOTHIXENE NAVANE

Classification Antipsychotic, thioxanthine derivative.

General Statement This thioxanthine derivative is closely related to the phenothiazines, especially chlorpromazine, as well as to chlorprothixene. It has CNS depressant, sedative, hypnotic, anticholinergic, and antiemetic properties. It is a more potent inhibitor of postural reflexes and motor coordination than chlorpromazine, but has less pronounced antihistaminic effects.

The margin between a therapeutically effective dose and one that causes extrapyramidal symptoms is narrow.

Uses Symptomatic treatment of acute and chronic schizophrenia, especially when condition is accompanied by florid symptoms.

Contraindication Children under 12 years of age.

Drug Interactions See *Chlorprothixene.*

Dosage **PO:** 2–5 mg t.i.d. Drug is initiated at lower dosage and increased gradually to a maximum of 60 mg daily. **IM:** 2–5 mg t.i.d. to a maximum of 30 mg daily. Switch to **PO** form as soon as possible.

Butyrophenone Derivatives

DROPERIDOL INAPSINE

Classification Antipsychotic, butyrophenone and antianxiety agent.

General Statement This butyrophenone derivative is closely related to haloperidol and the phenothiazines. It is only approved for use preoperatively and as an adjunct to anesthesia.

Its onset of action after IM or IV administration is rapid (3 to 10 minutes) and its effect lasts for 6 to 8 hours. For details about untoward reactions, see *Haloperidol* and *Phenothiazines.*

Dosage *Premedication:* 2.5–10 mg 30 to 60 minutes before anesthesia. *Adjunct to anesthesia:* 220–275 μg/kg. *Diagnostic procedures:* **IM** 2.5–10 mg 30 to 60 min prior to procedure; additional doses may be administered as necessary (usual 1.25–2.5 mg). **Pediatric,** *premedication:* 45–55 μg/kg; **2 to 12 years:** 88–165 μg/kg.

Additional Nursing Implications Monitor BP and pulse closely during the immediate postoperative period until stabilized at satisfactory levels.

HALOPERIDOL HALDOL

Classification Antipsychotic, butyrophenone.

General Statement The pharmacologic actions of this butyrophenone derivative are closely related to the phenothiazine tranquilizers. The mode of action of the drug is unknown. The margin between the therapeutically effective dose and one causing extrapyramidal symptoms is narrow. The compound has antiemetic effects. It causes less sedation, hypotension, and hypothermia than chlorpromazine. Its peak effect is attained in 30 to 45 minutes after IM injection. The drug is eliminated very slowly.

Uses   Tics and vocal utterances associated with Gilles de la Tourette's disease. Acute and chronic psychoses including schizophrenia, the manic phase of manic-depressive psychosis, and psychotic reactions in adults with brain damage and mental retardation.

Contraindications   Use with extreme caution, or not at all, in patients with parkinsonism.

Untoward Reactions   Extrapyramidal symptoms, especially akathisia and dystonias, occur more frequently than with the phenothiazines. Overdosage is characterized by severe extrapyramidal reactions, hypotension or sedation. The drug dose not elicit photosensitivity reactions like the phenothiazines.

Drug Interactions

Interactant	Interaction
Amphetamine	↓ Effect of amphetamine by ↓ uptake of drug at its site of action
Anticoagulants, oral	↓ Effect of anticoagulants due to ↑ breakdown by liver

Dosage   **PO (adults and children over 12 years), initial:** 1–15 mg daily in 2 to 3 divided doses. **Maintenance:** 2–8 mg daily. **IM:** 6–15 mg daily in divided doses. Switch to **PO** when feasible.

Elderly or debilitated patients should be started on lower dosage which should be increased more gradually.

MISCELLANEOUS ANTIPSYCHOTIC AGENTS

LITHIUM CARBONATE ESKALITH, LITHANE, LITHOBID, LITHONATE, LITHOTABS
LITHIUM CITRATE LITHIONATE-S

Classification   Antipsychotic agent, miscellaneous.

General Statement   Lithium carbonate is a psychotherapeutic agent used exclusively for manic-depressive patients.

The exact mode of action of the drug is unknown. The margin of safety between the therapeutic and toxic dose is narrow, and patients must be monitored by determination of their serum lithium levels that should not exceed 1.4 mEq/liter. Blood levels of 4 mEq/liter may be fatal. Tests should be made 1 to 2 times per week during initiation, and monthly thereafter, on samples taken 8 to 12 hours after dosage.

Full beneficial effect of lithium therapy is only noted 6 to 10 days after initiation. To reduce danger of lithium intoxication, sodium intake must remain at normal levels.

Uses   Control of manic episodes in manic-depressive patients. Prophylaxis.

Contraindications   Cardiovascular or renal disease. Brain damage.

Untoward Reactions These are related to the blood lithium level. Mild adverse reactions: nausea, diarrhea, malaise, thirst, polyuria, polydipsia, fatigue, and fine hand tremors. More severe adverse reactions are characterized by cardiac arrhythmias, and by anorexia, blurred vision, slurred speech, dry mouth, abdominal pain, weight loss, muscle hyperirritability, drowsiness, and other CNS disturbances. Very severe reactions (acute toxicity) are characterized by convulsions, oliguria, acute circulatory failure, coma, and death.

Hypothyroidism is also noted in some patients at all dosage levels.

Drug Interactions

Interactant	Interaction
Acetazolamine (Diamox)	↓ Lithium effect by ↑ renal excretion
Aminophylline	↓ Lithium effect by ↑ renal excretion
Diuretics	↑ Lithium effect due to ↓ excretion by kidney
Haloperidol	↑ Risk of neurological toxicity
Phenothiazines	Additive hyperglycemic effect
Sodium bicarbonate	↓ Lithium effect by ↑ renal excretion
Sodium chloride	Excretion of lithium is proportional to amount of sodium chloride ingested; if patient on salt-free diet, may develop lithium toxicity since less lithium excreted.
Thiazide diuretics	↓ Renal clearance of lithium
Urea	↓ Lithium effect by ↑ renal excretion

Laboratory Test Interference False + urinary glucose test (Benedict's), ↑ serum glucose, creatinine kinase. False − or ↓ serum protein bound iodine (PBI) and uric acid.

Dosage Individualized and according to lithium serum level (not to exceed 1.4 mEq/liter) and clinical response. *Usual,* **initial:** 600 mg t.i.d.; **elderly and debilitated patients:** 0.6–1.2 gm daily in 3 doses. **Maintenance:** 300 mg t.i.d.–q.i.d.

Administration of drug is discontinued when lithium serum level exceeds 1.2 mEq/liter and resumed 24 hr after it has fallen below that level.

Nursing Implications
1. Alert family that the patient must have blood tests at least weekly to check lithium levels (therapeutic serum concentrations usually 0.6–1.2 mEq/liter.
2. Warn patients and/or their families that should diarrhea, vomiting, drowsiness, muscular weakness, and lack of coordination occur, lithium therapy must be immediately discontinued, and patients must report to medical supervision.
3. Advise patients not to engage in physical activities that require alertness or physical coordination because these may be impaired while on therapy.
4. Advise the patient to eat a diet containing normal amounts of salt.
5. Advise the patient to maintain a fluid intake of 2.5–3 liters a day.
6. Advise the patient to report excessive sweating or diarrhea because this may indicate need for supplemental fluids or salt.

7. Be prepared to assist with gastric suction, parenteral administration of fluids and electrolytes to promote lithium excretion in case of toxicity.

LOXAPINE SUCCINATE DAXOLIN, LOXITANE

Classification   Antipsychotic, miscellaneous

General Statement   Loxapine belongs to a new subclass of tricyclic antipsychotic agents. Loxapine causes a high incidence of extrapyramidal symptoms, induces moderate sedation, has a low anticholinergic activity, and causes little orthostatic hypotension. Safe use in childhood or during pregnancy has not been established.

Use   Schizophrenia.

Additional Contraindications   History of convulsive disorders. Use with caution in patients with cardiovascular disease.

Additional Untoward Reactions   Tachycardia, hypertension, hypotension, lightheadedness, and syncope.

Dosage   **PO,** *individualized:* **initial,** 10 mg b.i.d. *Severe:* up to 50 mg daily. Increase dosage rapidly during 7 to 10 days until symptoms are controlled. **Range:** 60–100 mg up to 250 mg daily. **Maintenance:** If possible reduce dosage to 20–60 mg daily. Divide all daily dosages into 2 to 4 doses.

Administration   1. Measure the dosage of the concentrate *only* with the enclosed calibrated dropper.
2. Mix oral concentrate with orange or grapefruit juice immediately prior to administration to disguise unpleasant taste.

MOLINDONE LIDONE, MOBAN

Classification   Antipsychotic, miscellaneous.

Remarks   The drug is related to naturally occurring psychotropic substances like serotonin. The effect of molindone is similar to that of the phenothiazines.

Use   Schizophrenia.

Contraindications   Hypersensitivity to drug. Severe CNS depression caused by other agents.

Untoward Reactions   CNS symptoms: transient initial drowsiness, Parkinson-like reactions, akinesia, restlessness, insomnia, depression, blurred vision, hyperactivity, euphoria, dry mouth, headaches. Also nausea, postural hypotension, menstrual abnormalities, increased libido.

Dosage   Individualized and according to severity of symptoms: *Mild schizophrenia:* 5–15 mg t.i.d.–q.i.d.; *moderate schizophrenia:* 10–25 mg t.i.d.–q.i.d.; *severe schizophrenia:* 225 mg daily, up to maximum of 400 mg/day. Can be given once daily.

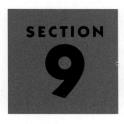

SECTION

9

antidepressants

Monoamine Oxidase (MAO) Inhibitors	Isocarboxazid Pargyline	Phenelzine Sulfate Tranylcypromine Sulfate
Tricyclic Antidepressants	Amitriptyline Hydrochloride Desipramine Hydrochloride Doxepin Hydrochloride Imipramine Hydrochloride	Imipramine Pamoate Nortriptyline Hydrochloride Protriptyline Hydrochloride

MONOAMINE OXIDASE (MAO) INHIBITORS

General Statement   This group of drugs is chiefly used to elevate the mood of depressed patients. Because of their relatively high toxicity, they are usually only prescribed when the tricyclic compounds are ineffective.

The exact mode of action of the MAO inhibitors is unknown. However, it is believed that they directly increase the concentration of norepinephrine and other chemical substances involved in nerve impulse transmission by interfering (inhibiting) with an enzyme called monoamine oxidase that breaks down norepinephrine. Thus, these drugs are called monoamine oxidase inhibitors. MAO inhibitors also lower blood pressure and interfere with the detoxification mechanisms (and thus metabolism of certain drugs) that take place in the liver.

Uses   Management of neuroses and psychoses characterized by depression, involutional melancholia, depressive phases of manic depressive psychoses. Occasionally used prophylactically for the treatment of hypertension.

Contraindications   Hypersensitivity to MAO inhibitors. History of liver disease, abnormal liver function tests, pheochromocytoma (tumor of the adrenal medulla), impaired renal function, hyperthyroidism, paranoid schizophrenia, epilepsy, cerebrovascular disease, hypertension, cerebral or generalized arteriosclerosis, hypernatremia, atonic colitis, and cardiovascular disease. MAO inhibitors may aggravate glaucoma. They may also suppress anginal pain, which may serve as a warning sign for patients with angina pectoris. Use cautiously in elderly patients.

Untoward Reactions   Restlessness, headache, dizziness, drowsiness, insomnia, constipation, anorexia, nausea, vomiting, dryness of mouth, urinary retention or increased urinary frequency, transient impotence, skin rash, orthostatic hypotension and paradoxical hypertension, peripheral edema, and anemia. Long-term therapy occasionally causes optic damage. Early optic changes affect color perception. MAO inhibitors also cause flushing, increased perspiration, appetite stimulation, weight gain, and hyperreflexia. High dosage may activate a latent schizophrenia and cause hyperexcitement.

Drug Interactions   MAO inhibitors potentiate both the pharmacologic actions and the toxic effects of a wide variety of drugs. Because of the long duration of action of MAO inhibitors, adverse drug reactions may also occur if any of the drugs listed below are given to patients within 2 to 3 weeks after the administration of MAO inhibitors have been terminated.

Interactant	*Interaction*
Alcohol, ethyl	Tyramine-containing beverages (e.g., Chianti wine) may result in hypertensive crisis
Amphetamine	See *Sympathomimetic Drugs*
Anticholinergic agents Atropine	MAO inhibitors ↑ effects of anticholinergic drugs
Antidepressants, tricyclics	Concomitant use may result in excitation, increase in body temperature, delirium, tremors, convulsions
Antidiabetic agents	MAO inhibitors ↑ and prolong hypoglycemic response to insulin and oral hypoglycemics
Barbiturates	↑ Effect of barbiturates due to ↓ breakdown by liver
Doxapram (Dopram)	MAO inhibitors ↑ adverse cardiovascular effects of doxapram (arrhythmias, increase in blood pressure)
Ephedrine	See *Sympathomimetic Drugs*
Guanethidine (Ismelin)	MAO inhibitors reverse the effects of guanethidine
Levodopa	Concomitant administration may result in hypertension, light headedness, and flushing
Metaraminol	See *Sympathomimetic Drugs*
Methoxamine	See *Sympathomimetic Drugs*
Methylphenidate (Ritalin)	See *Sympathomimetic Drugs*

Drug Interactions (Continued)	*Interactant*	*Interaction*
	Narcotic analgesics	Possible potentiation of either MAO inhibitor (excitation, hypertension), or narcotic (hypotension, coma) effects. Death has resulted.
	Phenothiazines	↑ Effect of phenothiazines by ↓ breakdown by liver. Also ↑ chance of severe extrapyramidal effects and hypertensive crisis.
	Phenylephrine	See *Sympathomimetic Drugs*
	Phenylpropanolamine	See *Sympathomimetic Drugs*
	Reserpine	Concomitant use may cause hypertensive crisis
	Succinylcholine	↑ Effect of succinylcholine by ↓ breakdown of drug in plasma by pseudocholinesterase
	Sympathomimetic drugs Amphetamine, ephedrine, metaraminol, methoxamine, methylphenidate, phenylephrine, phenylpropanolamine. (Many over-the-counter cold tablets and capsules, hayfever medications, and nasal decongestants contain one or more of these drugs)	All peripheral metabolic, cardiac, and central effects are potentiated up to two weeks after termination of MAO inhibitor therapy. Symptoms include acute hypertensive crisis with possible intracranial hemorrhage, hyperthermia, convulsions, coma. Death may occur
	Tyramine-rich foods, such as beer, broad beans, cheeses (brie, cheddar, Camembert, Stilton), Chianti wine, chicken livers, caffeine, cola drinks, figs, licorice, liver, pickled or kippered herring, tea, cream, yogurt, yeast extract, and chocolate	Severe headache, hypertension, intracranial hemorrhage, and even death have been reported if these foods are eaten by patient who is being treated with MAO inhibitor

Laboratory Test Interference ↑ BUN. May affect liver function tests.

Dosage All agents are administered orally. The effectiveness of the MAO inhibitors is cumulative and it may take days or even months for the drugs to reach their full effectiveness. The effects of the drugs also take 2 to 3 weeks to wane. Therefore, if switching from one MAO inhibitor to another, the second drug should not be given immediately after therapy until the first has been discontinued. Do not give second drug for 2 weeks. Also, all drug interactions between MAO inhibitors and other agents can occur up to 2 to 3 weeks after MAO inhibitor therapy has been discontinued. Rapid drug withdrawal in patients receiving high

TABLE 14 ANTIDEPRESSANT, MAO INHIBITOR-TYPE

Drug	Dosage	Remarks
Isocarboxazid (Marplan)	**PO: initial;** 30 mg daily as a single or divided dose. Reduce when clinical improvement is noted. **Maintenance:** 10–20 mg daily.	It may take 1 to 4 weeks for effect to become noticeable.
Pargyline (Eutonyl)		See *Antihypertensives*, p. 272.
Phenelzine sulfate (Nardil)	**PO: initial:** 15 mg t.i.d. for 2 to 6 weeks until beneficial effects are noted. Decrease dosage gradually over several weeks. Some patients can be maintained satisfactorily on as little as 15 mg every 2 days. **Maximum daily dose:** 75 mg.	
Tranylcypromine sulfate (Parnate Sulfate)	**PO:** 10 mg b.i.d. for 2 to 3 weeks until beneficial effect is noted. If no response is noted, increase to 30 mg daily **Maintenance:** Decrease dosage gradually to 10–20 mg daily. **Maximum daily dose:** 30 mg.	Onset of action more rapid than with other MAO inhibitors. More likely to cause hypertensive crisis. To be used for severely depressed, hospitalized patients.

doses may cause a rebound effect characterized by headache, CNS excitability, and occasional hallucinations. (For specific dosages, see Table 14 above.)

Nursing Implications

1. Advise patient and family that he/she is not to ingest any other drug while on MAO inhibitor therapy and for 2 to 3 weeks after discontinuance before consulting the physician.
2. Emphasize to the patient and family that foods rich in tyramine (see *Drug Interactions*) may be extremely harmful to patient and must be omitted from the diet. Give printed list of foods to be omitted.
3. Limit excessive drinking of coffee, tea, and cola beverages because excessive caffeine with MAO inhibitors may cause hypertensive crisis (characterized by marked elevation of BP, occipital headaches, palpitation, stiffness and soreness of neck, nausea, vomiting, sweating, photophobia, dilated pupils, tachycardia or bradycardia, and constricting chest pain).
4. Monitor BP and pulse when therapy is initiated and at regular

intervals thereafter so as to note hypertension that would necessitate discontinuance of the drug.

5. Warn patients against overexertion because drugs suppress anginal pain, a warning sign of myocardial ischemia.
6. Check for peripheral edema, which may be an early symptom of impending congestive heart failure.
7. Check on red-green vision for impairment as this may be the first indication of optic damage.
8. Observe diabetic patients for signs of hypoglycemia because MAO inhibitors potentiate the effect of insulin and sulfonylurea compounds.
9. Monitor intake and output and for bladder distention to check on possible urinary retention that may necessitate changes in medication.
10. Encourage the patient to rise slowly from supine position and to dangle feet before standing, to minimize orthostatic hypotension.
11. Advise the patient to lie down immediately if feeling faint.
12. Have on hand medication for treatment of overdosage: *Agitation* is treated with phenothiazine tranquilizers (IM). Excessive pressor response is treated with an *alpha*-adrenergic blocking agent (phentolamine) or a vasodilator-type drug.
13. Closely supervise patients for cues to suicide because patients on antidepressants are more prone to suicide when they emerge from deepest phase of depression than they were before therapy.

Tricyclic Antidepressants

General Statement This important group of antidepressant drugs includes: amitriptyline, desipramine, doxepin, imipramine, nortriptyline, and protriptyline (see Table 15, p. 390).

The drugs act on the CNS, but the mechanisms of their antidepressant effect have not yet been elucidated. The are thought to cause an increase in the levels of neurotransmitters (e.g. norepinephrine) at the synapse.

The compounds also have some anticonvulsant, peripheral atropinelike, antihistaminic, antiserotonin, anticholinergic, hypotensive, and sedative effects. The compounds are less effective for depressed patients in the presence of organic brain damage or schizophrenia.

They can also induce mania, and this should be kept in mind when given to patients with manic-depressive psychoses.

Therapeutic response usually takes several days or weeks to be fully established.

Leukocyte and differential counts and liver function tests are indicated in long-term therapy.

Uses Endogenous and reactive depressions. Sometimes used concomitantly with electroschock therapy (decreases the number of required treatments). Preferred over MAO inhibitors because they are less toxic. Enuresis in children.

TABLE 15 TRICYCLIC ANTIDEPRESSANTS

Drug	Dosage	Remarks
Amitriptyline hydrochloride (Amitril, Amitid, Elavil HCl, Endep, SK-Amitriptyline)	**PO** (*hospitalized patients*): 100–200 mg daily; (*outpatients*): 75 mg daily. Can be increased to 150 mg daily in divided doses. **Maintenance:** 40–100 mg daily. **IM: initial,** 20–30 mg q.i.d. After improvement (2 weeks usually) transfer to oral route.	Elderly and adolescent patients may have lower tolerance. Drug causes high degree of sedation *Additional Nursing Implications* Warn patient not to drive a car or operate hazardous machinery as drug causes high degree of sedation.
Desipramine hydrochloride (Desmethylimipramine Hydrochloride, Norpramin, Pertofrane)	**PO**, *individualized:* initial; 25–50 mg t.i.d. **Maximum daily dose:** 200 mg; **maintenance:** 50–100 mg daily; **geriatric and adolescent patients:** 25–100 mg/day. **Not recommended for children.**	Patients who will respond to drug usually do so within the first week. *Additional Untoward Reactions* Temperature elevation, "bad taste" in mouth.
Doxepin hydrochloride (Adapin, Sinequan)	**PO**, *individualized,* initial (*mild symptoms*): 10–25 mg t.i.d.; (*severe symptoms*): 50 mg t.i.d. **Maximum daily dose:** 300 mg. **Not recommended for children under 12 years of age.**	Drug is stable for 2 years. Check on expiration date. *Additional Contraindications* Glaucoma. *Additional Untoward Reactions* Drug has high incidence of side effects, including high degree of sedation, decreased libido, extrapyramidal symptoms, dermatitis, pruritus, fatigue, weight gain, edema, parasthesia, breast engorgement, insomnia, tremor, chills, tinnitus, and photophobia.
Imipramine hydrochloride (Antipress, Imavate, Janimine, Presamine, SK-Pramine, Tofranil, W.D.D.) Imipramine pamoate (Tofranil-PM)	**PO, IM**, *individualized (hospitalized patients):* 50 mg b.i.d. Can be increased by 25 mg every few days up to 200 mg daily. After minimum rest period of 2 weeks, dosage may again be increased gradually to	*Storage* Protect from direct sunlight and strong artificial light. High therapeutic dosage may increase frequency of seizures in epileptic patients

Drug	Dosage	Administration / Nursing Implications
	maximum of 250–300 mg/day. *Outpatients:* 75 mg daily in divided doses. Maximum dose for outpatients is 200 mg. Decrease when feasible to maintenance dosage: 30–150 mg daily. **Adolescent and geriatric patients: 30–40 mg/day PO,** up to maximum of 100 mg/day. *Childhood enuresis:* ages 6 and over, 25 mg/day 1 hr. before bedtime. Dose can be increased to 50 mg/day up to 12 years of age and 75 mg/day in children over 12 years of age.	and cause seizures in nonepileptic patients. Elderly and adolescent patients may have lower tolerance to the drug *Administration* Crystals which may be present in the injectable form can be dissolved by immersing closed ampuls into hot water for 1 minute. Total daily dose can be given once daily at bedtime. *Additional Nursing Implications* Report increase in frequency of seizures in epileptics and occurrence of seizures in nonepileptics.
Nortriptyline hydrochloride (Aventyl Hydrochloride, Pamelor)	**PO:** 25 mg t.i.d.–q.i.d. Dose individualized. **Doses above 100 mg not recommended. Not recommended for children. Elderly patients:** 30–50 mg/day in divided doses.	*Administration* After meals and at bedtime
Protriptyline hydrochloride (Vivactil Hydrochloride)	**PO,** *individualized,* **initial,** *severe depression:* 30–60 mg in 3 to 4 divided doses. After satisfactory response is obtained, decrease gradually to maintenance level of 15–40 mg daily in divided doses. **Not recommended for children. Elderly patients: initial,** 5 mg t.i.d., increase dose slowly.	Protriptyline causes more cardiovascular side effects than the other tricyclic antidepressants. Administer with caution to patients with myocardial insufficiency and those in whom tachycardia or a drop in blood pressure might lead to serious complications. Drug causes less sedation than other tricyclic antidepressants. *Administration* If drug causes insomnia give last dose no less than 8 hours before bedtime. *Additional Nursing Implications* Monitor V.S. at least b.i.d. during initiation of therapy

Contraindications   Severely impaired liver function. Use with caution in patients with epilepsy, cardiovascular diseases, glaucoma, benign prostatic hypertrophy, suicidal tendencies, a history of urinary retention, and the elderly. Do not use together with MAO inhibitors.

Untoward Reactions   Most frequent side effects are atropine-like reactions including dryness of mouth, blurred vision, constipation, urinary retention, and tachycardia. Headache and muscle tremors occur in 10% of all patients. Less frequent side effects are sweating, dizziness, insomnia, drowsiness, anorexia, heartburn, fatigue, weight gain, nausea, vomiting, urinary frequency, fine tremors (especially with high doses), orthostatic hypotension, angioneurotic edema, numbness and tingling of arms and legs, allergic reactions characterized by skin rash, swelling of face and tongue, itching, purpura and blood dyscrasias, allergic obstructive jaundice, manic excitement in certain patients, hallucinations, and delusions.

High dosage increases the frequency of seizures in epileptic patients and may cause epileptiform attacks in normal subjects. Has caused myocardial infarction and precipitated congestive heart failure and cardiac arrhythmias.

Drug Interactions

Interactant	Interaction
Acetazolamide (Diamox)	↑ Effect of tricyclics by ↑ renal tubular reabsorption of the drug
Alcohol, ethyl	Concomitant use may lead to ↑ GI complications and ↓ performance on motor skill tests. Death has been reported
Ammonium chloride	↓ Effect of tricyclics by ↓ renal tubular reabsorption of the drug
Anticholinergic drugs	Additive anticholinergic side effects
Anticoagulants, oral	↑ Hypoprothrombinemia due to ↓ breakdown by liver
Anticonvulsants	Tricyclics may ↑ incidence of epileptic seizures
Antihistamines	Additive anticholinergic side effects
Ascorbic acid	↓ Effect of tricyclics by ↓ renal tubular reabsorption of the drug
Barbiturates	Barbiturates ↑ adverse effects of toxic doses of tricyclic antidepressants
Chlordiazepoxide (Librium)	Concomitant use may cause additive sedative effects and/or additive atropinelike side effects
Clonidine (Catapres)	Tricyclics ↓ effect of clonidine by preventing up take at its site of action
Diazepam (Valium)	Concomitant use may cause additive sedative effects and/or additive atropinelike side effects
Ethychlorvynol (Placidyl)	Combination may result in transient delirium
Furazolidone (Furoxone)	Toxic psychoses possible
Glutethimide (Doriden)	Additive anticholinergic side effects

Drug Interactions (Continued)	*Interactant*	*Interaction*
	Guanethidine (Ismelin)	Tricyclics ↓ effect of guanethidine by preventing uptake at its site of action
	Meperidine (Demerol)	Tricyclics enhance narcotic-induced respiratory depression; also, additive anticholinergic side effects
	Methyldopa (Aldomet)	Tricyclics may block hypotensive effects of methyldopa
	Methylphenidate (Ritalin)	↑ Effect of tricyclics by ↓ breakdown by liver
	MAO inhibitors	Concomitant use may result in excitation, increase in body temperature, delirium, tremors, convulsions
	Narcotic analgesics	Tricyclics enhance narcotic-induced respiratory depression; also, additive anticholinergic effects
	Oxazepam (Serax)	Concomitant use may cause additive sedative effects and/or atropinelike side effects
	Phenothiazines	Additive anticholinergic side effects
	Phenylbutazone (Butazolidin)	↓ Effect due to ↓ absorption from GI tract of phenylbutazone
	Reserpine	Tricyclics ↓ hypotensive effect of reserpine
	Sodium bicarbonate	↑ Effect of tricyclics by ↑ renal tubular reabsorption of the drug
	Sympathomimetics	Potentiation of sympathomimetic effects → hypertension or cardiac arrhythmias
	Thyroid preparations	Mutually potentiating effects observed
	Vasodilators	Additive hypotensive effect

Laboratory Test Interferences

May alter liver function test, even causing jaundice. ↑ Blood glucose. False + or ↑ urinary catecholamines.

Nursing Implications

1. Advise patient and his/her family that patient is not to ingest any other drug while taking tricyclic antidepressants and for 2 weeks after therapy has been completed without consulting their medical supervisor.
2. Anticipate that dosage will be highly individualized according to patient's age, physical and mental condition, and response.
3. Anticipate that sedation and anticholinergic effects may be minimized by starting with small doses and then gradually increasing doses.
4. Advise patients and their families that it may take 2 to 4 weeks to achieve maximal clinical response.
5. Observe for allergic response manifested by skin rash, alopecia, eosinophilia, or other allergic-type response.
6. Monitor patient with a history of cardiovascular disorders for arrhythmia and tachycardia which may lead to increased anginal attacks, myocardial infarction, and stroke. Ascertain that a plan for periodic electrocardiograph evaluations is implemented.

7. Instruct patients to rise gradually from a supine position and not to remain standing in one place for any length of time, and to lie down if faint to minimize orthostatic hypotension. Provide appropriate safety measures.

8. Ascertain that drug is discontinued several days before surgery because tricyclic compounds may cause a hypertensive effect during surgery.

9. Observe for behavior manifesting further psychological disturbances that may require reducation in dosage or discontinuance of therapy.

10. Check with medical supervision before administering tricyclic compounds to patients on electroshock therapy because the combination may increase the hazard of therapy.

11. Warn patients performing hazardous tasks requiring mental alertness or physical coordination that the drug causes drowsiness and/ or ataxia.

12. Be aware that patient may have epileptiform seizures precipitated by drug. Practice seizure precautions.

13. Observe patients with a history of closed-angle glaucoma for acute attack often characterized by severe headache, nausea, vomiting, eye pain, dilation of the pupil, and halos.

14. Assess intake and output, abdominal distention, and bowel sounds that may indicate urinary retention, paralytic ileus, and constipation. These conditions may require reduction in dosage.

15. Reassure impotent patient that if condition is caused by tricyclic compound, adjustment of dosage by doctor will alleviate condition.

16. Ascertain that baseline blood and liver function tests are done before onset of therapy and that a plan for periodic evaluations is implemented.

17. Observe and report symptoms of blood dyscrasias, such as sore throat, fever, weakness and purpura, which necessitate withholding the drug and placing patient in reverse isolation until blood tests are reevaluated.

18. Assess for symptoms of cholestatic jaundice (indicating biliary tract obstruction), such as high fever, upper abdominal pain, nausea, diarrhea, rash, yellowing of skin, sclera, or mucous membranes. Withhold drug and report to medical supervision should these signs and symptoms be present.

19. Encourage rinsing oral cavity with water. Encourage increased fluid intake to relieve excessive dryness of mouth. If applicable, this also helps patient to retain dentures.

20. Be alert to adverse gastrointestinal reactions manifested by nausea, vomiting, anorexia, epigastric distress, diarrhea, constipation, peculiar taste, abdominal cramps, and black tongue. These symptoms necessitate adjustment of dosage.

21. Be alert to adverse endocrine reactions, such as increased or decreased libido, gynecomastia, testicular swelling, galactorrhea, interference with ADH secretion, and elevated or depressed blood sugar levels. Encourage diabetic patients to monitor urine carefully because drug may affect carbohydrate metabolism, and adjustments of hypoglycemic drugs and diet may be indicated.

22. Encourage photosensitive individuals to remain out of the sun.
23. Be alert to other adverse reactions that may be manifestations of the tricyclic compounds described under *Untoward Reactions*.
24. Closely supervise seriously depressed patients, particularly during the early therapy, because suicidal tendencies are increased when patients start recovering from depression. Also ascertain that such patients are ingesting drugs and not hoarding them.
25. Monitor patient with hyperthyroidism for cardiac arrhythmias precipitated by tricyclic compound.
26. On cessation of therapy, drug should be withdrawn gradually to prevent withdrawal symptoms, such as nausea, headache, and malaise.
27. Be aware that although MAO inhibitors are usually contraindicated with tricyclic antidepressants, they may be used in small dosages, under close medical supervision, for patients refractory to more conservative therapy.

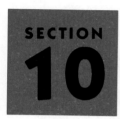

SECTION 10

central nervous stimulants: anorexiants, analeptics, and agents for minimal brain dysfunction

Psychomotor Stimulants: Anorexiants Amphetamines and Derivatives Miscellaneous Agents	Amphetamine Complex Amphetamine Sulfate Benzphetamine Hydrochloride Chlorphentermine Hydrochloride Clortermine Hydrochloride Dextroamphetamine Hydrochloride Dextroamphetamine Sulfate Dextroamphetamine Tannate Caffeine Caffeine and Sodium Benzoate	Diethylpropion Hydrochloride Fenfluramine Hydrochloride Mazindol Methamphetamine Hydrochloride Phendimetrazine Tartrate Phenmetrazine Hydrochloride Phentermine Hydrochloride Phentermine Resin Caffeine, Citrated
Analeptics	Doxapram Hydrochloride Nikethamide	Pentylenetetrazol

| **Agents for Minimal Brain Dysfunction** | Deanol Acetamidobenzoate
Methylphenidate Hydrochloride | Pemoline |

General Statement

The drugs that are grouped under the general heading of central nervous system stimulants are commonly classified according to their primary site of action into (1) cerebral or psychomotor stimulants (2) brain stem stimulants or analeptics, and (3) spinal cord stimulants or convulsants. Their effect often is not limited to the central nervous system. The cardiovascular system often becomes affected, and these side effects may become unwanted when central nervous system stimulation is the primary goal.

It is difficult to separate the central nervous system stimulants into rigid pharmacological classes because their effect is dose-dependent. For example any agent with primarily cerebral action will stimulate respiration, because respiratory control centers are located in the brain stem. Moreover, they can induce paradoxical reactions which are taken advantage of pharmacologically. For example, certain central nervous system stimulants have a quietening effect on children who suffer from hyperkinesia or other behavior problems of neurological rather than psychological origin. (These conditions are called minimal brain dysfunction or MBD for short.) These agents and other central nervous system stimulants can be beneficial for patients suffering from extrapyramidal motor symptoms and spasticity.

Even though there is a great deal of overlap among the indications for the various central nervous system stimulants, they have been divided according to their main clinical uses or pharmacological action, into *Psychomotor Stimulants; and Anorexiants; Analeptics*, and *Agents for Minimal Brain Dysfunction*. Spinal cord stimulants cause convulsions and are not used clinically; thus, they are not discussed.

Psychomotor Stimulants and Anorexiants

General Statement

The large number of anorexiant drugs consist principally of the amphetamines and derivatives. These general stimulants cause an increase in the activity of the nervous system. They are believed to act on the cerebral cortex and on the reticular activating system, including the medullary respiratory and vasomotor centers. They also have peripheral actions.

The amphetamines have pressor effects on the vascular system. They cause dilation of the pupil, bronchodilation and contraction of the urinary bladder sphincter. They also inhibit the enzyme monoamine oxidase (MAO).

Because of their stimulatory effects on the CNS, the drugs also cause an increase in motor activity and mental alertness, overcome fatigue, and have a mood-elevating and slightly euphoric effect. They also have an anorexigenic effect and are currently used as appetite suppressants for obese patients.

Response to amphetamines is very individualized. Their psychic stimulation is often followed by a rebound effect, manifested as fatigue.

A great number of different amphetamines are available today. The slight differences in their pharmacologic and untoward reactions (appetite suppression, respiratory stimulation, length of action) dictate their principal use.

Amphetamines are readily absorbed from the GI tract. They are distributed throughout most tissues, with highest concentrations in the brain and cerebrospinal fluid.

Uses

Appetite control, narcolepsy, hiccups. Also, postencephalitic parkinsonism, nocturnal enuresis, urinary incontinency, to counteract overdoses of depressants, to facilitate verbalization during psychotherapeutic interviews, mild mental disorders, chronic nervous exhaustion, psychoneurosis, the depressive phase of manic-depressive psychosis, hyperkinesia, and abnormal behavior patterns in children.

Contraindications

Hyperthyroidism, nephritis, diabetes mellitus, hypertension, narrow angle glaucoma, angina pectoris, cardiovascular disease and patients with hypersensitivity to drug. To be used with caution in patients suffering from hyperexcitability states; in elderly, debilitated, or asthenic patients; patients with psychopathic personality traits or a history of homicidal or suicidal tendencies. Contraindicated in emotionally unstable individuals susceptible to drug abuse.

Untoward Reactions

Nervousness, dizziness, headache, increased motor activity, chilliness, pallor, flushing, blurred vision, mydriasis, hyperexcitability, hypertension, hypotension, tachycardia, palpitation, cardiac arrhythmias. GI disturbances, including nausea, cramps, diarrhea, constipation, anorexia, metallic taste. Paradoxical increased depression and agitation in depressed patients.

Large doses may cause fatigue, mental depression, increased blood pressure, cyanosis, respiratory failure, disorientation, hallucinations, convulsions and coma. Long-term use results in psychic dependence as well as a high degree of tolerance.

Toxic Reactions There is a relatively wide margin of safety between the therapeutic and toxic doses of amphetamines. However, amphetamines can cause both acute and chronic toxicity. Amphetamines are excreted very slowly (5 to 7 days) and cumulative effects may occur with continued administration.

Acute toxicity (overdosage) is characterized by cardiovascular symptoms (flushing, pallor, palpitations, labile pulse, changes in blood pressure, heart block or chest pains), hyperpyrexia, mental disturbances (confusion, delirium, acute psychoses, disorientation, delusions and hallucinations, panic states, paranoid ideation).

Death usually results from cardiovascular collapse or convulsions.

Chronic toxicity due to abuse is characterized by emotional lability, loss of appetite, somnolence, mental impairment, occupational deterioration, a tendency to withdraw from social contact, teeth grinding, continuous chewing, and ulcers of the tongue and lips.

Prolonged use of high doses can elicit symptoms of paranoid schizophrenia, including auditory and visual hallucinations, and paranoid ideation.

Treatment of Acute Toxicity (Overdosage)

Have available equipment for symptomatic treatment of acute toxicity: sedatives, tourniquets, and ice packs (to be used after injection of sedative). After oral ingestion, emesis is to be induced and gastric lavage carried out. Saline cathartics may be given. Stimuli should be reduced so that patient can be maintained in a quiet dim environment. Patients who have ingested an overdosage of spansules should be treated for toxicity until all symptoms of overdosage have disappeared.

Note: At the present time the FDA is considering a recommendation that amphetamines be used for *only* narcolepsy or hyperactive syndrome in children.

Drug Interactions

Interactant	Interaction
Acetazolamide (Diamox)	↑ Effect of amphetamine by ↑ renal tubular reabsorption
Ammonium chloride	↓ Effect of amphetamine by ↓ renal tubular reabsorption
Ascorbic acid	↓ Effect of amphetamine by ↓ renal tubular reabsorption
Guanethidine (Ismelin)	↓ Effect of guanethidine by displacement from its site of action
Haloperidol (Haldol)	↓ Effect of amphetamine by ↓ uptake of drug at its site of action
Methyldopa (Aldomet)	↓ Hypotensive effect of methyldopa by ↑ sympathomimetic activity
MAO Inhibitors	All peripheral metabolic, cardiac, and central effects of amphetamine are potentiated up to 2 weeks after termination of MAO inhibitor therapy. Symptoms include hypertensive crisis with possible intracranial hemorrhage, hyperthermia, convulsions, coma. Death may occur
Phenothiazines	↓ Effect of amphetamine by ↓ uptake of drug into its site of action
Sodium bicarbonate	↑ Effect of amphetamine by ↑ renal tubular reabsorption
Thiazide diuretics	↑ Effect of amphetamine by ↑ renal tubular reabsorption

Laboratory Test Interferences

↑ Urinary catecholamines.

Dosage

Individualized. See Table 16, page 400. Many compounds are timed-release preparations.

Nursing Implications

1. Initial doses should be small and then increased gradually as necessary on an individual basis.

2. Administer last daily dose at least 6 hours before patient retires unless specified otherwise by physician.
3. As an appetite depressant, administer one-half hour before meals.
4. Caution patients on weight reduction programs that anorexiant effect is a short-term "crutch," usually lasting 4 to 6 weeks, and tolerance develops rapidly.
5. Assist patients on anorexiant therapy to curtail food intake. Help select appropriate diet.
6. Caution patients who have developed tolerance not to increase medication but rather to discontinue it.
7. Caution patients that amphetamines may mask extreme fatigue that can impair ability to perform potentially hazardous tasks such as operating a machine or an automobile.
8. Anticipate and teach diabetics on therapy that amphetamines may cause changes in insulin and dietary requirements.
9. Observe the patient for at least 14 days after receiving MAO inhibitors and then amphetamines as hypertensive crisis may occur.
10. Observe for acute toxicity as demonstrated by cardiovascular symptoms followed by psychotic syndrome. Be prepared to assist in treatment for overdosage as noted in general statement.
11. Observe for chronic toxicity manifested by emotional lability, loss of appetite, somnolence, mental impairment, and occupational deterioration. Drug should be discontinued.
12. Observe for marked psychological dependence and tolerance. Drug should be discontinued.
13. Amphetamines are regulated by the Controlled Substances Act. Availability and use are restricted in an attempt to prevent drug abuse.
14. Guide drug abusers to medical supervision and psychological counseling.
15. Weigh patients on amphetamines at least once a week as anorectic effect may occur in patients being treated for other problems. Note insomnia or restlessness in these patients.
16. Advise patients who discontinue drug after prolonged high dosage to seek medical supervision for management of extreme fatigue and depression.

Miscellaneous Agents

CAFFEINE NO DOZ, STIM TABS, VIVARIN

CAFFEINE AND SODIUM BENZOATE

CAFFEINE, CITRATED

Classification   CNS stimulant, miscellaneous.

TABLE 16 AMPHETAMINES AND DERIVATIVES

Drug	Dosage	Remarks
Amphetamine complex (Biphetamine)	**PO:** 7.5–20 mg daily (1 capsule). Product comes in 3 strengths (7½, 12½, 20 mg).	Resin complex of amphetamine and dextroamphetamine. *Administration* 10 to 14 hours before bedtime.
Amphetamine sulfate (Benzedrine sulfate)	*Narcolepsy,* **PO, adult:** 5–60 mg/day. **Pediatric 12 years or older:** 10 mg daily; **6–12 years:** 5 mg daily. *Hyperkinesis,* **PO, pediatric over 5 years:** 5 mg 1 or 2 times daily. May be increased to 20–30 mg daily in divided doses or as a single timed release form; **3–5 years: initial,** 2–5 mg daily. Increase dose until optimal response obtained. *Anorexia;* **PO, adult:** 5–10 mg t.i.d.	*Administration* As anorexiant: 30 to 60 minutes before meals. Last dose 6 hours before bedtime. IV injection should be made slowly. Switch to oral as soon as possible.
Benzphetamine hydrochloride (Didrex)	**PO:** 25–50 mg 1 to 3 times daily 1 hour before meals.	Long-term use of large doses may result in psychic dependence. *Administration* A single daily dose is preferably given in midmorning or midafternoon depending on eating habits of patient.
Chlorphentermine hydrochloride (Chlorophen, Pre-Sate, Teramine)	**PO:** 65 mg daily after first meal of the day.	*Administration* After breakfast.
Clortermine hydrochloride (Voranil)	**PO:** 50 mg daily at midmorning	*Administration* After breakfast.
Dextroamphetamine hydrochloride (Daro) Dextroamphetamine sulfate (Dexampex, Dexedrine, Diphylets, Ferndex) Dextroamphetamine tannate (Obotan)	Individualized, *anorexia,* **PO:** 5–10 mg 1 to 3 times daily one hr before meals or as single sustained release capsule. *Narcolepsy,* **PO, adult:** 5–60 mg daily. **Pediatric:** 5–10 mg daily. Give as 1 to 3 divided doses or as a single sustained release capsule. *Hyperkinesis,* **PO, 3–5 years:** 2.5 mg	Has stronger central action and weaker peripheral action than amphetamine and thus fewer undesirable cardiovascular effects *Administration* IM preferred to IV. When given IV, inject slowly. Switch to PO when feasible.

400

daily; **6 years or older:** 5 mg 1 or 2 times daily. Increase dose until optimal response obtained.

Administration

Give timed-release in midmorning.

Diethylpropion hydrochloride (Maruate, Ro-Diet, Tenuate, Tepanil)

PO: 25 mg t.i.d. 1 hr before meals or as a single, 75 mg extent-release tablet at mid-morning.

Fenfluramine Hydrochloride (Pondimin)

PO: 20 mg t.i.d. before meals. May be increased weekly to a maximum of 40 mg t.i.d.

This drug produces more CNS depression and less stimulation than standard amphetamine. If initial dose is not well tolerated, reduce to 40 mg daily, and increase very gradually.

Mazindol (Sanorex)

PO: 1 mg t.i.d. or 2 mg daily.

Take multiple doses 1 hour before meals, single dose 1 hour before lunch. In event of GI distress, take with meals.

Methamphetamine hydrochloride (Desoxyn, Desoxyephedrine, Methampex, Obedrin-LA)

Anorexia; **PO, adult:** 2.5–5 mg t.i.d. 30–60 minutes before meals or time release capsule 1 time daily *Hyperkinesis:* **pediatric over 5 years of age:** 2.5–5 mg initially. May be increased to 20–25 mg daily in divided doses.

When used to facilitate verbalization during psychotherapeutic interview, only give second dose if the first has proven effective

---

Phendimetrazine tartrate (Plegine, many others)

PO: 35 mg 2 to 3 times daily 1 hr before meals or one sustained release capsule in a.m. **Maximum:** 210 mg daily.

Phenmetrazine hydrochloride (Preludin Hydrochloride)

PO: *individualized:* 25 mg 2 to 3 times daily 1 hr before meals or as a single sustained release tablet (50–75 mg).

Phentermine hydrochloride (Adipex, Ambesa-LA, Anoxine-AM, Fastin, Obesamead, Panshape-M TP, Parmine, Phentercot TD, Phentrol, Rolaphent, Tora, Wilpowr Phentermine resin (Ionamin)

PO: HCl: 8 mg t.i.d. ½ hr before meals. Administer before breakfast. **Resin:** 15–30 mg given before breakfast.

Remarks Caffeine is an alkaloid that is a cerebral, respiratory, and cardiac stimulant and also acts as a diuretic.

Uses Although caffeine has been used to overcome "hangover" effects occuring during arousal from drug-induced coma such as that from intoxication with morphine, barbiturates, alcohol, and other CNS depressants, the use of caffeine for this purpose is neither advisable nor logical.

It is also rarely used for the treatment of Cheyne-Stokes respiration, paroxysmal nocturnal dyspnea, and other respiratory failures. In combination with ergotamine for treatment of migraine.

Drug Interactions

Interactant	Interaction
MAO inhibitors	Excessive caffeine may cause hypertensive crisis. Reduce intake of caffeine containing medication
Propoxyphene (Darvon)	Caffeine given to patients taking large doses of propoxyphene may cause convulsions
Xanthines (Caffeine)	↓ Effect of anticoagulants by ↑ plasma prothrombin and factor V

Laboratory Test Interferences ↑ Urinary catecholamines.

Dosage *Caffeine sodium benzoate:* **IM, IV, or SC.** *Usual route* **IM:** 0.5– 1 gm. *Caffeine citrate:* **PO,** 60– 120 mg.

Nursing Implications

1. Observe for high caffeine intake manifested by insomnia, irritability, tremors, cardiac irregularities, and gastritis.
2. Observe for psychological dependence on caffeine manifested by irritability and headache when drug is withheld.
3. Do not administer caffeine orally to patients sensitive to gastritis or having an ulcer because caffeine stimulates the flow of hydrochloric acid.
4. Administer an infusion of coffee as a retention enema in the treatment of acute alcholic intoxication if IM medication is not available.

Analeptics

General Statement Analeptic drugs act directly on the medulla located in the brain stem. At therapeutic doses, these agents are supposed to stimulate respiration. At higher doses, the analeptics stimulate the hindbrain and spinal cord. The drugs do not stimulate the myocardium. The analeptic agents are no longer considered a drug of choice in the treatment of central nervous system depression caused by an overdosage of sedatives and hypnotics. Current therapy for overdose of sedative-hypnotics relies largely on supportive therapy, such as establishing a patent airway, administering oxygen, assisting or controlling respiration when necessary and maintaining blood pressure and blood volume. Also, see *Agents for Minimal Brain Damage.*

Uses Adjunct in the treatment of preanesthetic and drug-induced respiratory depression.

Contraindications Respiratory arrest caused by overdosage of anesthetic, drowning, electrocution, anorexia, carbon dioxide accumulation, carbon monoxide poisoning, neuromuscular blockage, increased intracranial pressure or shock, to shorten the postanesthetic recovery period. Patients with a tendency towards convulsive states. The drugs are ineffective in the treatment of chronic lung disease, or cardiac arrest caused by an overdosage of CNS stimulation.

Untoward Reactions See individual agents. For all these agents, the difference between a therapeutic dose and a toxic (convulsive) dose is very narrow.

DOXAPRAM HYDROCHLORIDE DOPRAM

Classification CNS stimulant, analeptic, miscellaneous.

General Statement Stimulates entire CNS. Increases depth and rate of respiration by acting on medullary respiratory centers. Effect manifested 20 to 40 seconds after administration and lasts for 2 to 15 minutes. Also increases salivation, release of gastric acid, and epinephrine.

Uses Adjunct in treatment of postanesthetic respiratory depression induced by narcotic analgesics or anesthetics. However, artificial respiration is more effective and use of this drug for this purpose is neither advisable nor logical.

Contraindications Epilepsy, convulsive states, respiratory incompetence due to muscle paresis, pneumothorax, airway obstruction and extreme dyspnea, severe hypertension, and cerebrovascular accidents. Hypersensitivity. Use with caution in patients with cerebral edema, asthma, severe cardiovascular disease, hyperthyroidism and pheochromocytoma (cancer of adrenals), peptic ulcer, or gastric surgery.

Untoward Reactions Numerous, including: generalized CNS stimulation if dose is too high, respiratory disturbances, GI disturbances, urinary retention, spontaneous micturition, various cardiac disturbances, elevation of blood pressure, various central and autonomic nervous system effects, including dizziness, headache, convulsions, and confusion. Increased deep tendon reflexes, muscle twitching and spasticity, pupillary dilation, and other abnormal neurological reflexes have also been observed.

Overdosage
Characterized by respiratory alkalosis and by hypocapnia (too little CO_2 in blood) with tetany and apnea. Also excessive stimulation of CNS, which may result in convulsions.

Drug Interactions   MAO inhibitors increase the adverse cardiovascular effects of doxapram (arrhythmias, increase in blood pressure).

Laboratory Test Interference   False + protein, BUN

Dosage   **IV:** Amount is determined by the type of anesthetic used during surgery. Strive for minimum effective dosage. **Usual:** 0.5–1 mg/kg. **Maximum single dose:** 1.5 mg/kg. **Maximum total dose:** 2 mg/kg. Use lower dosage for patients who have or might develop hypertension.

Administration   Allow minimum of 10 minutes between the discontinuation of anesthetic administration and administration of doxapram. Doxapram can also be administered by IV drip (dextrose, isotonic saline) at an initial rate of 5 mg of doxapram/minute.

Nursing Implications

1. Monitor BP, heart rate, and deep tendon reflexes after administration of doxapram to prevent overdosage and to provide a guide for adjustment of rate of infusion.
2. After administration, observe the patient for at least ½ to 1 hour after he/she is alert, for possible poststimulation respiratory depression.
3. Administer oxygen along with the drug to patients suffering from chronic pulmonary insufficiency.
4. Have on hand short-acting barbiturates, oxygen, and resuscitative equipment to manage overdosage.
5. Use seizure precautions after administration of drug.

NIKETHAMIDE CORAMINE

Remarks   Currently this drug is not widely used. Acts directly on medulla as well as indirectly stimulating chemoreceptors in the periphery.

Uses   Respiratory depression, CNS depression, circulatory failure.

Dosage   **IV:** *narcotic depressant overdose, carbon monoxide poisoning,* 5–10 ml followed by 5 ml q 5 minutes for first hour, **then** 5 ml q 30 to 60 minutes if necessary. *Acute alcoholism:* 5–20 ml to overcome CNS depression. *Cardiac decompensation/coronary occlusion:* 5–10 ml **IM or IV.** *Electroshock therapy:* 5 ml with 5 ml sterile water in antecubital vein. Apply electrical stimulus when face of patient is flushed and respiratory rate increases noticeably. **PO, maintenance:** 3–5 ml oral solution q 4 to 6 hours.

Administration   Do not administer intra-arterially, because arterial spasm and thrombosis may result.

Nursing Implication   Have barbiturates on hand to treat overdosage.

PENTYLENETETRAZOL NIORIC, METRAZOL

Remarks   High doses may cause clonic convulsions.

Uses   Respiratory stimulant (parenteral); to increase mental and physical activity of geriatric patients (orally).

Laboratory Test Interference   False + pregnancy tests (Pregslide method).

Dosage   **IV:** up to 500 mg; **IM:** 100–200 mg. **PO: initial,** 200 mg t.i.d. **Maintenance:** 100 mg t.i.d.–q.i.d.

Administration   Administer IV dose rapidly. Repeat until patient is awake, then switch to IM.

Nursing Implications   Monitor pulse for arrhythmia and bradycardia and monitor B.P. for hypotension in cardiac patients receiving pentylenetetrazol.

AGENTS FOR MINIMAL BRAIN DYSFUNCTION

General Statement   Several mild CNS stimulants are currently used for the treatment of children suffering from hyperkinesia and other behavior problems, stemming from neurological and not psychological causes (minimal brain dysfunction). They are also used to treat senility in geriatric patients.

Before drug therapy of this ill-defined condition is undertaken in children, the child must undergo extensive evaluation including medical and psychological tests.

The mode of action of the agents used for the treatment of MBD is not fully understood. It is possible that the agents increase the concentration of choline, acetylcholine, and dopamine in the brain.

Some of the agents included in this group are used as a mild stimulant for geriatric patients.

DEANOL ACETAMIDOBENZOATE DEANER

Classification   CNS stimulant, used for MBD.

Remarks   Mild cerebral stimulant. Drug is thought to be converted in the brain to acetylcholine.

Uses   Behavioral problems, learning difficulties, and asocial behavior in children, including hyperkinesis and shortened attention span. Chronic fatigue, neurasthenia, and mild neurotic depression. Investigationally: Blepharospasm, dyskinesia associated with Huntington's chorea.

Contraindications   Use with caution in cases of grand mal and mixed epilepsy.

Untoward Reactions	Mild overstimulation, dull occipital headache, constipation, muscle tenseness, insomnia, pruritus, and transient rash. Rarely, postural hypotension. Most side effects disappear with usage.
Dosage	**PO: initial:** 500 mg daily; **maintenance:** 250–500 mg daily.
Administration	As single dose in morning.
Nursing Implications	Reassure the patient and family that side effects usually disappear with continued treatment or reduction in dosage.

METHYLPHENIDATE HYDROCHLORIDE RITALIN HYDROCHLORIDE

Classification	CNS stimulant, used for MBD.
Remarks	This piperidine derivative is a mild CNS stimulant. Its activity is intermediate between the amphetamines and caffeine.
Uses	To overcome depression and the depressive effects of chlorpromazine, meprobamate, reserpine, and other tranquilizing or anticonvulsant drugs although such use is neither advisable nor logical. Narcolepsy. To hasten recovery from anesthesia. A drug of choice in the management of hyperkinetic and perceptually handicapped children.
Contraindications	Marked anxiety, tension and agitation, glaucoma. Use with great caution in patients with history of hypertension or convulsive disease.
Untoward Reactions	Nervousness, insomnia, anorexia, nausea, headaches, palpitation, dizziness, and drowsiness. Symptoms usually disappear when dosage is decreased. Also tachycardia, abdominal pain, and weight loss, especially in children. Drug may cause psychological dependence.

Overdosage
Characterized by cardiovascular symptoms (hypertension, cardiac arrhythmias, tachycardia), mental disturbances, agitation, headaches, vomiting, hyperreflexia, hyperpyrexia, convulsions, and coma.

Drug Interactions	*Interactant*	*Interaction*
	Anticoagulants, oral	↑ Effect of anticoagulants due to ↓ breakdown by liver
	Antidepressants, tricyclic	Methylphenidate ↑ effect due to ↓ breakdown by liver
	Guanethidine (Ismelin)	↓ Effect of guanethidine by displacement from its site of action

	MAO inhibitors
	  Pargyline (Eutonyl)
	  Tranylcypromine (Parnate)
		Possibility of hypertensive crisis, hyperthermia, convulsions, coma

Drug	*Interactant*	*Interaction*
Interactions		
(Continued)	Phenytoin (Dilantin)	↑ Effect of phenytoin due to ↓ breakdown by liver
	Tricyclic Antidepressants	↑ Effect of antidepressant drug due to ↓ breakdown by liver

Dosage **PO,** individualized, **adults:** 20–60 mg/day in divided doses. *Hyperkinesis* 6 years and older: **initial,** 5 mg b.i.d.; **then** increase 5–10 mg/week to a maximum of 60 mg daily.

Administration Before 6 PM to avoid interference with sleep.

Nursing Implications
1. Monitor BP and pulse b.i.d. as changes may occur.
2. Weigh 2 times/week since patients tend to lose weight on drug.
3. Provide cooling procedures in event of hyperpyrexia associated with drug overdosage.
4. Be prepared to provide supportive measures for maintenance of adequate circulation and respiratory exchange in case of overdosage. Protect patient against self-injury and reduce possible external stimuli.

PEMOLINE CYLERT

Classification CNS stimulant used for MBD.

General Statement The actions of pemoline resemble those of the amphetamines.

Uses MBD. Investigational: fatigue, mental depression, chronic schizophrenia, mild stimulation of geriatric patients.

Contraindications Hypersensitivity to drug. Children under 6 years of age.

Untoward Reactions Insomnia, transient weight loss, gastric upset, skin rash, irritability, mild depression, nausea, dizziness, headache, drowsiness, and hallucinations, elevated SGOT and SGPT values.

Dosage **PO: initial,** 37.5 mg/day; increase at 1-week intervals by 18.75 mg until desired response is attained up to maximum of 112.5 mg/day. **Usual maintenance:** 56.25–75 mg daily.

Administration
1. Administer as a single dose each AM.
2. Interrupt treatment 1 or 2 times annually to determine whether behavioral symptoms still necessitate therapy.

Nursing Implications **Advise Parents to**
1. Measure height of child every month and weight 2 times/week. Record all measurements on a chart because drug may interfere with growth pattern. Instruct parents to bring chart to medical supervision.

2. Report weight loss or failure to grow to medical supervision.
3. Anticipate resumption of weight gain within 3 to 6 months.
4. Administer drug early in AM to minimize insomnia caused by drug.
5. Continue with therapy because behavior changes take 3 to 4 weeks to occur.
6. Interrupt drug administration, as recommended by medical supervision; then observe behavior to help doctor decide whether therapy should be resumed.
7. Periodically bring child for liver function tests in order to detect adverse reactions that would necessitate withdrawal of drug.
8. Note signs of overdosage, such as agitation, restlessness, hallucinations, and tachycardia. Should these symptoms occur, instruct parents to withhold drug, give supportive care, and report to medical supervision.

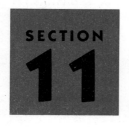

SECTION
11

nonnarcotic analgesics and antipyretics

Salicylates	Acetylsalicylic Acid	Salicylamide
	Calcium Carbaspirin	Salsalate
	Choline Salicylate	Sodium Salicylate
	Magnesium Salicylate	Sodium Thiosalicylate
Para-Aminophenol Derivatives	Acetaminophen	
	Phenacetin (Acetophenetidin)	
Miscellaneous Agents	Ethoheptazine Citrate	Propoxyphene Hydrochloride
	Mefenamic Acid	Propoxyphene Napsylate
	Methotrimeprazine	

General Statement

The nonnarcotic drugs for the relief of pain and fever are consumed in enormous amounts, especially since many can be obtained on a nonprescription basis. This, however, does not mean that their administration should be taken lightly. It is well to remember that aspirin is the agent most commonly responsible for the accidental poisoning of small children.

In addition to their analgesic and antipyretic effects, many of the drugs of this group have specific anti-inflammatory effects and are the drug of choice for rheumatic diseases. For these conditions the drugs are, however, prescribed at much higher dosage levels than for fever or simple analgesia.

The nonnarcotic analgesics fall into four groups according to their chemical structure: (1) the salicylates (e.g. aspirin), (2) the pyrazolone derivatives (e.g. phenylbutazone), (3) the para-aminophenol derivatives (e.g. acetaminophen), and (4) a few others that do not fit into any general classification.

The mechanisms of action of these agents are still poorly understood. Their anti-inflammatory and antipyretic effects may be related to a newly discovered group of physiological agents, the prostaglandins.

SALICYLATES

Classification Analgesics with antipyretic and anti-inflammatory action.

General Statement Salicylates have both a selective depressant effect on the CNS and depressant effect on peripheral pain receptors, which is responsible for their analgesic and antipyretic activity. At higher doses they have also an anti-inflammatory effect. The compounds also increase the excretion of uric acid in the urine (uricosuric effect). The drugs are readily absorbed from the GI tract. (See Table 17, p. 410.)

Uses Pain arising from integumental structures, myalgias, neuralgias, arthralgias, headache, dysmenorrhea, and similar types of pain. As antipyretics and antiinflammatories in conditions such as arthritis, systemic lupus erythematosus, acute rheumatic fever, and many other conditions. Gout. May be effective in less severe postoperative and postpartum pain; pain secondary to trauma and cancer. *Topical:* salicylic acid is used for its keratolytic activity. Methylsalicylate (oil of wintergreen) is used as a counterirritant.

Contraindications Hypersensitivity to salicylates. Patients with asthma, hay fever, or nasal polyps have a higher incidence of hypersensitivity reactions. Salicylates are to be used with caution in the presence of peptic ulcers, in conjunction with anticoagulant therapy, and in patients with cardiac disease. Salicylates can cause congestive failure in the large doses used for rheumatic diseases. Vitamin K deficiency and after surgery.

Untoward Reactions The toxic effects of the salicylates are dose related. *Low grade toxicity — called salicylism* —is characterized by skin reactions (redness, rashes and hives), edema, which may be laryngeal, GI reactions, headache, dizziness, ringing in the ears (most common symptom), visual and auditory disturbances, drowsiness, hyperventilation, sweating and thirst. Most patients exhibit symptoms of salicylism at plasma salicylate levels of 35 mg/100 ml.

Severe salicylate poisoning is characterized by skin eruptions, a disturbance of the acid-base and electrolyte balance, stimulation of the CNS followed by depression, incoherent speech, stupor, generalized convulsions, coma, respiratory insufficiency, and finally respiratory

TABLE 17 SALICYLATES

Drug	Uses	Dosage	Remarks
Acetylsalicylic acid (Aspergum, Aspirin, A.S.A., Decaprin, Ecotrin, others)	Analgesic, anti-inflammatory, antipyretic, rheumatic fever	*Analgesic, antipyretic,* **PO:** 5–10 gr q 3–4 hr; **pediatric:** check with physician. *Anti-inflammatory,* **PO:** 40–80 gr daily in divided doses. *Rheumatic fever;* up to 120 gr/day in divided doses.	
Calcium carbaspirin (Calurin)	Analgesic, antipyretic	**PO:** 300–600 mg q 4 hr; **pediatric 6–12 years:** 300 mg q 4 hr; **3–6 years:** 150 mg q 4 hr.	
Choline salicylate (Arthropan)	Analgesic, antipyretic, anti-inflammatory	*Analgesic, antipyretic,* **PO:** 870 mg q 4 hr but no more than 6 times/day; **pediatric 3–6 years:** 105–210 mg q 4 hr; **6–12 years:** 210–420 mg q 4 hr. *Anti-inflammatory:* 870–1740 mg up to 4 times daily.	May be preferred to sodium salicylate when sodium restriction is necessary. Administer syrup in ½ glass water to reduce aftertaste. Do not give antacids at the same time as choline salicylate is administered. If antacids are required, give choline salicylate before meals and antacid 2 hours after meal
Magnesium salicylate (Analate, Causalin, Lorisal, Mobidin, MSG-600, Magan, Triact	Analgesic, antipyretic, anti-inflammatory	*Analgesic, antipyretic,* **PO:** 600 mg t.i.d.–q.i.d. up to 3.6–4.8 gms daily *Anti-inflammatory/rheumatic fever:* up to 9.6 gm daily.	A sodium-free salicylate derivative. Not recommended for children under 12 years of age
Salicylamide	Antipyretic, analgesic, anti-inflammatory	*Antipyretic analgesics,* **PO: adults:** 325–650 mg q.i.d. *Anti-inflammatory:* 1–2 gm q 4 hr for 3–6 days *Uricosuric:* 1.8 gm daily	Compound less effective than aspirin. Overdosage does not produce metabolic acidosis but CNS symptoms, respiratory depression and convulsions.

Drug	Uses	Dosage	Remarks
Salsalate (Disalcid)	Analgesic, antipyretic	**PO:** 1000 mg t.i.d.	Patients allergic to aspirin may be able to tolerate salicylamide. Administer after meals or with fluids to minimize gastric irritation
Sodium salicylate (Uracel)	Antipyretic, analgesic, acute rheumatic fever, gout	*Antipyretic, analgesic,* **PO and IV:** 325–650 mg q 4–6 hr. *Acute rheumatic fever:* 10–15 gm daily in divided doses q 4–5 hr.	Insoluble in stomach. Slowly releases two molecules of salicylic acid in small intestine. Take last dose at bedtime.
Sodium Thiosalicylate (Arthrolate, Nalate, TH Sal, Thiodyne, Thiolate, Thiosul)	Rheumatic fever, gout, analgesic for muscle pain	**IM;** *analgesic:* 50–100 mg/day or on alternate days. *Acute gout:* 100 mg q 3–4 hr for 2 days, **then** 100 mg/day. *Rheumatic fever:* 100–150 mg q 4–6 hrs for 3 days, **then** 100 mg b.i.d. until no symptoms are present.	Do not give to patients on low sodium diet. One gram of menadione (vitamin K) should be given per gram of sodium salicylate during long-term therapy. Some physicians order concurrent administration of ½ gm sodium bicarbonate/gm sodium salicylate. This will reduce rate of elimination of drug. Do not infuse rapidly. Check frequently to avoid extravasation, as sloughing may occur

failure. Mental disturbances may simulate alcohol inebriation. Hemorrhages are also observed because salicylates increase prothrombin time.

Emergency treatment of salicylates (see *Nursing Implications* below).

Drug Interactions	*Interactant*	*Interaction*
	Alcohol, ethyl	↑ Chance of GI bleeding caused by salicylates
	Aminosalicylic acid (PAS)	Possible ↑ effect of PAS due to ↓ excretion by kidney or ↓ plasma protein binding
	Ammonium chloride	↑ Effect of salicylates by ↑ renal tubular reabsorption
	Anticoagulants, oral	↑ Effect of anticoagulant by ↓ plasma protein binding and plasma prothrombin
	Antidiabetic agents	↑ Effect of antidiabetics by ↓ plasma protein binding
	Ascorbic acid	↑ Effect of salicylates by ↑ renal tubular reabsorption
	Corticosteroids	Both are ulcerogenic. Also, corticosteroids may ↓ blood salicylate levels
	Heparin	Inhibition of platelet adhesiveness by aspirin may result in bleeding tendencies
	Indomethacin (Indocin)	Both are ulcerogenic and may cause ↑ GI bleeding
	Methotrexate	↑ Effect of methotrexate by ↓ plasma protein binding. Also, salicylates block renal excretion of methotrexate
	Phenylbutazone (Butazolidin)	Phenylbutazone inhibits uricosuric activity of salicylates
	Phenytoin (Dilantin)	↑ Effect of phenytoin by ↓ plasma protein binding
	Probenecid	Salicylates inhibit uricosuric activity of probenecid
	Pyrazinamide	Salicylates inhibit hyperuricemia produced by pyrazinamide
	Sulfinpyrazone (Anturane)	Salicylates inhibit uricosuric activity of sulfinpyrazone
	Sulfonamides	↑ Effect of sulfonamides by ↑ blood levels of salicylates

Laboratory Test Interference   False + or ↑: Amylase, SGOT, SGPT, uric acid, catecholamines, urinary glucose (Benedict's Clinitest), and urinary uric acid (at high doses) values. False − or ↓ CO_2 content, glucose (fasting), potassium and thrombocyte values.

Administration
1. Administer with meals or with milk or crackers to reduce gastric irritation.
2. If ordered by the doctor, sodium bicarbonate may be given concurrently to lessen irritation.
3. Enteric coated tablets or buffered tablets are better tolerated by some patients.

Nursing Implications

1. Check whether the patient has a history of hypersensitivity to salicylates before administration. Patients who have tolerated salicylates well for a long period of time may suddenly have an allergic or anaphylactoid reaction. Have on hand epinephrine for emergency treatment. Asthma caused by hypersensitive reaction to salicylates may be refractory to epinephrine so that antihistamines should also be available for parenteral and oral use.

2. Only administer salicylates to hospitalized patients at the express order of a physician and at the time scheduled. Advise patients against the indiscriminate use of aspirin at home.

3. Advise patients that sodium bicarbonate should only be taken with the knowledge of the physician as it may decrease serum level of aspirin sooner and thus reduce its effectiveness.

4. Administer salicylates for antipyretic effect only at the TPR ordered by the physician. After administering aspirin for antipyretic effect, monitor the patient's temperature at least once an hour and check the patient for marked diaphoresis. Use supportive nursing care measures, such as drying patient, changing linen, giving fluids, and preventing chilling after marked diaphoresis.

5. Teach patients about the therapeutic and toxic effects of the drug (noted in general statement).

6. Observe patients on anticoagulant therapy for bruises, bleeding of the mucous membranes, or bleeding from any orifice, because large doses of drugs may increase the prothrombin time.

7. Observe and teach diabetic patients that symptoms of hypoglycemia may occur because salicylates potentiate antidiabetic drugs.

8. Observe cardiac patients on large doses for symptoms of congestive failure.

Salicylate Toxicity

1. After repeated administration of large doses of salicylate, observe patients for symptoms of salicylism characterized by hyperventilation, auditory and visual disturbances and report promptly to physician.

2. Anticipate that severe salicylate poisoning, whether due to overdose or cumulation, will also have an exaggerated effect on the CNS and metabolic system. The patient sometimes develops a "salicylate jag" characterized by garrulous behavior as though inebriated. Convulsions and coma may follow.

3. Be aware that even topically applied salicylates, such as salicylic acid and methylsalicylate, are rapidly absorbed from intact skin, especially when applied in lanolin, and thereby can cause systemic poisoning.

4. Salicylate toxicity may occur in children when dosage exceeds 60 mg, for each year of age until a child is 5 years old, given five times a day.

5. Emergency supplies for treatment of acute salicylate toxicity should include:
   a. Apomorphine.
   b. Emetics, and equipment for gastric lavage (lavage for toxicity due

to methylsalicylate should continue until all odor of the drug is gone from the washings).

c. IV equipment and solution of dextrose, saline, potassium, and sodium bicarbonate; vitamin K.

d. Oxygen and respirator.

e. Short-acting barbiturates (for convulsions) such as pentobarbital or secobarbital.

6. Teach parents and those caring for children that:

a. Salicylates must be kept out of children's reach (4 ml of oil of wintergreen may be fatal for a child, 30 ml for an adult).

b. Aspirin should not be given routinely to children without consultation with a physician.

c. Children with fever and dehydration are particularly prone to intoxication from relatively small amounts of aspirin.

d. If a child refuses to take aspirin or vomits the medication, check with the doctor as to whether aspirin suppositories or acetaminophen may be used.

e. Report gastric irritation and pain to the doctor.

f. Caution parents to be alert for symptoms of hypersensitivity or toxicity.

PARA-AMINOPHENOL DERIVATIVES

General Statement The para-aminophenol derivatives (acetaminophen and phenacetin) resemble the salicylates in their antipyretic and analgesic activity but are devoid of anti-inflammatory and uricosuric effects. They do not cause GI irritation. They are readily absorbed from the GI tract. They are used much less frequently than the salicylates. The agents do not antagonize the uricosuric effects of drugs used for the treatment of gout.

Uses Control of fever and pain including headache, dysmenorrhea, arthralgia, myalgia, and so forth. Particularly suitable for patients who are allergic to salicylates.

Contraindications Renal insufficiency, anemia. Patients with cardiac or pulmonary disease are more susceptible to toxic effects of para-aminophenol derivatives.

Untoward Reactions Few when taken in small doses. Chronic and even acute toxicity can develop after long symptom-free usage. Symptoms include: methemoglobinemia (phenacetin only), hemolytic anemia (especially in patients with glucose-6-phosphate dehydrogenase deficiency), nephritis, mental confusion, dyspnea, vertigo, weakness and collapse, abnormal skin reactions, clammy sweat, and subnormal temperatures. Severe poisoning is characterized by CNS stimulation, excitement, and delirium. Massive doses affect the heart and blood vessels. Year-long usage may lead to psychological but not physical dependence.

Drug Interactions   Acetaminophen: When used concomitantly with anticoagulants, dosage of latter must be reduced to avoid possibility of hemorrhages.

Nursing Implications

1. Observe for symptoms of methemoglobinemia, such as bluish color of mucosa, and fingernails, dyspnea, vertigo, weakness, and headaches caused by anoxia.
2. Observe for signs of hemolytic anemia, such as pallor, weakness, and heart palpitations.
3. Observe for signs of nephritis such as hematuria and albuminuria.
4. Be on the alert for collapse with confusion, dyspnea, rapid weak pulse, cold extremities, clammy sweat, and subnormal temperatures all signs of chronic poisoning.
5. Observe for toxicity characterized by excessive CNS stimulation, excitement, and delirium.
6. Be alert for psychic disturbances that may accompany withdrawal of the drug.
7. Inform the patient that phenacetin may color urine dark brown or wine.
8. Inform patient that the long-term ingestion of headache remedies containing phenacetin or acetaminophen can result in toxic reactions.
9. Teach patients that so-called "headache and minor pain relievers" containing combinations of salicylates, para-amino derivatives, and caffeine may be no more beneficial than aspirin alone and that such combinations may be more dangerous.

ACETAMINOPHEN A'CENOL, ACEPHEN, ACETA, ACTAMIN, AMINODYNE, ANUPHEN, APAP, CAPITAL, DAPA, DATRIL, DOLANEX, DULARIN, FEBRIGESIC, FEBRINOL, G-1, LIQUIPRIN, NEOPAP, NILPRIN, PANEX, PANOFEN, PANPYRO, PARTEN, PEDRIC, PHENAPHEN, PIRIN, PROVAL, RELENOL, SK-APAP, ST. JOSEPH FEVER REDUCER, SUDOPRIN, TAPAR, TEMPRA, TENOL, TYLAPRIN, TYLENOL, VALADOL, VALDRIN

Dosage   **PO:** 325–650 mg q 4 hour. **Maximum daily dose:** 2.6 gm. **Pediatric, under 1 year:** 60 mg q 4–6 hours; **1–6 years:** 60–120 mg q 4–6 hours not to exceed 480 mg/day; **6–12 years:** 150–300 mg q 4 hours not to exceed 1.2 gm daily.

PHENACETIN (ACETOPHENETIDIN)

Dosage   Administer 300–600 mg q 3 hours. **Maximum daily dose:** 2.4 gm. For short periods of time, individual dose may be increased to 600 mg. During long-term therapy, one 300 mg dose should be omitted daily to prevent cumulative effect of drug. Used in combination with other drugs.

MISCELLANEOUS AGENTS

ETHOHEPTAZINE CITRATE ZACTANE

Classification Analgesic, nonnarcotic.

General Statement Drug is usually administered in combination with aspirin, or with aspirin, phenacetin, and caffeine. The drug does not seem to be habit-forming.

There are few side effects at ordinary doses. At higher doses the side effects of the other drug components must be taken into consideration. Use the combination with phenacetin cautiously in patients with renal insufficiency.

Uses Analgesia of mild-to-moderate pain. In combination with aspirin for arthritis.

Untoward Reactions GI irritation, drowsiness.

Dosage **PO:** 75–150 mg alone or in combination with aspirin or aspirin/phenacetin/caffeine t.i.d.–q.i.d.

Administration Administer with food or milk to minimize GI upset.

Nursing Implications Advise patient to use caution when driving a car or performing other tasks requiring mental alertness, because ethoheptazine citrate may cause drowsiness.

MEFENAMIC ACID PONSTEL

Classification Mild analgesic, antipyretic.

Remarks This drug is not superior to other mild analgesics and there is no rational indication for its use.

Use Short-term relief of mild to moderate pain such as that associated with toothache, tooth extraction, and musculoskeletal disorders.

Contraindications Ulceration or chronic inflammation of the GI tract, pregnancy or possibility thereof, children under 14, and hypersensitivity to drug.

To be used with caution in patients with impaired renal or hepatic function, asthma, or patients on anticoagulant therapy.

Untoward Reactions Neurological and GI effects, including headache, drowsiness, dizziness, GI cramps, diarrhea, GI hemorrhage, and blood dyscrasias.

Drug Interactions	Interactant	Interaction
	Anticoagulants	↑ Hypoprothrombinemia due to ↓ plasma protein binding
	Insulin	↑ Insulin requirement

Dosage PO: **initial,** 500 mg, followed by 250 mg q 6 hr. Length of therapy should not exceed 1 week.

Administration With food.

Nursing Implications
1. Withhold drug and report rash or diarrhea.
2. Observe the patient for any signs of bleeding, as drug lowers the prothrombin time.
3. Advise patient to use caution when operating potentially hazardous machinery as in driving because drug may cause dizziness, light-headedness or confusion.

METHOTRIMEPRAZINE LEVOPROME

Classification Analgesic, miscellaneous.

General Statement Methotrimeprazine is chemically related to the phenothiazines; the analgesic potency is approximately one-half that of morphine. It is not considered to be a narcotic since it does not produce psychological or physical dependence and will not suppress withdrawal symptoms from morphine. Maximal analgesic effect occurs in 20 to 40 minutes after IM administration and lasts for approximately 4 hours.

Uses Analgesic in nonambulatory patients. Obstetrical analgesia where respiratory depression is to be avoided. As preanesthetic for producing sedation and relief of anxiety and tension.

Contraindications This drug should be used with caution in geriatric patients or in individuals with heart disease. It should not be administered to patients in premature labor or with an antihypertensive agent as well as in severe myocardial, renal, or hepatic disease.

Untoward Reactions Orthostatic hypotension and sedation. Also dizziness, asthenia, slurred speech, blurred vision, nasal congestion, dry mouth, dysuria, chills, pain at site of injection. CNS symptoms include delirium and extrapyramidal symptoms.

Drug Interactions	Interactant	Interaction
	Alcohol, ethyl	Potentiation or addition of CNS depressant effects. Concomitant use may lead to drowsiness, lethargy, stupor, respiratory depression, coma, and possibly death

Drug Interactions (Continued)

Interactant	Interaction
Anticholinergic agents	Possibility of extrapyramidal symptoms with concomitant use
Antihypertensives	Additive hypotensive effect
CNS depressants	See *Alcohol, ethyl*
Antianxiety agents, barbiturates, narcotics, phenothiazines, sedative-hypnotics	
Guanethidine (Ismelin)	Additive hypotensive effect
Methyldopa	Additive hypotensive effect
Phenothiazines	*See Alcohol, ethyl.* Also, additive extrapyramidal effects
Reserpine	Additive hypotensive effect
Skeletal muscle relaxants, surgical	↑ Muscle relaxation
Succinylcholine	
Tubocurarine	

Dosage   **IM:** 10–20 mg q 4 to 6 hr. **Elderly: initial,** 5–10 mg. **Pediatric:** 0.2–0.3 mg/kg. *Postoperative analgesia:* **initially,** 2.5–7.5 mg due to residual effects of anesthetic. The drug should not be administered IV or SC.

Nursing Implications

1. Ambulation should be avoided for at least 6 hours following the initial dose as orthostatic hypotension, fainting, and dizziness may occur. Tolerance to these effects occurs with repeated administration.
2. Administer by deep IM injection into a large muscle mass. Rotation of sites is advisable.
3. Do not administer SC as irritation may occur.

PROPOXYPHENE HYDROCHLORIDE DARVON, DOLENE, PARGESIC-65, PROGESIC-65, PROXAGESIC, SK-65

PROPOXYPHENE NAPSYLATE DARVON-N

Classification   Analgesic, nonnarcotic

General Statement   Propoxyphene is structurally related to methadone although it is not considered a narcotic analgesic. Unlike aspirin, propoxyphene does not possess anti-inflammatory or antipyretic activity. As an analgesic, propoxyphene is approximately one-half to two-thirds as potent as codeine. Propoxyphene is often prescribed in combination with salicylates. In such instances, the information on salicylates should also be consulted. Because of the abuse potential of propoxyphene the drug has been placed under the provisions of the Controlled Substances Act.

Uses To relieve mild to moderate pain. Propoxyphene napsylate has been used experimentally to suppress the withdrawal syndrome from narcotics.

Contraindications Hypersensitivity to drug.

Untoward Reactions Nausea, vomiting, sedation, and dizziness are the most common reactions, especially in ambulatory patients. Other untoward reactions include constipation, abdominal pain, skin rashes, lightheadedness, headache, weakness, euphoria, dysphoria, and visual disturbances.

Propoxyphene can produce psychological dependence as well as physical dependence and tolerance.

Symptoms of overdosage are similar to those of narcotics and include respiratory depression, coma, pupillary constriction, and circulatory collapse. Treatment of overdosage consists of maintaining an adequate airway, artificial respiration, and the use of a narcotic antagonist (naloxone, levallorphan) to combat respiratory depression. Gastric lavage or the administration of activated charcoal may be helpful.

Drug Interactions

Interactant	Interaction
Carbamazepine	↑ Effect of carbamazepine due to ↓ breakdown by liver
CNS depressants	Additive CNS depression
Alcohol	Concomitant use may lead to drowsiness,
Antianxiety agents	lethargy, stupor, respiratory, depression, and
Antipsychotic agents	coma
Narcotics	
Sedative-hypnotics	
Orphenadrine (Norflex)	Concomitant use may lead to confusion, anxiety, and tremors

Dosage *Hydrochloride:* **Usual,** 65 mg q 4 hr. **Not recommended for use in children.** *Napsylate:* 100 mg q 4 hrs.

Nursing Implications
1. Advise patients to use caution when operating potentially hazardous machinery or while driving because drug may cause dizziness and sedation.
2. Ambulatory patients should be advised to lie down if dizziness, nausea, or vomiting occur.
3. Observe patient for growing dependence and tolerance.
4. Observe patient for early signs of toxicity as manifested by depressed respiration or constricted pupils.

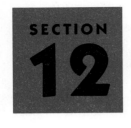

antirheumatic and anti-inflammatory agents

Non-Steroidal Anti-Inflammatories (Propionic acid derivatives and related compounds)	Fenoprofen Calcium Ibuprofen Indomethacin	Naproxen Sulindac Tolmetin Sodium
Pyrazolone Derivatives	Oxyphenbutazone Phenylbutazone	
Remitting Agents	Aurothioglucose Gold Sodium Thiomalate	Penicillamine

General Statement

Arthritis, which means inflammation of the joints, refers to about 80 different conditions also called rheumatic, collagen or connective tissue diseases. The most prominent symptoms of these conditions are painful, inflamed joints, but the cause for this joint inflammation varies from disease to disease. The joint pain of gout, for example, results from sodium urate crystals that are formed as a consequence of the overproduction or underelimination of uric acid. Osteoarthritis is caused by the degeneration of the joint; rheumatoid arthritis and systemic lupus erythematosus are autoimmune diseases. Immune factors trigger the release of corrosive enzymes in the joints in a complex manner. Infectious arthritis is the result of rapid joint destruction by microorganisms like gonococci that invade the joint cavity. Treatment must obviously be aimed at the cause of the particular form of arthritis, and a thorough diagnostic evaluation must, thus, precede the initiation of therapy. Gout is treated with urocosuric agents that alter uric acid metabolism (see next section); infectious arthritis responds to antibiotics (Chapter 1, Section 1); osteoarthritis is treated with analgesics and anti-inflammatories; rheumatoid arthritis, systemic lupus erythematosus (SLE), and ankylosing spondylitis respond to anti-inflammatories. Rheumatoid arthritis is also treated with two remitting agents: gold and penicillamine. Aspirin (Chapter 5, Section 11) is an important agent in the treatment of all rheumatic diseases. Corticosteroids are used, preferably for short-term therapy only, for some of the more recalcitrant cases of rheumatoid arthritis and SLE (Chapter 7, Section 7). Corticosteroids also are used for intraarticular injection. Antimalarials, especially hydroxychloroquine sulfate (Plaquenil Sulfate) are sometimes used for rheumatoid arthritis and SLE (Chapter 1, Section 7).

Drug therapy of the arthritides must be supplemented by a physical therapy program, as well as proper rest and diet. Total joint replacement therapy is also becoming an increasingly important mode of therapy to correct the ravages of arthritis.

NON-STEROIDAL ANTI-INFLAMMATORY AGENTS

General Statement Over the past decade, a growing number of non-steroidal anti-inflammatory agents have been developed. Chemically, these drugs are related to indene, indole, or propionic acid. As in the case of aspirin, the therapeutic actions of these agents are believed to result from the inhibition of prostaglandin synthesis. The agents are effective in reducing joint swelling, pain, and morning stiffness, as well as increasing mobility in arthritic patients. They do not alter the course of the disease, however. Their anti-inflammatory activity is comparable to aspirin. They also have analgesic activity; most have some antipyretic action.

The non-steroidal anti-inflammatory agents have an irritating effect on the GI tract. They differ from one another slightly with respect to their rate of absorption, length of action, anti-inflammatory activity and effect on the gastrointestinal mucosa. Some of the agents can be administered concurrently with aspirin. At present, all agents are approved for the treatment of rheumatoid arthritis. Some are also approved for osteoarthritis and ankylosing spondylitis, gout, and other musculoskeletal diseases. Some of the non-steroidal anti-inflammatory agents have been used for dysmenorrhea on an investigational basis.

Contraindications Most for children under 14 years of age. Hypersensitivity to any of these agents or to aspirin. Acute asthma, rhinitis, or urticaria. Use with caution in patients with a history of gastrointestinal disease, reduced renal function.

Untoward Reactions GI (most common): peptic ulceration and GI bleeding, reactivation of preexisting ulcers. Heartburn, dyspepsia (4%–16%), nausea, vomiting, anorexia, diarrhea, constipation, indigestion, stomatitis. CNS: dizziness, drowsiness, vertigo, headaches. Skin: pruritus, skin eruptions, sweating, ecchymoses, rashes, urticaria, purpura. Other: tinnitus, blurred and other vision disturbances. Blood dyscrasias: anemia, alteration of platelet function, increased bleeding time. Cardiovascular: edema, palpitations, tachycardia.

Nursing Implications
1. Encourage patients to take anti-inflammatory agents with meals, with milk, or with an antacid prescribed by their doctor to minimize gastric irritation.
2. Urge drug compliance because regular intake of medications is necessary for anti-inflammatory effect.
3. Urge regular medical supervision for adjustment of dosage based on patient's age, condition, and changes in disease activity.

4. Advise patients to report to the doctor signs and symptoms of GI irritation or bleeding, blurred vision or other eye symptoms, tinnitus, skin rashes, purpura, weight gain, or edema.
5. Advise patient to use caution in operating machinery or operating a car because medication may cause dizziness or drowsiness.

FENOPROFEN CALCIUM NALFON

Classification Nonsteroidal anti-inflammatory agent.

Use Rheumatoid arthritis (acute flares and long-term management).

Drug Interactions

Interactant	Interaction
Phenytoin Sulfonamides Sulfonylureas Also, See Ibuprofen	↑ Effect due to ↓ plasma protein binding

Dosage **PO: initial,** 600 mg q.i.d. Adjust dose according to response of patient; **maximum daily dose: 3200 mg.**

Administration
1. Drug should be given 30 minutes before or 2 hours after meals because food decreases the rate and extent of absorption of fenoprofen.
2. Concomitant administration with antacids does not interfere with the absorption of fenoprofen.

IBUPROFEN MOTRIN

Classification Anti-inflammatory, nonsteroidal.

Drug Interactions

Interactant	Interaction
Anticoagulants (Coumarin)	Concomitant use results in ↑ prothrombin time
Aspirin	↓ Effect of ibuprofen due to ↑ breakdown by liver
Phenobarbital	↓ Effect of ibuprofen due to ↑ breakdown by liver
Phenytoin (Dilantin)	↑ Effect of phenytoin due to ↓ plasma protein binding
Sulfonamides	↑ Effect of sulfonamides due to ↓ plasma protein binding
Sulfonylureas (oral hypoglycemics)	↑ Effect of sulfonylureas due to ↓ plasma protein binding

Dosage *Individualized:* 300–400 mg t.i.d. or q.i.d. When response is established (2 weeks), adjust dosage upward or downwards to maximum of 2400 mg daily.

INDOMETHACIN INDOCIN

Classification Anti-inflammatory, analgesic, antipyretic.

Remarks The antipyretic effect of this drug is exerted through the hypothalamus; its analgesic effect is due to its anti-inflammatory activity.

Uses Acute and moderate rheumatoid arthritis, rheumatic spondylitis, psoriatic arthritis, osteoarthritis, and in some cases of gouty arthritis. As an antipyretic in Hodgkin's disease with refractory fever.

Additional Contraindications To be used with caution in patients with history of epilepsy, psychiatric illness, parkinsonism, and in the elderly. Indomethacin should be used with extreme caution in the presence of existing, controlled infections.

Additional Untoward Reactions Reactivation of latent infections. More marked CNS manifestations than for other drugs of this group.

Drug Interactions

Interactant	Interaction
Anticoagulants, oral	↑ Effect of anticoagulants by ↓ plasma protein binding. Also indomethacin is ulcerogenic and may inhibit platelet function leading to hemorrhage
Corticosteroids	Increased chance of GI ulceration
Furosemide (Lasix)	↓ Diuretic and antihypertensive effect of furosmide
Probenecid	↑ Effect of indomethacin by ↓ kidney excretion
Salicylates	Both are ulcerogenic and cause ↑ GI bleeding
Sulfonamides	↑ Effect of sulfonamides by ↑ blood levels

Dosage **PO: initial,** 25 mg b.i.d.–t.i.d.; may be increased by 25 mg at weekly intervals according to condition, until satisfactory response is obtained. **Maximum daily dosage:** 150–200 mg. *Gouty arthritis:* 50 mg t.i.d. for 3 to 5 days. Reduce dosage rapidly until drug is withdrawn.

Administration/ Storage Store in amber-colored containers.

Additional Nursing Implications
1. Make every effort by observation, teaching, and reporting to help the physician establish the smallest effective dose for the individual patient because adverse reactions are dose related.
2. Withhold drug and report untoward reaction to physician because any one reaction may necessitate withdrawal of the drug.

3. Observe the patient for concurrent infection or reactivation of old infection because infectious symptoms may have been masked by indomethacin.
4. Teach the patient that medical supervision is essential during therapy with indomethacin. Ophthalmologic examinations and total blood counts are usually indicated during long-term therapy.
5. Advise patient to use caution operating potentially hazardous equipment because of possible light-headedness and decreased alertness.

NAPROXEN NAPROSYN

Classification Nonsteroidal, anti-inflammatory agent.

Remarks Longer acting than other drugs of this group.

Uses Rheumatoid arthritis (acute flares and long-term management).

Drug Interactions

Interactant	Interaction
Anticoagulants (Coumarin)	Concomitant use results in ↑ prothrombin time
Aspirin	↓ Effect of naproxen due to ↑ breakdown by liver
Phenobarbital	↓ Effect of naproxen due to ↓ breakdown by liver
Phenytoin	↑ Effect of phenytoin (Dilantin) due to ↓ plasma protein binding
Sulfonamides	↑ Effect of sulfonamides due to ↓ plasma protein binding
Sulfonylureas (oral hypoglycemics)	↑ Effect of sulfonylureas due to ↓ plasma protein binding

Laboratory Test Interference Naproxen may increase urinary 17-ketosteroid values.

Dosage **PO: initial,** 250 mg b.i.d. Adjust dose according to response of patient. **Maximum recommended daily dose:** 750 mg.

Administration
1. A morning and evening dose is recommended.
2. Clinical improvement may not be observed for 2 weeks.

SULINDAC CLINORIL

Classification Antirheumatic agent.

Remarks Indene derivative, particularly effective in treatment of ankylosing spondylitis. Sulindac undergoes biotransformation to the sulfide metabolite which is thought to be the active compound.

Uses Osteoarthritis, rheumatoid arthritis, ankylosing spondylitis, acute painful shoulder, acute gouty arthritis.

Drug Interaction

Interactant	Interaction
Aspirin	↓ Plasma levels of sulfide metabolite
Probenecid	Slight ↓ in uricosuric action of probenecid.

Dosage *Osteoarthritis, rheumatoid arthritis, ankylosing spondylitis:* 150 mg b.i.d. up to 400 mg daily. *Acute painful shoulder, acute gouty arthritis:* 200 mg b.i.d. for 7 to 14 days.

Administration For acute conditions, reduce dosage when satisfactory response is attained.

Additional Nursing Implications
1. Monitor intake and output closely of patient with impaired renal function because the drug is excreted by the kidneys.
2. Anticipate reduction of dosage to prevent excessive drug accumulation, should intake and output indicate renal dysfunction.
3. Teach patients not to take aspirin while they are on sulindac, as plasma levels of sulindac would be reduced.

TOLMETIN SODIUM TOLECTIN

Classification Nonsteroidal, anti-inflammatory agent.

Use Rheumatoid arthritis.

Drug Interactions

Interactant	Interaction
Anticoagulants (Coumarin)	Concomitant use results in ↑ prothrombin time
Aspirin	↓ Effect of tolmetin due to ↑ breakdown by liver
Phenobarbital	↓ Effect of tolemetin due to ↑ breakdown by liver
Phenytoin (Dilantin)	↑ Effect of phenytoin due to ↓ plasma protein binding
Sulfonamides	↑ Effect of sulfonamides due to ↓ plasma protein binding
Sulfonylureas (oral hypoglycemics)	↑ Effect of sulfonylureas due to ↓ plasma protein binding

Laboratory Test Interference Tolmetin metabolites give a false + test for proteinuria using sulfosalicylic acid.

Dosage **PO: initial,** 400 mg t.i.d. Adjust dose according to response of patient. **Maximum recommended daily dose:** 2000 mg/day. **Children 2 years and older: initial,** 20 mg/kg/day in 3 to 4 divided doses. **Maintenance:** 15–30 mg/kg/day.

Administration   1. One dose should be taken on arising, one during the day, and one dose at bedtime.
2. Administer with meals, milk, or antacids (other than sodium bicarbonate) if GI symptoms occur.
3. Beneficial effects may not be observed for several days to a week.

PYRAZOLONE DERIVATIVE

OXYPHENBUTAZONE OXALID, TANDEARIL

PHENYLBUTAZONE AZOLID, BUTAZOLIDIN, AZOLID-A, BUTAZOLIDIN ALKA

Classification   Anti-inflammatory, pyrazolone derivative.

General Statement   The pyrazolone derivatives have antipyretic, analgesic, and anti-inflammatory effects. The group includes antipyrine and dipyrone (no longer available in the United States), and phenylbutazone.

Drugs belonging to this group are potentially dangerous for a number of patients. The most serious toxic reactions are blood dyscrasias, including agranulocytosis, leukopenia, and thrombocytopenia. The untoward reactions are of a hypersensitivity nature and are not necessarily dose related. The effects can be developed by persons who have taken these drugs without ill effects for a number of years. Aim for the lowest dosage.

The onset of action of oxyphenbutazone and phenylbutazone is 30 to 60 minutes; effectiveness peaks at 2 hours, and the residual duration of action is 3 to 4 days. Azolid-A and Butazolidin Alka contain dried aluminum hydroxide gel and magnesium trisilicate to minimize gastric upset.

Uses   These drugs should only be used for short-term therapy due to possible severe toxic effects.

Acute gout, ankylosing spondylitis, psoriasis, rheumatoid arthritis, osteoarthritis, postoperative and posttraumatic inflammation, acute superficial thrombophlebitis.

Contraindications   Peptic ulcer or history thereof, edema, history of cardiac decompensation, drug allergies, blood dyscrasias, renal, hepatic or cardiac dysfunction, children under age 14. Reduce dosage for patients over 40 years of age. High dosage is contraindicated in glaucoma. The drug passes the placental barrier and appears in milk of nursing mothers.

Untoward Reactions   Agranulocytosis, nausea, vomiting, skin rash, GI disturbances, blood dyscrasias, sodium retention resulting in edema, pruritus, stomatitis, anorexia, urinary frequency, headaches, visual disturbances, vertigo, fever, hepatitis, nephritis, and peptic ulcer with hemorrhages or perforation. Hemogram blood tests should be done before initiation of therapy and at 1- to 2-week intervals during therapy.

Drug Interactions

Interactant	Interaction
Anabolic steroids	Certain androgens ↑ effect of phenylbutazone
Anticoagulants, oral	↑ Effect of anticoagulants by ↓ plasma protein binding. Phenylbutazone may also produce GI ulceration and therefore is ↑ chance of bleeding
Antidepressants, tricyclic	↓ Effect of phenylbutazone due to ↓ absorption from GI tract
Antidiabetic agents	↑ Hypoglycemic response due to ↓ breakdown by liver and ↓ plasma protein binding
Cholestyramine	Absorption of phenylbutazone delayed by cholestyramine. May ↓ effect.
Digitalis glycosides	↓ Effect of digitalis glycosides by ↑ breakdown by liver
Phenytoin (Dilantin)	↑ Effect of phenytoin due to ↓ breakdown by liver
Salicylates	Phenylbutazone inhibits uricosuric activity of salicylates
Sulfonamides	↑ Effect of sulfonamides by ↑ blood levels

Laboratory Test Interferences

May alter liver function tests. False + Coombs test. ↑ Prothrombin time.

Dosage

Initial: 300–400 mg (rarely 600 mg) daily in 3 to 4 equal doses. **Maintenance:** aim for minimum effective dose not to exceed 400 mg daily.

Administration

Administer before or after meals with a glass of milk to minimize gastric irritation.

Nursing Implications

1. Careful observation and teaching of the patient is essential during therapy.
2. Discontinue drug and notify the physician should the patient demonstrate any allergic manifestations to the drug such as rash, edema, or wheezing.
3. Be prepared for treatment of toxicity with equipment for gastric lavage, oxygen, and blankets for warmth.
4. Teach patient that drug must be immediately discontinued and the physician notified, should the patient develop skin reaction or fever, malaise, sore throat and ulcerated mucous membranes—symptoms of possibly irreversible agranulocytosis.
5. Emphasize the need for regular and frequent blood tests.
6. Teach patient to take only the dose ordered and not to increase the dose.
7. Practice reverse isolation technique in caring for patient, if agranulocytosis is severe.
8. Weigh patient daily and report weight gain.

9. Teach the patient how to check for edema and to report same.
10. Teach the patient to keep a written record of intake and output and to report a decrease in urinary excretion.
11. Teach the patient how to follow a low sodium or low salt diet, if ordered, to minimize edema.
12. Anticipate positive results of treatment by third to fourth day. Trial therapy is not usually continued beyond one week in the absence of favorable results.

REMITTING AGENTS

AUROTHIOGLUCOSE GOLD THIOGLUCOSE, SOLGANAL

GOLD SODIUM THIOMALATE MYOCHRYSINE

Classification Antirheumatic.

General Statement Gold injections have been used for the treatment of active rheumatoid arthritis for about 50 years. The mode of action of the drug is unknown.

Gold is a potentially toxic, heavy metal. Patients receiving gold injection must be watched very carefully. Dimercaprol (BAL), a heavy metal antagonist (see p. 762) should be on hand in case of severe toxic reaction.

Urine examination and CBC are indicated every 2 weeks during treatment.

Mild toxic symptoms or skin rash may indicate the need for a temporary discontinuation of drug. Gold therapy should be reinstituted carefully. Severe symptoms may necessitate discontinuation of therapy.

The beneficial effects of the drug are slow to appear (3 to 12 months). Most patients experience some transient side effects during initiation.

Uses Rheumatoid arthritis (active and progressive stages), nondisseminated lupus erythematosus.

Contraindications Severe diabetes, nephritis, hepatitis, marked hypertension, heart failure, history of agranulocytosis, angina, and hemorrhagic diathesis.

Untoward Reactions Skin reactions, mostly minor (pruritus and erythema), occasionally major (papular and vesicular dermatitis, exfoliative dermatitis). Also, stomatitis, irritations of the upper respiratory tract, blood dyscrasias, toxic hepatitis, acute yellow atrophy.

GI disturbances including diarrhea, colic and malaise. Headache. Untoward reaction of gold sodium thiomalate administered for active rheumatoid arthritis: flushing of face, giddiness, and vertigo.

Drug Interactions Concomitant use contraindicated with drugs known to cause blood dyscrasias (e.g. antimalarials, pyrazolone derivatives.)

Laboratory Test Interference Alters liver function tests. Urinary protein and RBCs, altered blood counts (indicative of toxic effect of drug).

Dosage *Gold sodium thiomalate, aurothioglucose — rheumatoid arthritis*, adults, **IM**, week 1 : 10 mg/week; weeks 2 and 3 : 25 mg/week. Thereafter, 50 mg/week until 0.8–1 gm total has been given. Thereafter according to individual response. *Usual:* 25 mg/week or 50 mg q 3 to 4 weeks. **Children:** Dose proportional to weight.

Administration
1. Shake vial well to insure uniform suspension before withdrawing medication.
2. Inject into gluteus maximus.

Nursing Implications
1. Have the patient continue lying down for at least 20 minutes after injection to prevent from falling caused by transient giddiness or vertigo that may occur.
2. Emphasize the need for close medical supervision during gold therapy.
3. Have on hand dimercaprol (BAL) to use as an antidote in case of severe toxicity.
4. Advise the patient that beneficial effects are slow to appear but that therapy may be continued up to 12 months in anticipation of relief.

PENICILLAMINE CUPRIMINE, D-PEN (OR DEPEN)

Classification Antirheumatic, heavy metal antagonist, cystinuria.

General Statement The drug, a degradation product of penicillin, is a chelating agent used as a heavy metal antagonist. (For this use, see *Heavy Metal Antagonists*.) Its mode of action in rheumatoid arthritis is not understood. It is believed to interfere with the release of lysosomal enzymes into the joint cavity. A positive response to therapy may take up to 6 months to become apparent (generally 3 months). Untoward effects usually respond to a decrease in dosage.

Uses Wilson's disease, cystinuria, and rheumatoid arthritis – severe active disease that does not respond to conventional therapy.

Contraindications Pregnancy, penicillinase-related aplastic anemia or agranulocytosis, hypersensitivity to drug. Patients allergic to penicillin may cross-react to penicillamine. Renal insufficiency or history thereof.

Untoward Reactions Hematologic toxicity: especially thrombocytopenia (4%) and leukopenia (2%). Renal damage: proteinuria (6%) and hematuria. Goodpasture's syndrome — a severe and ultimately fatal glomerulonephritis (rare), other allergic reactions, myasthenic syndrome, pemphigoid-type rash;

also transient drug fever and rash (1–2 weeks after initiation of therapy), early and late rashes indicative of allergic reactions. Positive antinuclear antibody (ANA) tests, oral ulcerations, stomatitis, glossitis, loss of taste (12%)—usually self-limiting. Increased skin friability. Tinnitus, reactivation of peptic ulcer, urticaria, and exfoliative dermatitis.

Drug Interaction

Interactant	*Interaction*
Isoniazid	↑ Effect of isoniazid
Antimalarials	
Cytotoxic Drugs	↑ Risk of blood dyscrasias and adverse renal
Gold therapy	effects
Pyrazolone derivatives	

Dosage

Wilson's disease Dosage is usually calculated on the basis of the urinary excretion of copper. One gram penicillamine promotes excretion of 2 mg copper. **PO, adults and older children:** *usual, initial,* 250 mg q.i.d. Dosage may have to be increased to 4–5 gm daily. A further increase does not produce additional excretion. **Pediatric, infants over 6 months:** 250 mg daily. Patient should also receive sulfurated potash (40 mg) or a cation exchange resin, such as Carbo-Resin (15–20 gm) with each meal. *Cystinuria:* individualized and based on excretion rate of cystine (100–200 mg/day in patients with no history of stones, below 100 mg with patients with history of stones or pain). Initiate at low dosage (250 mg/day) and increase gradually to minimum effective dosage. **PO, adult:** *usual,* 2 gm/day (range 1–4 gm); **children:** 30 mg/kg/day in 4 divided doses. If divided in less than 4 doses, give larger dose at night. *Rheumatoid arthritis,* **PO,** *individualized:* **initial,** 125–250 mg/day. Dosage may be increased at 12-week intervals by 250 mg increments until adequate response is attained. **Maximum:** 500–750 mg/day. Up to 500 mg/day can be given as a single dose, higher dosages should be divided.

Administration

Administer on an empty stomach at least 1 hour before meals and at least 1 hour apart from any drugs or food to permit maximum absorption of medication.

Nursing Implications

1. Ascertain that urinalysis and hematology tests are performed every 2 weeks for first 6 months of therapy and monthly thereafter.
2. Advise patient to report fever, sore throat, chills, bruising, or bleeding, early signs of granulocytopenia.
3. Teach patient to take temperature nightly during first few months of therapy because fever may be an indicator of hypersensitivity reaction.
4. Withhold penicillamine if WBC falls below 3500 per mm^3 and report platelet count below 100,000 per mm^3. If there is a progressive fall in WBC and platelet count during 3 successive lab tests, a temporary interruption of therapy is indicated.
5. Advise patient to observe urine for proteinuria (cloudy in appearance) and for hematuria, (smoky-brown in early state, slightly blood tinged later, and then grossly bloody).

6. Ascertain that liver function tests are done before initiation of therapy and q 6 months during first year and a half of therapy.
7. Advise oral care for stomatitis. This manifestation usually requires discontinuation of drug.
8. Advise patient with a blurring of taste perception that this may last 2 to 3 months or more, but that it is usually self-limiting. Encourage adequate nutrition in patient experiencing hypogeusia (loss of taste).
9. Stress necessity for a period of at least 2 hours to elapse between ingestion of penicillamine and therapeutic iron, because iron decreases cupruretic effects of penicillamine.
10. Alert patient (especially the elderly) to prevent excessive pressure on shoulders, elbows, knees, toes, and buttocks, because skin becomes more friable with penicillamine.
11. Rule out infection, if white papules appear at site of venipuncture and at surgical sites. Do not assume papules are due to penicillamine.
12. Anticipate reduction in dose to 250 mg/day prior to surgery and until wound healing is completed.
13. Note that a positive antinuclear antibody (ANA) test does not mandate discontinuation of drug, but suggests that a lupus-like syndrome may occur in the future.
14. Anticipate that pyridoxine will be ordered as a supplement, because penicillamine increases the body's need for this vitamin.
15. Encourage patients with rheumatoid arthritis to continue using other modalities to achieve relief of symptoms because the therapeutic response to penicillamine may take up to 6 months.
16. Advise women of childbearing age that use of penicillamine during pregnancy is contraindicated, because drug can cause fetal damage.
17. Advise women to report to medical supervision, if they miss a menstrual period or note other symptoms of pregnancy.
18. Advise patient with Wilson's disease to:
    a. Continue on low copper diet by excluding chocolate, nuts, shellfish, mushrooms, liver, molasses, broccoli, and cereals enriched with copper.
    b. Use distilled or demineralized water if drinking water contains more than 0.1 mg of copper/liter.
    c. Ingest sulfurated potash or Carbo-Resin with meals to minimize absorption of copper except when patient is also receiving supplemental iron.
    d. Continue therapy because it may take 1–3 months until there is an improvement of neurological symptoms.
    e. Check that any vitamin preparations ingested are copper free.
19. Advise patients with cystinuria to:
    a. Drink large amounts of fluid to prevent formation of renal calculi. Patients should drink 1 pint at bedtime and another pint during the night when urine tends to be the most concentrated and most acidic. Urine should have a specific gravity less than 1.010 and a pH of 7.5–8.
    b. Have yearly kidney x-rays performed to determine if renal calculi are present.

c. Continue on diet low in methionine, a major precursor of cystine, by excluding rich meat soups and broths, milk, eggs, cheeses, and peas.

d. That diet low in methione is contraindicated for children and during pregnancy because of its low protein content.

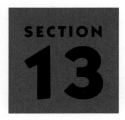

SECTION 13

antigout agents

Allopurinol
Colchicine

Probenecid
Sulfinpyrazone

General Statement   Gout or gouty arthritis is characterized by an excess of uric acid in the body. This excess results either from an overproduction of uric acid or from a defect in its breakdown or elimination.

When the concentration of uric acid in the blood exceeds a certain level (6 mg in 100 ml) it may start to form fine, needlelike crystals which can become deposited in the joints and cause an acute inflammatory response in synovial membrane. Hyperuricemia may also accompany other diseases such as leukemia or lymphomas. High levels of uric acid may also accompany treatment with certain antineoplastic agents or thiazide diuretics. In that case the excess acid may damage the kidney.

Therapy is aimed at reducing the uric acid level of the body to normal or near normal levels. Drugs used for the treatment of gout or hyperuricemia either promote the excretion of uric acid by the kidney or reduce the amount of uric acid formed. These drugs however have no analgesic or anti-inflammatory properties.

Previously, gout was often treated by dietary measures—reduced intake of purine-rich foods like meat. Dietary restrictions are seldom prescribed today, except for organ meats which have a high purine content.

Acute gout. As opposed to other forms of arthritis, acute gout has a dramatic onset. Maximum pain, joint swelling, and joint tenderness are reached within hours. An acute attack of gout is often accompanied by a low-grade fever and an increase in the WBC count.

In between attacks the patient with hyperuricemia is usually symptom free; however, since acute attacks usually recur in patients with hyperuricemia, patients are often kept on a maintenance dose of a uricosuric agent.

ALLOPURINOL ZYLOPRIM

Classification Antigout agent.

General Statement Allopurinol interferes with the production of uric acid by inhibition of xanthine oxidase, an enzyme that is involved in the formation of uric acid from hypoxanthine and xanthine. The effect of the drug on the blood uric acid level becomes noticeable after 24 to 48 hours, and is fully developed after 5 to 10 days. The drug is not useful for the treatment of *acute* attacks of gout, but is the drug of choice for *chronic* gouty arthritis.

Uses Gout, hyperuricemia associated with polycythemia vera, myeloid metaplasia or other blood dyscrasias, and certain cases of primary and secondary renal disease. Prophylaxis in hyperuricemia and as an adjunct in some antineoplastic therapy.

    Allopurinol is sometimes administered concomitantly with uricosuric agents in patients with severe tophaceous gout. (A tophus is a deposit of uric acid.)

Contraindications Hypersensitivity to drug. Patients with idiopathic hemochromatosis or relatives of patients suffering from this condition. Children except as an adjunct in treatment of neoplastic disease. Severe skin reactions on previous exposure. Use with caution in patients with liver or renal disease.

Untoward Reactions Most frequent: skin reactions including pruritic maculopapular skin rash which may be accompanied by fever and malaise. Exfoliative, urticarial, purpura type dermatitis and alopecia. Skin reaction may stop if drug is discontinued and then reinstated at lower dosages. Cataracts have developed occasionally in patients with dermatitis. Nausea, vomiting, anorexia, intermittent abdominal pain, diarrhea and drowsiness have been reported.

    Hypersensitivity or idiosyncracy to drug syndrome characterized by: fever, chills, leukopenia, eosinophilia, arthralgia, skin rash, pruritus, nausea and vomiting.

    Periodic blood counts are advised.

Drug Interactions

Interactant	*Interaction*
Ampicillin	Concomitant use may result in skin rashes
Azathioprine (Imuran)	↑ Effect of azathioprine due to ↓ breakdown by liver
Iron preparations	Allopurinol ↑ hepatic iron concentrations
Mercaptopurine	↑ Effect of mercaptopurine due to ↓ breakdown by liver

Laboratory Test Interferences Alters liver function tests. ↑ serum cholesterol. ↓ serum glucose levels.

Dosage
Gout, **PO:** 200–600 mg in divided doses. Adjust to response. **Average maintenance:** 100 mg t.i.d.

Transfer from colchicine, uricosuric agents and/or anti-inflammatory agents to allopurinol should be made gradually.

Prevention of uric acid nephropathy during therapy with antineo-plastic agents: 600–800 mg daily for 2 to 3 days. Then decrease to minimum effective level.

Pediatric: Hyperuricemia associated with neoplastic disease only: **6–10 years: initial,** 100 mg t.i.d. Adjust according to response; **under 6 years:** 50 mg t.i.d. *Note:* Allopurinol may cause an acute attack of gouty arthritis during initial administration. Give colchicine at the same time when therapy is begun to prevent this.

Nursing Implications
1. Inform patient that a skin rash even months after drug has been started may be caused by allopurinol.
2. Inform the patient who has an increased number of acute attacks of gout during initiation of therapy that these will subside.
3. In order to prevent kidney damage, maintain a fluid intake that will result in minimum excretion of 2 liters of urine daily unless other medical conditions contraindicate.
4. Anticipate that patients on uricosurics must be alkalinized by sodium bicarbonate or potassium citrate to reduce incidence of renal calculi.
5. Do not administer iron salts to patients on allopurinol therapy because of alteration in iron metabolism.
6. Advise patients to use caution driving a car or carrying out mechanical tasks that require mental alertness because drug may cause drowsiness.
7. Administer the drug in divided doses because the half-life of the drug is short.
8. Anticipate that during transfer of patient from uricosuric drug to allopurinol the dosage of the uricosuric is gradually decreased as the allopurinol dosage is gradually increased.

COLCHICINE COLSALIDE

Classification
Antigout agent.

Remarks
Colchicine is an alkaloid. It does not affect uric acid metabolism but is thought to decrease urate crystal deposition and decrease the inflammatory response. The drug is highly toxic.

Uses
Agent of choice in acute attacks of gout, either spontaneous or induced by allopurinol or uricosuric agents; diagnosis of gout. Prophylaxis of recurrent gouty arthritis.

Contraindications
Use with extreme caution for elderly, debilitated patients, especially in the presence of chronic renal, hepatic, GI, or cardiovascular disease.

Untoward Reactions Nausea, vomiting, diarrhea, abdominal cramping (discontinue drug at once and wait at least 48 hours before reinstating drug therapy). Prolonged administration can cause bone marrow depression, thrombocytopenia and aplastic anemia, peripheral neuritis, and liver dysfunction.

Acute colchicine intoxication is characterized at first by violent GI tract symptoms such as nausea, vomiting, abdominal pain, and diarrhea. The latter may be profuse, watery, bloody, and associated with severe fluid and electrolyte loss. Also burning of throat and skin, hematuria and oliguria, rapid and weak pulse, general exhaustion, muscular depression, and CNS involvement. Death is usually caused by respiratory paralysis. Treatment of acute poisoning involves gastric lavage, symptomatic support, including atropine and morphine, artificial respiration, hemodialysis, peritoneal dialysis and treatments of shock.

Drug Interactions

Interactant	Interaction
CNS depressants	Patients on colchicine may be more sensitive to CNS depressant effect of these drugs
Sympathomimetic agents	Enhanced by colchicine
Vitamin B$_{12}$	Colchicine may interfere with absorption from the gut

Laboratory Test Interferences Alters liver function tests. ↑ Alkaline phosphatase.

Dosage *Acute attack of gout*, **PO:** 1–1.2 mg followed by 0.5–0.6 mg q hr (or 1–1.2 mg q 2 hr) until pain is relieved or diarrhea occurs. **Total amount required:** 4–8 mg. **IV: initial,** 1–2 mg; *subsequently,* 0.5 mg q 3–6 hr until pain is relieved; give up to 4 mg. *Prophylaxis:* 0.5–0.6 mg/day for 3–4 days/week. Usually, oral route is used exclusively.

Administration/ Storage
1. Store in tight light-resistant containers.
2. Parenteral administration is only to be by IV route. Drug would cause severe local irritation if given SC or IM.

Nursing Implications
1. Instruct patient to always have colchicine on hand.
2. Instruct patient to start or increase dosage as ordered at first sign of joint pain or symptom of impending attack.
3. Withhold drug if GI side effects occur and check with physician because drug should be discontinued for 24 to 48 hours after such symptoms have disappeared.
4. Anticipate that paregoric may be ordered for treatment of severe diarrhea due to colchicine.

PROBENECID BENEMID, PROBALAN, PROBENIMEAD, ROBENECID

Classification Antigout agent, uricosuric agent.

**General
Statement** Probenecid promotes the elimination of urate salts by the kidney. It is neither analgesic nor anti-inflammatory. The drug is extremely long-lasting and also prolongs the activity of penicillin and aminosalicylic acid. Probenecid is not useful during an acute attack of gout, and therapy with the drug should not be initiated during such. However, when acute attacks do occur while patients are receiving probenecid, the drug should not be discontinued.

Colchicine is sometimes administered with probenecid during initiation therapy.

Uses Hyperuricemia in chronic gout. Adjunct in therapy with penicillin.

Contraindications Hypersensitivity to drug, blood dyscrasias, uric acid, and kidney stones. Administer with caution to patients with renal disease, and children below 3 years of age.

**Untoward
Reactions** Headaches. GI disturbances including: anorexia, nausea, vomiting, diarrhea, constipation, and abdominal discomfort. Hypersensitivity reaction characterized by skin rash or drug fever, and very rarely anaphylactoid reactions.

Initially, the drug may increase frequency of acute gout attacks.
Occasionally: Flushing, dizziness and anemia.

**Drug
Interactions**

Interactant	Interaction
Aminosalicyclic acid (PAS)	↑ Effects of PAS due to ↓ excretion by kidney
Cephalosporin	↑ Effect of cephalosporins due to ↓ excretion by kidney
Dapsone	↑ Effect of dapsone due to ↓ excretion by kidney
Indomethacin (Indocin)	↑ Effect of indomethacin due to ↓ excretion by kidney
Pyrazinamide	Probenecid inhibits hyperuricemia produced by pyrazinamide
Salicylates	Salicylates inhibit uricosuric activity of probenecid
Sulfinpyrazone (Anturane)	↑ Effect of sulfinpyrazone due to ↓ excretion by kidney
Sulfonamides	↑ Effect of sulfonamides due to ↓ plasma protein binding
Sulfonylureas, oral	↑ Action of sulfonylureas → hyperglycemia.

Dosage *Gout,* **PO: initial,** 250 mg b.i.d. for 1 week. **Maintenance:** 500 mg b.i.d. Dosage may have to be increased further (by 500 mg daily q 4 weeks to maximum of 2 gm) until urate excretion is less than 700 mg in 24 hr.

Adjuvant to penicillin or cephalosporin therapy: 500 mg q.i.d. Dosage is decreased for elderly patients with renal damage.

Pediatric 2 years and older: initial, 25 mg/kg, **then** 40 mg/kg q 6 hr. **Do not use in children less than 2 years of age.** Colbenemid (Merck Sharp & Dohme), a combination tablet containing colchicine (0.5 mg) and probenecid (500 mg), is available.

Nursing Implications

1. Encourage a liberal intake of fluids to help prevent the formation of uric acid stones.
2. Anticipate that urine must be alkalinized by sodium bicarbonate or potassium citrate to prevent urates from crystallizing out of acid urine and forming kidney stones.
3. Be alert to the possibility that medication may cause a false Benedict test.
4. Report gastric intolerance promptly so that dosage may be corrected without loss of therapeutic effect.
5. Be alert to hypersensitivity reactions that occur more frequently with intermittent therapy.
6. Advise the patient to note carefully whether there has been an increase in the number of attacks at the initiation of therapy as physician may decide to add colchicine to regimen.
7. Advise the patient to continue taking probenecid during acute attacks with colchicine as ordered unless specifically told by physician to discontinue use.

SULFINPYRAZONE ANTURANE

Classification Antigout agent, uricosuric.

General Statement Sulfinpyrazone promotes the excretion of uric acid by the kidney and inhibits the reabsorption of urate salts by the renal tubules. It is not effective during acute attacks of gout and may even increase the frequency of acute episodes during the initiation of therapy. However, drug should not be discontinued during acute attacks. Concomitant administration of colchicine during initiation of therapy is recommended.

Uses Prophylactic to reduce frequency and intensity of acute attacks of gout in hyperuricemic patients. Effective in treating acute gouty attacks if given at the time of the attack.

Contraindications Active peptic ulcer. Use with extreme caution in patients with impaired renal function and those with a history of peptic ulcers. Use with caution in pregnant women.

Untoward Reactions Upper GI tract disturbances including nausea, vomiting, abdominal discomfort. Skin rash which usually disappears with usage. Reactivation of peptic ulcer. Slight depression of WBC. Acute attacks of gout may become more frequent during initial therapy. Administer concomitantly with colchicine at this time.

	Interactant	Interaction
Drug Interactions	Anticoagulants	↑ Effect of anticoagulant due to effect on prothrombin.
	Probenecid	↑ Effect of sulfinpyrazone due to ↓ excretion by kidney
	Salicylates	Salicylates inhibit uricosuric effect of sulfinpyrazone
	Sulfonamides	↑ Effect of sulfonamides by ↓ plasma protein binding
	Sulfonylureas, oral	Potentiation of hypoglycemic effect

Dosage **Initial:** 200–400 mg/day in 2 divided doses with meals. Patients who are transferred from other uricosuric agents can receive full dose at once. **Maintenance:** 400 mg/day in 2 divided doses up to 800 mg/day, if necessary. Maintain full dosage without interruption even during acute attacks of gout.

Nursing Implications
1. Encourage liberal fluid intake to help prevent the formation of uric acid stones.
2. Anticipate the urine must be alkalinized by sodium bicarbonate to help prevent urates from crystallizing out of acid urine and forming kidney stones.
3. Administer with meals or with an antacid to minimize gastric distress.

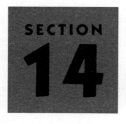

SECTION
14

antiparkinson agents

Cholinergic Blocking Agents	Benztropine Mesylate Biperiden Hydrochloride Biperiden Lactate Chlorphenoxamine Hydrochloride Cycrimine Hydrochloride	Ethopropazine Hydrochloride Orphenadrine Citrate Orphenadrine Hydrochloride Procyclidine Hydrochloride Trihexyphenidyl Hydrochloride
Other Antiparkinson Agents	Amantadine Hydrochloride Carbidopa/Levodopa	Diphenhydramine Hydrochloride Levodopa

Parkinson's disease is a progressive disorder of the nervous system, affecting mostly people over the age of 50.

Its main symptoms are slowness of motor movements (bradykinesia and akinesia), stiffness or resistance to passive movements (rigidity), muscle weakness, tremors, speech impairment, sialorrhea (salivation), and postural instability.

Parkinsonism is a frequent side-effect of certain antipsychotic drugs, including prochlorperazine, chlorpromazine and reserpine. Drug-induced symptoms usually disappear when the responsible agent is discontinued. Extrapyramidal parkinson-like symptoms can accompany brain injuries (strokes, tumors) or other diseases of the nervous system.

The cause of Parkinson's disease is unknown; however, it is associated with a depletion of the neurotransmitter dopamine in the nervous system. Administration of levodopa—the precursor of dopamine—relieves the symptoms in about one-half the patients. Anticholinergic agents also have a beneficial effect by reducing tremors and rigidity and improving mobility, muscular coordination, and motor performance. They are often administered together with levodopa. Certain antihistamines, notably diphenhydramine (Benadryl), are also useful in the treatment of Parkinsonism.

Patients suffering from Parkinson's disease need emotional support and encouragement because the debilitating nature of the disorder often causes depression. Comprehensive treatment includes physical therapy.

CHOLINERGIC BLOCKING AGENTS

General Statement The central nervous system effects of certain cholinergic blocking agents are beneficial for the treatment of parkinsonism. The drugs abolish or reduce the signs and symptoms of the disease, such as tremors and rigidity, and their administration produces improvement in mobility, muscular coordination, and motor performance. This central effect is attributed to interference with the action of acetylcholine on the central nervous system. The cholinergic blocking agents also have an antisalivary effect, which controls sialorrhea.

These agents have many untoward effects, related to their principal pharmacological action, on the autonomic nervous system. These can, however, often be controlled by a decrease in dosage. When properly adjusted, anticholinergic agents can be used satisfactorily for patients suffering from parkinsonism for extended periods of time.

Contraindications Glaucoma, tachycardia, partial obstruction of the GI and biliary tract, and prostatic hypertrophy. The drugs are to be used with extreme caution for patients with hypertension, cardiac disease, especially those with a tendency to develop tachycardia, and in the elderly with atherosclerosis or evidence of mental impairment.

Untoward Reactions GI and urinary tract: constipation (frequent), nausea, vomiting, urinary hesitancy, urinary retention, impotence. Cardiovascular system: tachycardia and palpitations. Central Nervous System: dizziness, drowsiness, lassitude, nervousness; disorientation; symptoms often may be mistaken for senility or mental deterioration. Excess dosage may cause agitation, psychotic reactions and hallucinations. Respiratory: decreased bronchial secretions, antihistamine effects. Ocular: blurred vision, acute glaucoma, photophobia. General: dryness of mouth that may cause difficulty in swallowing, suppression of perspiration, suppression of glandular secretions, scarlatiniform rash, loss of libido.

Drug Interactions

Interactant	Interaction
Amantidine	Additive anticholinergic side effects, especially with trihexyphenidyl and benztropine
Antidepressants, tricyclic	Additive anticholinergic side effects
MAO Inhibitors	MAO Inhibitors ↑ effects of anticholinergic drugs
Phenothiazines	↑ Risk of G.I. side effects including paralytic ileus
Procainamide	Additive anticholinergic side effects
Quinidine	Additive effect on blockade of vagus nerve action

Dosage

See individual agents. The agents are usually initiated at low dosage and increased gradually until optimum levels have been reached. Excessive untoward reactions can often be corrected by decrease in dosage. Agent should not be discontinued abruptly, but decreased gradually while another drug with the same effect is introduced slowly.

Nursing Implications

1. Be alert to a history of asthma, glaucoma, or duodenal ulcer which contraindicates the use of these drugs.
2. Check dosage and measure drug exactly because some of these antiparkinson agents are given in minute amounts and overdosage results in toxicity.
3. Inform the patient, family members, or other persons responsible for the patient, of side effects that may occur and advise them to report these to the physician who may alleviate side effects by reducing the dose or temporarily discontinuing the drug. Sometimes the patient will be asked to tolerate certain side effects (e.g., dry mouth, blurred vision) because of the overall beneficial effects of the drug.
4. Caution patients who improve with drug therapy to resume their normal activities gradually, taking other medical problems they may have into consideration.
5. Teach the patient or a responsible family member that antiparkinson drugs should not be withdrawn abruptly. When changing medication, one drug should be withdrawn slowly and the other started in small doses.
6. Relieve dry mouth by providing cold drinks (particularly postoperatively), hard candies, or chewing gum if permitted.

BENZTROPINE MESYLATE COGENTIN MESYLATE

Classification Antiparkinson agent, synthetic anticholinergic.

Remarks Drug also has antihistaminic and local anesthetic properties. Its effects are cumulative and it is long-acting. Full effects are established in 2 to 3 days. The drug rarely produces side effects.

Uses Paralysis agitans, tremors, parkinsonism, muscle rigidity, drug-induced parkinsonism associated with major tranquilizers. Useful primarily as an adjunct to other antiparkinsonism drugs. Useful at bedtime to provide relief through the night.

Dosage Patients can rarely tolerate full dosage. **PO (rarely by IV or IM).** *Parkinsonism:* 0.5–6 mg daily. *Drug-induced parkinsonism:* **initial,** 0.5 mg daily increased gradually to 1–4 mg 1 or 2 times daily.

Administration When used as replacement for or supplement to other parkinsonism drugs, substitute or add gradually.

Additional Nursing Implications
1. Inform the patient that it takes 2 to 3 days for drug to show effects.
2. Advise patient to use caution while driving or operating dangerous machinery because drug has a sedative effect.
3. Observe the patient for vomiting or excitement, which may require temporary withdrawal. Treatment may be resumed later at a lower dosage.

BIPERIDEN HYDROCHLORIDE AKINETON HYDROCHLORIDE

BIPERIDEN LACTATE AKINETON LACTATE

Classification Antiparkinson agent, synthetic anticholinergic.

Remarks Tolerance may develop and require an increase in dosage. Tremor may increase as spasticity is relieved.

Uses Parkinsonism, especially of the postencephalitic and idiopathic type. Drug-induced extrapyramidal manifestations.

Dosage *Hydrochloride,* **PO:** 2 mg t.i.d.–q.i.d. *Lactate, parenteral,* **IM, IV:** 2 mg, repeated if necessary up to a maximum of 8 mg daily, **pediatric; IM** (*dystonia*): 0.04 mg/kg up to q.i.d.

Administration Administer with meals to reduce gastric irritation.

Additional Nursing Implications
1. Have the patient supine during IV administration.
2. Dangle patient on edge of bed prior to walking after IV administration of drug to prevent transient hypotension, syncope, and falling.
3. Assist the patient in walking after IM or IV administration because of transient incoordination.

CHLORPHENOXAMINE HYDROCHLORIDE PHENOXENE HYDROCHLORIDE

Classification Antiparkinson agent, synthetic anticholinergic.

Remarks Onset of action, 30 minutes; duration, 4 to 6 hours. Drug also has antihistaminic activity.

Uses Adjunct to all types of parkinsonism.

Dosage **PO:** 50 mg or more t.i.d. Up to 400 mg daily can be given in severe cases.

Administration Administer after meals with milk to minimize gastric irritation.

Additional Nursing Implications
1. Advise patient to use caution driving a car or operating dangerous machinery because medication may cause drowsiness or dizziness.
2. Anticipate that prolonged use of the drug will result in slight tolerance which will necessitate increase in dosage of drug.

CYCRIMINE HYDROCHLORIDE PAGITANE HYDROCHLORIDE

Classification Antiparkinson agent, synthetic anticholinergic.

Remarks Side effects decrease with usage; if too severe, decrease dosage. Give with meals to minimize gastric distress.

Uses All types of parkinsonism.

Dosage **PO: initial,** 1.25 mg t.i.d. with meals. Increase gradually to 5 mg q.i.d. if required and tolerated. **Maximum dose:** 20 mg daily.

Administration Administer with meals to reduce gastric irritation.

Additional Nursing Implications
1. Observe for vertigo, disorientation or weakness, all of which indicate need to decrease dosage or discontinue drug.
2. Report dryness of mouth, blurring of vision, and epigastric distress to doctor.
3. Advise the patient to continue therapy explaining that these symptoms usually disappear with usage.

ETHOPROPAZINE HYDROCHLORIDE PARSIDOL HYDROCHLORIDE

Classification Antiparkinson agent, synthetic anticholinergic of the phenothiazine type.

General Statement Considered by some as drug of choice for treatment of major tremors of parkinsonism. Drug has strong atropinelike effect and some antihistaminic, local anesthetic, and CNS depressant effects. Onset: one-half hour; duration: 4 hours.

May require concomitant administration of CNS stimulants.

Drug produces a high incidence of side effects.

Uses Parkinsonism and drug-induced extrapyramidal symptoms.

Additional Untoward Reactions Drowsiness, dizziness, and lassitude. Prolonged use may cause adverse CNS stimulation, such as restlessness, delirium, hallucinations, paranoid psychosis, ataxia, and paresthesias. Potential toxicity requires close medical observation. Parkinsonian symptoms may become exacerbated.

Dosage **PO: initial,** 50 mg 1 or 2 times a day; increase by 10 mg per dose q 2 to 3 days until optimum effect or limit of tolerance. **Maintenance:** 100–600 mg daily.

Most patients, especially the elderly, cannot tolerate full therapeutic dosage.

Additional Nursing Implications 1. Observe patients for high incidence of side effects.
2. Anticipate that dosage for elderly will be less than full therapeutic dosage.

ORPHENADRINE CITRATE NORFLEX

ORPHENADRINE HYDROCHLORIDE DISIPAL

Classification Antiparkinson agent, anticholinergic.

Remarks Drug improves rigidity but not tremor. Peak effect, 2 hours; duration, 4 to 6 hours.

Uses Parkinsonism, especially of the postencephalitic type. Skeletal muscle spasms; drug-induced extrapyramidal reactions. Citrate used only as skeletal muscle relaxant. (see page 336).

Additional Untoward Reactions Adverse CNS manifestations (dizziness, drowsiness, increased tremor) may be present during initiation but will subside with continuation of usage or reduction in dose. Mild euphoria. Aplastic anemia occurs rarely.

Dosage *Parkinsonism (hydrochloride),* **PO:** *initial,* 50 mg t.i.d. Dosage up to 400 mg daily may be required.

Acute muscle spasms (citrate), **IM, IV:** 60 mg every 12 hr. **PO:** 100 mg b.i.d.

Additional Nursing Implications

1. Observe closely for increased tremor or adverse CNS effects that may require decrease in dosage.
2. Report side effects but encourage the patient to continue treatment since these may subside with continuous treatment.

PROCYCLIDINE HYDROCHLORIDE KEMADRIN

Classification   Antiparkinson agent, synthetic anticholinergic.

Remarks   Onset, 30 to 45 minutes; duration: 4 to 6 hours. Better tolerated by younger patients.

Uses   Parkinsonism, especially of postencephalitic type. Drug-induced extra-pyramidal symptoms.

Dosage   **PO: Initial,** 2.5 mg t.i.d. after meals; increase gradually to optimum level: 5–10 or more mg t.i.d. Lower dosage in conjunction with other antiparkinson drugs.

TRIHEXYPHENIDYL HYDROCHLORIDE ARTANE, HEXYPHEN, T.H.P., TREMIN, TRIHEXANE, TRIHEXIDYL

Classification   Antiparkinson agent, anticholinergic.

Remarks   Onset: 1 hour; duration: 6 to 12 hours. Relieves rigidity, little effect on tremor. High incidence of side effects.

Uses   Initial drug of choice for parkinsonism. Drug-induced extrapyramidal reactions.

Additional Contraindications   Arteriosclerosis and hypersensitivity to drug.

Additional Untoward Reactions   Serious CNS stimulation (restlessness, insomnia, delirium, agitation) and psychotic manifestations.

Dosage   Administer 1 mg on 1st day, 2 mg on 2nd day. Increase by 2 mg every 2 to 4 days. **Usual maintenance:** 6–10 mg as divided dose, given with meals.

Drug-induced extrapyramidal reactions: 1 mg initially. Usual total daily dose is 5–15 mg.

Additional Nursing Implications

1. Observe closely for high incidence of side effects and report to prevent overwhelming problems.
2. Observe for restlessness, delirium, and insomnia.

OTHER ANTIPARKINSON DRUGS

AMANTADINE HYDROCHLORIDE SYMMETREL

Classification Antiparkinson and antiviral agent.

General Statement Amantadine hydrochloride has been used successfully for the symptomatic treatment of parkinsonism. The drug decreases extrapyramidal symptoms including akinesia, rigidity, tremors, excessive salivation, gait disturbances, and total functional disability. Favorable results have been obtained in about 50% of the patients. Improvements can last up to 30 months, although some patients report that the effect of the drug wears off in 1 to 3 months. A rest period or increased dosage may reestablish effectiveness. For parkinsonism, amantadine hydrochloride is usually used concomitantly with other agents, such as levodopa, and anticholinergic agents.

Uses Symptomatic treatment of idiopathic parkinsonism and parkinsonian syndrome resulting from encephalitis, carbon monoxide intoxication, or cerebral arteriosclerosis (also see p. 163).

Contraindications Hypersensitivity to drug; history of epilepsy. Administer with caution to patients with liver and renal disease, congestive heart failure, peripheral edema, orthostatic hypotension, recurrent eczematoid dermatitis, severe psychosis, patients on CNS stimulant drugs, those exposed to rubella, and nursing mothers. Safe use for those who may become pregnant not established.

Untoward Reactions Most CNS manifestations such as nervousness, irritability, tremors, slurred speech, lethargy, and dizziness. Reversible livedo reticularis (mottling of skin of the extremities), congestive heart failure, edema, orthostatic hypotension, skin rash, dermatitis, visual disturbance, dry mouth, anorexia, nausea, vomiting, abdominal discomfort, constipation, and either urinary retention or increased frequency have also been noted.

Drug Interactions

Interactant	Interaction
Anticholinergics	Additive anticholinergic effects especially with trihexyphenidyl and benztropine
CNS stimulants	May ↑ CNS and psychic effects of amantadine. Use cautiously together
Levodopa	Potentiated by amantadine

Dosage *Antiparkinsonism;* **PO: initial,** 100 mg daily (after breakfast) for 5 to 7 days. In the absence of adverse reaction another 100 mg is given after lunch. To avoid exacerbations of parkinsonian symptoms, amantadine hydrochloride must be withdrawn gradually.

Administration Administer last daily dosage several hours before retiring to prevent insomnia.

Additional Nursing Implications
1. Anticipate that following loss of effectiveness of the drug, benefits may be regained by increasing the dosage or discontinuing the drug for several weeks and then reinstituting it.
2. Advise the patient not to drive a car after taking medication, since concentration and coordination may be affected.
3. Advise the patient to report patchy discoloration of the skin, but also that discoloration lessens when legs are elevated and usually fades completely within weeks after discontinuing drug.
4. Advise the patient to rise slowly from a prone position as orthostatic hypotension may occur.
5. Advise the patient to lie down if dizzy or weak to relieve the orthostatic hypotension.

CARBIDOPA/LEVODOPA SINEMET

Classification Antiparkinsonism agent.

Remarks Carbidopa inhibits metabolic deactivation of peripheral levodopa and thus makes more levodopa available for the brain (carbidopa does not cross the blood brain barrier).

Uses See *Levodopa*, page 447.
WARNING Levodopa must be discontinued at least 8 hours before carbidopa/levodopa therapy is initiated. Also, patients taking carbidopa/levodopa must not take levodopa concomitantly, because the former is a combination of carbidopa and levodopa.

Contraindications See *Levodopa*, page 447. History of melanoma. MAO inhibitors should be stopped 2 weeks before therapy. (See *PDR*.)

Untoward Reactions See *Levodopa*, page 447. Also, because more levodopa reaches the brain, dyskinesias may occur at lower doses with carbidopa/levodopa than with levodopa alone.

Drug Interactions See *Levodopa*, page 447. Pyridoxine (vitamin B_6) will *not* reverse the action of carbidopa/levodopa.

Dosage Individualized. Most patients can be maintained on 3 to 6 tablets daily of 25 mg carbidopa/250 mg levodopa in divided doses.

Additional Nursing Implications
1. Monitor patient closely during the dose-adjustment period for involuntary movement which may necessitate dosage reduction.
2. Observe for blepharospasm which is an early sign of excessive dosage in some patients.
3. Do not administer with levodopa.
4. Facilitate patient's adjustment to change of medication by adminis-

tering last dose of levodopa at bedtime and starting carbidopa/ levodopa when patient arises in A.M.

DIPHENHYDRAMINE HYDROCHLORIDE BENADRYL

Classification Antihistamine.

Remarks This antihistamine is useful in controlling tremors and is an excellent mild sedative for patients with parkinsonism who are sensitive to other sedatives.

Dosage **IM, IV:** 10–50 mg up to maximum of 400 mg/day. **PO:** 50 mg t.i.d.– q.i.d. For details, see *Antihistamines* Chapter 10, p. 685.

LEVODOPA BENDOPA, DOPAR, LARODOPA, L-DOPA

Classification Miscellaneous—antiparkinsonism agent.

General Statement Levodopa is a precursor of dopamine, a neurotransmitter that seems to be depleted in the CNS of patients suffering from parkinsonism. The drug is effective in more than half the patients. It, however, only provides symptomatic relief and does not alter the course of the disease. When effective it relieves rigidity, bradykinesia, tremors, dysphagia, seborrhea, sialorrhea and postural instability.

Periodic hepatic, hematopoietic, cardiovascular and renal function tests should be performed on patients receiving long-term therapy. Levodopa is often administered together with an anticholinergic agent.

Uses Parkinson's disease and parkinsonism.

Contraindications Hypersensitivity to drug, narrow angle glaucoma, blood dyscrasias, hypertension, coronary sclerosis. Use with extreme caution in patients with history of myocardial infarctions, convulsions, arrhythmias, bronchial asthma, emphysema, active peptic ulcer, psychosis or neurosis, wide angle glaucoma.

Untoward Reactions The side effects of levodopa are numerous and usually dose related. Some may abate with usage. They are also less marked when drug is given with meals.

GI effects: anorexia, nausea, vomiting, duodenal ulcer, GI bleeding, constipation, diarrhea, epigastric and abdominal distress, pain, flatulence, eructation, hiccups, sialorrhea, bitter taste, dry mouth, tightness of lips or tongue, difficulty in swallowing, burning sensation of the tongue.

Cardiac irregularities and orthostatic hypotension occur frequently. ECG abnormalities, palpitations, hypertension, flushing and phlebitis occur more rarely, but their appearance necessitates discontinuation of drug.

Neurological effects including grimacing, bruxism (grinding of teeth), twisting of tongue, waving of neck, hands, and feet, jerky and involuntary movements. Dizziness, sedation, dyskinesia, agitation, anxiety, confusion, depression, mental changes, antisocial behavior, ataxia, convulsions, torticollis and many other such neurological and psychological effects. Less frequently: suicidal tendencies, increased libido, and possibly associated antisocial behavior.

Also respiratory side effects, such as cough, hoarseness, bizarre breathing patterns; increased urinary frequency, retention, incontinence, hematuria, dark urine, and nocturia. Blurred vision, diplopia, changes in blood cells, fever, hot flashes, and changes in many laboratory parameters.

Levodopa interacts with many other drugs (see below) and must be administered cautiously.

Drug Interactions

Interactant	Interaction
Amphetamines	Levodopa potentiates the effect of indirectly-acting sympathomimetics
Anticholinergic drugs	Possible ↓ effect of levodopa due to ↑ breakdown of levodopa in stomach (due to delayed gastric emptying time)
Ephedrine	Levodopa potentiates the effect of indirectly-acting sympathomimetics
Guanethidine	↑ Hypotensive effect of guanethidine
Hypoglycemic drugs	Levodopa upsets diabetic control with hypoglycemic agents
Methyldopa (Aldomet)	Inhibits effect of levodopa
Monoamide Oxidase Inhibitors Pargyline (Eutonyl) Tranylcypromine (Parnate)	Concomitant administration may result in hypertension, light headedness, and flushing
Phenothiazines	↓ Effect of levodopa in Parkinson patients
Phenylephrine	Levodopa ↓ mydriasis following topical phenylephrine
Phenytoin (Dilantin)	Phenytoin antagonizes the effect of levodopa
Propranolol (Inderal)	Propranolol may antagonize the hypotensive and positive inotropic effect of levodopa
Pyridoxine	Pyridoxine reverses levodopa-induced improvement in Parkinson's disease
Reserpine	Reserpine inhibits response to levodopa by ↓ dopamine in the brain
Thioxanthines	↓ Effect of levodopa in Parkinson patients

Laboratory Test Interference

False + or ↑ SGOT values. False + Coombs test.

Dosage

PO with meals. Individualized. **Usual initial:** 0.5–1 gm daily in 2 or more divided doses. Increases by 100 to 500 mg q 2 to 3 days until maximum response is obtained. **Usual optimum dose:** 4–6 gm daily in 3 or more divided doses. This dose is attained in 4 to 6 weeks. **Maximum daily dose:** 8 gm.

Administration

Administer to patients unable to swallow tablets or capsules by crushing tablets or emptying capsule into a small amount of fruit juice at time of administration.

Additional Nursing Implications

1. Instruct the patient not to take multivitamin preparations containing 10–25 mg of vitamin B_6 which rapidly reverses the antiparkinson effect of levodopa.
2. Check with medical supervision whether drug is to be stopped 24 hours prior to surgery and ascertain when the drug is to be reinstituted.
3. Emphasize to the patient and family that dosage of drug is not to exceed 8 gm daily.

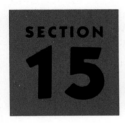

SECTION 15

anesthetics

Local Anesthetics	Benoxinate Hydrochloride Benzocaine Bupivacaine Hydrochloride Butamben Picrate Chlorprocaine Hydrochloride Cocaine Cyclomethycaine Sulfate Dibucaine Hydrochloride Dimethisoquin Hydrochloride Diperodon Dyclonine Hydrochloride	Etidocaine Hydrochloride Hexylcaine Hydrochloride Lidocaine Hydrochloride Mepivacaine Hydrochloride Piperocaine Hydrochloride Pramoxine Hydrochloride Prilocaine Hydrochloride Procaine Hydrochloride Proparacaine Hydrochloride Tetracaine Hydrochloride
General Anesthetics Volatile Liquids	Diethyl ether Enflurane Halothane	Methoxyflurane Trichloroethylene
General Anesthetics Gases	Nitrous oxide Cyclopropane	Ethylene
Miscellaneous General Anesthetics	Innovar	Ketamine

General Statement

Since local and general anesthetics are often administered to patients they are reviewed here briefly in tabular form. Note their duration of action and other characteristics since they interfere with the other drugs a patient is receiving.

LOCAL ANESTHETICS

General Statement Local anesthetics stabilize the nerve membrane and thus prevent the initiation and transmission of impulses; this leads to the anesthetic action. The use of epinephrine in conjunction with local anesthetics decreases systemic absorption and prolongs the duration of action.

Use See Table 18.

Contraindications Hypersensitivity. Large doses should not be used in patients with heart block. **Preparations containing preservatives should not be used for spinal or epidural anesthesia.**

Untoward Reactions Swelling and paresthesia of lips and oral tissue. Systemic reactions occur when plasma levels are high, and in rare cases such reactions can be fatal. Systemic symptoms include CNS excitation with tremors, shivering, and convulsions; cardiovascular effects, including hypotension, intraventricular conduction defect, or AV block which may lead to cardiac and respiratory arrest; eczematoid dermatitis.

Epinephrine in local anesthetic preparations may result in anginal pain, tachycardia, tremors, headache, restlessness, palpitations, dizziness, and hypertension.

Drug Interactions

Interactants	Interaction
Local anesthetics containing vasoconstrictors with monoamine oxidase inhibitors, tricyclic antidepressants, phenothiazines	Severe hypo- or hypertension
Local anesthetics containing vasoconstrictors and oxytocic drugs	Excess hypertensive response
Local anesthetics containing vasoconstrictors and chloroform, halothane, cyclopropane, trichloroethylene	↑ Chance of cardiac arrhythmias

Administration/ Storage
1. Do not use preparations of local anesthetics containing preservatives for spinal or epidural anesthesia.
2. Store local anesthetics containing *epinephrine* separately from those which do not.
3. Store local anesthetics containing *preservatives* separately from those which do not.
4. Clearly mark each container indicating exactly which local anesthetics are stored in the compartment.
5. Autoclave vials of anesthetics, which are not destroyed by heat for sterile handling.
6. Use antiseptic or detergent with dye as a solution in which to store

anesthetics that cannot be autoclaved but which must be sterile and ready for use. The dye will indicate if there is a crack in the vial and if the sterilizing solution is seeping into the anesthetic.

7. Read label three times to ascertain that the correct local anesthetic is being prepared or provided to the doctor for administration.

8. Discard preparations without preservatives following initial use.

9. *Do not use epinephrine* in nerve block of digits in which blood supply can be compromised and tissue damage result.

Nursing Implications

1. Have resuscitative equipment and drugs available whenever local anesthetics are used.

2. Remember patient is awake when local anesthesia is used. Minimize anxiety provoking noise and conversation.

3. Assess patient for CNS excitation symptoms, such as nervousness, dizziness, blurred vision, and tremors and for depression symptoms, such as drowsiness, respiratory distress, convulsions, and unconsciousness. The initial symptoms may be depressive.

4. Have available for treatment of patient with convulsions ultra-

TABLE 18 LOCAL ANESTHETICS

Generic Name (Trade Name)	Duration of Action	Indications
Benoxinate HCl (Dorsacaine HCl)		*Ophthalmology:* Anesthesia, Removal of foreign bodies, Tonometry (0.4% solution).
Benzocaine (Aerocaine, Aerocaine-5, Anbesol, Americaine, B-B, Ben-Caine, Benzocol, Col-Vi-Nol, Hurricaine, Morusan, Solarcaine, Urolocaine, Burntame, Ora-Jel)		*Topical:* Anesthetic for skin disorders (0.5%–6.37% as aerosol, cream, liquid, lotion, ointment, spray). *Mucous Membrane Anesthesia:* dental procedure (22%); toothache (7.5%); Anesthetic for pharyngeal and nasal catheters and airways, naso-gastric or endoscopic tubes, urinary catheters, laryngoscopes, proctoscopes, sigmoidscopes, vaginal specula (all 10%–20% as gel or liquid).
Bupivacaine HCl (Marcaine HCl)	4–5 hr	Local infiltration, caudal block, peripheral block, sympathetic block (all 0.25% or 0.5%); epidural block (0.25%–0.75%).
Butamben Picrate (Butesin Picrate)		*Topical:* Anesthetic for skin disorders (1% ointment).
Chlorprocaine HCl (Nescaine, Nescaine-CE)	1 hr	Infiltration and nerve block (1%–2%); Caudal and epidural block (2%–3%).

TABLE 18 LOCAL ANESTHETICS (*Continued*)

Generic Name (Trade Name)	Duration of Action	Indications
Cocaine		*Mucous Membrane Anesthesia:* nose, throat, ear, rectum, vagina (all 1%–2% solution).
Cyclomethycaine Sulfate (Surfacaine)		*Topical:* Anesthetic for skin disorders (0.5% cream or 1% ointment). *Mucous Membrane Anesthesia:* mouth, respiratory tract, or urethra prior to endoscopy (0.5%–1% solution); Pain associated with oral or ano-genital lesions (0.5% solution).
Dibucaine HCl (Nupercaine, Nupercainal)	3 hr	Isobaric spinal anesthesia (1 : 200); Hypobaric spinal anesthesia (1 : 1500); Low spinal anesthesia (2.5 mg with 5% dextrose); *Topical:* for skin disorders (0.25%–1% as cream, ointment, spray).
Dimethisoquin HCl (Quotane)		*Topical:* anesthetic for skin disorders (0.5% cream or 1% ointment).
Diperodon (Diothane)		*Topical:* anesthetic for skin disorders (1% ointment).
Dyclonine HCl (Dyclone)		*Mucous Membrane Anesthesia:* mouth, respiratory tract or urethra prior to endoscopy (all 0.5%–1% solution); pain associated with oral or anogenital lesions (0.5% solution).
Etidocaine HCl (Duranest)	5–10 hr	Percutaneous infiltration (0.5%), Peripheral nerve block (0.5%–1%), Central nerve block (0.5%–1.5%), Caudal block (0.5%–1%).
Hexylcaine HCl (Cyclaine)		*Mucous Membrane Anesthesia:* respiratory, upper GI, or urinary tracts (5% solution).
Lidocaine HCL (Anestacon, Dilocaine, Dolicaine, L-Caine, L-Caine E, Lida-Mantle, Nervocaine, Nulicaine, Octocaine, Ultracaine, Xylocaine, Xylocaine Viscous)	1–1½ hr	Infiltration (0.5%–2%); Peripheral nerve block (1%–2%); Sympathetic nerve block (cervical or lumbar, 1%); Central nerve block, epidural: thoracic (1%) or lumbar (1%–2%); Caudal block (1%–1.5%); Spinal anesthesia (5% with glucose); Low spinal anesthesia (1.5% with dextrose). *Mucous Membrane*

TABLE 18   LOCAL ANESTHETICS (*Continued*)

Generic Name (*Trade Name*)	Duration of Action	*Indications*
		Anesthesia: oral and nasal cavities, endotracheal intubation, urethritis, for urethral procedures (all 2%–5% as jelly, ointment, solution). *Topical:* anesthetic for skin disorders (2.5%–5% as cream or ointment)
Mepivacaine HCl (Carbocaine, Isocaine)	2–2½ hr	Nerve block (1%–2%); Transvaginal block (1%) Paracervical block (Obstetrics, 1%); Caudal and Epidural (1%–2%); Infiltration (0.5%–1%); Management of pain (1%–2%); Dental (infiltration or nerve block 3%).
Piperocaine HCl (Metycaine)	1–2 hr	Infiltration (0.5%–1%); Nerve block (0.5–2%) *Ophthalmology:* with merthiolate for infections of cornea or conjunctiva (ointment).
Pramoxine HCl (Tronothane)		*Topical:* anesthetic for skin disorders (1% cream or jelly)
Prilocaine HCl (Citanest)	2–2½ hr	Infiltration (1%–2%); Peripheral nerve block: intercostal or paravertebral (1%–2%), brachial plexus or sciatic/femoral (2%–3%); Central nerve block: epidural or caudal (1%–3%); Dental (4%).
Procaine HCl (Anduracaine, Anuject, Durathesia, Novocain)	1 hr	Infiltration (0.25%–0.5%); Nerve block (1%–2%); Spinal anesthesia (10%); Rectal in proctology (1.25%–1.5%).
Proparacaine HCl (Alcaine, Ophthetic, Ophthaine)		*Ophthalmology:* Anesthesia for cataract removal, Removal of foreign bodies or sutures, Tonometry (all 0.5% solution)
Tetracaine HCl (Anacel, Pontocaine, Pontocaine Eye)	Up to 3 hr	Spinal anesthesia (0.5%–2%). *Topical:* for skin disorders (0.5% ointment or 1% cream). *Ophthalmology:* Anesthesia, Removal of foreign bodies, Tonometry (all: 0.5% ointment, 1–2 drops of 0.5% solution). *Mucous Membrane Anesthesia:* nose or throat in preparation for bronchoscopy or other procedures (2% solution).

short-acting barbiturates (i.e., thiopental, thiamylal) or short-acting barbiturates (i.e., secobarbital, pentobarbital). Since CNS depressants should not be administered when cardiac or respiratory depression is present, have available a short-acting muscle relaxant (succinylcholine) to administer IV.

5. Assess patient for depressant cardiovascular reactions characterized by hypotension (monitor BP), myocardial depression, bradycardia (monitor pulse), and possibly cardiac arrest (assess BP, PR, EKG monitor, and appearance of patient).
6. Have available for treatment of patient with cardiovascular reaction vasopressors (i.e., ephedrine, metaraminol) and IV fluids. *Do not administer epinephrine* when patient is anoxic, because ventricular fibrillation may occur.
7. Support respiratory efforts by maintaining a patent airway and supplying oxygen by assisted or controlled ventilation methods.
8. Assess patient for allergic reactions characterized by cutaneous lesions, urticaria, edema, or anaphylaxis.
9. Have available for treatment of patient with allergic reaction oxygen, epinephrine, corticosteroids, and antihistamines.
10. Assess for local reactions characterized by burning, tenderness, swelling, tissue irritation, sloughing, and tissue necrosis. Report immediately and implement appropriate therapy ordered.

Additional Nursing Implications

Administration of Anesthetic Eye Drops
1. Administer as noted on page 13 (Part One, Division D).
2. Do not allow dropper to come into contact with eyelid and surrounding tissue during administration.
3. Administer precisely the number of drops ordered since excess dosage causes serious side effects and retards wound healing in surgical conditions of the eye.
4. Rinse tonometer (instrument used for measuring intraocular pressure) with sterile distilled water prior to use to avoid introducing foreign bodies into the anesthetized eye.
5. Protect eye from irritating chemicals, foreign bodies, and rubbing of eye while eye is anesthetized. Cover eye with a patch following procedure because blink reflex is temporarily absent.
6. Teach patient:
   a. Not to touch or rub anesthetized eye.
   b. Not to touch eyelid and surrounding tissue with dropper when self-administering medication.
   c. To use medication sparingly, as ordered.

Administration of Anesthetic to Nasopharynx
Advise patient not to eat food or drink fluids for at least one hour following use of topical anesthetic, as the second stage (pharyngeal) of swallowing is interfered with and aspiration may occur.

Administration of Anesthetic to Rectum and Anus
1. Teach patient to use the lowest possible dose to minimize systemic toxicity.
2. Examine anal area for break in skin, if patient complains of burning on administration.

Administration of Anesthetic by Nerve Block

Oral Cavity Block (1) Advise patient not to eat food for at least 1 hour after injection, because swallowing reflex is depressed. Aspiration and loss of sensation in tongue may result in injury during chewing. (2) Observe for swelling of lips and oral tissue, which may necessitate use of cold compresses.

Epidural Block (1) Assess for diminished cardiac and respiratory function, which may result inadvertently from the anesthesia itself. (2) Monitor pulse, BP, and skin color. (3) Constantly monitor the progress of labor because patient will have diminished sensation of contractions. (4) Palpate bladder for urinary retention. Catheterization may be indicated. (5) Check for fecal incontinence and cleanse perineal area as necessary while patient is in labor.

Paracervical Block Monitor fetal heart closely, preferably with a fetal monitor because local anesthesia by paracervical block may cause fetal bradycardia and acidosis.

Spinal Anesthesia (1) Maintain patient flat in bed supine for 8 hours after anesthesia to reduce occurrence of headache. (2) Apply ice bag to head if headache occurs. (3) Protect patient from burns because patient's bodily sensations are absent. (4) Chart when motion and sensation are recovered. When patient can move toes, sensation is completely recovered. (5) Provide analgesics and sedatives ordered as needed. (6) Hydrate adequately to prevent hypotension. (7) Assist in exercising lower limbs to prevent thrombophlebitis.

GENERAL ANESTHETICS

The objectives of general anesthesia are to produce: (1) a state of unconsciousness and amnesia, (2) analgesia, (3) hyporeflexia, and (4) skeletal muscle relaxation.

There are two types of general anesthetics: inhalation anesthetics that include gases, such as nitrous oxide and cyclopropane, and highly volatile liquids, such as halothane, methoxyflurane, and ether; and intravenous, or fixed-dose anesthetics. This group includes the ultra short-acting barbiturates, such as methohexital and thiopental.

Since general anesthetics should be used only by those with specialized training and experience, only general information on special uses, advantages, and disadvantages of general anesthetics currently in use will be presented. Since the nurse is largely responsible for patient care after anesthesia, extensive nursing implications have been included.

Nursing Implications

1. Obtain a complete report (diagnosis, surgery, or procedure done, anesthetic administered, and time of administration, response to surgery anesthetic, current condition, and level of consciousness) prior to accepting responsibility for patient from the anesthetist.
2. Assess for adequate airway. Attach a ventilator, with the assistance

TABLE 19   GENERAL ANESTHETICS

Generic/ Trade Name	Special Use	Advantages	Disadvantages	Additional Nursing Implications
		Volatile Liquids		
Diethyl ether	Rarely used drug	With overdose respiration stops before heart; reversible with artificial respiration Inexpensive, safe	Slow, unpleasant induction and recovery Irritation of mucous membranes Explosive Causes nausea and vomiting	
Enflurane (Ethrane)		Induction and recovery are rapid Does not stimulate salivation, bronchial secretion, or affect bronchomotor tone Usually provides sufficient muscle relaxation for abdominal surgery	As depth of anesthesia increases, hypotension increases Sensitizes myocardium to epinephrine leading to serious arrhythmias	Monitor cardiac function more closely if epinephrine is administered because arrhythmias are more likely to occur
Halothane (Fluothane)	Most widely used anesthetic	Rapid, pleasant induction and recovery Little nausea/vomiting Nonexplosive Not an irritant and thus no increase in secretions	Hypoxia, acidosis, or apnea may occur during deep anesthesia Sensitizes heart to epinephrine with possible serious arrhythmias Has been said to cause hepatic damage with repeated doses Produces only moderate muscle relaxation May produce hypotension	Have available methylphenidate (Ritalin) to combat shivering which occurs frequently at recovery and is caused by neurological response rather than by loss of body heat. Monitor cardiac function more closely if epinephrine is administered concurrently because of increased likelihood of arrhythmias
Methoxyflurane (Penthrane)	May be combined with nitrous oxide for surgery expected to	Analgesia and drowsiness persist so need for narcotics in immediate	Induction and recovery are slow Does not produce	Have available methylphenidate (Ritalin) to combat shivering which tends

Drug	Uses	Advantages	Disadvantages	Nursing implications
	last 4 hr or less. Also may be used alone or in comb. with N$_2$O for analgesia in OB or minor surgery	post-op period reduced Nonexplosive	appreciable muscle relaxation when used alone	to occur in very ill patients when methoxyflurane is administered alone. Expect a prolonged recovery to consciousness and a delayed need for analgesia.
Trichloroethylene (Trilene)	Analgesia and light anesthesia—used in childbirth	Rapid induction and recovery No liver or kidney damage	Possibility of cardiac arrhythmias Causes rapid, shallow respiration	Monitor cardiac function closely for arrhythmias. Monitor for hyperventilation.
Gases				
Nitrous oxide	Used for analgesia Used in dentistry	Rapid, pleasant induction and recovery Non-explosive gas	With 100% gas which is necessary for anesthesia, hypoxia and anoxia occur; with 80% gas + 20% oxygen, get good analgesia but poor anesthesia Does not cause skeletal muscle relaxation	
Cyclopropane	Induction of anesthesia	Induction is rapid Skeletal muscle relaxation in full anesthetic doses	Sensitizes heart to epinephrine leading to arrhythmias Difficult to detect planes of anesthesia May produce laryngospasms Postanesthetic nausea, vomiting, and headache are frequent Cyclopropane/oxygen mixtures are explosive	Monitor cardiac function more closely if epinephrine is administered because arrhythmias are more likely to be precipitated
Ethylene		Rapid onset and recovery Little bronchospasms and laryngospasms; little post-anesthetic vomiting Nontoxic	Adequate analgesia but poor muscle relaxant properties Must be administered in high concentrations (80%) with oxygen (20%) Hypoxia can occur	

(Continued)

TABLE 19 GENERAL ANESTHETICS (*Continued*)

Generic/ Trade Name	Special Use	Advantages	Disadvantages	Additional Nursing Implications
		Miscellaneous		
Innovar	A combination of a narcotic analgesic (fentanyl) and an antipsychotic (droperidol)	Produces general quiescence, reduced motor activity, and excellent analgesia; complete loss of consciousness usually does not occur Used to produce tranquilization and analgesia for surgical or diagnostic procedures or for anesthetic premedication		Observe closely for hypoventilation during immediate post recovery phase since patient may have to be encouraged to breathe. Anticipate that postoperative narcotic orders will be reduced to ⅓ to ¼ of the usual dose because Innovar contains a narcotic and an antipsychotic agent.
Ketamine (Ketalar)	In children for analgesia during painful procedures—burns, cystoscopy	Rapid acting; procedures good analgesia No effect on pharyngeal-laryngeal reflexes Used to supplement low-potency agents as nitrous oxide	Cardiovascular and respiratory stimulation Inadequate skeletal muscle relaxation In adults—vivid, unpleasant dreams during recovery	To prevent dreams likely to occur with ketamine: Place patient in a quiet area after anesthesia. Do not disturb during emergence phase. Take vital signs gently. Avoid making noises, bumping bed, or vigorously rousing patient. Anticipate that a low dose of a barbiturate sedative may be required if patient is excessively active during recovery phase.

of the anesthetist, if the endotracheal tube is still in place and adjust it as ordered to maintain adequate ventilation.

3. Keep patient on side at least until conscious, unless contraindicated, to prevent aspiration of vomitus.

4. Note excessive mucus in nasopharynx and oral cavity and suction as needed.

5. Monitor BP, pulse, respiration, and patient's appearance as ordered. Assessments usually may be decreased in frequency as vital signs are stabilized.

6. Note which anesthetic the patient received and whether a short or long recovery to consciousness is anticipated. Plan care accordingly.

7. Monitor parameters by CVP, arterial pressures, cardiac monitor, and urinary drainage as ordered.

8. Remember that the first sense to return is hearing and that anxiety provoking noise or conversation should be minimized. Orientation and positive encouragement should be provided by the nurse.

9. Help patient reestablish normal physiologic balance with the least anxiety possible.

10. Administer analgesic ordered if patient complains of pain after exhalation of anesthetic.

11. Assess patient experiencing hypotension and pain, because the pain may, in fact, cause the hypotension. Report assessment to doctor and determine with him/her whether analgesia should be administered though patient is hypotensive.

12. Cover patient adequately to prevent vasodilation and subsequent heat loss, which tends to occur after administration of anesthetic agents.

13. Note that temperature is not a reliable vital sign for 1 or 2 hours after surgery because the patient is adjusting to different environmental conditions.

14. Refer to Medical-Surgical Nursing text for complete care of the postoperative patient.

15. *Prevent Fire and Explosive Hazards.* Follow the protocols for preventing fire and explosive hazard associated with general anesthesia in the institution in which it is administered.

a. Learn which gases are explosive.

b. Avoid using explosive gases when electrocautery and electric dessication are to be used.

c. Wear conductive shoes or boots.

d. Do not wear nylon uniforms where anesthetic gases may be used.

e. Do not use wool blankets in area.

f. Ascertain that all electrical equipment used is adequately grounded.

g. Check with anesthesiologist before activating any electrical equipment in the operating room.

h. Matches are not to be used in the operating room.

CHAPTER 6

DRUGS AFFECTING THE AUTONOMIC NERVOUS SYSTEM

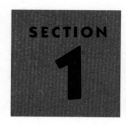

introduction: the autonomic nervous system

The system that automatically regulates the basic physiological functions of the body is called the autonomic, involuntary, or visceral nervous system (ANS).

Among the important functions regulated by the ANS are respiration, perspiration, body temperature, carbohydrate metabolism, digestion, bowel motility, pupil size, blood pressure, heart rate, and glandular secretions such as salivation.

The ANS is a composite of two opposing subsystems—the sympathetic and the parasympathetic divisions—that interact with one another to maintain the body in physiological equilibrium. Even though it is difficult to separate the exact functions of the sympathetic and the parasympathetic system, since both play a role in all major physiological processes, the sympathetic system is more closely associated with the quick regulation of the expenditure of energy during emergencies (fight or flight response), whereas the parasympathetic system is more directly involved in the storage and conservation of energy (e.g., digestion and absorption of food).

The manner in which the two divisions of the ANS work together can best be illustrated by looking at a major organ like the heart. Impulses transmitted via the *sympathetic* division will have a tendency to *increase* the heart rate, the contractibility of the muscle, and the speed at which the impulse is transmitted. The *parasympathetic* system will *decrease* the rate of contractibility and conduction.

Normally the two divisions of the ANS are in balance. In an emergency situation, however, when there is an increased need for rapidly circulating blood, the sympathetic system dominates. Impulses are sent that increase the rate of the heart. Blood pressure rises. The small arterioles that supply the skin and outlying parts of the body constrict, and blood supply to the GI tract decreases. When the situation returns to normal the parasympathetic division returns the body to more normal housekeeping functions.

Each nerve pathway in the ANS is composed of two nerve cells. The preganglionic cell is located in the spinal cord, and the axon of this cell (preganglionic fiber) travels to a nerve cell outside the cord where there is a neurojunction or synapse. This nerve cell outside the cord is in a nerve ganglion and the neurojunction is the ganglionic synapse. Most of the sympathetic ganglia are located in the paravertebral ganglionic chain. The parasympathetic ganglia are located near the effector organ. The axon of the ganglionic cell (postganglionic fiber) then travels to the effector organ where there is a second synapse at the organ or effector structure. The nerve impulses at the ganglia and effector organ synapses are transmitted by means of chemical *mediators* or *neurohormones*.

When a nerve impulse reaches any of these synapses, it releases the chemical mediator, a neurohormone, from special storage sites in the nerve terminal. The chemical mediator flows across the synapse and combines with a part of the cell called a receptor site. This then initiates a specific response of the effector organ. Once this is accomplished (the entire sequence of events is almost instantaneous), the remaining hormone is either destroyed by a specific enzyme or taken back up into the special storage sites of the cell. Also, a small amount of the hormone is carried away in the blood. Then the entire system is ready to respond again.

Three neurohormones are presently known to transmit the nerve impulse at the synapses of the ANS: *acetylcholine, epinephrine* (also known as adrenalin, which is also found in the adrenal gland) and *norepinephrine* (noradrenaline).

Acetylcholine is found at both *synapses* (preganglionic and postganglionic) of the *parasympathetic* nervous system as well as the ganglionic synapses of the sympathetic nervous system. Drugs whose actions reinforce or mimic acetylcholine are called cholinergic, or parasympathomimetic. Furthermore, drugs which act at the junction of the post ganglionic fiber and effector organ are called "muscarinic," while drugs which act at the ganglia are called "nicotinic."

Norepinephrine and/or epinephrine (adrenalin) are the chemical mediators at the postganglionic sympathetic nerve endings (junction at the effector organ). Norepinephrine combines with sites called *alpha* receptors. Epinephrine combines with *alpha-* and *beta*-receptors. In the heart both norepinephrine and epinephrine combine with *beta* receptor sites. Drugs whose actions reinforces or mimic these chemical mediators are called adrenergic or sympathomimetic.

Drugs which interfere with the enzymes that destroy the excess neurohormone after it is released from its storage vessels also increase the effectiveness of the neurohormones. Such drugs are also called *cholinergic* or *adrenergic*.

The other types of drugs that act on the ANS interfere with or block ANS nerve transmission. They are referred to as cholinergic blocking agents (*parasympatholytic*) and adrenergic blocking agents (*sympatholytic*).

From an anatomical point of view, the sweat glands and some of the salivary glands belong to the sympathetic system. However, since acetylcholine is found at both their neurojunctions, they respond to some of the drugs effective for the parasympathetic system.

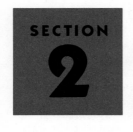

adrenergic (sympathomimetic) drugs

Dobutamine Hydrochloride
Dopamine Hydrochloride
Ephedrine
Ephedrine Sulfate
Epinephrine
Epinephrine Bitartrate
Epinephrine Borate
Epinephrine Hydrochloride
Ethylnorepinephrine Hydrochloride
Hydroxyamphetamine Hydrobromide
Isoetharine Hydrochloride
Isoetharine Mesylate
Isoproterenol Hydrochloride

Isoproterenol Sulfate
Levarterenol Bitartrate
Mephentermine Sulfate
Metaproterenol Sulfate
Metaraminol Bitartrate
Methoxamine Hydrochloride
Methoxyphenamine Hydrochloride
Nylidrin Hydrochloride
Phenylephrine Hydrochloride
Phenylpropanolamine Hydrochloride
Protokylol Hydrochloride
Pseudoephedrine Hydrochloride
Terbutaline Sulfate

Theophylline Derivatives

Aminophylline
Dyphylline
Oxtriphylline

Theophylline
Theophylline Monoethanolamine
Theophylline Sodium Glycinate

Nasal Decongestants

Epinephrine Hydrochloride
Ephedrine Sulfate
Naphazoline Hydrochloride
Oxymetazoline Hydrochloride
Phenylephrine Hydrochloride
Methyl Hexan Amine

Propylhexedrine
Tetrahydrozoline Hydrochloride
Tuaminoheptane
Tuaminoheptane Sulfate
Xylometazoline Hydrochloride

General Statement

These drugs supplement, mimic, and reinforce the messages transmitted by the natural neurohormone (norepinephrine) that transmits nerve impulses at the postganglionic neurojunctions of the sympathetic nervous system. They also mimic the effects of epinephrine (adrenalin) produced by the adrenal gland. Epinephrine increases blood pressure, stimulates the heart muscles, increases oxygen consumption, and reduces peripheral circulation. The word "adrenergic" is derived from adrenalin.

The adrenergic drugs work in two ways: (1) by acting like the natural neurohormones—norepinephrine, epinephrine; (2) by causing the release of additional amounts of the natural neurohormones from their storage sites at the proximal (near) end of the nerve terminals. Some drugs exhibit a combination of effects 1 and 2.

The distal (far) end of the neurojunction is equipped with special receptors for the neurohormones. These receptors have been classified into two types: α (alpha) and β (beta) according to whether they respond to norepinephrine, epinephrine, or isoproterenol and to certain blocking agents. Alpha adrenergic receptors are blocked by phenoxybenzamine and phentolamine whereas beta adrenergic receptors are blocked by propranolol. Certain adrenergic drugs stimulate both alpha and beta receptors; however, most have a greater affinity for one or the other.

The adrenergic drugs affect the cardiac muscle in the heart and the smooth muscle that controls the tone (elasticity) of the blood vessels.

The drugs also affect the muscles surrounding the bronchi, the gut, the sphincter of the genitourinary tract, the exocrine glands, the salivary glands, the ocular musculature, and the CNS system.

There is a considerable difference in the specific pharmacologic action of the adrenergic drugs, and there is some difficulty in balancing the desirable therapeutic effect and the undesirable side effects.

Before considering the specific effects of each drug, examine Table 20, page 467, to get an overview of the general physiological effects of the adrenergic drugs.

Contraindications Angina pectoris, hypertension, hyperthyroidism, tachycardia, psychoneuroses, nervous and hyperexcitability states. Use with caution in the presence of heart disease and obstructions of the urinary tract.

Untoward Reactions Cerebral hemorrhage, cardiac arrhythmias, palpitations, precordial pain. CNS (not all adrenergic drugs affect CNS): excess stimulation, insomnia, throbbing headache, nervousness, palpitations, vertigo, sweating, nausea, restlessness, tremor, weakness, dizziness, pallor, respiratory difficulties. Also difficulties in urinating, urinary retention.

Drug Interactions

Interactant	Interaction
Beta-adrenergic blocking agents	Inhibit adrenergic stimulation of the heart and bronchial tree. Cause bronchial constriction; asthma, not relieved by adrenergic agents
Anesthetics	Halogenated anesthetics sensitize heart to adrenergics—causes cardiac arrhythmias
Anticholinergics	Concomitant use aggravates glaucoma
Antidiabetics	Hyperglycemic effect of epinephrine may necessitate ↑ in dosage of insulin or oral hypoglycemic agents
Corticosteroids	Used chronically with sympathomimetics may result in or aggravate glaucoma; aerosols containing sympathomimetics and corticosteroids may be lethal in asthmatic children
Digitalis glycosides	Combination may cause cardiac arrhythmias

MAO inhibitors
  Pargyline (Eutonyl)
  Tranylcypromine
  (Parnate)
	All effects of monoamine oxidase inhibitors are potentiated. Symptoms include hypertensive crisis with possible intracranial hemorrhage, hyperthermia, convulsions, coma. Death may occur

Drug Interactions (*Continued*)

Interactant	*Interaction*
Methylphenidate	Potentiates pressor effect of sympathomimetics; combination hazardous in glaucoma
Oxytocics	↑ Chance of severe hypertension
Trycyclic antidepressants	Potentiation of pressor response of sympathomimetics

Nursing Implications

1. Plan to have patients receiving IV administration of adrenergic drugs constantly attended and closely monitored for BP and pulse.
2. Discard colored solutions.
3. Do not administer maintenance doses of these drugs at bedtime because they may cause insomnia.
4. Teach patient on maintenance doses and responsible family member the untoward side effects of drugs and the need to report these to physician should they occur.
5. Caution the patient on maintenance dose and a responsible family member not to increase or administer the medication more frequently. If symptoms become more severe, consult the physician.

Special Nursing Implications for Adrenergic Bronchodilators

See Administration by Inhalation—Part One, Division D.

1. Monitor BP before and after patient uses bronchodilator for the first time to evaluate cardiac response.
2. Continue to provide oxygen mixture and ventilating assistance for patients with status asthmaticus and abnormal blood gases, even though symptoms appear relieved by bronchodilator.
3. Use the method and the amount of oxygen per minute ordered. This is based on evaluation of clinical symptomatology and blood gases of the individual patient and is geared to preventing depression of respiratory effort.
4. Further treatment with the same agent is inadvisable if 3–5 aerosol treatments within the last 6 to 12 hours have only produced minimal relief.
5. Be prepared to assist with alternative therapy, if patient's dyspnea worsens after repeated excessive use of inhalator, as paradoxical airway resistance may occur.
6. Teach patient and/or family member
   a. That a single aerosol treatment is usually enough to control an asthma attack.
   b. To contact medical supervision if the patient requires more than 3 aerosol treatments within a 24-hour period.
   c. That overuse of adrenergic bronchodilators may result in reduced effectiveness, possible paradoxical reaction, and cardiac arrest.
   d. To consult a doctor if bronchodilator causes dizziness, chest pain, or lack of therapeutic response to usual dose.
   e. To initiate inhalation therapy on arising in the morning and before meals to improve lung ventilation and to reduce fatigue that accompanies eating.
   f. That increased fluid intake is an aid in the liquefication of secretions.

TABLE 20 OVERVIEW OF EFFECTS OF ADRENERGIC DRUGS*

Action	*Therapeutic Use*
Heart Excitation resulting in increase in heart rate and force of contraction. Dilation or constriction of coronary vessels. Results in increase in stroke volume and cardiac output, strengthening of pulse	Cardiogenic shock, heart block, Stokes-Adams disease, cardiac slowing (bradycardia), resuscitation
Blood Vessels, Systemic Vasoconstriction Blood supply to abdominal viscera, cerebrum, skin, and mucosa is sharply reduced (vasoconstriction of peripheral blood circulation). Blood pressure in large vessels is increased (pressor effect) and regulated	Increase in blood pressure in drug-induced acute hypotension during anesthesia or after myocardial infarction or hemorrhage. Isoproterenol causes vasodilation of vessels in skeletal muscle accompanied by increase in cardiac output. Increased blood flow. Nasal decongestion, certain dermatoses, nose-bleeds, migraine headaches, all types allergic reaction, anaphylactic reaction
GI and Genitourinary Tracts Inhibition of glandular secretion. Constriction of sphincters. Decrease of muscle tone and motility in GI tract, urinary bladder. Increase of muscle tone and motility in ureter	To relieve spasms during ureteral and biliary colic, dysmenorrhea, and labor. Enuresis
Lungs Relaxes muscles of bronchial tree	Acute and chronic asthma, pulmonary emphysema and fibrosis, chronic bronchitis
Eyes Dilates iris, increases ocular pressure, relaxes ciliary muscle	
CNS Stimulation Excitatory action, respiratory stimulation, wakefulness	Appetite control, overdosage with CNS depressant drugs, narcolepsy
Metabolism Increase in glycogenesis (sugar metabolism). Increase in lipolysis (release of free fatty acids)	
Miscellaneous Stimulates salivary glands	
Sex Organs Ejaculation	

* Not all drugs are useful under all circumstances.

    g. To accomplish postural drainage, cough productively and clap and vibrate for good respiratory hygiene.

    h. Other adrenergic medications are not to be taken by patient, unless expressly prescribed by medical supervision.

    i. Regular consistent use of drug as ordered is essential for maximum benefit.

DOBUTAMINE HYDROCHLORIDE DOBUTREX

Classification   Adrenergic (sympathomimetic) agent, synthetic.

General Statement   Dobutamine stimulates the beta receptors of the heart, increasing cardiac function. The drug increases heart output and stroke volume and has little effect on the heart rate. Dobutamine has a rapid onset of action (1 to 2 minutes) and has a very short span of activity (half-life 2 minutes).

Uses   Short-term treatment of cardiac decompensation.

Contraindications   Idiopathic hypertrophic subaortic stenosis. Safe use during pregnancy, childhood, or following acute myocardial infarctions not established.

Untoward Reactions   Marked increase in heart rate, blood pressure, and ventricular ectopic activity. Also, nausea, headache, anginal and nonspecific chest pain, palpitations, and shortness of breath (1%–3%).

Additional Drug Interactions

Interactant	Interaction
Nitroprusside	↑ Cardiac output and ↓ pulmonary wedge pressure
Oxytocics	Severe hypertension

Dosage   **IV infusion:** *individualized,* **usual,** 2.5–10 μg/kg/minute. Sometimes up to 40 μg/kg/minute. Rate of administration and duration of therapy are determined by response of patient as determined by heart rate, presence of ectopic activity, blood pressure, and urine flow.

Administration/ Storage
1. Reconstitute solution according to direction provided by manufacturer. Dilution process takes place in two stages.
2. The more concentrated solution may be stored in refrigerator for 48 hours and at room temperature for 6 hours.
3. Before administration, the solution is diluted further according to the fluid needs of patient. This more dilute solution should be used within 24 hours.
4. Dilute solutions of dobutamine may darken. This does not affect the potency of the drug when used within the time spans detailed above.
5. The drug is incompatible with alkaline solutions.

Nursing Implications
1. Monitor ECG and BP continuously during administration.
2. Be prepared to monitor central venous pressure to assess vascular volume and efficiency of cardiac pumping of the right side of the heart. The normal range is 5 to 8 mm H_2O. An elevated CVP is indicative of disruption in cardiac output as in pump failure or pulmonary edema. A low CVP is indicative of hypovolemia.
3. Be prepared to monitor pulmonary artery wedge pressure to determine the pressure in the left atrium and left ventricle and measure efficiency of cardiac output. The mean pressure ranges between 4–12 mm Hg.
4. Have IV equipment readily available to infuse volume expanders before therapy with dobutamine hydrochloride is initiated.
5. Report overdosage as evidenced by excessive alteration of BP or tachycardia and be prepared to reduce rate of administration or temporarily discontinue.
6. Monitor intake and output.

DOPAMINE HYDROCHLORIDE INTROPIN

Classification Adrenergic (sympathomimetic) agent.

General Statement This natural biological substance (a catecholamine) is the immediate precursor of norepinephrine in the body. The effect of exogenously administered dopamine is short-lived. Its onset of action is rapid (5 minutes) and its lasts for 10 minutes. It is not effective orally.

The drug acts mostly on the adrenergic receptors of the sympathetic nervous system. It also seems to release norepinephrine from its storage sites. In pharmacologic terms the drug augments the cardiac output by increasing myocardial contractibility and stroke volume. Dopamine usually has little effect on blood pressure. It induces fewer cardiac arrhythmias than isoproterenol. Dopamine also increases renal blood flow, promotes sodium excretion, and causes peripheral vasoconstriction.

Uses Cardiogenic shock, especially in myocardial infarctions associated with severe congestive heart failure. Also shock associated with trauma, septicemia, open heart surgery, renal failure and congestive heart failure. Especially suitable for patients who react adversely to isoproterenol.

Additional Contraindications Pheochromocytoma, uncorrected tachycardia or arrhythmias. Pediatric patients.

Additional Untoward Reactions Ectopic heart beats, tachycardia, anginal pain, palpitations, vasoconstriction, hypotension, dyspnea, nausea, vomiting, and headache.
Overdosage causes hypertension and decreased urinary output.

Additional Drug Interactions

Interactant	Interaction

MAO inhibitors
  Pargyline (Eutonyl)
  Tranylcypromine (Parnate)
	MAO inhibitors potentiate dopamine. Adjust dosage of dopamine if MAO inhibitors were taken during 2–3 weeks prior to initiation of dopamine therapy

Oxytocin	Severe hypertension; possibility of stroke
Phenytoin	Hypotension and bradycardia
Propranolol	↓ Effect of dopamine

Dosage

IV infusion: 1–5 μg/kg/minute. Severely ill patients can receive more (up to 50 μg/kg/minute.)

Administration/ Storage

1. Follow directions for dilution on package insert.
2. Diluted solution stable for 24 hours.
3. In order not to overload system with excess fluid, patients receiving high doses of dopamine may receive more concentrated solutions than average. Be prepared to make such adjustment when so instructed by physician.
4. Protect dopamine from light.

Additional Nursing Implications

1. Monitor BP, ECG, cup and pulmonary wedge pressure, and urine flow of patients receiving dopamine very closely. Report changes to physician.
2. Be prepared to adjust rate of flow of infusion.
3. Check infusion frequently for extravasation.

EPHEDRINE I-SEDRIN PLAIN

EPHEDRINE SULFATE BOFEDROL, ECTASULE MINUS, EPHEDSOL-1%, NASDRO, SLO-FEDRIN

Classification

Adrenergic agent.

Remarks

More stable and longer lasting than epinephrine. This drug acts in part by releasing neurohormones from storage sites at synapses.

Uses

Asthmatic conditions (bronchodilator), angioneurotic edema, hay fever, maintenance of blood pressure during spinal anesthesia, control of postural hypotension, including after heart block, overdosage with CNS depressants, enuresis, narcolepsy, carotid sinus syncope, myasthenia gravis, nasal decongestion (may also be used topically for this purpose).

Drug Interactions

Interactant	Interaction
Guanethidine (Ismelin)	↓ Effect of guanethidine by displacement from its site of action
Methyldopa (Aldomet)	Effect of ephedrine ↓ in methyldopa treated patients
Reserpine	Effect of ephedrine ↓ in reserpine-treated patients

Dosage   *Bronchodilator:* **PO:** 25–50 mg q 3 to 4 hr. *Parenteral:* 25–50 mg. **Pediatric 6–12 years:** 6.25–12.5 mg q 4 to 6 hr; **2–6 years:** 0.3–0.5 mg/kg q 4 to 6 hr. *Topical:* 2–3 gtts of 1.0%–3.0% solution no more than 4 times/day. *Vasopressor,* **SC, IM, IV:** 25–50 mg. **Maximum dose** should not exceed 150 mg/24 hr.

Additional Nursing Implications

1. Take baseline BP and pulse before initiating therapy and monitor frequently until stabilized when drug is given for hypotension. During anesthesia, BP and pulse should be monitored frequently.
2. Teach the patient, when appropriate, to count radial pulse and to report elevated or irregular pulse.
3. Caution older male patient to report difficulty in voiding which may be caused by drug-induced urinary retention.
4. After prolonged usage of ephedrine, observe the patient for resistance to the drug. This may necessitate a rest period of 3 to 4 days. Patient usually will again respond to drug.

EPINEPHRINE ASMOLIN, MICRO NEFRIN, PRIMATENE MIST, SUS-PHRINE

EPINEPHRINE BITARTRATE BRONITIN MIST, MEDIHALER-EPI, EPITRATE, LYOPHRIN, MUROCOLL, MYTRATE OPHTHALMIC SOLUTIONS

EPINEPHRINE BORATE EPINAL AND EPPY OPHTHALMIC SOLUTIONS

EPINEPHRINE HYDROCHLORIDE ADRENALINE CHLORIDE, EPIFRIN, GLAUCON, VAPONEFRIN

Classification   Adrenergic agent.

Remarks   The neurohormone epinephrine, a catecholamine, is the active principle of the adrenal medulla. Both synthetic epinephrine and epinephrine isolated from animal adrenal glands can be used for therapeutic purposes. Epinephrine has an exceedingly rapid onset of action (onset 3–10 minutes; maximum effect 20 minutes) when administered parenterally, intranasally, or by inhalation. (The drug is ineffective when given orally.)

The drug acts directly on both alpha and beta receptors, and its effect resembles stimulation of the sympathetic nervous system (see p. 464 and 465). Epinephrine is a widely used therapeutic agent as a sympathomimetic, pressor agent, cardiac stimulant, bronchodilator, decongestant, and for the treatment of shock and glaucoma. Extreme caution must be taken *Never to Inject* 1:100 solution for inhalation; accidental injection of this concentration has caused death.

Laboratory Test Interferences   False + or ↑ BUN, fasting glucose, lactic acid, urinary catecholamines, glucose (Benedict's), ↓ in coagulation time. The drug may affect electrolyte balance.

Dosage   Epinephrine injection is a premixed 1 : 1,000 (0.1%) sterile solution of epinephrine hydrochloride. *Bronchial asthma,* **SC, adult:** 0.2– 1.0 mg; **pediatric:** 0.01 mg/kg or 0.3 mg/m² to a maximum of 0.5 mg. Repeat q 4 hr. *Vasopressor;* **IM, SC:** 0.2– 1.0 ml of 1 : 1,000 solution. *Cardiac Resuscitation,* **IV:** 0.1– 0.4 mg; *intracardiac,* 0.1– 0.2 mg. *Use with local anesthetic:* 1 : 20,000 to 1 : 100,000. *Inhalation:* Aqueous solution is administered from nebulizer with least number of inhalations that produce relief. *Mucosal Decongestant:* 1– 2 drops of 0.1% solution in nose q 4 to 6 hr. **Not used in children under 6 years of age.** *Glaucoma:* 1 drop of 0.25%– 2.0% solution in each eye.

Overdosage is characterized by a sharp increase in systolic and diastolic blood pressure, transient bradycardia followed by tachycardia, and potentially fatal cardiac arrhythmias. Treatment is mostly supportive in view of the short duration of action of epinephrine. If necessary the pressor effects of the drug can be counteracted with trimethaphan camsylate or phentolamine.

Administration/
Storage
1. *Never administer* 1 : 100 solution IV. Utilize 1 : 1000 solution for IV administration.
2. Preferably use a tuberculin syringe to measure epinephrine as the parenteral doses are very small and the drug is very potent. An error in measurement may be disastrous.
3. Administer epinephrine IV by a double bottle setup so that rate of administration may be easily adjusted.
4. For IV administration to adults the drug must be well diluted as a 1 : 1,000 solution and quantities of 0.05 ml to 0.1 ml of the solution should be injected cautiously and very slowly, taking about a minute for each injection, noting the response of the patient (BP and pulse). Dose may be repeated several times if necessary.
5. Briskly massage site of SC or IM injection to hasten the action of the drug. Do not expose epinephrine to heat, light, or air as this causes deterioration of the drug.
6. Discard solutions that have a reddish-brown color.
   Discard after expiration date.

Additional
Nursing
Implications
1. For IV administration, take initial reading of BP and pulse before initiation of therapy and then monitor closely, every minute, until desired effect is achieved, then every 2 to 5 minutes until patient has stabilized and then monitor blood pressure every 15 to 30 minutes.
2. Observe and report the rate and character (regularity and force) of the pulse.
3. Plan for patient to be constantly attended while receiving epinephrine IV.
4. Observe patients for signs of shock such as cold, clammy skin, cyanosis, and loss of consciousness.
5. Be prepared to assist with the administration of IV fluids and blood to patients in hypovolemic shock.
6. Check where epinephrine and syringes are stored on the unit so that in case of emergency the drug can be readily administered.

ETHYLNOREPINEPHRINE HYDROCHLORIDE BRONKEPHRINE

Classification Adrenergic agent.

Remarks Sympathomimetic amine resembling epinephrine. Has little effect on blood pressure and may be safer than epinephrine. Especially suitable for children and diabetic asthmatics.

Use Relief of spasms in bronchial asthma especially in those who do not respond to isoproterenol or epinephrine.

Additional Contraindications Sensitivity to drug. Use with caution in cardiovascular disease.

Additional Untoward Reactions Changes in blood pressure, increased pulse rate, palpitations, dizziness, nausea.

Dosage **IM, SC:** 1–2 mg (0.5–1 ml of 0.2% solution); **pediatric:** 0.2–1 mg (0.1–0.5 ml of 0.2% solution).

HYDROXYAMPHETAMINE HYDROBROMIDE PAREDRINE

Classification Adrenergic agent.

Remarks This compound releases neurohormones from storage sites at synapses and thus stimulates alpha- and beta-receptors.

Uses Topical: ophthalmic agent (pupillary dilation).

Additional Contraindications Hypersensitivity to drug, narrow-angle glaucoma.

Additional Untoward Reactions Ventricular tachycardia and arrhythmias; increased blood pressure, palpitations, precordial pain, redness, headache, or browache. Transitory stinging on initial instillation. Conjunctival allergy.

Dosage *Pupillary dilatation:* 1–2 drops of 1% solution in each eye. Preparation contains 1 : 50,000 thimerosal.

ISOETHARINE HYDROCHLORIDE BRONKOSOL

ISOETHARINE MESYLATE BRONKOMETER

Classification Adrenergic agent—bronchodilator.

General Statement Isoetharine is a sympathomimetic, which acts preferentially on the beta-adrenergic receptors of the bronchial tree, causing relaxation and relieving bronchospasms. The drug has a rapid onset and a relatively long duration of action (4 hours).

Uses Bronchial asthma, chronic bronchitis, emphysema.

Contraindications Hypersensitivity to sympathomimetic amines. Use with caution in the presence of cardiac disease, hyperthyroidism, and hypertension.

Untoward Reactions Tachycardia, palpitations, nausea, headache, changes in blood pressure, anxiety, and other neurological manifestations.

Dosage *Bronkometer inhalation:* 1 or 2 inhalations (each metered dose contains approximately 340 μg isoetharine mesylate). Bronkosol is used in hand nebulizer (**usual dose: 4** inhalations, undiluted of 1% solution) or **oxygen aerosolization** or **IPPB** (0.25–1.0 ml of the solution—1.0% isoetharine—diluted 1 : 3 with saline or other diluent)

Administration 1. One or two inhalations are usually sufficient. Wait 1 minute following initial dose to insure necessity of another dose.
2. Treatment usually needs not be repeated more than q 4 hours. See also *Nursing Implications* for *Administration by Inhalation*, page 466.

Nursing Implications See *Nursing Implications for Adrenergic Bronchodilators*, page 466.

ISOPROTERENOL HYDROCHLORIDE IPRENOL, ISUPREL HYDROCHLORIDE, NORISODRINE AEROTROL, PROTERNOL, VAPO-ISO

ISOPROTERENOL SULFATE MEDIHALER-ISO, NORISODRINE SULFATE

Classification Adrenergic, synthetic.

General Statement The drug acts almost exclusively on beta-receptors of the sympathetic system.
    The chief effect of isoproterenol is cardiac excitation, relaxation of the muscles surrounding the bronchial tree and the GI tract. Causes decrease in blood pressure, which is unlike the increase caused by other adrenergic agents. Causes less hyperglycemia than epinephrine, but causes an equal amount of CNS excitation.
    The onset of action of the drug is rapid and varies with the route of administration: within minutes after inhalation (duration 30 to 60 minutes) or IV administration (duration 1 to 2 hours). The effect of

timed-release tablet starts within 30 minutes and lasts 6 to 8 hours. The drug is often dispensed from metered aerosol dispensers for asthma.

Uses
Bronchodilator in asthma, chronic pulmonary emphysema, bronchitis, and other conditions involving bronchospasms. Adjunct in cardiogenic and other types of shock. Adams-Stokes and carotid sinus syndrome, adjunct in anesthesia. Certain cardiac arrhythmias.

Additional Contraindications
Tachycardia, cardiac arrhythmias. Timed-release tablets are contraindicated in central hyperexcitability states, coronary sclerosis, or hypertension. Use with caution in the presence of tuberculosis, cardiovascular disease, and diabetes.

Additional Untoward Reactions
Tachycardia, palpitations, bronchial edema, bronchial inflammation, flushing of skin. Swelling of the parotid gland, which may occur after prolonged usage necessitates discontinuation of therapy. Excessive inhalation causes refractory bronchial obstruction. Sublingual administration may cause buccal ulceration. Side effects of drug are less severe after inhalation.

Additional Drug Interaction
Isoproterenol: propranolol blocks the pharmacologic effects of isoproterenol.

Dosage
Isoproterenol HCl, **Inhalation** (*Oral*): 1–2 inhalations of 0.25–1% solution. Do not exceed more than 6 inhalations/hr. *Bronchospasm;* **IV:** 0.01–0.02 mg (repeat as necessary); **sublingual:** 10–20 mg. Not to exceed 60 mg daily. **Pediatric:** not to exceed 30 mg daily; not to be used more often than q 3 to 4 hr or more than 3 times daily. *Shock:* infusion of 0.5–5.0 µg/min of 1 mg in 500 ml diluent. *Cardiac standstill/cardiac arrhythmias:* **adult, IV, initial:** 0.02–0.06 mg; **infusion** 5 µg/minute; **IM, SC:** 0.2 mg; *intracardiac;* 0.02 mg. *Heartblock/ventricular arrhythmias:* **adult, initial, sublingual,** 10 mg; **rectal,** 5 mg. **Pediatric:** Initially, one half of the adult dose. Subsequent doses in adult or children depend on response. *Isoproterenol sulfate* dispersed from metered aerosol dispensor: 70–150 µg; or one or two inhalations of 1:500 solution, up to maximum of 6 inhalations/hr.

Additional Nursing Implications
1. Observe the patient and report if respiratory problems seem worse after administration of drug. Refractory reaction may be occurring and this necessitates withdrawal of the drug.
2. Encourage the patient to rinse with water to minimize dryness after inhalation therapy.
3. Warn the patient that sputum or saliva may appear pink after inhalation therapy; this is due to the drug.
4. Advise the patient not to use inhalation therapy more frequently than prescribed because severe cardiac and respiratory problems have occurred due to excessive use.
5. Withhold drug and report parotid gland enlargment that may occur after prolonged use and necessitates stopping the drug.
6. See *Nursing Implications for Adrenergic Bronchodilators* page 466.

LEVARTERENOL BITARTRATE LEVOPHED BITARTRATE, NOREPINEPHRINE BITARTRATE

Classification	Adrenergic agent.
General Statement	Levarterenol primarily activates alpha-receptors. Drug does not affect cardiac output but increases blood pressure by vasoconstriction. Has only slight hyperglycemic effect and can be given to diabetics. Dextrose protects drug from destruction by preventing oxidation.
Uses	Maintenance of blood pressure in acute hypotensive states caused by trauma, central vasomotor depression, and myocardial infarctions.
Additional Contraindication	Do not use in conjunction with cyclopropane anesthesia because of the possibility of fatal arrhythmias.
Additional Untoward Reaction	Drug may cause bradycardia that can be abolished by atropine.
Dosage	**IV infusion only** (effect on BP determines dosage): **average,** 2–4 μg/min or 0.5–1 ml of a 0.004 mg/ml solution/minute.

Administration/ Storage

1. Discard solutions that are brown or have precipitate.
2. Do not administer through same tube as blood products.

Additional Nursing Implications

1. Take baseline reading of BP and pulse before initiation of therapy.
2. Check BP every 2 minutes from start of drug until desired level is obtained, and then every 5 minutes during administration of drug. Following administration, check BP frequently to ascertain that desired level is being maintained.
3. Check rate of flow constantly.
4. Administer levarterenol by IV using a double bottle setup so that the rate of administration may be easily adjusted.
5. Plan for patient to be constantly attended while receiving levarterenol.
6. Check frequently for extravasation as ischemia and sloughing may occur.
7. Have on hand phentolamine which may be used at site of extravasation to dilate local blood vessels.
8. Observe for blanching along the course of the vein for this would indicate permeability of the vein wall, permitting leakage that would necessitate changing site of IV.
9. Anticipate that IV will be given via a large vein preferably the antecubital and not in a limb demonstrating poor circulation.
10. Check pulse frequently for bradycardia. Have atropine on hand for treatment of bradycardia should this occur.

MEPHENTERMINE SULFATE WYAMINE SULFATE

Classification Adrenergic agent.

General Statement The observed increase in blood pressure is mainly due to an increase in cardiac output. The drug increases the peripheral resistance only slightly. CNS stimulation is very slight. Mephentermine prolongs the action of epinephrine. Onset, after IV, is immediate, and lasts 30 to 45 minutes. Onset, after IM, is 15 minutes, and lasts 1 to 2 hours.

Uses Hypotensive states after myocardial infarction, prophylactic vasopressor agent during anesthesia, nasal decongestant, extrasystoles, and conversion of flutter or fibrillation to sinus rhythm.

Additional Contraindications Do not use in shock associated with hemorrhage, concealed hemorrhage, or decrease in blood pressure due to phenothiazines.

Dosage **IV** (*preferred in shock*): 15–30 mg given slowly in 50–100 ml dextrose injection. **SC, IM:** 10–30 mg.
Preanesthetic prophylaxis; **IM:** 15–45 mg 10 minutes before anesthesia. *Postoperative hypotension and postmyocardial infarction:* 15–30 mg. Give first dose **IV**, then maintain blood pressure by **IM. Children, IV, IM:** 0.4 mg/kg.

Additional Nursing Implications Take an initial reading of BP and pulse before initiation of therapy, and then every 5 minutes until stable, and then every 15 to 30 minutes beyond the duration of the drug's action to check that BP is stabilized at a satisfactory level.

METAPROTERENOL SULFATE ALUPENT, METAPREL

Classification Adrenergic agent—bronchodilator.

General Statement This sympathomimetic resembles isoproterenol, having somewhat fewer side effects and a more prolonged duration of action. Metaproterenol stimulates the beta-adrenergic receptors of the sympathetic nervous system, causing the relaxation of smooth muscles of the bronchial tree and the peripheral vasculature. It has a very rapid onset of action: one minute after oral inhalation and 15 minutes after PO administration. Effects often persist for 4 hours or more.

Uses Bronchodilator in asthma, bronchitis, emphysema, and other conditions associated with reversible bronchospasms.

Contraindications Preexisting cardiac arrhythmias associated with tachycardia. Safe use in pregnancy not established. Use with caution in patients with hypertension, coronary artery disease, congestive heart failure, hyperthyroidism, or diabetes mellitus.

Untoward Reactions   Tachycardia, palpitations, tremor, dizziness, hypertension, nervousness, headaches, nausea, vomiting, and bad taste.

Drug Interactions   Possible potentiation of adrenergic effects if used before or after other sympathomimetic bronchodilators.

Dosage   **Inhalation** *via metered dose inhaler:* 1.30–1.95 mg (2 to 3 inhalations) of the micronized powder. A minimum of 2 minutes should elapse between inhalations, and dose should not be repeated more often than q 3 or 4 hr. **Maximum dose:** 7.8 mg (12 inhalations) in 24 hr. **Inhaler not recommended for children under 12 years of age. PO, adults:** 20 mg t.i.d. or q.i.d.; **children 6 to 9 years or less than 60 pounds:** 10 mg t.i.d. or q.i.d. **Not recommended for children under 6 years of age.**

Administration   1. Instruct patient to shake the container.
2. See *Nursing Implications for Administration by Inhalation.* p. 11

Nursing Implications   See *Nursing Implications for Adrenergic Bronchodilators.* p. 466

METARAMINOL BITARTRATE ARAMINE BITARTRATE

Classification   Adrenergic agent.

General Statement   This drug has a long duration of action. It causes peripheral vasoconstriction and cardiac stimulation. It is slower acting than levarterenol but with a "smoother" more general effect on blood pressure. IV onset: 1 to 2 minutes; IM onset: 10 minutes; SC onset: 5 to 10 minutes. Duration (all modes): 20 minutes to 1 hour.

Uses   Hypotension associated with surgery, anesthesia, hemorrhages, trauma, infections, and adverse drug reactions.

Additional Contraindication   Do not use with cyclopropane anesthesia because of the possibility of fatal arrhythmias.

Additional Drug Interaction   Concomitant use with oxytocic drugs, reserpine or guanethidine may result in hypertensive crisis.

Dosage   Whenever feasible, use test dose and determine pressor response before administering more drug. **IV infusion: (preferred for treatment of shock):** only sodium chloride injection or 5% dextrose injection should be used as a diluent. *Prevention of hypotension,* **IM SC:** 2–10 mg: **pediatric:** 0.1 mg/kg. **IV infusion:** 15–100 mg in 500 ml diluent. *Severe shock;* **IV:** 0.5–5.0 mg followed by **IV infusion.**

Administration   Do not inject IM in areas that seem to have poor circulation as sloughing has occurred with extravasation.

Additional Nursing Implications

1. Determine blood pressure before administering drug and at frequent intervals thereafter for at least 2 hours until BP is stabilized at satisfactory level.
2. Check site of IV administration frequently as extravasation followed by sloughing may occur.

METHOXAMINE HYDROCHLORIDE VASOXYL HYDROCHLORIDE

Classification   Adrenergic agent.

Remarks   This drug has no cardiac stimulant effect. The increase in blood pressure is due only to constriction of the arteries and arterioles. IV onset: immediate; duration 1 hour. IM onset: 15 minutes; duration 90 minutes.

Uses   Hypotensive states associated with surgery, anesthesia, hemorrhages, trauma, drug reactions. Myocardial shock. Prior to and after spinal anesthesia and for hypotensive surgical patients, paroxysmal supraventricular tachycardia.

Additional Untoward Reactions   Avoid overdosage, which may cause persistant elevated blood pressure and severe headaches. IV administration may cause bradycardia, pilomotor erection, headache, urinary urgency, and vomiting.

Dosage   **IM:** 10–15 mg. **IV** (*emergency*): 3–5 mg by slow injection or infusion as directed. **Pediatric; IM:** 0.25 mg/kg; **IV:** 0.08 mg/kg slowly in divided doses.

Additional Nursing Implications

1. Observe pulse closely for reduction in pulse rate as bradycardia may be an untoward effect.
2. Position comatose patient on side as vomiting may occur. Have suction available.
3. Have bedpan or urinal readily available for urinary urgency.
4. Report BP readings promptly as drug must be discontinued when desired pressor response is achieved.

METHOXYPHENAMINE HYDROCHLORIDE ORTHOXINE HYDROCHLORIDE

Classification   Adrenergic agent.

Remarks   Methoxyphenamine is similar to ephedrine. It has a long duration (3 to 4 hours) and is used for patients susceptible to pressor effects of ephedrine. PO onset: 30 minutes.

Uses Bronchodilation in asthma, allergic rhinitis, acute urticaria, and GI allergy.

Dosage **PO:** 50–100 mg q 4 to 6 hr; **pediatric:** 25–50 mg q.i.d.

NYLIDRIN HYDROCHLORIDE ARLIDIN HYDROCHLORIDE

Classification Adrenergic agent.

Remarks Nylidrin is a direct acting vasodilator affecting mostly the blood vessels of the skeletal muscles. The drug increases cardiac output. Its beneficial effects may take several weeks before becoming apparent.

Uses Intermittent claudication associated with endoarteritis obliterans, Raynaud's disease, diabetic vascular disease, thrombophlebitis, thromboangiitis (Buerger's disease), night leg cramps, and ischemic ulcers.

Additional Contraindications Use with caution in patients with myocardial lesions, thyrotoxicosis, or severe angina pectoris.

Additional Untoward Reaction Palpitations.

Dosage **PO:** 3–6 mg t.i.d.–q.i.d. May be increased to 12 mg 3 to 4 times daily.

Additional Nursing Implications
1. Be alert to complaint of palpitations because this is the chief side effect of the drug. This may require reduction in dosage if palpitations do not subside.
2. Observe for beneficial effect of the drug such as relief of pain, increase in temperature, improvement in color of affected part, and healing of tissues.
3. Encourage and support patients early during course of therapy because response to drug may take several weeks to become apparent.

PHENYLEPHRINE HYDROCHLORIDE ALCONEFRIN, ALLEREST NASAL, CORICIDIN NASAL, EFRICEL, ISOPHRIN, NEO-SYNEPHRINE HCL, OCUSOL, PREFRIN, PYRACORT-D, RHINALL, SINAREST, SINOPHEN, SUPER ANAHIST, TEAR-EFRIN, VACON

Classification Adrenergic agent.

Remarks Phenylephrine resembles epinephrine with more prolonged action and less effect on the heart.

Uses Acute hypotensive states caused by peripheral circulatory collapse; adjunct in spinal anesthesia; paroxysmal tachycardia; nasal decongestion, allergies; ophthalmologic examination (mydriasis); selected cases of glaucoma.

Additional Untoward Reactions   Overdosage may cause ventricular extrasystoles and short paroxysm or ventricular tachycardia, tingling of the extremities and a sensation of "heavy head."

Drug Interactions

Interactant	Interaction
Guanethidine (Ismelin)	↑ Response of phenylephrine in guanethidine-treated patients
Levodopa	Levodopa ↓ mydriasis following topical phenylephrine

Dosage   *Hypotension:* **IM or SC: initial,** 1–10 mg (no more than 5 mg initial). Administer as a 1% solution. **Total:** 1–10 mg (minimum interval between doses: 10 min). **Children:** 0.1 mg/kg. **IV:** 0.25–0.5 mg diluted and given slowly.
   Tachycardia: **IV,** 500 μg within 20–30 seconds in form of 0.2% solution. Adjust depending on blood pressure up to additional maximum of 200 μg.
   Shock: 100–180 drops/min of 1:50,000 solution. If no response concentration can be increased. *Nasal decongestant:* 0.25–1% solution q 3 to 4 hr; **children 6 years and older:** 0.25% q 3 to 4 hr; **infants:** 0.125%–0.2% q 2 to 4 hr. *Glaucoma:* 1 gtt of 10% solution. *Refraction of eye:* use 2.5% solution.

Administration/ Storage
1. Store drug away from light in a brown bottle.
2. Anticipate that before administering neosynephrine ophthalmic solution, a drop of local anesthetic will be necessary.

Additional Nursing Implications
1. Monitor the patient for "fullness in head" or tingling of extremities as these are untoward effects peculiar to drug and indicate overdosage.
2. Tell the patient to blow nose before administration, when drug is used as a nasal decongestant.

PHENYLPROPANOLAMINE HYDROCHLORIDE PROPADRINE HYDROCHLORIDE

Classification   Adrenergic agent.

Remarks   The drug resembles ephedrine. It affects the CNS. Often found in over-the-counter products for weight control.

Uses   Hay fever, allergic rhinitis.

Dosage   **PO:** 25 mg q 3 to 4 hr or 50 mg q 6 to 8 hr; **children 6–12 years:** 12.5 mg q 4 hr or 25 mg q 8 hr; **2–6 years:** 6.25 mg q 4 hr or 12.5 mg q 8 hr.

Additional Nursing Implication Caution older male patients to report difficulties in voiding because they are more susceptible to drug-induced urinary retention.

PROTOKYLOL HYDROCHLORIDE VENTAIRE

General Statement Protokylol resembles isoproterenol but is more effective after PO administration. It stimulates beta adrenergic receptors. The drug relaxes the smooth muscles of the bronchial tree and improves pulmonary function. Onset: PO: 30 minutes, lasting for 3 to 4 hours.

Uses Bronchodilator, bronchial asthma.

Additional Contraindications Cardiac arrhythmias, insufficient coronary circulation, pregnancy or possibility thereof. Administer with caution to patients with cardiovascular disorders, diabetes mellitus, hyperthyroidism, prostatic hypertrophy, or glaucoma.

Additional Untoward Reactions Tachycardia, palpitations, CNS stimulation (insomnia, tremulousness, tenseness, dizziness, vertigo).

Dosage *Individualized.* **PO: usual;** 2–4 mg q.i.d.; **pediatric:** 1–2 mg 3 to 4 times daily.

Additional Nursing Implications
1. Discontinue drug immediately if anginal or precordial pain occurs.
2. Do not administer in evening because it may cause insomnia.
3. Advise the patient to report rapid palpitations as they are usually dose related and may indicate need for dosage adjustment.

PSEUDOEPHEDRINE HYDROCHLORIDE D-FEDA, NEOFED, NOVAFED, PSEUDO-BID, SUDADRINE, SUDAFED, SUDECON

Classification Adrenergic agent.

General Statement This drug, like epinephrine, acts at the sympathetic nerve endings, but also acts directly on smooth muscle. It has fewer side effects than epinephrine. It can be administered systemically (PO) as a nasal decongestant, which eliminates possible damage to the nasal mucosa. It has fewer side effects than epinephrine. Antihistamines can be given concurrently.

Use with caution in hypertensive patients.

Uses Nasal congestion associated with sinus conditions, otitis, allergies. Asthma.

Dosage   **PO, adults:** 60 mg t.i.d.–q.i.d.; **pediatric 6–12 years:** 30 mg q 4 hr; **2–3 years:** 15 mg q 4 hr.

Additional Nursing Implications
1. Avoid taking drug at bedtime because it causes stimulation that may result in insomnia.
2. Observe the patient with hypertension for increase in symptoms due to elevation of BP, such as headache or dizziness. Alert the patient that these symptoms should be reported because they may be drug related.

TERBUTALINE SULFATE BRETHINE, BRICANYL SULFATE

Classification   Adrenergic agent—bronchodilator.

General Statement   This sympathomimetic drug resembles isoproterenol. Its main effect is relaxation of the muscles surrounding the bronchial tree and peripheral vasculature. The drug is rapidly effective after SC administration (15 minutes). Its effect peaks within 30 to 60 minutes and lasts for 90 minutes to 4 hours.

Uses   Bronchodilator in asthma, bronchitis, emphysema, and other conditions associated with reversible bronchospasms.

Contraindications   Hypersensitivity to sympathomimetic agents. To be used with caution in patients with diabetes mellitus, hypertension, hyperthyroidism, or cardiac disease, especially when accompanied by arrhythmias. Safe use during pregnancy or childhood not established.

Untoward Reactions   Increased heart rate, nervousness, tremors, palpitations, dizziness, and other neurologic and GI manifestations characteristic of sympathomimetic agents.

Dosage   **PO, adult:** 5 mg t.i.d. q 6 hr during waking hr, not to exceed 15 mg/24 hr. If disturbing side effects are observed, dose can be reduced to 2.5 mg t.i.d. without loss of beneficial effects. Anticipate use of other therapeutic measures, if patient fails to respond after second dose. **Children 12–15 years:** 2.5 mg t.i.d., not to exceed 7.5 mg/24 hr. **SC:** 250 μg. May be repeated 1 time after 15 to 30 minutes, if no significant clinical improvement was noted. **Pediatric** (*investigational*): 3.5–5 μg/kg. A total dose of 0.5 mg should not be exceeded in 4 hrs.

Nursing Implications   See *Nursing Implications for Adrenergic Bronchodilators.* p. 466

THEOPHYLLINE DERIVATIVES

AMINOPHYLLINE

DYPHYLLINE

OXTRIPHYLLINE

THEOPHYLLINE

THEOPHYLLINE MONOETHANOLAMINE

THEOPHYLLINE SODIUM GLYCINATE

General Statement   Theophylline, aminophylline, and other methylxanthines relax the smooth muscles of the bronchi and of the pulmonary blood vessels. They also stimulate the CNS, produce diuresis (see diuretics), and affect the myocardium. Response to the drugs is highly individualized; the rather prolonged action of the drugs (half-life 7–8 hours, 3.5 hours in children) varies from patient to patient. The drugs are excreted mostly unchanged by the kidneys.

Uses   Relief of acute bronchial asthma, reversible bronchospasms associated with chronic bronchitis, and emphysema.

Contraindications   Hypersensitivity to drug, hypotension, coronary artery disease, angina pectoris. Safe use in pregnancy has not been established. Xanthines usually are not tolerated by small children because of excessive CNS stimulation. Use with caution in the presence of peptic ulcer, acute cardiac diseases, hypoxemia, severe renal and hepatic disease, severe hypertension, severe myocardial damage, hyperthyroidism, glaucoma, the elderly, and neonates.

Untoward Reactions   GI irritation: nausea, vomiting, epigastric pain, hematemesis, diarrhea. CNS effects: irritability, restlessness, headaches, insomnia, reflex hyperexcitability, muscle twitching, convulsions, agitation. Cardiovascular effects: palpitations, sinus tachycardia, ventricular tachycardia, extra systoles, and circulatory failure. Renal: albuminuria, increased excretion of red blood cells, diuresis resulting in dehydration. Other: tachypnea, respiratory arrest, fever, hyperglycemia, and inappropriate ADH syndrome.

Rectal suppositories and enemas may cause local irritation.

Overdosage: Early signs of toxicity include anorexia, nausea, vomiting, wakefulness, restlessness, irritability. Later symptoms include agitated, manic behavior, frequent vomiting, extreme thirst, delirium, convulsions, hyperthermia, vasomotor collapse. Serious toxicity can develop without earlier signs of toxicity. Toxicity is usually associated with parenteral administration only.

Drug Interactions

Interactant	Interaction
Ephedrine and other sympathomimetics	↑ CNS stimulation
Erythromycin ⎱ Troleandomycin ⎰	↑ Action of xanthines because of reduced renal excretion

Dosage   See Table 21 below. Individualized. Initially dosage should be adjusted according to plasma level of drug. Usual: between 10–20 μg/ml plasma.

TABLE 21   THEOPHYLLINE DERIVATIVES*

Drug	Dosage	Remarks
Aminophylline (Aminodur, Lixaminol, Rectalad-Aminophylline, Somophyllin, Theophylline Ethylenediamine)	**PO:** *Acute asthmatic attacks,* **adults:** 500 mg **STAT; pediatric:** 7.5 mg/kg **STAT. Maintenance, adults:** 200–315 mg q 6–8 hr; **pediatric:** 3–6 mg/kg q 6–8 hr. **Rectal, adults:** 300 mg 1 to 3 times/day or 450 mg b.i.d.; **pediatric:** 5 mg/kg no more than q 6 hr. **IM:** 500 mg as required (painful). **IV:** Use only 25 mg/ml preparations. **Loading dose:** 5.6 mg/kg over 30 min. **Maintenance:** Up to 0.9 mg/kg/hr by infusion.	Drug of choice when one cannot differentiate between bronchospasms and pulmonary edema *Administration* Dilute in 10–20 ml diluent and inject slowly over period of 5–10 min to avoid severe hypotension. Do not give PO to children. *Additional Nursing Implications* 1. Monitor BP closely during IV administration because drug may cause a transitory lowering of BP that requires immediate dosage and flow rate adjustment. 2. Encourage administration by other than IM injection because this route is painful.
Dyphylline (Airet, Dilin, Dilor, Dyflex, Emfabid, Lufyllin, Neothylline)	**PO:** 200–400 mg q 6–8 hr; **pediatric (PO only):** 4.5–5.8 mg/kg b.i.d.–t.i.d. **IM:** 250–500 mg; repeat as necessary.	Less irritating than theophylline or aminophylline
Oxtriphylline (Choledyl)	**PO:** 200 mg t.i.d.–q.i.d.; **pediatric 2–12 years:** 3.6 mg/kg q.i.d.	Choline salt of theophylline. Less irritating than aminophylline. Preferentially give after meals and at bedtime

* Used as bronchodilators for acute bronchospasm.

(Continued)

TABLE 21   THEOPHYLLINE DERIVATIVES (*Continued*)

Drug	*Dosage*	*Remarks*
Theophylline (Aerolate, Bronkodyl, Elixophyllin, Theolair, others)	**PO:** 200–250 mg q 6 hr; **pediatric:** 100 mg q 6 hr. **Rectal:** 250–500 mg q 8–12 hr; **pediatric:** 10 mg/kg in divided doses.	
Theophylline monoethanolamine (Fleet Theophylline)	**Rectal (retention enema):** 250–500 mg q 12 hr.	*Administration* Eight hours should elapse before dose is repeated. No more than 2 doses should be given per day.
Theophylline sodium glycinate (Glynazan, Panophylline Forte, Synophylate, Theofort)	**PO:** 330–660 mg q 6 to 8 hr; **pediatric 6–12 yr:** 220–330 mg; **under 6 yr:** 18.2–36.4 mg/kg q 6–8 hr.	IV injection for emergency only. **Inject very slowly**

Nursing Implications

1. Monitor closely for clinical response and signs of toxicity.
2. Check that serum levels of theophylline are in the 10–20 μg/ml range. Levels above 20 μg/ml require dosage adjustments.
3. Teach patient to notify doctor if nausea, vomiting, GI pain, or restlessness occurs.
4. Observe small children particularly for excessive CNS stimulation because they are unable to report side effects.
5. Dilute drugs properly and maintain proper infusion rates to minimize problems of overdosage.
6. Wait to initiate oral therapy at least 4 to 6 hours after switching from IV therapy.
7. Have available a respirator, oxygen, diazepam (Valium), and IV fluids for treatment of overdosage.

NASAL DECONGESTANTS

General Statement   The most commonly used agents for relief of nasal congestion are the adrenergic drugs. They act by constricting the arterioles in the nasal mucosa and thus reduce the blood flow to the area.

Use   Symptomatic relief of acute rhinitis associated with colds or other respiratory infections, allergic rhinitis, acute and chronic sinusitis, and hay fever.

Contraindications   Hyperthyroidism, diabetes, ischemic heart disease, hypertension. Also, patients receiving MAO inhibitors may manifest hypertensive crisis following the use of oral nasal decongestants.

Untoward Reactions   Stinging and burning with mucosal dryness may be manifested following topical administration. Rebound congestion following termination of drug effects. Systemic effects due to absorption from the GI tract when excess solution trickles down the throat and is swallowed. Systemic effects include nervousness, nausea, dizziness, CNS stimulation, transient increase in blood pressure. A severe shocklike syndrome (hypotension, coma) has been reported in children.

Dosage   See Table 22, below.

TABLE 22   TOPICAL NASAL DECONGESTANTS

Drug	Dosage	Remarks
Epinephrine hydrochloride (Adrenalin Chloride)	1–2 gtts in each nostril q 4–6 hr.	1. Available as 1 : 1000 aqueous solution. 2. Because of presence of sodium bisulfite as a preservative, there may be slight stinging after administration.
Ephedrine sulfate	2–4 gtts in each nostril up to q.i.d. Do not use for more than 3 to 4 days.	Available as a 1% or 3% solution.
Naphazoline hydrochloride (Privine)	2 gtts of 0.05%–0.1% solution q 4 to 6 hr.	Available as a 0.05% and 0.1% solution and a 0.05% spray.
Oxymetazoline hydrochloride (Afrin, Duration, St. Joseph Decongestant for Children)	*Solution:* 2–4 gtts b.i.d. in each nostril. *Spray:* 2 to 3 squeezes b.i.d.; **children 2–5 years:** 2–3 gtts of 0.025% solution in each nostril b.i.d.	1. Available as a 0.05% solution or spray or 0.025% solution. 2. Not recommended for children under 6 years of age.
Phenylephrine hydrochloride (Alconefrin, Allerest Nasal, Biomydrin, Coricidin Nasal, Coryban-D Nasal, Isohalant, Isophrin, Neo-Synephrine, Rhinall, Pyracort-D, Sinarest Nasal, Sinutab, Sinophen, Super Anahist, Vacon, Zemphrine)	Several gtts of the 0.25% or 1% solution in each nostril as needed. **Children over 6 yr:** 0.25% in each nostril q 3 to 4 hr. **Infants:** 0.125–0.2% in each nostril q 2 to 4 hr. Nasal spray or small amount of the jelly may be placed in each nostril and inhaled.	1. Available as a 0.125%, 0.16%, 0.2%, 0.25%, 0.5%, and 1% solution. As a 0.2%, 0.25%, and 0.5% spray and as a 0.5% water-soluble jelly. 2. For infants the 0.125% or 0.16% solution should be used.

(Continued)

TABLE 22   TOPICAL NASAL DECONGESTANTS (*Continued*)

Drug	Dosage	Remarks
Methyl Hexane Amine (Forthane)	Used as an inhaler.	
Propylhexedrine (Benzedrex)	Used as an inhaler.	
Tetrahydrozoline hydrochloride (Tyzine)	**Adults and pediatric over 6 yr:** 2–4 gtts of 0.1% solution in each nostril no more than q 3 hr. **2–6 years:** 2–3 gtts of 0.05% solution in each nostril no more than q 3 hour.	1. Available as 0.05% pediatric solution and 0.1% spray. 2. Not recommended for children less than 2 years of age.
Tuaminoheptane (Tuamine)	Used as an inhaler.	
Tuaminoheptane sulfate (Tuamine Sulfate)	**Adults:** 4–5 gtts in each nostril q 3–4 hr; **pediatric 1–6 years:** 2–3 gtts in each nostril q 3–4 hr. **Infants under 1 year:** 1–2 gtts in each nostril q 3 to 4 hr	1. Drug should not be used more than 5 times daily and no longer than 3–4 days. 2. Available as a 1% solution.
Xylometazoline hydrochloride (4-Way Long Acting, Neo-Synephrine II, Otrivin, Sine-Off Once-A-Day, Sinex L.A.)	**Adults:** 2–3 gtts of 0.1% solution in each nostril or 1–2 inhalations of 0.1% spray q 8 to 10 hr; **pediatric under 12 years:** 2–3 gtts of 0.05% solution in each nostril or 1 inhalation of 0.05% spary q 8 to 10 hr. **Infants under 6 months:** 1 gtt q 6 hr.	1. Available as a 0.1% solution and spray and as a 0.05% pediatric solution. 2. Should not be used in atomizers made of aluminum.

Administration   1. Most nasal decongestants are used topically in the form of sprays, drops, or solutions.
2. Drugs should be instilled with the patient in the lateral head-low position.
3. Solutions of topical nasal decongestants may become contaminated with use and result in the growth of bacteria and fungi. Thus, the dropper or spray tip should be rinsed in hot water after each use.

adrenergic blocking (sympatholytic) drugs

Dihydroergotamine Mesylate	Phentolamine Hydrochloride
Ergotamine Tartrate	Phentolamine Mesylate
Methysergide Maleate	Timolol Maleate
Phenoxybenzamine Hydrochloride	Tolazoline Hydrochloride

**General
Statement**

The neurohumor, norepinephrine, transmits nerve impulses across the postganglionic neuroeffector organ junction of the sympathetic division of the autonomic nervous system (ANS). Each neurojunction also responds to epinephrine (adrenalin), which is secreted by the medulla of the adrenal gland.

Impulses that are transmitted through these nerves and then by norepinephrine increase the resistance to peripheral blood flow, increase heart rate and contractile force, inhibit motility of the GI tract, cause dilation of the pupil of the eye, and have many other effects.

At the distal end of the postganglionic sympathetic neurojunction, located on the effector organ that receives the nerve impulse, are receptor sites to which norepinephrine binds, thus stimulating the organ to respond. These receptors are of two types: alpha and beta.

As a rule, the action of norepinephrine or epinephrine on alpha-receptors results in an excitatory response. For example, activation of the sympathetic nerves to peripheral arterioles releases norepinephrine at the neurojunctions of the smooth muscle in the arterioles. The norepinephrine combines with the alpha-receptors, causing the smooth muscle to contract thereby decreasing the diameter of the vessel and increasing peripheral resistance.

On beta-receptors, the action of norepinephrine or epinephrine results in an inhibitory response. Activation of the sympathetics to the intestine releases norepinephrine, which acts on beta-receptors in the smooth muscles, causing them to relax and thereby decreases intestinal motility. However, there is a major exception to the above: in the heart there are no alpha-receptors, only beta-receptors. Stimulation of the beta-receptors in the heart by norepinephrine or epinephrine causes an excitation response manifested as an increase in heart rate and force of contraction.

Two classes of adrenergic blocking drugs act to prevent the combination of norepinephrine or epinephrine with the receptors at the postjunctional sites: alpha-adrenergic blocking drugs and beta-adrenergic blocking drugs. By preventing epinephrine or norepinephrine from combining with the receptors, these drugs prevent the response normally seen when the sympathetic nerves are stimulated. For example, alpha-adrenergic drugs prevent contraction of peripheral arterioles in response to the norepinephrine released by sympathetic activation. They do not affect the action of norepinephrine on beta-receptors of the GI tract or on the heart. Beta-adrenergic blocking agents prevent the inhibitory effect of norepinephrine on the GI tract or its excitatory effect on the heart.

Some of the adrenergic blocking agents have a direct systemic cardiac effect in addition to their peripheral vasodilating effect. The fall in blood pressure that accompanies their administration may trigger a compensatory tachycardia (reflex stimulation). The cardiac blood vessels of a patient with arteriosclerosis may be unable to dilate rapidly enough to accommodate these changes in blood volume and the patient may experience an acute attack of angina pectoris or even cardiac failure.

Adrenergic blocking agents have many undesirable effects which, although not toxic, limit their use. Treatment should always be started at low doses, to be increased gradually.

Alpha-Adrenergic Blocking Agents

Most of the adrenergic blocking agents currently available are of the alpha-blocking type. They reduce the tone of muscles surrounding peripheral blood vessels and consequently increase peripheral blood circulation and decrease blood pressure.

Beta-Adrenergic Blocking Agents

These drugs block the nerve impulse transmission to the beta-type receptors of the sympathetic division of the ANS. These receptors are particularly numerous at the postjunctional terminals of the nerve fibers that control the heart muscle and reduce muscle tone.

Uses Alpha-adrenergic blocking agents have proven useful in the diagnosis and temporary treatment of secondary hypertension caused by pheochromocytoma—a tumor of the adrenal gland that produces large quantities of epinephrine. This excess epinephrine causes an increase in blood pressure. Small amounts of alpha-blocking agents reverse this type of hypertension.

These drugs are also useful in the treatment of peripheral vascular disease with a strong vasospastic component (e.g., Raynaud's disease) and in selected cases of shock and glaucoma as well as pulmonary congestion and edema. Also, selected drugs are used for migraine headaches.

The beta-type blocking agents decrease heart rate as well as force of contraction. Propranolol, the most important of the beta-adrenergic blocking agents, is used as an antiarrhythmic in angina pectoris and as an antihypertensive. It is presented under the antiarrhythmic drugs (p. 284).

Contraindications Coronary artery disease and conditions in which a sudden change in blood pressure may be detrimental or even dangerous. Use with extreme caution in patients with asthma, respiratory disease, or peptic ulcer.

**Untoward
Reactions**

1. When used as vasodilators: postural hypotension, headache, dizziness, weakness, faintness, fatigue, and reflex tachycardia. Nasal congestion, dryness of mouth, and drug fever. Inhibition of ejaculation.
2. When used as headache remedies: long-term use and overdosage may cause peripheral vascular constriction, including tingling and numbness of the extremities, muscle pain, gangrene, tachycardia, and bradycardia.

DIHYDROERGOTAMINE MESYLATE D.H.E. 45

Classification   Adrenergic blocking agent, alpha-type.

**General
Statement**

The drug resembles ergotamine but does not have an oxytocic effect. It is more effective when given early in the course of a migraine attack. Like ergotamine (see below), the drug has a direct stimulating effect on vascular smooth muscles, causing the vessels to constrict and preventing the onset of a migraine attack.

Uses   Migraine and vascular headaches.

Contraindications   See *Ergotamine*. This drug, however, can be used during pregnancy.

**Untoward
Reactions**   See *Ergotamine*. However, side effects of this drug are milder.

Dosage   **SC, IM, IV:** 1–2 mg repeated every 1 to 2 hr to a total of 3 mg, if necessary. **Total weekly dose should not exceed 6 mg.**

**Nursing
Implication**   Encourage patient to take drug at onset of migraine headache because this drug is most effective when administered early in an attack.

ERGOTAMINE TARTRATE ERGOMAR, ERGOSTAT, GYNERGEN TARTRATE, MEDIHALER-ERGOTAMINE

Classification   Alpha-adrenergic blocking agent.

**General
Statement**

Ergot alkaloids have an alpha-blocking effect. However, their effectiveness as a headache remedy results from their direct stimulatory action on vascular smooth muscle, which causes the vessels to constrict. This action prevents or aborts migraine and vascular headaches. However, these agents are much more effective when given before the start of an attack of migraine.

Ergotamine tartrate also has an oxytocic effect. It is often combined with caffeine, which is said to potentiate ergotamine.

Uses   Drug of choice for treating acute attacks of migraine. Also for cluster headache.

Contraindications Pregnancy, peripheral vascular disease, coronary heart disease, hypertension, impaired hepatic or renal function, sepsis, hypersensitivity, or malnutrition.

Untoward Reactions Numbness and tingling of fingers and toes, muscle pain in extremities, weakness in legs, precordial pain, transient tachycardia, bradycardia, nausea, vomiting, localized edema, and itching. Prolonged use of overdose may cause gangrene.

Drug Interaction Triacetyloleandomycin potentiates ergotamine. May cause ergot toxicity.

Dosage **Sublingual:** 2 mg at start of migraine attack followed by 2 mg every 30 minutes if necessary but not more than 6 mg in 24 hours and 10 mg in 1 week. **Oral:** Same as sublingual. **IM, SC:** 0.25 mg initially but not more than 0.5 mg in 24 hour, and 10 mg/week. **Inhalation:** 0.36 mg in a single inhalation at start of attack. Can take up to 6 doses in 24 hr. **Maximum dose** for 1 week is 12 mg. Combination with caffeine: **Initial,** 2 mg ergotamine and 200 mg caffeine repeated q 30 minutes if necessary, up to maximum of 6 mg ergotamine.

Nursing Implications
1. Alert the patient on long-term use to check for coldness of extremities or tingling of fingers and toes. These symptoms appear before onset of gangrene.
2. Alert female patient of childbearing age not to take ergotamine if she believes she is pregnant because drug has an oxytocic effect.

METHYSERGIDE MALEATE SANSERT

Classification Adrenergic blocking agent, alpha-type.

General Statement Although this drug is an adrenergic blocking agent, its therapeutic effect is due to its direct stimulatory action on vascular smooth muscle surrounding blood vessels in the brain. It is to be used only for patients refractory to other antimigraine drugs. It is not useful for the treatment of ongoing migraine or muscle contraction (tension) headaches. Effects of this drug may be delayed and it should be tried for 3 to 4 weeks before being abandoned.

Discontinue the drug gradually to avoid migraine headache rebound.

Use Prophylaxis of migraine or other vascular headache.

Contraindications Severe renal or hepatic disease, severe hypertension, coronary artery disease, peripheral vascular disease, or tendency toward thromboembolic disease, cachexia (profound ill health or malnutrition), infectious disease, or peptic ulcer.

Untoward Reactions   The drug is associated with a high incidence of side effects including GI disturbances, such as nausea, vomiting, and epigastric pain; circulatory effects, such as claudication, leg cramps, anginal pain, coldness and numbness, tingling and edema of the extremities, vascular insufficiency, as well as cardiac murmurs, pleural and pulmonary inflammation, cardiac infarction in patients apparently free of heart disease, and obstruction of the urinary tract (retroperitoneal fibrosis). CNS disturbances, including drowsiness, dizziness, vertigo, headaches, weakness, paresthesias, and insomnia may occur as well as severe psychic reactions, such as depersonalization, depression, and confusion.

Miscellaneous side effects include sweating, flushing, tachycardia, postural hypotension, arthralgia, myalgia, nasal stuffiness and dermatitis, weight gain, and excessive hair loss.

Drug Interaction   Narcotic analgesics are inhibited by methysergide.

Dosage   Administer 4–8 mg daily, in divided doses. Continuous administration should not exceed 6 months. Drug may be readministered after a 3 to 4 week rest period.

Administration   Administer drug with meals or milk to minimize irritation due to increased hydrochloric acid production.

Nursing Implications

1. Advise patient to check weight daily, keep a record of weights, and to report unusually rapid weight gain.
2. Teach patient how to check extremities for edema.
3. Teach the patient how to maintain a low salt intake.
4. Assist the patient in adjusting caloric intake if weight gain is excessive, or to select proper diet if ordered to reduce edema.
5. Instruct the patient that chest girdle or flank pain, dyspnea, cold, numb, or painful extremities and dysuria must be reported immediately.
6. Teach the patient to rise slowly from a supine position and to dangle feet for a few minutes before standing erect.
7. Advise the patient to lie down with legs elevated if feeling faint.
8. Observe the patient's behavior and use interviewing techniques to check whether "hallucinatory experiences" or other untoward CNS symptoms are occurring.
9. Caution the patient against abruptly discontinuing medication because migraine headache rebound may occur. Discontinue gradually.

PHENOXYBENZAMINE HYDROCHLORIDE DIBENZYLINE

Classification   Alpha-adrenergic blocking agent.

Remarks   The drug is an alpha-receptor blocking agent with some antihistaminic activity. As a long-acting drug, its maximum effects may not become manifest for 2 to 4 weeks.

Uses   Pheochromocytoma, peripheral vascular disease, Raynaud's disease, acrocyanosis, chronic ulceration of the extremities, frostbite sequelae, and diabetic gangrene.

Dosage   **PO: initial,** 10 mg daily, may be increased by 10 mg daily q 4 days, up to maximum of 60 mg daily.

Nursing Implications
1. Monitor BP every 4 hours to check for excessive hypotension both in supine and erect position.
2. Warn the patient to rise slowly from a supine position and to dangle feet for a few minutes before standing erect.
3. Advise the patient to lie down immediately and elevate legs if feeling faint.
4. Teach the patient how to monitor radial pulse and to report tachycardia as it is a sign of autonomic blockade.
5. Monitor BP, pulse, quality of peripheral pulses, and extremities for increased warmth for 4 days after a change in dosage to assist in evaluation as to whether patient needs an adjustment in dosage.
6. Anticipate that the symptoms of respiratory infections may be aggravated by the drug. The patient will then require more supportive care.
7. Have levarterenol on hand to treat overdosage. Epinephrine is ineffective and may increase heart rate as well as cause further peripheral dilatation.
8. Keep the patient flat for 24 hours after overdosage and apply Ace bandage to legs as well as an abdominal binder, unless contraindicated.

PHENTOLAMINE HYDROCHLORIDE REGITINE HYDROCHLORIDE

PHENTOLAMINE MESYLATE REGITINE MESYLATE

Classification   Alpha-adrenergic blocking agent.

General Statement   Phentolamine is an alpha-adrenergic blocking agent with direct effects on vascular smooth muscle and the heart. The drug has a histaminelike effect and stimulates gastric secretion. It is somewhat more potent than tolazoline as an alpha-adrenergic blocker.

Uses   Hypertension associated with pheochromocytoma and diagnosis thereof.

Untoward Reactions   Acute and prolonged hypotension especially after parenteral administration. Use with great caution in the presence of gastritis, ulcers, and history thereof. Overdosage, characterized by excessive hypotension, can be treated with norepinephrine.

Drug Interactions	*Interactant*	*Interaction*
	Epinephrine	Antagonized by phentolamine. Do not use epinephrine to overcome shock induced by phentolamine.
	Levarterenol	Suitable antagonist to treat overdosage induced by phentolamine. Phentolamine ↓ hyperthermia induced by levarterenol
	Norepinephrine	See *Epinephrine*
	Propranolol	Concomitant use during surgery for pheochromocytoma is indicated

Dosage   **PO:** 50 mg 4 to 6 times daily; **pediatric:** 25 mg 4 to 6 times daily. **IM or IV** (*preoperatively to reduce blood pressure*): 5 mg; **pediatric:** 1 mg. *Diagnosis of pheochromocytoma:* **IV, adults,** 5 mg; **children,** 1 mg. **IM, adults:** 5 mg; **children,** 3 mg.

Nursing Implications
1. Monitor BP and pulse prior to and after parenteral administration until stabilized at satisfactory level.
2. Avoid postural hypotension after parenteral administration by keeping the patient supine for at least 30 minutes after injection. Then have patient rise slowly and dangle feet before standing to avoid orthostatic hypotension.
3. Treat overdosage by placing the patient in Trendelenburg position, assisting with administration of parenteral fluids, and having levarterenol available for use to minimize hypotension. *Do not use epinephrine.*

TIMOLOL MALEATE TIMOPTIC

Classification   Ophthalmic agent, beta-adrenergic blocker.

General Statement   This beta-adrenergic blocking agent reduces elevated and normal intraocular pressure. The effect becomes apparent 30 minutes after administration, is maximal 1 to 2 hours thereafter, and persists for 24 hours. Compared to pilocarpine, timolol does not reduce pupil size or visual acuity. It also does not cause night blindness. The drug has little sympathomimetic, local anesthetic, or myocardial depressant activity.

Uses   Chronic open angle glaucoma, selected cases of secondary glaucoma, ocular hypertension, aphakic (no lens) patients with glaucoma.

Contraindications   Hypersensitivity to drug. Use with caution in patients for whom systemic beta-adrenergic blocking agents are contraindicated. Safe use in pregnancy and in children not established.

Untoward Reactions   Few. Occasionally, ocular irritation, local hypersensitivity reactions, slight decrease in resting heart rate.

Drug Interactions Possible potentiation with systemically administered beta-adrenergic blocking agents.

Dosage One drop of 0.25%–0.50% solution in each eye, b.i.d. When patient is transferred from other antiglaucoma agent, continue old medication on day 1 of timolol therapy (one drop of 0.25%). Thereafter, discontinue former therapy. Initiate with 0.25% solution. Increase to 0.50% solution if response is insufficient. Further increases in dosage are ineffectual.

Administration Teach patient to apply finger lightly on lacrymal sac for 1 minute following administration.

Nursing Implication Emphasize need for continued regular intraocular measurements by an ophthamologist because ocular hypertension may recur and/or progress without overt signs or symptoms.

TOLAZOLINE HYDROCHLORIDE PRISCOLINE HYDROCHLORIDE, TOLZOL

Classification Alpha-adrenergic blocking agent.

Remarks Tolazoline produces a moderately effective alpha-adrenergic blockade. It stimulates the heart and is available in both oral and parenteral forms.

Uses Spastic peripheral vascular disease, endarteritis, diabetic arteriosclerosis, gangrene, postthrombotic conditions, scleroderma, Raynaud's disease, Buerger's disease, and frostbite sequelae.

Contraindications Following cerebrovascular accidents and in patients with coronary artery disease.

Untoward Reactions Tolazoline stimulates gastric secretions. Use with caution in patients with gastritis, peptic ulcer, or history thereof.

Drug Interaction Alcohol causes hazardous symptoms of acetaldehyde poisoning (Antabuselike reaction) when tolazoline is ingested before or during alcohol ingestion.

Dosage *Individualized.* **PO: usual,** 25 mg 4 to 6 times daily. May be increased to 50 mg 6 times daily. *Long-acting tablet:* 1 tablet (80 mg) every 12 hr. **SC, IM, IV:** 10–50 mg q.i.d. **Intra-arterial: initial,** 25 mg test dose then 50–75 mg 1 or 2 times daily. Eventually 2 to 3 times weekly with **PO** tolazoline.

Administration
1. Administer PO medication with meals or milk to minimize gastric irritation due to excessive production of hydrochloric acid in stomach.
2. Administer parenteral drugs only to hospitalized patients.
3. Position patient supine for intra-arterial injection.

Nursing Implications

1. Check BP and pulse at least b.i.d. as patients are subject to either hypertensive or hypotensive reactions.
2. Check that the patient is experiencing a feeling of warmth in the affected limb and not a feeling of increased cold due to a paradoxical reaction.
3. Observe affected extremity for flushing and piloerection (hair erected) after drug is administered because these indicate optimal dosage.
4. Keep the patient warm to increase effectiveness of drug.
5. Avoid postural hypotension after injection by keeping patient supine for at least 30 minutes after administration. Then have patient rise slowly and dangle feet before standing.
6. Warn the patient not to ingest alcohol before or after ingestion of drug, as poisoning may occur.
7. Treat overdosage by placing patient in Trendelenburg position, assisting with administration of parenteral fluids, and having ephedrine available for use to minimize hypotension. (*Do not use epinephrine or norepinephrine.*)

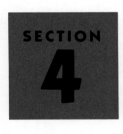

SECTION 4

cholinergic (parasympathomimetic) drugs

	Neostigmine Methylsulfate
Ambenonium Chloride	Physostigmine Salicylate
Bethanechol Chloride	Pyridostigmine Bromide
Edrophonium Chloride	
Neostigmine Bromide	

Ophthalmic Cholinergic (Miotic) Agents

Acetylcholine Chloride	Physostigmine Salicylate
Carbachol	Physostigmine Sulfate
Demecarium Bromide	Pilocarpine Hydrochloride
Echothiophate Iodide	Pilocarpine Nitrate
Isoflurophate	Pilocarpine Ocular Therapeutic System
Physostigmine	Timolol Maleate

General Statement

The cholinergic drugs mimic the action of acetylcholine. They do this either by acting like acetylcholine (direct-acting drugs) or by increasing the available amount of acetylcholine at the synapses by partially inhibiting the enzyme acetylcholinesterase that destroys acetylcholine after nerve transmission (indirect-acting drugs).

The cholinergic drugs have some effect on all neurojunctions at which acetylcholine is the neurohormone. However, some of these synapses do not respond readily to exogenous acetylcholine. Acetylcholine and other cholinergic drugs particularly enhance nerve impulse transmission to the cardiac and smooth muscles and the exocrine glands.

Cholinergic drugs have the following pharmacologic effects on various structures:

GI Tract
Enhance secretion by gastric and other glands (may cause belching, heartburn, nausea, and vomiting). Increase smooth muscle tone and stimulate bowel movement.

Genitourinary System
Stimulation of ureter and relaxation of urinary bladder results in micturition.

Cardiac Muscle
Slowing of heart rate (bradycardia), decrease in atrial contractility, impulse formation, and conductivity.

Blood Vessels
Vasodilation, resulting in increased skin temperature and local flushing.

Respiration
Increased mucus secretion and bronchial constriction, which causes coughing, choking, and wheezing, especially in patients with history of asthma.

Eyes
Contraction of radial and sphincter muscles of iris (pupillary constriction or miosis). Contraction of the ciliary body producing spasm of accommodation of the lens, which then no longer adjusts to see at various distances. Reduction of intraocular pressure.

Skin
Sweat and salivary glands: Activation, increased pilomotor response.

It is to be noted that some of these effects are more pronounced with some drugs than with others. Also, the cholinergic drugs are rather nonspecific because they affect so many different parts of the body and thus have many side effects.

The direct-acting drugs can be divided into synthetic choline esters and cholinomimetic alkaloids.

Most of the indirect-acting drugs are either quaternary ammonium salts or organophosphate compounds.

Uses   Prophylaxis of postoperative constipation, drug-induced constipation, postoperative and postpartum urinary retention, management of neurogenic bladder, abdominal distention, selected cases of peripheral vascular disease, scleroderma, myasthenia gravis, gastric atony and retention following bilateral vagotomy, glaucoma.

Diagnostic: testing of pancreatic function, diagnosis of nerve injury, counteraction of dry mouth, glaucoma (topical application only). Diagnosis of pheochromocytoma. Diagnosis of atropine poisoning.

Contraindications Severe cardiac disease, bradycardia, hypotension, vagotonia, mechanical intestinal or urinary tract obstruction, peptic ulcer, asthma, allergies, hyperthyroidism, coronary occlusions, Addison's disease, and vesical neck obstruction of urinary bladder.

Untoward Reactions Abdominal cramps, diarrhea, spontaneous bowel movements, sweating, flushing, increased urinary frequency and salivation, incontinence, malaise, headache, nausea, vomiting, asthmatic attacks, substernal pain, bradycardia, lowered blood pressure, atrioventricular block, cardiac arrest, miosis, and muscular weakness. These effects can usually be reversed by parenteral administration of 0.6 mg of atropine sulfate, which should be readily available.

Administration Never give IM or IV. Preferred route is PO. Can be given SC (use small "test" dose to determine reaction of patient). A syringe containing 0.6 mg atropine sulfate should always be on hand to combat excess cholinergic effect whenever drug is administered SC.

Nursing Implications Atropine and epinephrine for parenteral use should always be readily available for treatment of cholinergic overdose. Epinephrine is also valuable in overcoming severe cardiovascular or bronchoconstrictor reactions to cholinomimetic drugs.

AMBENONIUM CHLORIDE MYTELASE CHLORIDE

Classification Indirectly acting cholinergic-acetylcholinesterase inhibitor.

Remarks Onset PO: 20 minutes; duration: 3 to 4 hours. When daily dose equals 200 mg, watch closely for signs of toxicity. Discontinue other cholinergic drugs before initiating ambenonium.

Uses Myasthenia gravis, postoperative abdominal distention, and urinary retention.

Dosage **PO: initial,** 5 mg increased gradually as required. **Maintenance:** 5–25 or more mg t.i.d.-q.i.d.; **pediatric: initial,** 0.3 mg/kg every 24 hr. Maintenance dose can be increased to 1.5 mg/kg every 24 hr in 3 to 4 divided doses.

Additional Nursing Implications
1. Observe closely for side effects as they are an indication of overdosage with this drug.
2. Have on hand 0.5–1 mg of atropine sulfate as an antidote to be administered slowly IV, and be prepared to administer supportive therapy such as artificial respiration and oxygen inhalation.

3. Observe for reactions peculiar to this cholinergic drug, such as jitteriness, dizziness, headache, and mental confusion.
4. Observe patient's response to initial and subsequent doses as dosage is highly individualized and based on patient's response.

BETHANECHOL CHLORIDE DUVOID, MICTROL, MYOTONACHOL, URECHOLINE CHLORIDE, UROLAX, VESICHOLINE

Classification Cholinergic (parasympathomimetic), direct acting.

General Statement Drug of choice for paralytic ileus. Bethanechol chloride is a choline ester with actions like acetylcholine but resistant to destruction by acetylcholinesterase. Major action, after subcutaneous or oral doses, is to increase peristaltic movement of GI tract, to stimulate secretions in glands of GI tract, and to stimulate the bladder. Bethanechol, when given by this route, has very little conspicuous cardiovascular effect. There may be a slight transient fall in diastolic blood pressure which is accompanied by a minor reflex tachycardia.

Additional Uses Postoperative abdominal distention, urinary and gastric retention especially after vagotomy (severance of vagus nerve), test for pancreatic enzymatic function.

Additional Contraindications Asthma, hypothyroidism, and vesical neck obstruction of urinary bladder. Peptic ulcer or mechanical intestinal or urinary obstruction.

Dosage Never give **IM or IV. PO** (*preferred*): 10–50 mg 2 to 4 times daily. **Maximum:** 120 mg. **SC** (*test dose*): 2.5 mg. Repeated after 15 to 30 minutes if necessary up to maximum of 10 mg.

Additional Nursing Implication Have on hand a syringe containing 0.6 mg of atropine whenever drug is given SC.

Drug Interactions

Interactant	Interaction
Cholinergic Inhibitors	Additive cholinergic effects
Ganglionic Blocking Agents	Critical hypotensive response
Procainamide	Antagonism of cholinergic effects
Quinidine	Antagonism of cholinergic effects

EDROPHONIUM CHLORIDE TENSILON CHLORIDE

Classification Indirectly acting cholinergic-acetylcholinesterase inhibitor.

General Statement When used as diagnostic agent for myasthenia gravis, edrophonium increases muscle strength. At high doses the drug may potentiate curariform drugs. When using as an antidote for curariform drug overdosage, use only with artificial respiration and oxygen therapy.

Additional Uses Antidote for curariform drugs. Diagnosis of myasthenia gravis.

Dosage **IV** (*diagnosis of myasthenia gravis*): 2 mg initially; if no reaction in 45 seconds, additional 8 mg given. If patient is over 50 years of age, 0.4 mg atropine SC should be given before edrophonium to prevent bradycardia and hypotension; **pediatric:** 0.2 mg/kg (¹/₅ dose given within 1 minute; if no response occurs, remainder of dose given). **IM, adults:** 10 mg.

Additional Nursing Implications
1. Observe for side effects such as increased salivation, bronchiolar spasm, bradycardia, and cardiac dysrhythmia in older patients.
2. Note the effect of each dose of drug when it is used as antidote for curare before next dose is given.

NEOSTIGMINE BROMIDE PROSTIGMIN BROMIDE

NEOSTIGMINE METHYLSULFATE PROSTIGMIN METHYLSULFATE

Classification Indirectly acting cholinergic-acetylcholinesterase inhibitor.

General Statement Drug is shorter acting than ambenonium chloride and pyridostigmine, which are also used for myasthenia gravis. Atropine is often given concurrently to control side effects. Neostigmine bromide is given PO; neostigmine methylsulfate is given parenterally.

Uses Myasthenia gravis—diagnosis and management. Amenorrhea. Emergency treatment of angle-closure glaucoma; open-angle glaucoma. Urinary retention.

Dosage *Neostigmine bromide, Myasthenia gravis,* **PO:** 15–375 mg/day. **Usual,** 150 mg/day; **pediatric:** 7.5–15 mg t.i.d.-q.i.d. *Neostigmine Methylsulfate, Myasthenia gravis,* **IM, SC:** 0.5 mg (use 1 ml of 1:2000 solution). *Antidote for tubocurarine,* **IV** (with atropine, 0.6–1.2 mg): 0.5–2 mg slowly. Can repeat if necessary up to total dose of 5 mg. *Glaucoma,* see Table 23.

Additional Nursing Implications
1. Observe for toxic reaction demonstrated by generalized cholinergic stimulation.
2. Check for vaginal bleeding when medication is used for treatment of functional amenorrhea or as a test for pregnancy.
3. Assist in ventilation of the patient and maintenance of a patent airway when medication is used as an antidote for tubocurarine.
4. Have atropine available to be used with neostigmine when it is used as an antidote.
5. Anticipate the use of atropine before the administration of neo-

stigmine if there is bradycardia. Pulse rate should be increased to 80/minute before giving neostigmine.

PHYSOSTIGMINE SALICYLATE ANTILIRIUM

Classification Indirectly acting cholinergic-acetylcholinesterase inhibitor.

General Statement This drug was previously used for the treatment of myasthenia gravis. It is now used for glaucoma (see Table 23) and as an antidote for belladonna poisoning or tricyclic antidepressant overdosage. Doses of 1–4 mg abolish delirium coma of 200 mg atropine. It has the typical therapeutic properties and side effects of cholinergic agents.

Dosage *Belladonna poisoning,* **IM, IV:** 0.5–2 mg no faster than 1 mg/minute. Since drug is of shorter duration than atropine, dose may have to be repeated q 2 hr.

PYRIDOSTIGMINE BROMIDE MESTINON BROMIDE

Classification Indirectly acting cholinergic-acetylcholinesterase inhibitor.

General Statement This drug has longer action and fewer side effects than neostigmine, which is also used for treatment of myasthenia gravis. Atropine is often given concurrently to control side effects. It should, however, be given sparingly because it may mask symptoms of cholinergic overdosage.

Use Myasthenia gravis.

Dosage **PO,** *individualized:* **usual,** 600 mg daily; range: 0.36–1.5 gm daily, or 1 to 3 80-mg sustained release tablets 1 to 2 times a day. There should be a minimum of 6 hr between administrations. **IM, IV** (*slow*): *during myasthenic crisis, pre- and post-operatively, during labor and postpartum:* 1/30 oral dose.

Additional Nursing Implications
1. Observe for toxic reaction demonstrated by generalized cholinergic stimulation.
2. Observe for muscular weakness, which may be a sign of impending myasthenic crisis and cholinergic overdose.
3. Explain to patient how extended release tablets work and caution them not to take these tablets more often than q 6 hours.
4. Explain to patient that conventional tablets may be taken with extended release tablets if ordered.

OPHTHALMIC CHOLINERGIC (MIOTIC) AGENTS

General Statement Cholinergic agents are commonly used for the treatment of glaucoma and less frequently for the correction of accommodative (nonparalytic) convergent strabismus and ocular myasthenia gravis.

The drugs are directly instilled into the conjunctival sac of the eye.

The ophthalmic cholinergic drugs fall into two classes: Direct-acting (carbachol, pilocarpine) and indirect-acting (demecarium, echothiophate, isoflurophate, neostigmine, physostigmine), which inhibit the enzyme cholinesterase. In the treatment of glaucoma, the drugs lead to an accumulation of acetylcholine that stimulates the ciliary muscles and increases contraction of iris sphincter muscle. This opens the angle of the eye and results in increased outflow of aqueous humor and consequently in a decrease of intraocular pressure. This effect is of particular importance in narrow angle glaucoma. Hourly tonometric measurements are recommended during initiation of therapy. The drugs also cause spasms of accommodation. (For individual agents and dosages, see Table 23, p. 504.)

Uses   Glaucoma: primary acute narrow angle glaucoma (acute therapy) and primary chronic wide angle glaucoma (chronic therapy). Selected cases of secondary glaucoma. Accommodative (nonparalytic) convergent strabismus (squint). Ocular myasthenia gravis. Antidote against harmful effects of atropinelike drugs in patients suffering from glaucoma. Alternately with a mydriatic drug to break adhesions between lens and iris.

Contraindications   *Direct-acting drugs:* Inflammatory eye disease (iritis), asthma, hypertension.

Indirect-acting drugs: As above and acute angle glaucoma, history of retinal detachment, ocular hypotension accompanied by intraocular inflammatory processes, intestinal or urinary obstruction, peptic ulcer, epilepsy, parkinsonism, spastic GI conditions, vasomotor instability, severe bradycardia or hypotension, and recent myocardial infarctions.

Untoward Reactions   *Local:* Painful contraction of ciliary muscle, pain in eye, blurred vision, spasms of accommodation, darkened vision, failure to accommodate to darkness, twitching, headaches, painful brow. Most of these symptoms lessen with prolonged usage. Iris cysts and retinal detachment (indirect-acting drugs only).

Systemic: Systemic absorption of drug may cause nausea, GI discomfort, diarrhea, hypotension, bronchial constriction, and increased salivation.

Dosage   *Individualized,* see Table 23.

Nursing Implications   1. Caution the patient not to drive for 1 to 2 hours after administration of drugs.
2. Advise the patient that pain and blurred vision usually will diminish with prolonged usage.
3. Side effects can be minimized by administering dose at bedtime.
4. Prevent overflow of solution into nasopharynx after topical instillation of gtts by exerting pressure on the naso-lacrimal duct for 1 to 2 minutes before allowing lid to close.
5. Have epinephrine and atropine available for emergency treatment of increased intraocular pressure.

TABLE 23 OPHTHALMIC CHOLINERGIC DRUGS (MIOTICS)

Drug	Uses	Dosage	Remarks
Acetylcholine chloride (Miochol)	Rapid, intense-miosis during eye surgery	0.5–2 ml of 1% solution.	Irrigate slowly to avoid atrophy of iris. Rapid acting, short duration. Since aqueous solutions of acetylcholine are unstable, prepare immediately before use.
Carbachol, Topical (Carbacel Ophthalmic, Isopto Carbachol)	Glaucoma	1 drop of 0.75%–3% solution 1 to 4 times/day.	Administered together with wetting agent. Long-acting miotic effect reversible by atropine. *Side Effects* Slight hyperemia during first few days, aching of eyes and head which usually passes after third day of treatment. *Nursing Implications* After instillation of gtts, absorption may be improved by gentle massage of the lids.
Demecarium bromide (Humorsol Ophthalmic)	Chronic simple and selected cases of secondary glaucoma	1 drop of 0.125%–0.25% solution 2 times/week–2 times/day.	Long-acting miotic. *Nursing Implications* Initial instillation should be made by a physician after it has been confirmed that the angle of the eye is open.
Echothiophate Iodide (Echodide, Phospholine Iodide)	Accommodative (nonparalytic) convergent strabismus, ocular myasthenia gravis, antidote against harmful effect of atropinelike drugs in patients with glaucoma	*Glaucoma:* 1 drop of 0.03%–0.06% solution every 12 to 48 hr. *Accommodative Esotropia:* **initial,** 1 drop of 0.125% solution/day in both eyes for 2 to 3 weeks, **then,** one drop of 0.125% solution every other day or 0.06% solution daily.	Long-acting miotic. Miotic effect reversible by atropine. Enhanced by concomitant administration of Diamox.

Drug	Indication	Dosage	Comments
Isoflurophate (DFP, Diisopropyl-flurophosphate, Floropryl)	Glaucoma, strabismus	¼" strip of ointment in eye q 8–72 hour.	Drug should be refrigerated. Long-acting miotic. Miotic effect irreversible by atropine. Accidental systemic ingestion treated with atropine; if severe also with MgSO₄
Physostigmine salicylate (Isopto Eserine) Physostigmine sulfate (Eserine Sulfate)	Glaucoma, especially after cataract extrusion	1–2 drops of 0.25%–0.5% solution (salicylate) b.i.d.-q.i.d.; 0.25% ointment (sulfate) used at night.	Short-acting miotic. Short-onset miotic (2 minutes) lasting 12 to 36 hr.
Pilocarpine hydrochloride (Adsorbocarpine, Almocarpine, Isopto Carpine, Pilocar, Pilocel, Pilomiotin) Pilocarpine nitrate (P.V. Carpine Liquifilm)	Commonly used agent for management of glaucoma	*Usual:* 1–2 drops of 0.5%–4% solution 1 to 6 times/day. Solutions up to 10% are available.	Onset of action: 15 minutes, lasting 20 hr.
Pilocarpine Ocular Therapeutic System (Ocusert Pilo-20 and -40)	Glaucoma responsive to pilocarpine	A unit designed to be placed in cul-de-sac of eye for release of pilocarpine at rate of 20 or 40 μg/hr for 1 week.	Patient should check for presence of unit before bed and upon arising.
Timolol Maleate (Timoptic)	Chronic simple and selected cases of secondary glaucoma and ocular hypertension	1 drop 0.25%–0.50% solution in each eye b.i.d.	This beta-blocking agent is used for the treatment of chronic simple glaucoma. The drug does not affect pupil size or visual acuity. Onset of action: 30 minutes, lasting 24 hr.

6. Report redness around the cornea as epinephrine or phenylephrine hydrochloride (10%) may be ordered with demecarium bromide, echothiophate iodide, and isoflurophate to minimize this type of reaction.
7. Stress to the patient the need for regular medical supervision while on drug therapy.
8. Teach the patient that painful eye spasms may be relieved by application of cold compresses (ice cube).

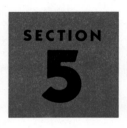

SECTION

5 cholinergic blocking (parasympatholytic) agents

Anisotropine Methylbromide
Atropine Sulfate
Belladonna Alkaloids
Belladonna Extract
Belladonna, Levorotatory Alkaloids of
Clidinium Bromide
Dicyclomine Hydrochloride
Diphemanil Methylsulfate
Glycopyrrolate
Hexocyclium Methylsulfate
Homatropine Methylbromide
Hyoscyamine Sulfate

Isopropamide Iodide
Mepenzolate Bromide
Methantheline Bromide
Methixene Hydrochloride
Methscopolamine Bromide
Oxyphencyclimine Hydrochloride
Oxyphenonium Bromide
Propantheline Bromide
Scopolamine Hydrobromide
Thiphenamil Hydrochloride
Tridihexethyl Chloride

Mydriatics & Cycloplegics

Atropine Sulfate
Cyclopentolate Hydrochloride
Homatropine Hydrobromide

Scopolamine
Tropicamide

General Statement

This group of drugs prevents acetylcholine from transmitting nerve impulses across the junction between the postganglionic parasympathetic nerve terminal and the effector organ (muscarinic site). The drug accomplishes this by competing for the receptor site normally occupied by acetylcholine at the distal (far) end of the neurojunction. In this manner acetylcholine cannot transmit the nerve impulses and the intended "message" does not get across. In therapeutic doses, these drugs have very little, if any, effect on acetylcholine transmissions of nerve impulses in ganglia ("nicotinic site").

The main effects of cholinergic blocking agents are to:

1. Reduce spasms of smooth muscles like those controlling the urinary bladder or spasms of bronchial and intestinal smooth muscle.
2. Block vagal impulses to the heart, resulting in an increase in the rate and speed of impulse conduction through the atrioventricular conducting system.
3. Suppress or decrease gastric secretions, perspiration, salivation, and secretion of bronchial mucus.
4. Relax the sphincter muscles of the iris and cause pupillary dilation (mydriasis) and loss of accommodation for near vision (cycloplegia).
5. They also have diverse effects on the central nervous system, such as depression (scopolamine) or stimulation (toxic doses of atropine). Many of the anticholinergic drugs also have antiparkinsonism effects. They abolish or reduce the signs and symptoms of Parkinson's disease, such as tremors and rigidity and result in some improvement in mobility, muscular coordination, and motor performance. These effects may be due to blockade of the effects of acetylcholine in the central nervous system. This chapter also discusses miscellaneous synthetic antispasmodics related to anticholinergic drugs. Agents used primarily for Parkinson's disease are presented in Chapter 5, Section 12.

Contraindications Glaucoma, tachycardia, partial obstruction of the GI and biliary tract, and prostatic hypertrophy. The drugs are to be used with extreme caution for patients with cardiac disease, especially those with a tendency to develop tachycardia, and in the elderly with atherosclerosis or evidence of mental impairment.

Untoward Reactions These are desirable in some conditions and undesirable in others. Thus, the anticholinergics have an antisalivary effect that is useful in parkinsonism. This same effect is unpleasant when the drug is used for spastic conditions of the GI tract.

Most untoward reactions are dose related and decrease when dosage decreases. Sometimes it helps to discontinue the medication for several days. With this in mind, anticholinergic drugs have the following untoward reactions:

GI and urinary tract: constipation, nausea, vomiting, urinary hesitancy, urinary retention, impotence.

Cardiovascular system: tachycardia and palpitations.

Central nervous system: dizziness, drowsiness, lassitude, nervousness, disorientation. Atropine fever. Symptoms often may be mistaken for senility or mental deterioration in parkinsonism patients caused by progression of the disease. If dosage of drug is not reduced or discontinued, patient may become agitated, psychotic, and develop hallucinations.

Respiratory: decreased bronchial secretions, antihistaminic effect.

Ocular: blurred vision, dilated pupils, photophobia, may precipitate acute glaucoma.

Also, dryness of mouth that may cause difficulty in swallowing, suppression of perspiration (drug or atropine fever), suppression of glandular secretions, scarlatiniform rash, loss of libido, nausea, vomiting. Not all side effects are associated with all drugs.

Drug Interactions

Interactant	Interaction
Amantadine	Additive anticholinergic side effects
Antacids	↓ Absorption of anticholinergics from GI tract
Antidepressants, Tricyclic	Additive anticholinergic side effects
Antihistamines	Additive anticholinergic side effects
Cyclopropane	↑ Chance of ventricular arrhythmias
Guanethidine	Reversal of inhibition of gastric acid secretion caused by anticholinergics
Histamine	Reversal of inhibition of gastric acid secretion caused by anticholinergics
Levodopa	Possible ↓ effect of levodopa due to ↑ breakdown of levodopa in stomach (due to delayed gastric emptying time)
Meperidine (Demerol)	Additive anticholinergic side effects
Methotrimeprazine (Levoprome)	Possibility of extrapyramidal symptoms with concomitant use
Methylphenidate (Ritalin)	Potentiation of anticholinergic side effects

Monoamine oxidase inhibitors
    Pargyline (Eutonyl)
    Tranylcypromine (Parnate)
	MAO inhibitors ↑ effects of anticholinergic drugs

Nitrates, Nitrites	Potentiation of anticholinergic side effects
Orphenadrine (Norflex)	Additive anticholinergic side effects
Phenothiazines	Additive anticholinergic side effects
Procainamide (Pronestyl)	Additive anticholinergic side effects
Propranolol (Inderal)	Anticholinergics are used to counteract excessive bradycardia produced by propranolol
Quinidine	Additive effect on blockade of vagus nerve action
Reserpine	Reversal of inhibition of gastric acid secretion caused by anticholinergics
Sympathomimetics	↑ Bronchial relaxation
Thioxanthines	Potentiation of anticholinergic side effects

Dosage See individual agents.

Nursing Implications

1. Be alert to a history of asthma, glaucoma, or duodenal ulcer that contraindicates use of the drug.
2. Check dosage and measure drug exactly because some drugs are given in minute amounts and overdosage leads to toxicity.
3. Inform the patient that certain side effects are to be expected and advise to report these to the physician who may alleviate symptoms by reducing the dose or temporarily stopping the drug. Sometimes

the patient will be expected to tolerate certain side effects (e.g., dry mouth, blurred vision) for other beneficial effects.

4. Emphasize to the patient the importance of maintaining the dietary regimen prescribed by the physician. Help the patient to understand and plan diet.
5. Teach the patient or a responsible family member that antiparkinsonism drugs are not to be withdrawn abruptly. If there is to be a change in medication, one drug should be withdrawn slowly and the other started in small doses.
6. Relieve dry mouth by providing cold drinks (particularly postoperatively), hard candies, or chewing gum if permitted.

Additional Nursing Implications Related to Pathologic Condition for Which Drug is Administered

Cardiovascular

Note alterations in pulse rate and whether patient is having palpitations.

Ocular

1. Assist patients on ward who are experiencing dizziness or blurred vision and caution them to use safety precautions.
2. Inform patients using anticholinergic drops how long vision will be affected so that activities can be planned.
3. Advise patients experiencing photophobia that dark glasses will be helpful.
4. Teach patients to report marked visual changes.

GI

1. Administer medication for treatment of GI pathology early enough before a meal so that medication will be effective when needed.
2. Teach patients with GI pathology how to maintain their prescribed diets and to continue taking other medication as ordered.

GU

1. Note that if the patient (particularly a middle-aged male) is voiding infrequently he may be experiencing urinary retention.
2. Ascertain that young men on an atropinelike blocking agent understand the drug may cause impotence.

Belladonna Poisoning

Infants and children are especially susceptible to the toxic effects of atropine and scopolamine. Poisoning (dose dependent) is characterized by dryness of the mouth, burning sensation of the mouth, difficulties in swallowing and speaking, blurred vision, photophobia, rash, tachycardia, increased respiration, increased body temperature (fever up to 109°F (42.7°C)), restlessness, irritability, confusion, muscle incoordination, dilated pupils, hot dry skin, respiratory depression and paralysis, and death.

Treatment of Belladonna Poisoning

After PO intake: gastric lavage with a solution containing precipitants such as tannic acid or iodine.

Systemic antidote: physostigmine (Eserine) IM, IV, or SC in doses of 1–4 mg. Effect of this drug lasts only 1 to 2 hours and administration of antidote may thus have to be repeated. Small doses of short-acting barbiturate, given at frequent intervals, may be required. Care should be taken not to aggravate depression stage of belladonna poisoning. Depression can be controlled by caffeine sodium benzoate or picrotoxin and oxygen inhalation.

ANISOTROPINE METHYLBROMIDE VALPIN 50

Classification Synthetic antispasmodic and anticholinergic.

Remarks Quaternary ammonium compound. Onset of action of drug is 1 hour; duration, 4 to 6 hours.

Uses Adjunct for treatment of GI spasms and peptic ulcers.

Dosage **PO:** 50 mg t.i.d.-q.i.d. before meals and at bedtime.

ATROPINE SULFATE

Classification Anticholinergic (antispasmodic, mydriatic).

Remarks Anticholinergic of choice for certain diseases. Has spasmolytic and CNS effects (medulla), causes an increase in heart rate and respiration.

Uses Effectiveness in parkinsonism due to action on CNS rather than peripheral action. Antidote for poisoning by insecticides containing anticholinesterases and pilocarpine, physostigmine, isoflurophate, choline esters, and mushroom (*Amanita* species) poisoning. During anesthesia for control of excessive salivation, bronchial secretions, and rhinorrhea. Certain instances of acute myocardial infarction, which are accompanied by severe sinus bradycardia or heart block. Pupillary dilatation, cycloplegia, common cold, bronchial asthma, hypertonicity of uterus, and peptic ulcer.

Additional Untoward Reactions Flushing, dry and warm skin, scarlatiniform rash. Overdosage (belladonna poisoning) is characterized by tachycardia, excessively increased respiration, restlessness, irritability, disorientation, incoherence, depression, and ultimately medullary paralysis, and death.

Treatment of Overdosage Stomach lavage: 1–2 ml of strong iodine solution, which will precipitate atropine and prevent absorption, are added to lavage. For systemic antidote, see *Treatment of Belladonna Poisoning,* above.

Dosage   **PO, adults:** 0.4–0.6 mg; **pediatric over 90 lbs:** same as adult; **65–90 pounds:** 0.4 mg; **40–65 pounds:** 0.3 mg; **24–40 pounds:** 0.2 mg; **17–24 pounds:** 0.15 mg; **7–16 pounds:** 0.1 mg.

Additional Nursing Implications
1. Explain to patients that atropine flush is due to vasodilation. It is an expected effect of the drug and does not indicate infection or fever.
2. Be alert to the development of hot, dry flushed skin, tachycardia, increased respirations, CNS changes, and scarlatiniform rash, signs of atropine poisoning.
3. Have neostigmine methylsulfate and short-acting barbiturates, such as secobarbital, available for treatment of poisoning.
4. Have on hand strong iodine solution and equipment for stomach lavage for treatment of poisoning.

BELLADONNA ALKALOIDS PRYDON

BELLADONNA EXTRACT BELAP SE

LEVOROTATORY ALKALOIDS OF BELLADONNA BELLAFOLINE

Classification   Mixture of natural alkaloids.

Uses   Often prescribed in fixed combination with phenobarbital. Adjunct in treatment of gastric, duodenal, and intestinal ulcers, excess motor activity, pylorospasms, spastic constipation, or ulcerative colitis.

Dosage   *Alkaloids:* 0.4–0.8 mg q 12 hr. *Extract:* 10.8–21.6 mg t.i.d.-q.i.d.; *Levorotatory alkaloids,* **PO, adults:** 0.25–0.5 mg t.i.d.; **pediatric over 6 yrs:** 0.125–0.25 mg t.i.d.; **SC, adults:** 0.125–0.5 mg 1 or 2 times/day. **Parenteral use not recommended for children.**

CLIDINIUM BROMIDE QUARZAN

Classification   Synthetic anticholinergic.

Uses   Adjunct in the treatment of peptic ulcer, irritable bowel syndrome.

Dosage   **Adults, PO:** 2.5–5 mg t.i.d. to q.i.d. before meals and at bedtime. *Geriatric or debilitated patients:* 2.5 mg t.i.d. before meals.

DICYCLOMINE HYDROCHLORIDE ANTISPAS, BENTOMINE, BENTYL, DIBENT, DI-SPAZ, OR-TYL, NOSPAZ, SPASTYL

Classification   Synthetic antispasmodic, miscellaneous.

Remarks Does not reduce excess gastric secretions or salivation. Has local anesthetic properties. Antacids and sedatives may be given concurrently.

Uses Hypermotility and spasms of GI tract associated with irritable colon and spastic colitis, ulcerative colitis, diverticulitis, and peptic ulcers.

Additional Untoward Reactions Brief euphoria, slight dizziness, and feeling of abdominal distention. Not contraindicated in glaucoma.

Dosage **PO, adults:** 10–20 mg t.i.d.-q.i.d.; **children:** 10 mg t.i.d.–q.i.d.; **infants:** 5 mg (as liquid) t.i.d.–q.i.d. **IM only, adults:** 20 mg q 4 to 6 hr. **Not for IV use.**

DIPHEMANIL METHYLSULFATE PRANTAL METHYLSULFATE

Classification Synthetic anticholinergic, antispasmodic (quaternary ammonium compound).

Remarks Available as timed-release preparation. Onset: 1 to 2 hours; duration: 4 hours. Oral absorption is poor.

Uses Adjunct in management of peptic ulcer, gastritis, pylorospasm, selected cases of bronchial asthma, hyperhidrosis, and excess sweating associated with dermatoses.

Dosage **PO:** 100–200 mg or more every 4 to 6 hr up to total maximum of 1.2 gm daily. **Maintenance:** 50–100 mg q 4 to 6 hr.

Administration Administer 2 hours before meals.

GLYCOPYRROLATE ROBINUL

Classification Synthetic anticholinergic, antispasmodic (quaternary ammonium compound).

Remarks PO: onset, 1 hour; duration of action, 6 hours. IV: onset, 10 minutes. Parenteral administration may retard emptying of stomach and cause pain at injection site. Drug not indicated for children less than 12 years old or pregnant women.

Uses Adjunct in management of peptic ulcer and other suitable GI conditions characterized by hypermotility, hypersecretion, and spasm.

Additional Contraindications Acute glaucoma, cardiospasms, prostatic hypertrophy, pyloric or duodenal obstruction, stenosis, peptic ulcer, urinary or gastric retention. Children under 12 years old.

Drug Interaction Do not add to IV solutions containing sodium chloride or bicarbonate.

Dosage *Individualized:* morning, early evening, bedtime. **PO:** 1–2 mg t.i.d.; **SC, IM, IV:** when rapid onset is required, 0.1–0.2 mg every 4 or more hours for GI disorders. Do not mix with sodium chloride or bicarbonate. *Preanesthetic medication,* **adults: IM:** 0.0044 mg/kg 30–60 minutes prior to induction; **pediatric less than 12 yrs: IM:** 0.0044–0.0088 mg/kg. *Reversal of neuromuscular blockade:* **IV:** 0.2 mg for each 1 mg neostigmine or equivalent dose of pyridostigmine.

Additional Nursing Implications
1. Have nasogastric tube available when more than two doses are given parenterally as it may be utilized to prevent gastric distention or vomiting.
2. Anticipate that the patient may complain of burning sensation at site of parenteral injection.

HEXOCYCLIUM METHYLSULFATE TRAL

Classification Synthetic anticholinergic, antispasmodic (quaternary ammonium compound).

Remarks Onset, 1 hour; duration, 3 to 4 hours.

Uses Peptic ulcer. GI conditions associated with hyperacidity, hypermotility, and spasms.

Dosage **PO:** 25 mg q.i.d. Give before meals and at bedtime. Special time-release tablets (50 or 75 mg b.i.d.) before lunch and bedtime. **Not for use in children.**

HOMATROPINE METHYLBROMIDE RU-SPAS NO. 2, SED-TENS SE

Classification Quaternary ammonium derivative of belladonna alkaloids.

Remarks Less active and less toxic than belladonna alkaloids.

Uses Spasmolytic: GI spasms, hyperacidity, and mild spasticity of bile ducts, gallbladder, and uterus.

Dosage **PO, adults:** 2.5–10 mg t.i.d.-q.i.d. before meals and at bedtime; **infants** (*colic*): 0.3–1 mg dissolved in H_2O 4 to 6 times a day before feeding.

HYOSCYAMINE SULFATE ANASPAZ, CYSTOSPAZ-M, LEVAMINE, LEVSIN, LEVSINEX

Classification Belladonna alkaloid.

Remark   This drug is one of the principal alkaloids of belladonna.

Uses   Antispasmodic and anticholinergic therapy. For the management of peptic ulcer, gastric hypersecretions, intestinal hypermotility, abdominal cramps, diarrhea, parkinsonism, and poisoning by anticholinesterase agents.

Dosage   **PO:** 0.125–0.25 mg t.i.d.-q.i.d. or 0.375 mg sustained release q 12 hrs. **IM, SC, IV:** 0.25–0.5 mg q 6 hr. **Pediatric, PO, 2–10 years:** ½ of adult dosage; **up to 2 years:** ¼ of adult dosage.

ISOPROPAMIDE IODIDE DARBID

Classification   Synthetic anticholinergic antispasmodic (quaternary ammonium compound).

Remarks   Long-acting, up to 12 hours. Sedatives and antacids may be given concurrently.

Uses   Peptic ulcer and GI conditions associated with hyperacidity.

Dosage   **PO,** *individualized:* 5 mg every 12 hr; some may require 10 mg b.i.d. **Not for use in children under 12 years of age.**

MEPENZOLATE BROMIDE CANTIL

Classification   Synthetic anticholinergic antispasmodic (quaternary ammonium compound).

Uses   Inflammatory conditions of colon.

Dosage   **PO:** 25–50 mg q.i.d. before meals and at bedtime. Initiate therapy with 25 mg q.i.d., increase gradually until therapeutic response is obtained or until side effects appear.

Additional Nursing Implication   Carefully observe for side effects while dosage is being increased. Maintenance dosage is attained when maximum therapeutic response or side effects appear.

METHANTHELINE BROMIDE BANTHINE

Classification   Synthetic anticholinergic antispasmodic (quaternary ammonium compound).

Remarks   PO: onset, 30 minutes; duration 6 hours; IM: duration, 2 to 4 hours. Drug also has some ganglionic blocking effect.

Uses   Peptic ulcer, pylorospasm, spastic colon, spasms of ureter or bladder, biliary dyskinesia, pancreatitis, selected cases of gastritis and bronchial asthma, preanesthetic antisecretory agent, control of sweating, and urinary frequency and enuresis.

Additional Untoward Reactions   Postural hypotension, impotence. Overdosage may cause respiratory paralysis and tachycardia.

Dosage   **PO, adults:** 50–100 mg q.i.d.; **pediatric, over 1 year:** 12.5–50 mg q.i.d.; **infants 1–12 months:** 12.5 mg q.i.d. up to 25 mg q.i.d.

Additional Nursing Implications   1. Initiate therapy in patients with duodenal ulcer while they are on liquid diet.
2. Observe ulcer patients for abdominal distention, epigastric distress, and vomiting because drug reduces gastric motility.
3. Assist the patient to rise slowly from supine position because of possibility of postural hypotension.
4. Alert patients to possibility of drug-induced impotence.

METHIXENE HYDROCHLORIDE TREST

Classification   Synthetic antispasmodic, miscellaneous.

Remarks   This drug has a direct relaxant effect on smooth muscles and some antihistaminic and CNS stimulant effect. It has no effect on gastric secretion.

Uses   GI conditions associated with hypermotility or spasms.

Dosage   **PO:** 1–2 mg t.i.d.

METHSCOPOLAMINE BROMIDE HYOSCINE METHYLBROMIDE, PAMINE BROMIDE, SCOPOLAMINE METHYLBROMIDE

Classification   Anticholinergic; quaternary ammonium derivative of belladonna alkaloids.

Remarks   Onset: PO, 1 hour; duration, 4 to 6 hours. Side effects are dose related. Reduction in dose for 5 to 7 days may relieve side effects.

Uses   Adjunctive for treatment of peptic ulcer, hyperhidrosis, excess salivation. Selected spastic conditions of GI tract (hypermotility).

Dosage   **PO:** 2.5–5 mg q.i.d. 30 minutes before mealtime and at bedtime; **infants up to 3 mo:** 0.5–1 mg daily; **6–12 mo:** 2–3 mg daily. **IM or SC** (*acute condition*): 0.25–1 mg every 6 to 8 hr.

OXYPHENCYCLIMINE HYDROCHLORIDE DARICON

Classification Anticholinergic antispasmodic, tertiary amine type.

Remarks Sedatives and antacids may be given concurrently. High doses may cause CNS stimulation. Have neostigmine available for treatment of toxicity.

Uses Peptic ulcer, pylorospasms, spastic and inflammatory condition of GI tract (colon), ureter, bladder, or biliary tract.

Dosage **PO: initial,** 10 mg b.i.d. in AM and before bedtime. May be increased up to maximum of 50 mg daily. **Not recommended for use in children under 12 years of age.**

OXYPHENONIUM BROMIDE ANTRENYL

Classification Anticholinergic antispasmodic (quaternary ammonium compound).

Remarks Large incidence of side effects. Onset, 30 minutes; duration, 6 hours. Have neostigmine on hand for treatment of toxic effects.

Uses Peptic ulcer; GI conditions associated with spasms and hyperacidity. Bronchial asthma, and control of perspiration.

Dosage *Highly individualized.* **PO:** 10 mg q.i.d. before meals and at bedtime. **Not for use in children.**

PROPANTHELINE BROMIDE PRO-BANTHINE, NORPANTH, ROPANTH

Classification Anticholinergic antispasmodic (quaternary ammonium compound).

Uses Peptic ulcer, spastic and inflammatory disease of GI tract, urethral, and bladder spasms, control of salivation and perspiration, and enuresis.

Dosage **PO: Usual,** 15 mg t.i.d. plus 30 mg at bedtime. **Extreme:** 30 mg q 8 hr. **IM or IV:** 30 mg q 6 hr. Safe use in children not established.

Administration Mix just before parenteral administration.

Additional Nursing Implication A liquid diet is recommended during initiation of therapy for patients with edematous duodenal ulcer.

SCOPOLAMINE HYDROBROMIDE HYOSCINE HYDROBROMIDE

Classification Anticholinergic.

Remarks   CNS depressant. When administered with morphine or meperidine, it produces amnesia. Tolerance may develop if scopolamine is given alone; in the presence of pain, it may produce delirium.

Uses   Sedative; salivary inhibitor; parkinsonism; paralysis agitans and other spastic states; preanesthetic; motion sickness; mydriatic; cycloplegic.

Contraindications   Hepatitis, asthma, and toxemia of pregnancy.

Additional Untoward Reactions   Disorientation, delirium, increased heart rate, and decreased respiration.

Dosage   **PO:** 0.4–0.8 mg t.i.d.-q.i.d.; **SC, IM, IV,** *preanesthetic:* 0.32–0.65 mg. **SC, pediatric,** *preanesthetic,* **6 mo–3 years:** 0.1–0.15 mg; **3–6 years:** 0.15–0.2 mg; **6–12 years:** 0.2–0.3 mg.

Additional Nursing Implications
1. Do not administer drug alone for pain as it is likely to cause delirium.
2. Observe for tolerance after a long course of therapy.
3. Orient and reassure patient who has experienced amnesia after receiving drug.

THIPHENAMIL HYDROCHLORIDE TROCINATE

Classification   Synthetic antispasmodic, miscellaneous; related to local anesthetics. More effective and less toxic than cocaine.

Remarks   Very low incidence of side effects. May be used in the presence of glaucoma.

Uses   Hypermotility and spasms of GI tract.

Dosage   **PO:** 400 mg q 4 hours. **Not for use in children.**

TRIDIHEXETHYL CHLORIDE PATHILON CHLORIDE

Classification   Anticholinergic, antispasmodic (quaternary ammonium compound).

Remark   Neostigmine should be on hand for toxic reactions.

Uses   Peptic ulcer, spastic and irritable colon, and pylorospasms and GI conditions associated with hyperacidity, hypermotility, and spasms.

Dosage   *Highly individualized.* **PO: initial,** 25–50 mg t.i.d. before meals, 50 mg at bedtime or 75 mg sustained release q 12 hr. **IV, IM, SC:** 10–20 mg q.i.d. Switch to **PO** therapy as soon as possible.

MYDRIATICS AND CYCLOPLEGICS

General Statement

These agents dilate the pupil (mydriasis) and paralyze the muscles required to accommodate for close vision (cycloplegia). This enables the physician to examine the inner structure of the eye including the retina. The cycloplegic action of the drug permits the physician to examine for refractive errors of the lens without the patient automatically accommodating. (For individual agents and dosages, see Table 24, below.)

Uses

Diagnostic ophthalmoscopic examination, refraction in children, pre- and postoperative mydriasis during eye surgery, provocative test for

TABLE 24 MYDRIATICS AND CYCLOPLEGICS

Drug	Dosage	Remarks
Atropine Sulfate (Atropisol, Buf-Opto Atropine, Isopto Atropine)	*Refraction,* **adults:** 1–2 gtts in eye 1 hr before examination; **children:** 1–2 gtts, 0.5% solution in eyes b.i.d. for 1 to 3 days prior to examination and 1 hr prior to examination. *Uveitis,* **adults:** 1–2 gtts in eye up to t.i.d.; **children:** 1–2 gtts of 0.5% solution in eye up to t.i.d.	*Remarks* Prolonged duration (up to 12 days in children). Drug particularly prone to have systemic effects such as contact dermatitis, allergic conjunctivitis. Available in 0.25%–4% solutions or 0.5% or 1.0% ointment.
Cyclopentolate hydrochloride (Cyclogyl)	*Refraction:* 1–2 gtts of 0.5%–2% solution.	Rapid onset (25–75 minutes); medium duration (24 hours).
Homatropine hydrobromide (Homatrocel, Isopto Homatropine)	*Refraction:* 1–2 gtts; repeat in 5 to 10 minutes if necessary. *Uveitis:* 1–2 gtts q 3 to 4 hours.	Short acting. Onset 60 minutes. Persisting for 36 to 48 hours. Available as 1%, 2% or 5% solution.
Scopolamine (Isopto Hyoscine)	1–2 gtts of 0.2%–0.25% solution.	Shorter acting with fewer side effects than atropine.
Tropicamide (Mydriacyl)	*Refraction:* 1–2 drops of 0.5%–1% solution repeated after 20 to 25 minutes if necessary. Maximum cycloplegia occurs in 20 to 35 minutes when a second drop is given 5 minutes after first.	Rapid onset: 20–35 minutes; duration, 2 to 6 hr. Drug particularly likely to cause systemic side effects.

angle-closure glaucoma, selected cases of secondary angle-closure glaucoma, malignant glaucoma, and anterior uveitis.

Contraindication Angle-closure glaucoma.

Untoward Reactions Blurred vision. Systemic reactions (rarely): those characteristics of all cholinergic blocking agents, including dryness of mouth and skin, flushing, fever, rash, thirst, tachycardia, irritability, hyperactivity, ataxia, confusion, somnolence, hallucinations and delirium. These reactions occur more frequently in children, elderly patients, and in case of damage to the corneal epithelium.

Dosage See Table 24.

Administration Drops are instilled in conjunctival sac.

Nursing Implications
1. Warn the patient that these drugs will temporarily impair vision and that he/she should not do close work, operate machinery, or drive a car until the effects have worn off.
2. Before administering, check whether the patient has a history of angle-closure glaucoma because the drug may precipitate an acute crisis.

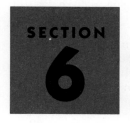

SECTION 6

neuromuscular blocking agents

Decamethonium Bromide
Gallamine Triethiodide
Hexafluorenium Bromide
Metocurine Iodide

Pancuronium Bromide
Succinylcholine Chloride
Tubocurarine Chloride

General Statement The drugs considered in this section do not act on the CNS but interfere locally with nerve transmission between the motor endplate and the receptors of the skeletal muscles. Normally, these muscles contract when acetylcholine is released from storage sites embedded in the motor endplate. Release occurs when the motor nerve is stimulated appropriately.

The drugs fall into two groups: competitive (nondepolarizing) agents, like tubocurarine, and depolarizing agents like succinylcholine and decamethonium. The competitive agents compete with acetylcholine for the receptor sites in the muscle cells. They are also often referred to as curariform agents because their mode of action is similar to that of the poison curare in which ancient hunters dipped arrows to paralyze their prey. The depolarizing agents prolong depolarization of the muscle and prevent the receptors from responding to acetylcholine, thus keeping the muscle from responding.

The muscle paralysis caused by the neuromuscular blocking agents is sequential. Therapeutic doses produce muscle depression in the following order: heaviness of eyelids, difficulty in swallowing and talking, diplopia, progressive weakening of the extremities and neck, followed by relaxation of the trunk and spine. The diaphragm (respiratory paralysis) is affected last. The drugs do not affect consciousness, and their use, in the absence of adequate levels of general anesthesia, is frightening.

There is a narrow margin of safety between a therapeutically effective dose causing muscle relaxation and a toxic dose causing respiratory paralysis. **The neuromuscular blocking agents are always administered by a physician.** However, the nurse must be prepared to maintain a patient's respiration until the drug wears off.

Uses   Skeletal muscle relaxation during anesthesia. This usually permits use of a lighter level of anesthesia. The drugs also facilitate endotracheal intubation and prevent laryngospasms.

As adjunct when muscle relaxation is required in tetanus, encephalitis, poliomyelitis, and electroshock therapy. Diagnosis of myasthenia gravis.

Contraindications   The neuromuscular blocking agents should be used with caution in patients with myasthenia gravis; renal, hepatic, or pulmonary impairment; respiratory depression; and in elderly or debilitated patients.

Depolarizing agents should be used with caution for patients with electrolyte imbalance, especially hyperkalemia, and in patients on digitalis.

Untoward Reactions   **Respiratory Paralysis**
Some neuromuscular blocking agents cause hypotension, bronchospasms, cardiac disturbances, hyperthermia.

Drug Interactions   Some drugs interfere with either competitive blockers or depolarizing agents.

Interactant	Interaction
Aminoglycoside antibiotics	↑ Muscle relaxation
Gentamicin	
Kanomycin	
Neomycin	
Streptomycin	
Amphotericin B	↑ Muscle relaxation
Colistin	↑ Muscle relaxation

Drug Interactions (Continued)

Interactant	Interaction
Furosemide (Lasix)	Furosemide ↑ effect of skeletal muscle relaxants
Magnesium salts	↑ Muscle relaxation
Methotrimeprazine (Levoprome)	↑ Muscle relaxation
Narcotic analgesics	↑ Respiratory depression and ↑ muscle relaxation
Phenothiazines	↑ Muscle relaxation
Polymyxin B	↑ Muscle relaxation
Procainamide	↑ Muscle relaxation
Procaine	↑ Muscle relaxation by ↓ plasma protein binding
Quinidine	↑ Muscle relaxation
Thiazide diuretics	↑ Muscle relaxation

Nursing Implications

1. Monitor respiration, BP, and pulse very closely for the duration of action of the drug, and report untoward signs.
2. Observe the patient for signs of respiratory embarrassment or apnea and be prepared to assist with artificial respiration and provision of oxygen.
3. Observe and report excessive bronchial secretions or respiratory wheezing.
4. Have oxygen, a respirator, neostigmine, atropine, and epinephrine available for emergency use.
5. Be aware that the respiratory depression caused by nondepolarizing type may be relieved by anticholinesterase drugs, such as neostigmine, which increase the body's production of acetylcholine, but that the antidote for depolarizing drugs is oxygen under pressure followed by whole blood or plasma if apnea is prolonged.

DECAMETHONIUM BROMIDE SYNCURINE

Classification Depolarizing blocker.

General Statement Acts directly on motor endplate. No CNS effect. Onset, 8 to 20 minutes. Duration of action is longer than succinylcholine—complete recovery may take 20 minutes.

Overdosage causes complete respiratory paralysis for which oxygen is the only antidote. Patients should be routinely intubated when drug is used.

Uses Muscle relaxation during anesthesia, endotracheal intubation, and electroshock therapy.

Additional Contraindications Preexisting respiratory depression. Use with caution in the very old and the very young.

Dosage IV: 0.5–3 mg at a rate of 1 mg/minute. Subsequent doses of 0.5–1 mg may be given at 10- to 30-minute intervals up to maximum of 10 mg.

GALLAMINE TRIETHIODIDE FLAXEDIL I.V.

Classification   Competitive blocker (non depolarizing).

Remarks   Similar to tubocurarine. Always induces tachycardia. Onset: immediate; duration: 20 minutes. Effect of drug is cumulative.

Uses   Muscle relaxant during surgery, electroshock therapy, and manipulative procedures like laryngoscopy.

Additional Contraindications   Cardiac disease, especially for patients in whom tachycardia may be dangerous. Also in presence of hypertension, hyperthyroidism, impaired renal function or respiratory depression, and hypersensitivity to iodine.

Dosage   **IV (after general anesthesia has been introduced):** *highly individualized.* **Initial,** 1 mg/kg body weight up to maximum of 100 mg; an additional dose of 0.5–1 mg/kg body weight may be given at 30- to 50-minute intervals.

Dose should be reduced if used with cyclopropane, ether, halothane, or methoxyflurane.

HEXAFLUORENIUM BROMIDE MYLAXEN

Classification   Plasma cholinesterase inhibitor.

Remarks   Only used in conjunction with succinylcholine to prolong action. Permits reduction of dosage of succinylcholine and thus decreases side effects of the latter. Has no muscle relaxing effect by itself.

Main Use   Adjunct muscle relaxant during surgery.

Dosage   **IV:** 0.4 mg/kg body weight to be followed after 3 minutes by 0.2 mg/kg body weight succinylcholine.

Administration   Drug is administered after anesthetization and prior to surgery.

METOCURINE IODIDE METUBINE IODIDE INJECTION

Classification   Competitive blocker, curare type (nondepolarizing).

Remarks   Similar to tubocurarine with lower incidence of respiratory paralysis. Initial dose provides relaxation for 25 to 90 minutes.

Uses   Muscle relaxation during surgery, manipulative procedures, electroshock therapy, certain CNS injuries, diagnosis of myasthenia gravis.

Dosage   **IV:** Dose depends on type of anesthetic used. For example, with *ether anesthesia:* 1.5–3.0 mg; with *nitrous oxide anesthesia:* 4–7 mg; with *cyclopropane anesthesia:* 2–4 mg. Drug is injected over a period of 30 to 90 sec. Additional doses of 0.5–1.0 mg may be given as required. *Electroshock therapy:* range of 1.75–5.5 mg (usual 2–3 mg).

Additional Nursing Implications
1. Have neostigmine methylsulfate on hand during IV administration to combat respiratory depression.
2. Do not give neostigmine when respiratory depression is associated with fall in blood pressure as it may aggravate shock.

PANCURONIUM BROMIDE PAVULON

Classification Competitive blocker, curare type (nondepolarizing).

Remarks Drug is about 5 times as potent as *d*-tubocurarine chloride.

Use Muscle relaxation during anesthesia and for endotracheal intubation.

Additional Contraindications Hypersensitivity to bromide, tachycardia, children under 10 years of age, and patients in whom increase in heart rate is undesirable.

Dosage **IV: initial,** 40–100 μg/kg. Additional doses of 10 μg/kg may be administered at 25- to 60-minute intervals. Dosage requirements for children are the same as adults. **Neonates:** a test dose of 20 μg/kg should be administered first to determine responsiveness.

SUCCINYLCHOLINE CHLORIDE ANECTINE CHLORIDE, QUELICIN CHLORIDE, SUCOSTRIN CHLORIDE, SUX-CERT

Classification Depolarizing blocker.

Remarks Short-acting muscle relaxant. Onset, 1 minute; duration, 2 to 4 minutes.

Uses Muscle relaxant during surgery, endotracheal intubation, endoscopy and short manipulative procedures; electroshock therapy.

Additional Contraindications Use with caution in patients with severe liver disease, severe anemia, malnutrition, or impaired cholinesterase activity (i.e. insecticide poisoning). May cause severe, persistent respiratory depression.

Drug Interactions

Interactant	Interaction
Aminoglycoside antibiotics Kanamycin, Gentamicin, Neomycin, Streptomycins	Additive skeletal muscle blockade
Colistin	Additive skeletal muscle blockade
Cyclophosphamide	↑ Effect of succinylcholine by ↓ breakdown of drug in plasma by pseudocholinesterase
Diazepam (Valium)	↓ Effect of succinylcholine
Digitalis glycosides	↑ Chance of cardiac arrhythmias

Interactant	*Interaction*
Echothiophate Iodide	↑ Effect of succinylcholine by ↓ breakdown of drug in plasma by pseudocholinesterase
Lidocaine	↑ Effect of succinylcholine by ↓ plasma protein binding
Magnesium salts	Additive skeletal muscle blockade

Monoamide oxidase inhibitors
  Pargyline (Eutonyl)
  Tranylcypromine
  (Parnate)
	↑ Effect of succinylcholine by ↓ breakdown of drug in plasma by pseudocholinesterase

Narcotic analgesics	↑ Neuromuscular blockade due to CNS depressant effects
Neostigmine	↑ Effect of succinylcholine by ↓ breakdown of drug in plasma by pseudocholinesterase
Polymyxin	Additive skeletal muscle blockade
Procaine	↑ Effect of succinylcholine by ↓ plasma protein binding
Quinidine	Additive skeletal muscle blockade
Thiotepa	↑ Effect of succinylcholine by ↓ breakdown of drug in plasma by pseudocholinesterase

Dosage   **IV: Usual,** an initial test dose of 10 mg should be given to assess sensitivity and recovery time. For surgical procedures, dose range is 25–75 mg. **Pediatric:** 1–2 mg/kg. For prolonged procedures, use **IV drip:** 2.5 mg/minute for adults. **IM,** 2.5 mg/kg up to maximum of 150 mg total dose.

Administration/ Storage
1. For IV infusion, use 1 or 2 mg/ml solution of drug in 5% dextrose injection, 0.9% sodium chloride, or other suitable IV solution.
2. Alter degree of relaxation by altering rate of flow.
3. Store in refrigerator.
4. Do not mix with anesthetic.

TUBOCURARINE CHLORIDE *d*-TUBOCURARINE CHLORIDE

Classification   Natural curare alkaloid. Competitive blocker (non-depolarizing).

General Statement   Narrow margin between therapeutic dose and toxic dose. Overdosage chiefly treated by artificial respiration, although neostigmine, atropine, and edrophonium chloride should be on hand.

Uses   Muscle relaxant during abdominal surgery, setting of fractures and dislocations; spasticity caused by injury to or disease of CNS; electro-shock therapy; diagnosis of myasthenia gravis.

Additional Contraindications   Use with extreme caution in patients with renal dysfunction, liver disease, or obstructive states. Drug may cause excessive secretion and circulatory collapse.

Additional Drug Interaction   Combination with diazepam (Valium) may cause malignant hyperthermia.

Dosage   **IV, IM:** initial dose should be 20 units *less* than the calculated amount. *Surgery*, **IV:** usually 1.1 unit/kg (40–60 units at time of incision followed by 20–30 units in 3 to 5 minutes, if necessary). *Electroshock therapy:* 1.1 units/kg **IV** over 60–90 sec. *Diagnosis of myasthenia gravis*, **IV:** 0.07–0.22 units/kg.

<table>
<tr><td rowspan="2">CHAPTER
7</td></tr>
</table>

| CHAPTER **7** | # HORMONES AND HORMONE ANTAGONISTS |

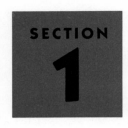
insulin and oral antidiabetics

Insulins	Extended Insulin Zinc Suspension	Insulin Zinc Suspension
	Globin Zinc Insulin Injection	Isophane Insulin Suspension
	Insulin Injection	Prompt Insulin Zinc Suspension
	Insulin Injection Concentrated	Protamine Zinc Insulin Suspension
Oral Antidiabetic Agents	Acetohexamide	Tolbutamide
	Chlorpropamide	Tolbutamide Sodium
	Tolazamide	
Insulin Antagonists	Diazoxide	
	Glucagon	

INSULINS

General Statement

In 1922, the isolation of the hormone insulin, which is naturally produced by the islets of Langerhans in the pancreas, marked the beginning of hormone therapy. Insulin, isolated from cattle or hog pancreas, can effectively replace human insulin in insulin-deficiency diseases. Deficient insulin secretion results in the inadequate utilization of sugar by body tissues, which, in turn, results in diabetes.

Insulin enables all tissues, including the liver, to utilize carbohydrates. Insulin also participates in the metabolism of fats and proteins and is necessary for the transport of glucose through the cell walls. Regular administration of this hormone to diabetic patients maintains their blood sugar levels within the normal range (80– 120 mg/100 ml) and keeps the urine free of sugar and acetone bodies. Insulin prevents the development of diabetic acidosis and coma.

Since insulin is a protein, it is destroyed in the GI tract. It must be administered parenterally and is readily absorbed into the bloodstream.

In recent years, insulin preparations having different times of onset, peak activity, and duration of action have been developed. These preparations permit the physician to select the preparation best suited to the lifestyle of patient.

Three different types of insulin are available today. They are all obtained from cattle or hogs, but they are prepared in such a manner that the insulin is absorbed by the body at different rates.

The action of a preparation that is absorbed rapidly has a rapid onset and is of short duration. By contrast, that of a preparation absorbed slowly has a slower onset and is more prolonged.

The three available types of insulin are classified as: fast acting; intermediate acting; and long acting.

Fast-Acting Insulin

1. Insulin injection (Regular Insulin, Crystalline Zinc Insulin, Regular Iletin)
2. Prompt insulin zinc suspension (Semilente Insulin, Semilente Iletin)

Insulin injection is a noncrystalline (amorphous) form of insulin that is rapidly absorbed into the bloodstream from the site of subcutaneous injection.

Its onset of action is one-half to 1 hour and its effect lasts from 5 to 16 hours. It usually is given in an emergency and 15 to 30 minutes before meals. If necessary, insulin injection can be given IV.

Because of its rapid onset of action and short duration of effect, fast-acting insulin is usually used to stabilize newly diagnosed diabetic patients. At a later date, these patients usually are transferred to a long-acting preparation.

Intermediate-Acting Insulin

1. Globin zinc insulin injection
2. Isophane insulin suspension (NPH Insulin, NPH Iletin)
3. Insulin zinc suspension (Lente Iletin, Lente Insulin)

When insulin is precipitated in the presence of zinc chloride, it forms large crystals. This form of insulin has a slightly slower onset of action (2 hours) and a slightly longer duration of action (18 to 24 hours).

Most patients with maturity-onset diabetes can be maintained on a single daily dose of intermediate-acting insulin, especially if it is coupled with a sound diet.

Other patients may require additional doses of another form of insulin (prompt-acting) later in the day. A long-acting insulin to prevent nocturnal increase in blood sugar may be required by some patients.

Long-Acting Insulin

1. Protamine zinc insulin suspension (Protamine, Zinc and Iletin; PZI)
2. Extended insulin zinc suspension (Ultralente Iletin, Ultralente Insulin)

This type of insulin consists of a combination of insulin, zinc chloride, and the protein protamine. The latter makes the insulin relatively insoluble so that it is absorbed slowly from the site of injection. These preparations have a slow onset of action (7 hours) and are active for approximately 24 to 36 hours.

Long-acting insulin is never prescribed for diabetic emergencies and is most suitable for patients whose blood sugar increases during the night.

It is rarely used as the sole antidiabetic agent. *Note:* Insulin preparations with various times of onset and duration of action are often mixed to obtain optimum control of diabetic patients.

Compatibilities and characteristics of various preparations are listed in Table 25, p. 530.

TABLE 25 INSULINS

	Trade Name	Appearance	Dosage**	Onset	Peak (Hours)	Duration	Compatible With
Fast Acting							
Insulin injection	Regular Insulin Regular Iletin	Clear	*Individualized* 5–100 USP units 1 to 4 times daily	½–1	2–3	5–8	All preparations
Prompt insulin zinc suspension	Semilente Iletin Semilente Insulin*	Cloudy suspension	*Individualized* 10–80 USP units	½–1	3–9	12–16	All preparations
Intermediate Acting							
Globin zinc insulin suspension		Clear	*Individualized* 10–80 USP units	1–4	6–16	16–24	All preparations
Insulin zinc suspension	Lente Iletin Lente Insulin*	Cloudy suspension	*Individualized* 10–80 USP units	1–4	7–12	24–30	All preparations
Isophane insulin suspension	NPH Iletin NPH Insulin	Cloudy suspension	*Individualized* 10–80 USP units	1–2	7–12	24–30	All preparations
Long Acting							
Extended zinc insulin suspension	Ultralente Iletin Ultralente Insulin*	Cloudy suspension	*Individualized*	4–8	10–18	30–36	All preparations
Protamine zinc insulin suspension	PZI Protamine, Zinc, and Iletin	Cloudy suspension	*Individualized* 10–80 USP units	4–8	12–24	30–36	All preparations

* Contains only beef insulin.
** Number of times drug is given is highly individualized.
Remarks: These preparations are derived from cattle and/or hogs. Also see Insulin concentrate.

Uses Replacement therapy in the treatment of diabetes mellitus, juvenile onset diabetes, brittle diabetes, as a substitute for oral antidiabetic therapy for patients with maturity onset diabetes complicated by acidosis, ketosis, diabetic coma, major surgery, fever, severe trauma, infections, impaired renal or hepatic function, thyroid or other endocrine dysfunction, gangrene, Raynaud's disease, and during pregnancy of diabetic patients. Insulin has been used for shock therapy in the treatment of mental depression and is occasionally used during hyperalimentation. In the latter case, excess insulin results in the increased utilization of sugar.

Diet The dietary control of diabetes is as important as medication with appropriate drugs. The role of the nurse in teaching the patient how to eat properly cannot be underestimated.

As a first step the physician must determine the individual patient's dietary requirements. Since there is a very close relationship between carbohydrate (CHO), fat (F), and protein (P), intake of each of these nutrients must be regulated. The prescribed amount of CHO, P, and F eaten at each meal must remain constant.

The nurse must teach the patient how to calculate exchange values of various foods. Food lists and food exchange values published by the American Diabetes Association and the American Dietetic Association are valuable teaching aids.

Diabetic patients should adhere to a regular meal schedule. Patients taking large amounts of insulin will frequently be better controlled when they have four to six small meals daily rather than three large ones. The frequency of meals and the overall caloric intake vary with the type of drug taken. Diabetic children may be on a "free diet."

Contraindication Hypersensitivity to insulin.

Untoward Reactions Hypoglycemia or insulin shock due to hyperinsulinism (excess insulin). Even carefully controlled patients may occasionally develop signs of insulin overdosage characterized by hunger, weakness, fatigue, nervousness, pallor or flushing, profuse sweating, headache, palpitations, numbness of mouth, tingling in the fingers, tremors, blurred and double vision, hypothermia, excess yawning, mental confusion, incoordination, tachycardia, and loss of consciousness.

Symptoms of hypoglycemia may mimic psychic disturbances. Severe prolonged hypoglycemia may cause brain damage and in the elderly may mimic stroke.

Mild hypoglycemia can be relieved by PO administration of carbohydrates (orange juice, candy, sugar).

Extreme hypoglycemia responds to the IV administration of dextrose solutions. Glucagon (0.5–1 mg SC, IM, or IV; repeat after 25 minutes if response of patient is unsatisfactory) or epinephrine (SC: 0.25–0.50 ml of 1 : 1000 epinephrine hydrochloride solution) can be used in an emergency.

Localized allergic reactions, which disappear with continued use, are seen in about one fourth of the patients started on insulin. Symptoms usually appear 1 to 3 weeks after the onset of therapy.

Generalized allergic reactions (generalized urticaria, angioneurotic edema, and anaphylaxis) occur rarely and then usually after intermittent insulin therapy or IV administration of large amounts to insulin-resistant patients.

Symptoms usually can be relieved with antihistamines.

Severe allergic reactions can be treated with corticosteroids. These compounds, however, induce insulin resistance and should be discontinued as soon as possible.

Patients who are highly allergic to insulin and cannot be treated with oral hypoglycemics can be desensitized by the SC administration of small doses of the hormone as directed by the physician.

Resistance to insulin rarely develops; it can be induced by chronic overdosage, however.

Some patients may be selectively resistant to one particular form of insulin and in these patients, insulin derived from another animal species should be tried.

Atrophy and hypertrophy of subcutaneous tissue may appear at frequently used injection sites.

Changes in vision occur occasionally while insulin therapy is being initiated or in patients who have been uncontrolled for a long period of time.

Diabetic Coma and Hypoglycemic Reaction (Insulin Shock)

Coma in diabetes may be caused by uncontrolled diabetes (high sugar content in blood or urine, ketoacidosis) or by too much insulin (insulin shock, hypoglycemia).

Diabetic coma and insulin shock can be differentiated in the following manner:

Diagnostic Feature	Hyperglycemia (Diabetic Coma)	Hypoglycemia (Insulin Shock)
Onset	Gradual (days)	Sudden (24–48 hours)
Medication	Insufficient insulin	Excess insulin
Food intake	Normal or excess	Probably too little
Overall appearance	Extremely ill	Very weak
Skin	Dry and flushed	Moist and pale
Infection	Frequent	Absent
Fever	Frequent	Absent
Mouth	Dry	Drooling
Thirst	Intense	Absent
Hunger	Absent	Occasional
Vomiting	Common	Absent
Abdominal pain	Frequent	Rare
Respiration	Increased, air hunger	Normal
Breath	Acetone odor	Normal
Blood pressure	Low	Normal
Pulse	Weak and rapid	Full and bounding
Vision	Dim	Diplopia

Diagnostic Feature	Hyperglycemia (Diabetic Coma)	Hypoglycemia (Insulin Shock)
Tremor	Absent	Frequent
Convulsions	None	In late stages
Urine sugar	High	Absent in 2nd specimen
Ketone bodies	High	Absent in 2nd specimen
Blood sugar	High	Less than 60 mg/100 ml

Adapted from *Merck Manual*.

Diabetic coma is usually precipitated by the patient's failure to take insulin. Hypoglycemia is often precipitated by the patient's unpredictable response, excess exertion, stress due to illness or surgery, errors in calculating dosage, or failure to eat.

Treatment of Diabetic Coma or Severe Acidosis

Administer 30 to 60 units of insulin. This is followed by doses of 20 units or more every 30 minutes. To avoid a hypoglycemic state, 1 gm of dextrose is administered for each unit of insulin given. Treatment is often supplemented by electrolytes and fluids. Urine samples are collected for analysis and vital signs monitored as ordered.

Treatment of Hypoglycemia (Insulin Shock)

Glucose is administered PO or IV (25–50 ml of 25% solution). If this is not possible, epinephrine, hydrocortisone, or glucagon is given SC (see p. 548). When the patient regains consciousness, he/she should continue taking carbohydrates, especially if the hypoglycemia was caused by a long-acting antidiabetic agent.

Dosage Insulin is usually administered SC. Insulin injection (regular insulin) is the only preparation that may be administered IV. This route should only be used for patients with severe ketoacidosis or diabetic coma.

Dosage for insulin is always expressed in USP units.

Dosage is established and monitored by blood glucose, urine glucose, and acetone tests. Dosage is highly individualized. Furthermore, since the requirements of patients may change with time, dosage must be checked at regular intervals. It is usually advisable to hospitalize patients while their daily insulin and caloric requirements are being established.

In pregnancy, insulin requirements may increase suddenly during the last trimester. After delivery, there may be a sudden drop in requirement to prepregnancy levels. To prevent the development of hypoglycemia, insulin is often discontinued on the day of delivery and glucose is administered IV.

The various insulin preparations and their onset, peak effect, and length of action are detailed in Table 25. They can be mixed to obtain the preparation best suited for the individual patient. However, mixing must be done according to the directions received from the physician and/or pharmacist.

Drug Interactions

Interactant	Interaction
Alcohol, ethyl	Additive hypoglycemia may lead to low blood sugar and coma
Anabolic steriods	Additive hypoglycemia
Chlorthalidone (Hygroton)	Antagonizes hypoglycemic effect of antidiabetics
Contraceptives, oral	May impair glucose tolerance and thus change requirements for antidiabetics
Corticosteriods	Hyperglycemic effect of corticosteroids may necessitate ↑ in dose of antidiabetic agent
Cyclophosphamide	Cyclophosphamide inhibits insulin antibody formation leading to hypoglycemia
Dextrothyroxine (Choloxin)	Hyperglycemic effect of dextrothyroxine may necessitate ↑ in dose of antidiabetic agent
Epinephrine	Hyperglycemic effect of epinephrine may necessitate ↑ in dose of antidiabetic agent
Estrogens	May impair glucose tolerance and thus change requirements for antidiabetics
Ethacrynic acid (Edecrin)	Antagonizes hypoglycemic effect of antidiabetics
Furosemide (Lasix)	Antagonizes hypoglycemic effect of antidiabetics
Glucagon	Hyperglycemic effect of glucagon antagonizes hypoglycemic effect of antidiabetics
MAO Inhibitors Pargyline (Eutonyl) Tranylcypromine (Parnate)	MAO inhibitors ↑ and prolong hypoglycemic response to antidiabetics
Oxytetracyclines	↑ Effect of insulin
Phenothiazines	↓ Effect of antidiabetic agents since phenothiazines ↑ blood glucose
Propranolol (Inderal)	Propranolol inhibits the rebound of blood glucose following insulin-induced hypoglycemia
Thiazide diuretics	Antagonizes hypoglycemic effect of antidiabetics
Thyroid preparations	Hyperglycemic effect of thyroid preparations may necessitate ↑ in dose of antidiabetic agent
Triamterene (Dyrenium)	Antagonizes hypoglycemic effect of antidiabetics

Laboratory Test Interference

Alters liver function tests and thyroid function tests. False + Coombs test, ↑ serum protein, ↓ serum amino acids, calcium, cholesterol, potassium, and urine amino acids.

Administration/ Storage

1. Read the product information brochure and any important notes inserted into package of prescribed insulin.
2. Discard open vials that have not been used for several weeks or any whose expiration date has passed.
3. Refrigerate stock supply of insulin but avoid freezing. Freezing

destroys the manner in which insulin is suspended in the formulation.

4. Store insulin vial in use at room temperature avoiding extremes of temperature or exposure to sunlight.
5. Store compatible mixtures of insulin for no longer than 1 month at room temperature or 3 months at 2°–8°C (36°–46°F).
6. To ensure a constant amount of precipitate in each dose, invert the vial several times to mix before the material is withdrawn. Avoid vigorous shaking and frothing of the material. (Regular and globin insulin are the only two insulins that do not have a precipitate.)
7. Discard any vial in which the precipitate is clumped or granular in appearance or which has formed a solid deposit of particles on the side of the vial.
8. To insure correct preparation check that the top of the insulin vial matches the color of the needle cap on the syringe.

   Red is for U-40 insulin
   Green is for U-80 insulin
   Orange is for U-100 insulin

9. Procedure for preparing injection of mixture of an intermediate-acting insulin with a short-acting one.
   a. Inject an amount of air into the vial of intermediate-acting insulin equal to the prescribed insulin dosage.
   b. Inject an amount of air into the vial of short-acting insulin equal to the dose prescribed.
   c. Withdraw the dose of short-acting insulin.
   d. Remove the needle from the vial and check to make sure you have the proper amount of fluid without air bubbles.
   e. Turn the vial of intermediate-acting insulin upside down and roll it in your hands until it becomes cloudy.
   f. Insert the needle into the vial of intermediate-acting insulin and withdraw dosage into syringe.
   g. Withdraw needle from vial of insulin and make a final check for air bubbles before administering.

10. When preparing a mixture of regular and modified insulin, draw the regular insulin up *first* in the syringe to avoid transferring modified insulin into vial of regular insulin.
11. Administer at a 90° angle when using a ½ inch needle and a 45° angle when using a ⅝ inch needle for subcutaneous injection.
12. Provide an automatic injector for patients who are fearful of injecting themselves.
13. Assist the visually impaired diabetic to obtain information and devices for self-administration of insulin by writing to: New York Diabetes Association, 104 East 40th Street, New York, N.Y. 10016, for *Devices for Visually Impaired Diabetics*, and to The New York Association for the Blind, 111 East 59th Street, New York, N.Y. 10022, for *An Evaluation of Devices for Insulin Dependent Visually Handicapped Diabetics*.
14. Rotate the sites of SC injections of insulin to prevent local atrophy (appears as mild dimpling of skin to deep pits seen mostly on girls and young women) and hypertrophy (appears as well-developed

muscle on anterior and lateral thigh mostly in boys and young men).

    a. Encourage patient to keep a chart indicating injection sites. (See Figure 3)

    b. Allow 3–4 cm between injection sites.

    c. Do not inject same site for at least 1 month.

    d. Avoid 1 cm around the umbilicus because area has vascularity.

    e. Avoid waistline, as area has a sensitive nerve supply.

    f. For selfinjection, teach patient to brace arm to be injected against a hard surface such as a wall or a chair.

    g. See Figure 3 for recommended sites for insulin injection.

    h. Prevent further lipodystrophy by utilizing insulin at room temperature.

15. Always have an extra vial of insulin and equipment for administration on hand when the patient is in the hospital, at home, or travelling.

16. Have regular insulin available for emergency use.

17. Apply pressure for a minute after injection but do not massage after injection since this may interfere with rate of absorption.

18. Delay administration of insulin if breakfast is delayed for tests.

19. Care of reusable syringes and needles.

    a. Do not use heavily chlorinated water or water with a high chemical content for sterilizing syringes. For sterilization, boil the syringe and needle for 5 minutes.

    b. If the syringe and needle are sterilized by keeping them in alcohol for 24 hours, the alcohol must evaporate before equipment is used to prevent reduction in strength of insulin.

    c. Clean syringes covered by a precipitate with a cotton tipped swab soaked in vinegar; then, thoroughly rinse syringe in water and sterilize it. Clean needles with a wire and sharpen with a pumice stone.

Nursing Implications

1. *Applicable to all diabetic patients controlled by medication whether insulin or an oral hypoglycemic.*

Teach the patient and responsible family members:

    a. The nature of diabetes mellitus—signs and symptoms.

    b. Necessity for regular medical examinations.

    c. How to test urine for sugar and acetone.

    d. How to administer insulin. Explain equipment, care of equipment, provision and storage of medication, and the technique and time of administration.

    e. The importance of adhering to prescribed diets, with emphasis on weight control and ingestion of food relative to peak period of the medication being taken and the use of the food exchange list.

    f. The effects of exercise in raising carbohydrate needs.

    g. The necessity for good hygienic practices to prevent infection.

    h. To observe for hypoglycemic symptoms, such as fatigue, headache, drowsiness, tremulousness, or nausea.

    i. To observe for symptoms of hyperglycemia (leading to ketoaci-

Setting Up An Easy Rotation Cycle

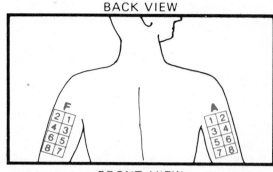

BACK VIEW

FRONT VIEW

Figure 3. Pattern for varying insulin injection sites.

If you follow the sketch, you'll see that the right arm is marked A, the right side of the abdomen is B, and the right thigh is C. Crossing to the left side of the body, the left thigh is marked D, the abdomen E, and the left arm F.

Each of these areas can be thought of as a rectangle which may be divided, as shown, into eight different squares more than one inch on each side. These squares are numbered, starting from the upper and outside corner, which is number one, to the lowest corner, which is number eight, with all even numbers toward the middle of the body.

If you select square number one and inject into it at each of the six Areas A through F, it will take you six days to return again to A. Then selecting square number two and injecting into it at each of the six areas again rotates you around your body, returning in six days to Area A. Follow with square number three, and so forth. It is easy to see that this procedure provides 48 different places in which to make your injections. If you make one injection daily, it will be that many days before you return to the A-1 square . . . almost seven weeks.

Figure and legend courtesy of Becton Dickinson and Company.

Injection Log

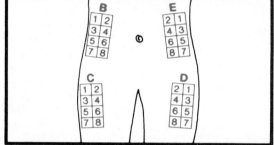

SITE		1	2	3	4	5	6	7	8
right arm	A								
right abdomen	B								
right thigh	C								
left thigh	D								
left abdomen	E								
left arm	F								

dosis), thirst, polyuria, drowsiness, flushed dry skin, fruity odor of breath, unconsciousness or diabetic coma.

j. Procedures to follow in hypo- and hyperglycemia and other emergency situations, as noted in the following.

k. Necessity for patient to carry candy or a lump of sugar to counteract hypoglycemia.

l. Importance of reporting hypo- and hyperglycemic reactions to medical supervision for adjustment of dosage of medication.

m. The advisability of patients carrying a card or wearing a Medic Alert bracelet, (see Appendix) indicating that they are diabetic.

2. Reassure the patient that allergic reactions, such as itching, redness, swelling, stinging, or warmth at the injection site, usually disappear after a few weeks of therapy.

3. Test urine for glycosuria with Clinitest Tablets, Tes-Tape, Diastix, or Clinistix, as recommended by the physician. Test a fresh second voided specimen. Instruct patient to empty bladder by urinating about 1 hour before mealtime. As soon as the patient can void again, obtain the specimen and test. ·

4. Observe the patient for symptoms of hypoglycemia, such as fatigue, headache, drowsiness, lassitude, tremulousness, or nausea. More marked symptoms, such as weakness, sweating, tremor, or nervousness may occur. Observe the patient at night for excessive restlessness and profuse sweating.

5. Administer carbohydrate promptly to a hypoglycemic patient and notify the physician. Orange juice, candy, or a lump of sugar are helpful, if the patient is conscious. If the patient is unconscious, honey or karo syrup may be applied to the buccal membrane or glucagon administered if available. If the patient is on long-acting insulin, also administer slow digestible carbohydrate, such as corn syrup or honey with bread. Provide additional carbohydrate for the next 2 hours. Milk and crackers would be suitable. In the hospital, have available for IV therapy 10–20 gm of dextrose in a vial.

6. Be alert for Symogi effect when the patient is being treated for hypoglycemia. Even though the hypoglycemia will trigger the release of epinephrine, glucocorticoid, and growth hormone that stimulate glucogenesis and a higher blood sugar, less insulin is indicated in treating the patient.

7. Obtain medical supervision as rapidly as possible for patient showing signs of hyperglycemic reaction. Have insulin injection available for administration. After administration of insulin, monitor patient closely. As a guide for continued therapy utilize clinical observations and laboratory data.

8. Advise the patient experiencing blurred vision during initiation of insulin therapy that the condition will subside in 6 to 8 weeks, and to delay eye examination until that time. The effect is caused by the fluctation of blood glucose levels which produce osmotic changes in the lens and within the ocular fluids.

9. If a meal is skipped because of illness (fever, nausea, or vomiting), omit the next dose of insulin, unless the urine test indicates that there is sugar present. Test urine every 4 hours and report to physician for insulin regulation.

10. Replace foods omitted by the patient using insulin by a similar amount of carbohydrate in the form of orange juice, or some other form of easily absorbed carbohydrate.
11. If the supply of insulin is exhausted or equipment unavailable, and the patient must skip medication, he/she should be told to decrease food intake by one third and drink plenty of fluids. It is most important that supplies be obtained immediately and that the patient continue with dosage and diet.
12. If the patient becomes ill, notify the physician. Maintain adequate hydration to prevent coma by providing 1 cup or more/hour of noncaloric fluids (coffee, tea, water, and broth). Test urine more frequently.
13. Juvenile diabetics are more susceptible to insulin shock and have a more limited response to glucagon.
14. Observe juvenile diabetics closely for infection or emotional disturbances since insulin requirements may be increased under these circumstances and make these patients more susceptible to diabetic coma.
15. Refer the patient and family to a public health agency to ensure continued health supervision in the home.

EXTENDED INSULIN ZINC SUSPENSION ULTRALENTE ILETIN, ULTRALENTE INSULIN

Classification   Antidiabetic agent, long-acting insulin.

Remarks   Large crystals of insulin and a high content of zinc are responsible for the slow-acting properties of this preparation.

Not suitable for the treatment of diabetic coma or emergency situations.

Dosage   SC, *individualized*. **Do not administer IV.**

GLOBIN ZINC INSULIN INJECTION

Classification   Antidiabetic agent, intermediate-acting insulin.

Remarks   Insulin modified by addition of zinc chloride and globin. Clear yellowish solution. Not suitable for treatment of diabetic coma or emergency situations requiring rapid action. Useful in patients sensitive to protamine.

Dosage   SC, *individualized*.

INSULIN INJECTION BEEF REGULAR ILETIN, PORK REGULAR ILETIN, REGULAR ILETIN, REGULAR INSULIN

Classification   Antidiabetic agent, fast-acting insulin.

Remarks   Fresh solutions are clear. Do not use cloudy, colored solutions.

Only insulin preparation suitable for IV administration.

Suitable for treatment of diabetic coma, acidosis, or other emergency situations. Especially suitable for the patient suffering from labile diabetes.

During acute phase of diabetic acidosis or for the patient in diabetic crisis, patient is monitored by serum glucose and serum ketone levels.

INSULIN INJECTION, CONCENTRATED REGULAR (CONCENTRATED) ILETIN

Remarks   This very concentrated preparation (500 units/ml) of Insulin Injection (see above) is indicated for patients with a marked resistance to insulin requiring more than 200 units/day. Patients must be kept under close observation until dosage is established. Depending on response, dosage may be given SC or IM as a single or as 2 or 3 divided doses. Not suitable for IV administration because of possible allergic or anaphylactoid reactions.

Additional Untoward Reactions   Deep secondary hypoglycemia 18 to 24 hours after administration.

Administration
1. Administer only water clear solutions (concentrated insulin may appear straw colored).
2. Use a tuberculin type syringe for accuracy of measurement.
3. Do not administer IV.
4. Keep cool or refrigerated.

Additional Nursing Implications   (See *Nursing Implications* under *Insulin*).

1. Observe patients closely for signs and symptoms of hyper- or hypoinsulinism during period when correct dosage is being established. Monitor urine q hour.
2. Be prepared to assist with treatment for deep secondary hypoglycemia 18 to 24 hours after injection with glucagon injection and/or glucose. Administer by IV injection or gavage.
3. Encourage patient to carefully monitor urine as ordered by medical supervision and to be alert to signs of hypoglycemia because these may indicate responsiveness to insulin has been regained, and that a reduction in dosage is warranted.

INSULIN ZINC SUSPENSION BEEF LENTE ILETIN, LENTE ILETIN, LENTE INSULIN, PORK LENTE ILETIN

Classification   Antidiabetic agent, intermediate-acting insulin.

General Statement   Contains 30% prompt and 70% extended insulin zinc suspension. Principal advantage is the absence of a sensitizing agent such as protamine or globin.

Useful in patients allergic to other types of insulin, and for patients disposed to thrombotic phenomena in which protamine may be a factor.

Patients on NPH can be transferred to insulin zinc suspension on a unit for unit basis.

Zinc insulin is not a replacement for regular insulin and is not suitable for emergency use.

Dosage   In new cases, insulin (10 units) is given before breakfast. Dosage is then increased by increments of 3 to 5 units until satisfactory readjustment is established.

For patients who are already being treated with protamine or unmodified insulin or both, dosage should be approximately 20% lower than that required with other insulin preparations. The dose is then adjusted as necessary.

ISOPHANE INSULIN SUSPENSION (NPH) BEEF NPH ILETIN, ISOPHANE INSULIN, NPH ILETIN, NPH INSULIN, PORK NPH ILETIN

General Statement   Contains zinc insulin crystals modified by protamine. Many more patients can be controlled on one dose of NPH than was possible with other insulin preparations. Not recommended for emergency use. Not suitable for IV administration. Not useful in the presence of ketosis. Most often the choice for previously untreated diabetic patients.

Dosage   SC, *individualized.*

PROMPT INSULIN ZINC SUSPENSION SEMILENTE ILETIN, SEMILENTE INSULIN

Classification   Antidiabetic agent, fast-acting insulin.

Remarks   Contains small particles of zinc insulin in suspension. Not suitable for emergency use. Cannot be injected IV. Mix only with lente preparations.

PROTAMINE ZINC INSULIN SUSPENSION BEEF PROTAMINE, ZINC AND ILETIN; PORK PROTAMINE, ZINC AND ILETIN; PROTAMINE, ZINC, AND ILETIN

Classification   Antidiabetic agent, long-acting insulin.

Remarks   Contains protamine, zinc, and insulin in a suspension of minute particles. Not suitable for use in emergency situations.

ORAL ANTIDIABETIC AGENTS

General Statement
Several oral antidiabetics agents are available for patients with the milder forms of diabetes. These are used chiefly for patients with maturity-onset, mild, nonketotic diabetes, usually associated with obesity, whose condition cannot be controlled by diet alone but who do not require insulin. The oral antidiabetics should not be used in unstable or brittle diabetes, whatever the patient's age.

Most oral antidiabetic drugs belong to a group of chemicals called sulfonylureas. They are not a substitute for insulin but act by stimulating the release of endogenous insulin from islet tissue of the pancreas. The mechanism by which these oral antidiabetics stimulate the release of insulin is unknown. They are ineffective in the complete absence of functioning islet (beta) cells.

Patients whose condition is to be controlled by oral antidiabetics should be subjected to a 7-day therapeutic trial. A fall in blood sugar, decrease in glucosuria, and disappearance of pruritus, polyuria, polydipsia, and polyphagia are indicative that the patient can probably be managed on oral antidiabetic agents. These drugs should not be used in patients with ketosis.

If the patient is transferred from insulin to an oral antidiabetic drug, the hormone should be discontinued gradually over a period of several days. This is not true for acetohexamide.

Peak effects occur within 5 to 8 hours and the total duration of action is between 10 and 12 hours. The effects of chlorpropamide may last several days. Two to six weeks of therapy may be required before satisfactory control is achieved.

Use
Maturity onset type diabetes, after age 40, requiring less than 20 units of insulin daily.

Contraindications
Stress prior to and during surgery, severe trauma, fever, infections, pregnancy, diabetes complicated by recurrent episodes of ketoacidosis or coma, juvenile, growth onset or brittle diabetes, impaired endocrine, renal or liver function. Use with caution in debilitated, malnourished patients. Not indicated for patients whose diabetes can be controlled by diet alone. Relapse may occur with the sulfonylureas in undernourished patients.

Untoward Reactions
Dose-related GI disturbances characterized by anorexia, nausea, vomiting, epigastric distress, abdominal cramps, constipation, diarrhea. Adverse GI effects can usually be alleviated by decreasing dosage. Other rarely seen side effects include blood dyscrasias, hypoglycemia, liver dysfunction, weakness, fatigue, dizziness, vertigo, malaise, photosensitive reactions (especially after ingestion of alcohol), headache, confusion, tinnitus, ataxia, and paresthesia.

Resistance to drug action develops in a small percentage of patients.

Dosage
PO, See individual preparations. Adjust dosage according to weekly blood sugar determinations.

Sulfonylureas are often used in conjunction with other antidiabetic agents.

Transfer from Insulin

(1) Patients receiving 20 or less units of insulin daily: Institute maintenance dosage of oral hypoglycemic agents. Insulin may be discontinued abruptly. (2) Patients receiving 20–40 units of insulin daily: Institute maintenance dosage of oral hypoglycemic agent and reduce insulin dose by 50%. Discontinue insulin gradually, using absence of sugar in urine as a guide. (3) Patients receiving more than 40 units of insulin daily: Institute maintenance dosage and reduce insulin by 25%. Discontinue insulin gradually, using sugar in urine as a guide. It might be advisable to transfer patients on such high doses of insulin while they are hospitalized.

Patients should test their urine for sugar and ketone bodies regularly (1 to 3 times daily) during the transfer period. Positive results must be reported to the physician.

Mild symptoms of hyperglycemia may appear during the transfer period. No transition period is needed when patient is transferred from one sulfonylurea to another.

Therapeutic Failure of Hypoglycemic Agents

Diabetic patients who do not respond to the sulfonylureas are said to be "primary failures." Patients may respond to the sulfonylureas during the initial months of therapy but may fail to respond thereafter. These patients are referred to as "secondary failures."

Drug Interactions

Interactant	Interaction
Acetazolamide (Diamox)	↑ Blood sugar in prediabetics and diabetics on oral hypoglycemics
Alcohol	Additive hypoglycemia, "Antabuse-like" reaction
Anticoagulants, oral	↑ Effect of oral hypoglycemics by ↓ breakdown by liver and ↓ plasma protein binding
Barbiturates	Oral hypoglycemics ↑ effects of barbiturates
Chloramphenicol (Chloromycetin)	↑ Effect of oral hypoglycemics by ↓ breakdown by liver
Phenylbutazone (Butazolidin)	↑ Effect of oral hypoglycemics due to ↓ breakdown by liver and ↓ plasma protein binding.
Phenyramidol (Analexin)	↑ Effect of oral hypoglycemics by ↓ breakdown by liver
Probenecid (Benemid)	↑ Effect of oral hypoglycemics by ↓ excretion through kidney
Salicylates	↑ Effect of oral hypoglycemics by ↓ plasma protein binding
Sulfonamides	↑ Effects of oral hypoglycemics by ↓ plasma protein binding
Thiazides	↑ Requirements for sulfonylureas

Nursing Implications

1. See *Nursing Implications* for all diabetic patients receiving medication to control the disease (see page 536).
2. Observe the patient very closely during the first seven days of treatment with a sulfonylurea because this is a trial period during which the therapeutic response must be evaluated.
3. Advise and plan with patient for close medical supervision during the first six weeks of therapy, with complete medical evaluation at least once weekly.
4. Be prepared to begin treatment with IV dextrose solution if severe hypoglycemia develops. Close medical supervision will be required during the following 3 to 5 days.
5. *Teach patient and/or family member:*
   a. To observe for symptoms of hypoglycemia such as fatigue, headache, drowsiness, tremulousness, or nausea.
   b. If hypoglycemia occurs, to ingest an easily absorbed carbohydrate such as orange juice, candy, or sugar.
   c. To observe for symptoms of hyperglycemia such as thirst, polyuria, drowsiness, flushed dry skin, fruity odor of breath, or unconsciousness.
   d. If hyperglycemia occurs, report immediately to medical supervision for adjustment of medication.
   e. Test urine for sugar and ketone bodies at least three times a day during transition period.
   f. The need to adhere to prescribed diet so that sulfonylurea may be effective. Most secondary failures are due to poor dietary practices.
   g. That any unusual exercise will increase his/her need for food.
   h. To self-administer insulin since it may be necessary should complications occur.
   i. To report to medical supervision if he/she does not feel as well as usual or notes pruritis, skin rash, jaundice, dark urine, fever, sore throat, or diarrhea.
   j. To report sulfonylurea medication if he/she is to have a thyroid test because the drug interferes with the uptake of radioactive iodine.

ACETOHEXAMIDE DYMELOR

Classification   Oral antidiabetic agent, sulfonylurea.

Remarks   Withdraw medication if ketonuria, acidosis, increased glycosuria, unsatisfactory or persistent rise in blood pressure, or serious side effects (GI upset with nausea, vomiting, diarrhea, blood dyscrasias, jaundice, change in liver function tests) develop.

Additional Untoward Reaction   Hair loss.

Dosage **PO Range:** 0.25–1.5 gm daily. *Newly diagnosed or elderly*, 250 mg daily before breakfast, adjusting by 250–500 mg increments every 5 to 7 days. *Moderately severe diabetes*, 1.5 gm on day 1; 1.0 gm on day 2, **then** 0.5 gm daily, adjusting dosage thereafter until optimum control is achieved.

CHLORPROPAMIDE DIABINESE

Classification Oral antidiabetic, sulfonylurea.

Additional Untoward Reactions Occur frequently with this drug and may be severe. Severe diarrhea is occasionally accompanied by bleeding in the lower bowel. Severe GI distress may be relieved by dividing total daily dose in half. Intolerance to alcohol, vague neurological symptoms, and paresthesia have been reported; also, occasionally photosensitivity reactions. Hypersensitivity reactions have been observed, especially during the first 6 weeks of therapy. Cholestatic jaundice has been reported rarely—drug should be given with extreme caution to patients with hepatic dysfunction. In older patients hypoglycemia may be severe. May cause hyponatremia.

Dosage **PO: initial** (*middle-aged patients*), 250 mg daily as a single or divided dose. **Geriatric: initial,** 100–125 mg daily. Adjust by increments of 50–125 mg q 3 to 5 days. **Maintenance:** 100–500 mg daily as a single or divided dose up to maximum of 750 mg daily.

Transfer from insulin <40 units insulin/day: Insulin may be withdrawn abruptly. >40 mg insulin/day: Transfer gradually by decreasing insulin by 50% daily. Patient can be transferred from other sulfonylureas abruptly.

TOLAZAMIDE TOLINASE

Classification Oral antidiabetic agent, sulfonylurea.

Remarks Drug is effective in some patients with a history of coma or ketoacidosis. Duration of action is 10 to 14 hours. Use with insulin is not recommended for maintenance.

Additional Contraindication Renal glycosuria.

Dosage **PO: initial,** 100 mg/day if fasting blood sugar is less than 200 mg %, or 250 mg/day if fasting blood sugar is greater than 200 mg %. Adjust dose to response. If more than 500 mg/day required, the dose should be given in 2 divided doses. **Elderly or debilitated patients:** 100 mg/day with breakfast, adjusting dose by increments of 50 mg daily each week. Doses greater than 1 gm daily will probably not improve control.

TOLBUTAMIDE ORINASE

TOLBUTAMIDE SODIUM ORINASE DIAGNOSTIC

Classification   Oral antidiabetic agent sulfonylurea.

Remarks   May be used as a supplement to insulin therapy in some cases of labile diabetes. Duration of action is 6 to 12 hours. It is most useful for patients with poor general physical status who should receive a short-acting compound.

Special Use   Tolbutamide sodium is used to diagnose pancreatic islet cell tumors. It causes blood glucose, in presence of a tumor, to quickly drop after IV administration and remain low for 3 hours.

Additional Untoward Reactions   Melena (dark, bloody stools) in some patients with a history of peptic ulcer. It should therefore be used with caution in such cases. Tolbutamide may cause photosensitivity, weakness, tinnitus, transient hyperopia, and alcohol intolerance accompanied by tachycardia, tachypnea, and a drop in blood pressure. Relapse or secondary failure may occur a few months after therapy has been started. May cause hyponatremia.

    Patients receiviang 20– 40 units of insulin daily should be transferred gradually.

Additional Drug Interactions   Tolbutamide causes an initial increase in effect of anticoagulants by decreasing plasma protein binding. This is followed by a decreased effect of anticoagulants due to increased breakdown in liver. Also, increased effect of tolbutamide by decreased breakdown in liver.

Dosage   **PO,** administered as a single dose before breakfast or divided doses with meals. *Dosage schedule:* day 1 = 3 gm; day 2 = 2 gm; days 3 and 4 = 1 gm. Adjust to maintenance dose of 0.5– 2.0 gm daily based on maintenance dose required for satisfactory control. *Alternate dosage technique:* 0.5 gm b.i.d. initially, adjusting to minimum control.

INSULIN ANTAGONISTS

DIAZOXIDE PROGLYCEM

Classification   Insulin antagonist, hypotensive agent.

General Statement   Diazoxide is a thiazide that produces a prompt dose-related increase in blood glucose levels caused primarily by inhibiting the release of insulin from the beta (islet) cells of the pancreas. The effect of the drug becomes apparent after 1 hour and lasts for 8 hours when kidney function is normal.

    Optimum dosage is usually established within 2 to 3 days. Blood glucose levels must be monitored carefully until the patient has stabilized, which usually takes 1 week. The drug is discontinued if a satisfactory effect has not been established within 2 to 3 weeks.

The drug causes sodium, potassium, uric acid and water retention. The drug is also commonly used as an antihypertensive agent (see p. 273).

Uses Hypoglycemia caused by insulin overdosage, or overproduction of insulin by malignant beta cells.

Contraindications Functional hypoglycemia, hypersensitivity to drug or thiazides. Use with extreme caution in patients with history of gout or those in whom edema presents a risk (cardiac disease).

Untoward Reactions Frequent and serious: sodium and fluid retention. Infrequent but serious: Diabetic ketoacidosis and hyperosmolar nonketonic coma. Other: Hirsutism, hyperglycemia or glycosuria (may require adjustment of dosage), gout, G.I. intolerance, transient loss of taste, tachycardia, palpitations, increased levels of uric acid (frequent), thrombocytopenia (may require discontinuation of drug), neutropenia, skin rash, headaches, weakness, malaise, hypotension, various hematological, hepatorenal and neurological manifestations. Transient cataracts and other ophthalmological manifestations, monilial dermatitis, herpes, premature aging of bone, alopecia, fever, lymphadenopathy, acute pancreatitis, pancreatic neurosis, galactorrhea, enlargement of lump in breast.

Drug Interactions

Interactant	Interaction
Anticoagulants, oral	↑ Effect of anticoagulant due to ↓ plasma protein binding
Antihypertensives	Excessive ↓ blood pressure due to additive effects
Thiazide Diuretics	↑ Hypoglycemic and hyperuricemic effects

Dosage *Individualized,* based on blood glucose level and response of patient. **PO, adults and children: initial,** 3 mg/kg/day in 3 equal doses q 8 hr; **usual,** 3–8 mg/kg daily divided into 2 or 3 equal doses q 8 to 12 hr. **PO, infants and newborns: initial,** 10 mg/kg/day in 3 equal doses q 8 hr; **usual,** 8–15 mg/kg daily divided into 2 or 3 equal doses q 8 or 12 hr.

Administration/ Storage
1. Shake suspension well before withdrawing drug.
2. Protect drug from light.

Nursing Implications
1. Assess patient's clinical response, which together with results of laboratory tests, is the basis of the dosage adjustments.
2. Observe patient with a history of congestive heart failure for fluid retention which may precipitate failure.
3. Assess B.P. for potentiation of antihypertensive effect when patient is already taking an antihypertensive agent.

4. Reassure patient with hirsutism that the condition will subside with discontinuation of the drug.
5. Assess for echymosis, petechiae, or frank bleeding, symptoms that will require discontinuation of drug.
6. Have insulin and IV fluids available to counteract possible ketoacidosis.
7. Monitor closely up to 7 days after overdosage until blood sugar is within normal range. (80–120 mg/100 ml).

GLUCAGON

Classification Insulin antagonist.

General Statement Glucagon is a protein produced by the alpha cells of the pancreas. It is instrumental in mobilizing glucose stored in the liver and also stimulates the manufacture of neoglucose from fats. The drug is only effective in overcoming hypoglycemia when the liver has a reserve of glycogen. Glucagon is convenient for use at home when IV dextrose cannot be administered. Carbohydrates should be given as soon as the patient awakens to prevent secondary hypoglycemic reactions.

Uses Also used to terminate insulin-induced shock in psychiatric patients. Patient usually regains consciousness 5 to 20 minutes after the parenteral administration of glucagon. The drug should only be used under medical supervision or in accordance with strict instructions received from the physician. Failure to respond may be an indication for IV administration of glucose.

Contraindications Use with caution in patients with renal or hepatic disease or in those who are undernourished and emaciated.

Untoward Reactions Nausea, vomiting, circulatory collapse, and hypersensitivity.

Drug Interactions

Interactant	Interaction
Anticoagulants, oral	↑ Effect of anticoagulants by ↑ hypoprothrombinemia
Antidiabetic agents	Hyperglycemic effect of glucagon antagonizes hypoglycemic effect of antidiabetics
Hyperglycemic agents Corticosteroids Epinephrine Estrogens Phenytoin	Additive hyperglycemic effect

Dosage **SC, IM, IV** (*hypoglycemia or coma in insulin shock therapy*): 0.5–1 mg. Repeat after 25 minutes if response of patient is unsatisfactory.

Nursing Implications

1. Refer to Chart, p. 532 to differentiate between diabetic coma and insulin shock (reaction).
2. Administer carbohydrate after the patient awakens following administration of glucagon. Rapidly available sugar such as that in orange juice and Karo syrup in water should be given. If shock was caused by a long-acting medication, give a more slowly digestible carbohydrate such as bread and honey.
3. Teach responsible family members how to administer glucagon SC or IM in the event of a hypoglycemic reaction with loss of consciousness by the patient.
4. Emphasize the need to family members and to the patient of informing the physician of hypoglycemic reactions so that the dose of insulin can be adjusted.

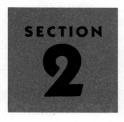

SECTION 2

thyroid and antithyroid drugs

Thyroid Preparations
Levothyroxine Sodium
Liothyronine Sodium
Liotrix

Thyroglobulin
Thyroid Desiccated
Thyrotropin

Antithyroid Drugs
Methimazole
Potassium Iodide
Propylthiouracil

Sodium Iodide
Strong Iodine Solution

Radioactive Agent
Sodium Iodide I[131]

General Statement

The thyroid manufactures two active hormones: thyroxine and triiodothyronine, both of which contain iodine. These thyroid hormones are released into the bloodstream where they are bound to protein. The protein, however, is not essential for their activity.

The exact mechanism of action of the thyroid hormones is not known. They affect many physiological processes. They regulate the rate of metabolism in almost all body cells; affect protein, carbohydrate, and lipid (fat) metabolism; and assist in the development of bones and teeth, playing an important role in growth, especially that of the long bones, and in bone calcification.

The hormones also have a definite cardiostimulatory effect and can increase renal blood flow as well as glomerular filtration rate (diuresis). The thyroid gland is under the control of the hypothalamus and pituitary gland, which produce thyroid-stimulating hormone releasing factor and thyrotropin (thyroid-stimulating hormone, TSH) respectively. Like other hormone systems, the thyroid, pituitary, and hypothalamus work together in a feedback (see-saw) mechanism. Excess thyroid hormone causes a decrease in TSH and a lack of thyroid hormone causes an increase in the production and secretion of TSH.

Diseases involving the thyroid fall into two groups:

(1) Hypothyroidism or diseases in which little or no hormone is produced. These can be subdivided into cretinism, resulting from a deficiency of thyroid hormone during fetal and early life, and myxedema, a deficiency of thyroid hormone in the adult. Cretinism is characterized by arrested physical and mental development with dystrophy of the bones and soft parts and lowered basal metabolism. Myxedema is characterized by a dry waxy type swelling, with abnormal deposits of mucin in the skin. The edema is nonpitting, and the facial changes are distinctive, with swollen lips and a thickened nose. Primary myxedema results from atrophy of the thyroid gland. Secondary myxedema may result from hypofunction of the pituitary gland or prolonged administration of antithyroid drugs.

(2) Hyperthyroidism or conditions associated with an overproduction of hormones as in Graves' or Basedow's disease (diffuse enlargement of the thyroid gland; often characterized by protruding eyes), and Plummer's disease in which extra thyroid hormone is produced by a single "hot" thyroid nodule. These conditions are usually characterized by hypertrophy and hyperplasia of the thyroid and a state of extreme nervousness.

Euthyroid or Simple, Nontoxic Goiter (Endemic Goiter)
In these states, a normal or near normal amount of hormone is produced by an enlarged thyroid gland. This condition can occur when the dietary intake of iodine is below normal. Today, the disease is much rarer because iodine is added as a matter of routine to cooking salt. The thyroid, in such patients, tends to become enlarged, especially during adolescent growth and pregnancy. Surgery may be necessary to alleviate the pressure on the trachea caused by the enlarged thyroid and from preventing the oxygen supply from being cut off.

Drugs used in the treatment of thyroid disease fall into two groups: (1) thyroid preparations used to correct thyroid deficiency diseases, and (2) anti-thyroid drugs that cut down production of hormones by an overactive gland.

Thyroid preparations are also administered for certain ob-gyn disorders, including menstrual disorders, premenstrual tension, and infertility.

The external supply of thyroid hormones usually results in a reduction in the amount of natural hormone produced by the thyroid gland.

The accurate determination of thyroid function is crucial for the treatment of thyroid disease. Thyroid function can be evaluated by (1) basal metabolism rate (BMR) determination, which measures the rate at which the patient utilizes oxygen (normal value: 10); (2) radioactive iodine uptake (I^{131}), which measures the ability of the thyroid to take up iodine (normal value: 25% to 50%). Hypothyroid patients take up too little iodine; hyperthyroid patients take up too much iodine; and (3) protein bound iodine (PBI), which measures the actual amount of thyroid hormone circulating in the blood (normal value: 4.8 μg/100 ml). The results of some of the tests are at times skewed by medications the patient is taking so that the effect of these drugs must be considered when evaluating the test.

Thyroid conditions are often treated by fixed combinations of levothyroxine sodium and liothyronine sodium in a ratio of 4:1. Such a preparation is liotrix (Euthroid, Thyrolar). For all information regarding these drugs, see *Thyroid Preparations, General Statement,* and drug entries for levothyroxine sodium and liothyronine sodium.

THYROID PREPARATIONS

Uses   Replacement therapy in primary and secondary myxedema, myxedemic coma, nontoxic goiter, hypothyroidism, some thyroid tumors, chronic thyroiditis, sporadic cretinism, and thyrotropin-dependent tumors.

Contraindications   Uncorrected adrenal insufficiency, myocardial infarction, hyperthyroidism, and thyrotoxicosis. Use with extreme caution in the presence of angina pectoris, hypertension, and other cardiovascular disease, renal insufficiency, and ischemic states.

Untoward Reactions   The thyroid preparations are cumulative, and overdosage is a constant danger. The following side effects, which can appear within 24 hours but also much later, may be an indication of chronic overdosage: palpitations, angina, dyspnea, headache, excessive warmth, diarrhea, cramps, vomiting, continued weight loss, hyperhidrosis, intolerance to heat, nervousness, mental agitation, hyperirritability, insomnia, twitching, tremors, increased cardiac output, tachycardia, cardiac arrhythmias, increased pulse, increased blood pressure, cardiac decompensation, and collapse.

In infants and children, the earliest manifestations of thyroid overdosage may be an accelerated rate of bone maturation. Thyroid preparations may also alter a patient's response to insulin.

Drug Interactions

Interactant	Interaction
Anticoagulants	↑ Effect of anticoagulants by ↑ hypoprothrombinemia
Antidepressants, tricyclic	Mutually potentiating effects observed
Antidiabetic agents	Hyperglycemic effect of thyroid preparations may necessitate ↑ in dose of antidiabetic agent
Cholestyramine (Cuemid, Questran)	↓ Effect of thyroid hormone due to ↓ absorption from GI tract

Drug	*Interactant*	*Interaction*
Interactions		
(Continued)	Corticosteroids	Thyroid preparations increase tissue demands for corticosteroids. Adrenal insufficiency must be corrected with corticosteroids before administering thyroid hormones. In patients already treated for adrenal insufficiency, dosage of corticosteroids must be increased when initiating therapy with thyroid drug
	Digitalis compounds	Toxic effects of digitalis may be potentiated by thyroid preparations. May be necessary to ↑ dose of digitalis when thyroid hormone therapy is initiated
	Epinephrine	Cardiovascular effects ↑ by thyroid preparations
	Indomethacin (Indocin)	Concomitant use may cause cardiac arrhythmias
	Ketamine	Concomitant use may result in severe hypertension and tachycardia
	Levarterenol	Cardiovascular effects ↑ by thyroid preparations
	Phenytoin (Dilantin)	↑ Effect of thyroid hormone by ↓ plasma protein binding

Laboratory Test Interferences

Alter thyroid function tests. ↑ Prothrombin time. ↓ Serum Cholesterol.

Dosage

Thyroid drugs are started with a low initial dose that is gradually increased until a satisfactory response is achieved within safe dose limits.

When necessary, a decrease in dosage and a more gradual upward adjustment relieves severe side effects.

Nursing Implications

1. Anticipate that treatment is usually begun with a small dose which is gradually increased.
2. Follow specific instructions to prevent overdose or relapse when changing from one thyroid drug to another.
3. Stress to patient that drug must be taken only with medical supervision and that the drug must be taken regularly.
4. Teach the patient to report promptly to physician excessive weight loss, palpitations, leg cramps, nervousness, diarrhea, or abdominal cramps, headache, insomnia, intolerance to heat, and fever. Symptoms are most likely to occur from 1 to 3 weeks after therapy for hypothyroidism is started.
5. Observe for positive results of medication characterized by reduction in weight, improvement in appearance of skin and hair, and increased mental alertness.
6. Caution diabetic patients to test urine at least three times a day for sugar and acetone because thyroid preparations may require adjustment of insulin dosage.

7. Observe and caution patients on anticoagulant therapy to report bleeding from any orifice or purpura since anticoagulants are potentiated by thyroid preparations.

LEVOTHYROXINE SODIUM (T4) CYTOLEN, LETTER, LEVOID, RO-THYROXIN, SYNTHROID, L-THYROXINE SODIUM

Classification Thyroid preparation.

Remarks Synthetic sodium salt of the levoisomer of thyroxine (tetraiodothyronine). Drug is well absorbed from the GI tract and has a slower onset but longer duration than sodium liothyronine. It is more active on a weight basis than thyroid.

Dosage *Individualized.* **PO: initial,** 25– 100 μg daily increased by 50– 100 μg q 1 to 4 weeks until desired clinical response is attained. **Maintenance:** 100– 400 μg daily.

Myxedematous coma, **IV: initial,** 200– 400 μg. If there is no response in 24 hr, 100– 300 μg more may be given; **pediatric, PO: initial,** 50 μg, daily, maximum increase same as adult.

Cretinism, **Children:** 300– 400 μg daily.

Administration Prepare solutions for injection immediately before administration. Solution is made by adding prescribed amount of NaCl solution to powder and shaking solution until it is clear. Discard unused portion of IV medication.

Additional Nursing Implications
1. Transfer from liothyronine to levothyroxine—administer replacement drug for several days before discontinuing liothyronine.
2. Transfer from levothyroxine to liothyronine—discontinue levothyroxine before starting patient on low daily dose of liothyronine.

LIOTHYRONINE SODIUM (T3) CYTOMEL, RO-THYRONINE, SODIUM-L-TRIIODOTHYRONINE

Classification Thyroid preparation.

Remarks Synthetic sodium salt of levoisomer of triiodothyronine. Drug has a rapid onset and short duration of action.

Use Drug of choice for IV use in myxedematous coma.

Dosage *Mild hypothyroidism, individualized.* **PO:** 25 μg daily. Increase by 12.5– 25 μg q 1 to 2 weeks until satisfactory response has been obtained. **Usual maintenance:** 25– 100 μg daily. Use lower initial dosage (5 μg/day) for the elderly, children, and patients with cardiovascular disease. Increase gradually as adult dosage.

Myxedema, **PO: initial,** 5 μg/day increased by 5– 10 μg daily q 1 to 2 weeks. **Usual maintenance:** 50– 100 μg/day.

Cretinism: **initial,** 5 μg daily; increase by 5 μg weekly to a total daily dose of 25 μg; 50 μg/day may be required for children 1 year of age; full adult dosage may be necessary for children 3 years of age or older.

Additional Nursing Implications

1. Transfer from other thyroid preparations to liothyronine—discontinue old preparation before starting on low daily dose of liothyronine.
2. Transfer from liothyronine to other thyroid preparation—start therapy with replacement drug several days prior to complete withdrawal of sodium liothyronine.

LIOTRIX EUTHROID, THYROLAR

Classification   Thyroid preparation.

Remarks   Mixture of synthetic levothyroxine sodium (T4) and liothyronine sodium (T3). The mixture contains the products in a 4:1 ratio by weight and in a 1:1 ratio by biological activity. The two commercial preparations contain slightly different amounts of each component. Because of this discrepancy, a switch from one preparation to the other must be made cautiously. The dosage content of the two preparations are as follows:

Tablets #	T4	T3	Thyroid Equivalency
Euthroid			
½	30 μg	7.5 μg	30 mg
1	60 μg	15 μg	60 mg
2	120 μg	30 μg	120 mg
3	180 μg	45 μg	180 mg
Thyrolar			
¼	12.5 μg	3.1 μg	15 mg
½	25 μg	6.25 μg	30 mg
1	50 μg	12.5 μg	60 mg
2	100 μg	25 μg	120 mg
3	150 μg	37.5 μg	180 mg
5	250 μg	62.5 μg	300 mg

Dosage   **PO, adults and children: initial,** Tablet # ½ (*Euthroid:* 30 μg levothyroxine and 7.5 μg of liothyronine; *Thyrolar* 25 μg levothyroxine and 6.25 μg of liothyronine). In adults, dosage is increased by Tablet # ½ at 1- or 2-week intervals and in children by Tablet # ½ at 2-week intervals, until satisfactory response has been attained.

Administration/ Storage

1. Give as single dose before breakfast.
2. Protect tablets from light, heat, and moisture.

THYROGLOBULIN PROLOID

Classification Thyroid preparation, containing levothyroxine (T4) and liothyronine (T3) in a ratio of 2.5 to 1.

Remarks Drug is a natural product purified from hog thyroid glands. It has no clinical advantage over thyroid, and has a slow onset of action that makes it unsuitable for the treatment of myxedematous coma.

Dosage **PO: initial,** 15–60 mg or more, increased gradually until control is established. **Usual maintenance:** 32–200 mg daily.
Cretinism, **pediatric, infants:** 45–60 mg daily; **6 months–1 year:** 60–90 mg daily. Some physicians prefer to reach above dosage gradually.
Dosage calculated on body weight. **Young children:** 2–12 mg/kg daily. Older children receive less. Therapy is aimed at maintaining 5–9 μg/100 ml protein-bound iodine.

Additional Nursing Implication Transfer from and to sodium liothyronine should be made gradually.

THYROTROPIN THYTROPAR, THYROID STIMULATING HORMONE

Classification Thyroid preparation.

Remark Highly purified thyroid stimulating hormone from bovine pituitary glands.

Uses Diagnostic agent to evaluate thyroid dysfunction. Certain types of thyroid cancer.

Dosage **IM, SC:** Administer 10 International Units daily for 3 to 8 days.

THYROID DESICCATED ARMOUR THYROID, DELCOID, S-P-T, THYRAR, THYROCRINE, THYROGLANDULAR, THYROID U.S.P., THYRO-TERIC

Classification Thyroid preparation.

Remarks Thyroid is cleaned, dried powdered animal (usually hog) thyroid gland. The active ingredient of the powder is mainly levothyroxine and l-triiodothyronine. The drug has a slow onset of action that makes it unsuitable for the treatment of myxedematous coma.

Dosage *Myxedema, individualized.* **PO: initial,** 15 mg daily, increased gradually q 2 weeks until dose is 60 mg/day after 4 weeks. **Maintenance, range:** 60–180 mg/day.

Cretinism: therapy is aimed at maintaining serum thyroxine levels in the upper half of the normal range. **Infants 1–4 months:** 15– 30 mg daily initially; **then,** maintain at 30– 45 mg daily; **4–12 months:** 30– 60 mg daily. Older children require approximately the same amount as adults (60– 180 mg/day).

Storage   Store protected from moisture and light.

Additional Nursing Implications
1. Transfer from liothyronine: start thyroid several days before withdrawal.
2. When transferring from thyroid discontinue thyroid before starting with low daily dose of replacement drug.

ANTITHYROID DRUGS

General Statement   Antithyroid drugs interfere with the synthesis of thyroid hormones by the thyroid gland. They do not interfere with the release of preformed hormones already present in the gland. Thus, it may take up to several weeks for the therapeutic effect to become established. The most effective members of this class of drugs are the thiouracil derivatives. Large amounts of iodide also have an antithyroid effect.

Uses   Hyperthyroidism and preparation for thyroid surgery.

Contraindications   Lactation. Use with caution during pregnancy and in the presence of cardiovascular disease.

Untoward Reactions   Agranulocytosis, leukopenia, and thrombopenia, early signs of which are sore throat and fever. Also skin rash, salivary gland and lymph node enlargement, GI disturbances, hepatic damage, arthralgia, visual disturbances, headache, drowsiness, vertigo, edema, loss of taste, vascular purpura, paresthesias, neuropathy, hair loss, cutaneous pigmentation, and hypoprothrombinemia.

Drug Interaction

Interactant	Interaction
Anticoagulants, oral	Potentiated by propylthiouracil. Dose of anticoagulant may have to be reduced

Nursing Implications
1. Encourage the patient to take drug regularly, exactly as directed. If this is not done, hyperthyroidism may recur, whereas if the drug is taken as ordered for 1 or more years, more than half of the patients achieve permanent remission.
2. Teach the patient to report any symptoms of illness to his/her physician promptly: sore throat, enlargement of cervical lymph nodes, GI disturbances, fever, rash, or jaundice. These symptoms may necessitate either a reduction of dosage or withdrawal of the drug.

POTASSIUM IODIDE

SODIUM IODIDE

STRONG IODINE SOLUTION LUGOL'S SOLUTION

(Commercial preparations usually contain 5% iodine and 10% potassium iodide.)

Classification	Antithyroid drug.
General Statement	Today, iodine is generally used together with other antithyroid drugs. Iodine specifically produces involution of a hyperplastic thyroid gland, making it less friable and less vascular prior to surgery. Iodine also shortens the time required by other antithyroid drugs to reduce the output of natural hormone.
	Strong iodine solutions are ineffective for the treatment of postoperative thyroid crisis.
	Acute iodine poisoning is characterized by vomiting, diarrhea, and gastroenteritis. Hypersensitivity is characterized by dermatitis, largyngeal edema, swelling of the salivary glands, or increased salivation.
Uses	Prophylaxis of simple and colloid goiters, exophthalmic goiter. Preparation of thyrotoxic patients for thyroidectomy, and in combination with antithyroid drugs for thyrotoxic crises.
Contraindications	Iodine is contraindicated in tuberculosis because it may cause breakdown of healing of lesions. Also contraindicated in patients hypersensitive to iodine.
Dosage	*Preoperatively,* **PO:** 6 mg iodine daily for 2 to 3 weeks but doses up to 500 mg iodine/day have been used. *Thyroid crisis:* 1 gm by **IV infusion.**
Administration	1. Measure iodine solution very carefully with a dropper because medication is very potent. 2. Dilute, preferably in 60 ml of milk or orange juice, because medication is very bitter.
Additional Nursing Implications	1. Teach patients symptoms of acute iodide poisoning. (See *General Statement*.) 2. Check with the physician regarding use of iodized salt by the patient.

METHIMAZOLE TAPAZOLE

Classification	Antithyroid preparation.
Remarks	Acts more rapidly but less consistently than propylthiouracil. Iodine is usually administered concomitantly for 7 to 10 days prior to surgery.

Uses   Hyperthyroidism, preoperatively, or when thyroidectomy is contraindicated. Thyroid crisis.

Dosage   **PO: initial,** 15– 60 mg daily in 3 divided doses. Initial dose is usually maintained for about 2 months. **Maintenance:** 5– 15 mg daily. **Pediatric 6–10 years:** 5– 15 mg daily in divided doses every 8 hr; **maintenance:** approximately one-half initial dose.

Storage   Store in light-resistant containers.

PROPYLTHIOURACIL PROPACIL

Classification   Antithyroid preparation.

Uses   Drug of choice for hyperthyroidism, preoperatively, or when thyroidectomy is contraindicated. Treatment of thyroid crisis. Iodine (Lugol's solution or potassium iodide solution) usually is given as an adjunct 7 to 10 days preoperatively so as to overcome the propylthiouracil-induced vascularity and friability of the gland.

Drug Interaction   Propylthiouracil may produce hypoprothrombinemia, adding to the effect of anticoagulants.

Dosage   **PO: initial,** 100– 600 mg daily in 3 to 6 divided doses for about 2 months. After symptoms are controlled, maintenance dose is established from BMR data. **Usual maintenance:** 100– 150 mg daily. **Children 6–10 years:** 50– 150 mg daily in divided doses q 8 hr; **10 years and older: initial,** 150– 300 mg daily. **Maintenance:** determined by response.

RADIOACTIVE AGENT

SODIUM IODIDE I[131] IODOTOPE I-131, ORIODIDE-131, SODIUM-RADIO-IODIDE, THERIODIDE-131

Classification   Radioactive agent.

General Statement   Sodium iodide contains radioactive iodine. Like iodine, the radioactive salt is selectively absorbed by the thyroid gland when the iodine is incorporated into the thyroid hormone.

Radioactivity can be detected in the thyroid within minutes after administration. Release of radioactivity destroys thyroid tissue. After a therapeutic dose, it takes about 8 to 10 weeks for thyroid function to return to normal.

Uses   Diagnosis: evaluation of thyroid function and detection of malignancies involving the thyroid gland. Therapeutic: hyperthyroidism, selected cases of thyroid cancer.

Contraindications   Therapeutic: extreme tachycardia. Recent episodes of coronary thrombosis, myocardial infarction, or large nodular goiters.
Pregnancy, lactation, persons younger than 18 years of age.

Untoward Reactions   Therapeutic: transient gastritis, nausea, vomiting, inflammation of salivary glands, decrease in leukocyte counts, transient and permanent alteration of thyroid function, blood dyscrasias.

Dosage   *Diagnostic*, **PO, IV:** 1–25 microcuries. *Therapeutic,* **PO, IV,** *hyperthyroidism:* 4–10 millicuries. *Thyroid cancer or metastases:* 50–150 millicuries.

Administration
1. Therapeutic dose only given to hospitalized patients.
2. Upon standing solution and glass storage containers may darken as a result of radiation. This does not affect efficacy of the product.

Nursing Implication   For radiation protection, observe hospital procedure.

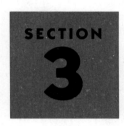

SECTION 3
parathyroid, calcitonin, and calcium salts

Calcitonin
Parathyroid Injection

Dihydrotachysterol

Calcium Salts   Calcium Carbonate
Calcium Chloride
Calcium Gluconate

Calcium Gluceptate
Calcium Lactate
Calcium Levulinate

Miscellaneous   Etidronate Disodium

General Statement   Calcium ions participate in many fundamental processes such as blood coagulation, regulation of heart rhythm, and neuromuscular activity.

The parathyroid hormone regulates calcium metabolism in the body and maintains the calcium ion concentration in the extracellular fluid.

Blood calcium ion concentration and parathyroid secretion regulate each other by feedback mechanism.

Total parathyroidectomy results in hypocalcemic tetany, convulsions, and death.

Administration of either parathyroid hormone extracted from cattle or a synthetic compound with similar actions restores calcium levels to normal values when the disorder is due to parathyroid malfunction.

Because the physiological response is slow (4 hours for parathyroid, days for dihydrotachysterol), calcium salts are usually administered concurrently.

Recently a second hormone, calcitonin, whose function is to promote a decrease of excess extracellular calcium, was discovered.

CALCITONIN CALCIMAR

General Statement

Calcitonin is a polypeptide hormone produced in mammals by the parafollicular cells of the thyroid gland. Its effects oppose the parathyroid hormone. Calcitonin decreases serum calcium levels by inhibiting calcium and phosphorus reabsorption by the renal tubules. The hormone also inhibits bone resorption. When used for therapeutic purposes, calcitonin is isolated from salmon. Except for a higher potency per milligram and a somewhat longer duration of action, salmon calcitonin appears to have the same actions as calcitonin derived from mammalian sources.

Calcitonin is ineffective when administered orally. Its onset of action, after parenteral administration, has been estimated at 2 hours, and peak and duration of action at 6 and 12 hours respectively. Calcitonin is excreted essentially unchanged in the urine. Clinical improvement becomes apparent within the first months after treatment. To gauge effectiveness of drug, periodic determinations of alkaline phosphatase and 24-hour urinary excretion of hydroxyproline are indicated. Reduction in these levels indicates beneficial effect of therapy. Urine should also be examined for casts, indicative of kidney damage.

Uses

Moderate to severe Paget's disease characterized by polyostotic involvement with elevation of serum alkaline phosphatase and urinary excretion of hydroxyproline.

Contraindications

Allergy to salmon calcitonin or its gelatin diluent. Pregnancy, lactation. Safe use in children not established.

Untoward Reactions

Systemic allergic ("foreign protein") reaction to salmon calcitonin or gelatin diluent, possibility of hypocalcemic tetany. Nausea, vomiting, local inflammation at injection site (10% of patients). Facial flushing. Antibody formation to salmon calcitonin, which renders drug ineffective.

Dosage

SC or IM: initial, 100 MRC units/day. In some patients improvement can be maintained through administration of 50 MRC every day or every other day, but long-term effectiveness of such low doses has not yet been established.

Nursing Implications

1. Check that skin testing is completed and that the response is negative before administering medication.
2. Observe patient for systemic allergic reaction and be prepared to provide emergency care with oxygen, epinephrine, and steroids.

3. Observe patient for hypocalcemic tetany during initial (several) administrations of calcitonin and have calcium available for emergency use. (Progressive signs of hypocalcemic tetany are muscular fibrillation, twitching, tetanic spasms, and finally convulsions.)
4. Inform patient experiencing nausea and vomiting at the onset of treatment that GI distress tends to disappear as treatment is continued.
5. Observe and report local inflammatory reaction at the site of injection.
6. Report facial flushing which may occur with treatment.
7. Evaluate patient compliance with drug regimen if a relapse occurs.
8. Ascertain that patients who have a good initial clinical response, but then relapse, are evaluated for antibody formation in response to salmon calcitonin.
9. Help patient understand that if hypocalcemic action of calcitonin is lost administration of further medication is not effective.
10. Ascertain that periodic urine sediment tests are done to check for casts indicating possible kidney damage.
11. Teach patient:
    a. Aseptic method of reconstituting solution.
    b. Injection technique.
    c. Importance of alternating injection sites.

PARATHYROID INJECTION

Classification   Parathyroid hormone, calcium regulator.

General Statement   This is a sterile, aqueous extract of natural parathyroid hormone obtained from cattle parathyroid tissue. The standard preparation contains 100 units/ml.

The hormone helps mobilize calcium from bone, and promotes the excretion of phosphorus and reabsorption of calcium by the renal tubules. Effect of hormone becomes noticeable 4 hours after administration.

Use   Parathyroid tetany. Use only if calcium level is demonstrably low. (Normal values are 10 mg/100 ml serum. Values above 15 mg calcium/100 ml may be dangerously high.)

Contraindication   Tetany not caused by low calcium levels from parathyroid dysfunction.

Untoward Reactions   The only adverse effect is overdosage leading to hypercalcemia. Mild hypercalcemia is characterized by thirst, headache, vertigo, tinnitus, anorexia, exanthema. More severe manifestations are vomiting, diarrhea, muscle atony, and uremic coma.

Frequent blood serum and urine calcium determinations are indicated. Prolonged usage is undesirable because parathyroid may stimulate production of antihormone antibodies.

Drug Interactions

Interactant	Interaction
Androgens	↓ Effect of parathyroid
Calciferol	↓ Effect of parathyroid
Corticosteroids	↓ Effect of parathyroid

Dosage   **IM, SC, IV (usually best route):** 20–40 units (0.2–0.4 ml) q 12 hr with calcium gluconate and oral calcium. **Infants: initial,** 10–20 units (0.1–0.2 ml) maximum. For *chronic parathyroid tetany,* dihydrotachysterol or calciferol are drugs of choice since patients become refractory to parathyroid hormone within a few days.

Nursing Implications

1. Observe patients with a history of parathyroid insufficiency for signs of hypocalcemia demonstrated by muscular fibrillation, twitching, tetanic spasms, and finally convulsions. Report the earliest signs of hypocalcemia.
2. Provide seizure precautions, such as padded siderails and padded tongue blade, for patient with hypocalcemia.
3. Reduce sound and light stimulus to the patient by placing him/her in a quiet room and by dimming the lights.
4. Anticipate that the effects of parathyroid will take about 4 hours to take effect and that the effect will wear off in 20 to 24 hours. The patient will be most susceptible to hypocalcemia before and after these times.
5. Observe and report symptoms of hypercalcemia which may occur during therapy, such as muscular weakness, lethargy, headache, anorexia, nausea, vomiting, abdominal cramps, vertigo, tinnitus, ataxia, diarrhea or constipation, and cardiac arrhythmias.

DIHYDROTACHYSTEROL HYTAKEROL

Classification   Calcium regulator.

General Statement   Dihydrotachysterol increases calcium levels in the serum mainly by promoting excretion of phosphate by the renal tubules. This, in turn, promotes the mobilization of phosphate and calcium from bone.

The onset of action of dihydrotachysterol is slow. Its effect on calcium level is only noticeable after 7 to 10 days. In this manner it is very different from parathyroid hormone. It is usually administered concurrently with calcium salts or calciferol.

Uses   Hypocalcemia, hypoparathyroidism, pseudohypoparathyroidism, premenstrual tetany, tetany during pregnancy, tetany in infants with severe diarrhea, vitamin D-resistant rickets.

Contraindications   Hypocalcemia associated with renal insufficiency or hyperphosphatemia.

Untoward Reactions The margin between the therapeutic dose and toxic dose of dihydrotachysterol is narrow, and the drug must be used with great care.

Therapy is aimed at maintaining a blood calcium level of 9–10 mg/100 ml.

Toxic effects are due to hypercalcemia. Early warning signs include headache, exanthema. More severe effects include nausea, albuminuria, thirst, ataxia of the lower extremities, and stupor. Hypercalcemia necessitates withdrawal of drug, a light diet, and plenty of fluids and laxatives. In critical cases, patient may receive 250 ml of a 2.5% solution of sodium citrate IV every 4 hours.

Dosage *Pseudohypothyroidism,* **PO:** 0.75–2.5 mg daily for several days. **Maintenance:** 0.25–1.75 mg q week plus 10–15 gm calcium lactate or calcium gluconate. *Prophylaxis after parathyroid surgery:* 0.25 mg together with 6 gm calcium lactate. *Premenstrual tetany:* 0.25 mg daily. Increase to 0.375 mg daily during week before menstruation. *Infants with severe diarrhea:* 0.25 mg daily with 3 or more gm calcium lactate.

Nursing Implications
1. Observe for early warning signs of hypercalcemia, such as thirst, headache, vertigo, tinnitus, anorexia. More severe effects may include nausea, vomiting, abdominal cramps, polyuria, albuminuria, ataxia of the lower extremities, and stupor.
2. Withhold drug if symptoms of hypercalcemia are noted and report to the physician.
3. Explain to the patient the necessity for light diet, plenty of fluids, and laxatives to facilitate the elimination of excessive calcium from the body.
4. Have available for emergency use 2.5% solution of sodium citrate which may be administered q 4 hours for the critically ill patient.

CALCIUM SALTS

Classification Electrolyte, mineral

General Statement Calcium is an essential mineral. Ninety percent of the total calcium content of the body is present in the skeleton as calcium phosphate and calcium carbonate. Small amounts of calcium are however present in the extracellular fluid. Calcium ions participate in many important metabolic processes including regulation of the heart rhythm, blood coagulation, the proper function of nerves and muscles, and electrolyte balance.

When the calcium level of the extracellular fluid falls below a certain level (10 mg/100 ml), calcium is first mobilized from bone. However, eventually blood calcium depletion may be so great as to become openly manifest.

Hypocalcemia is characterized by muscular fibrillations, twitching, skeletal muscle spasms, leg cramps, tetanic spasms, cardiac arrhythmias, smooth muscle hyperexcitability, mental depression, and anxiety states.

Extreme chronic hypocalcemia is characterized by brittle, defective nails, poor dentition, and brittle hair.

The normal calcium requirement for adults is 1 gm daily; for children, 1–1.4 gm daily. Requirement may be doubled during pregnancy and lactation. Calcium deficiency can be corrected by the administration of various calcium salts.

Calcium is well absorbed from the upper GI tract. However, severe low calcium tetany is best treated by IV administration of calcium gluconate.

The presence of vitamin D is necessary for maximum calcium utilization. The hormone of the parathyroid gland is necessary for the regulation of the calcium level.

Uses Malnutrition, malabsorption syndromes, tetany in newborn, steatorrhea, hypoparathyroidism, osteomalacia, surgical short-circuiting of bowel, vitamin D insuffciency, acute pancreatitis, pancreatic insufficiency, renal failure, hyperphosphatemia.

Contraindications History of hypercalcemia or lithiasis. Cancer patients with bone metastases. Give with great caution to patients receiving digitalis glycosides.

Untoward Reactions Excess calcium may cause hypercalcemia characterized by lassitude, fatigue, depression of nervous and neuromuscular function (emotional disturbances, confusion, skeletal muscle weakness and constipation), impairment of renal function (polyuria, polydipsia and azotemia), renal calculi, arrhythmias, and bradycardia.

Drug Interactions

Interactant	Interaction
Cephalocin	Incompatible with calcium salts
Corticosteroids	Interfere with absorption of calcium from GI tract
Digitalis	Increased digitalis arrhythmias and toxicity. Death has resulted from combination of digitalis and IV calcium salts
Milk	Excess of either agent may cause hypercalcemia, renal insufficiency with azotemia, alkalosis, and ocular lesions
Tetracyclines	↓ Effect of tetracyclines due to ↓ absorption from GI tract
Vitamin D	Enhances intestinal absorption of dietary calcium

Dosage See Table 26.

Administration **Oral**

1. Administer 1–1½ hours p.c. because alkalies and large amounts of fats decrease absorption of calcium.
2. Advise patients who have difficulty swallowing large pills that calcium in water suspension may be obtained from the pharmacist

TABLE 26 CALCIUM SALTS®

Drug	Uses	Dosage	Percent of Calcium in Preparation, Which Indicates Efficacy
Calcium carbonate	Mild hypocalcemia, latent hypocalcemic tetany	**PO:** 1–2 gm t.i.d. with meals.	Calcium content: 40%
Calcium chloride	Mild hypocalcemia, latent tetany, severe hypocalcemic tetany, magnesium intoxication, cardiac resuscitation	**PO:** 6–8 gm daily in divided doses given with demulcent. **Children, PO:** 300 mg/kg daily of a 2% solution in divided doses. **IV,** *hypocalcemia:* 0.5–1 gm q 1–3 days; *magnesium intoxication:* 0.5 gm, observe for recovery before other doses given; *cardiac resuscitation:* 0.2–0.8 gm into ventricular cavity. **Never administer IM.**	27%
Calcium gluconate	Latent hypocalcemic tetany, severe hypocalcemic tetany	**PO:** 1–2 gm t.i.d.; **children:** 500 mg/kg in divided doses. **IV:** 0.5–2.0 gm. **Children:** 500 mg/kg/day in divided doses. Rate of injection should not exceed 0.5 ml/minute.	9%
Calcium glucetptate	Hypocalcemia, tetany, extransfusion in newborns	**IM and IV:** 2–5 ml (0.44–1.1 gm containing 36–90 mg calcium). *In newborns for exchange transfusions:* 0.5 ml (0.11 gm) after every 100 ml of blood exchanged	22%
Calcium lactate	Latent hypocalcemic tetany, hyperphosphatemia	**PO, adult:** 0.325–1.3 gm t.i.d. with meals. **Pediatric:** 500 mg/kg daily in divided doses.	13%
Calcium levulinate	Hypocalcemia, tetany	**IM, IV, or SC, adults:** 1 gm (equivalent to 130 mg calcium). **Children:** 0.2–0.5 gm	10%

® Other calcium salts may also be prescribed.

565

or be made by diluting medication with *hot* water because calcium goes into suspension six times more readily in hot water than cold water. Solution may then be cooled before drinking.

IV

1. Administer very slowly, observing vital signs closely for bradycardia and hypotension.
2. Prevent leakage of medication into tissues because these salts are highly irritating.

IM

1. Rotate sites of injection because medication may cause sloughing.
2. Do not administer IM calcium gluconate to children.

Nursing Implications

1. Teach the patient that calcium requirements are best met by milk in diet.
2. Advise the patient that multivitamin and mineral preparations do not contain sufficient calcium to meet their needs.
3. Prevent patient in hypocalcemic tetany from injuring him/herself by providing safety precautions.

ETIDRONATE DISODIUM DIDRONEL

Classification Bone growth regulator.

General Statement At present, etidronate disodium is used almost exclusively for the treatment of Paget's disease, also called osteitis deformans. This condition is characterized by bone resorption, compensatory new bone formation, and increased vascularization of the bone. The disease affects mostly persons over 45 years of age. Etidronate disodium slows bone metabolism and thus decreases bone resorption, bone turnover, and new bone formation. It also reduces vascularization of bone. Results with drug are variable, but beneficial effects often persist for 3 months to 1 year after discontinuation.

Uses Paget's disease, especially of the polyostotic type accompanied by pain and increased urine levels of hydroxyproline and serum alkaline phosphatase. Heterotopic ossification due to spinal cord injury.

Contraindications Enterocolitis: use with caution in the presence of renal dysfunction. Safe use during pregnancy and lactation not established.

Untoward Reactions (Dose-Related) Increased incidence of fractures, increased and recurrent bone pain. GI manifestations: diarrhea, nausea. Drug should be discontinued if fracture occurs and until healing takes place.

Dosage *Paget's disease,* **PO: usual,** 5 mg/kg/day for 6 months or less. 10 mg/kg up to a maximum of 20 mg/kg/day for patients when bone metabolism suppression is highly advisable; treatment at this dose level should not exceed three months. Another course of therapy may be instituted after rest period of 2 months. *Heterotopic ossification due to spinal cord injury:* 20 mg/kg/day for 2 weeks; **then** 10 mg/kg/day for 10 weeks.

Administration

1. Give as single dose 2 hours before meals with juice or water.
2. Advise patient not to eat for 2 hours after taking medication because foods high in calcium may reduce absorption.

Nursing Implications

1. Monitor urinary hydroxyproline excretion and serum alkaline phosphatase because reduction in these levels are first indication of a beneficial therapeutic response. Reduced levels usually occur 1 to 3 months after initiation of therapy.
2. Encourage patient to maintain a well-balanced diet with adequate intake of calcium and vitamin D.

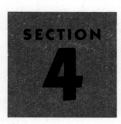

SECTION 4

adrenocorticosteroids and analogs

Beclomethasone Dipropionate
Betamethasone
Betamethasone Acetate and
  Betamethasone Sodium Phosphate
Betamethasone Benzoate
Betamethasone Dipropionate
Betamethasone Sodium Phosphate
Betamethasone Valerate
Corticotropin
Corticotropin Repository
Corticotropin Gel
Cortisone Acetate
Desonide
Desoximetasone
Desoxycorticosterone Acetate
Desoxycorticosterone Pivalate
Dexamethasone
Dexamethasone Acetate
Dexamethasone Sodium Phosphate
Fludrocortisone Acetate
Flumethasone Pivalate
Fluocinolone Acetonide
Fluocinonide
Fluorometholone
Fluprednisolone
Flurandrenolide

Halcinonide
Hydrocortisone
Hydrocortisone Acetate
Hydrocortisone Cypionate
Hydrocortisone Sodium Phosphate
Hydrocortisone Sodium Succinate
Hydrocortamate Hydrochloride
Meprednisone
Methylprednisolone
Methylprednisolone Acetate
Methylprednisolone Sodium Succinate
Paramethasone Acetate
Prednisolone
Prednisolone Acetate
Prednisolone Acetate and Prednisolone
  Sodium Phosphate
Prednisolone Sodium Phosphate
Prednisolone Tebutate
Prednisone
Triamcinolone
Triamcinolone Acetonide
Triamcinolone Diacetate
Triamcinolone Hexacetonide

General Statement

The adrenocorticosteroids are a group of natural hormones produced by the adrenal cortex (outer shell of the adrenal gland). They are used for a variety of therapeutic purposes. Many slightly modified synthetic variants are available today, and some patients may respond better to one substance than to another.

The hormones of the adrenal gland influence many metabolic pathways and all organ systems. They are essential for survival and have the ability to maintain the constant "inner environment" of humans and other mammals.

The release of adrenocorticosteroids is controlled by hormones such as corticotropin releasing factor and ACTH, produced by the hypothalamus and anterior pituitary, respectively. The adrenocorticosteroids play an important role in most major metabolic processes. They have the following effects:

1. **Carbohydrate metabolism.** Deposition of glucose as glycogen in the liver and the conversion of glycogen to glucose when needed. Gluconeogenesis, i.e., the transformation of protein into glucose.
2. **Protein metabolism.** The stimulation of protein loss from many organs (catabolism). This is characterized by a negative nitrogen balance.
3. **Fat metabolism.** The deposition of fatty tissue in facial, abdominal, and shoulder regions.
4. **Water and electrolyte balance.** Alteration of glomerular filtration rate; increased sodium and consequently fluid retention. Also affect the excretion rate of potassium, calcium, and phosphorus. Urinary excretion rate of creatine and uric acid increases.

The hormones also have a marked anti-inflammatory effect and aid the organism to cope with various stressful situations (trauma, severe illness). The adrenocorticosteroids also suppress the lymphatic system, decreasing the number of circulating lymphocytes and eosinophils, shrinking the lymph nodes, and atrophying the thymus. The production of immunoglobulins (antibodies) is depressed.

According to their chemical structure and chief physiological effect, the adrenocorticosteroids fall into two subgroups:

1. Those, like cortisone and hydrocortisone, that mainly regulate the metabolic pathways involving protein, carbohydrate, and fat. This group is often referred to as *glucocorticoids*.
2. Those, like aldosterone and desoxycorticosterone, that are more specifically involved in electrolyte and water balance. These are often referred to as *mineralocorticoids*.

There is considerable functional overlap between the two groups.

Uses

1. **Replacement Therapy.** Acute and chronic adrenal insufficiency, including Addison's disease, congenital adrenal hyperplasia, adrenal insufficiency secondary to anterior pituitary insufficiency. However, not all drugs can be used for replacement therapy; some lack glucocorticoid effects, others lack mineralocorticoid effects. For replacement therapy, drugs must possess both effects.

2. **Collagen Diseases.** Rheumatoid arthritis, rheumatic fever, especially in the presence of carditis, systemic lupus erythematosus, dermatomyositis, scleroderma, periarteritis nodosum, and pemphigus.
3. **Allergic States, Allergic Dermatoses.** Serum sickness, bronchial asthma, acute allergic rhinitis, angioneurotic edema, intractable hay fever, and exfoliative dermatitis.
4. **Various Eye Conditions.** Allergic blepharitis, purulent conjunctivitis, corneal inflammation, uveitis, acute choroiditis, sympathetic ophthalmia, and retrolental fibroplasia.
5. **Hematologic and Neoplastic Conditions.** The leukemias, especially those involving the lymphatic system, such as chronic lymphatic leukemia, Hodgkin's disease, and lymphosarcoma. Nonneoplastic blood dyscrasias, such as aplastic anemia, autoimmune hemolytic anemia, and agranulocytosis, and various solid tumors.
6. **Acute Emergencies.** Shock, emergency conditions involving the CNS, such as encephalitis, meningitis. Also for fulminating bacterial infections caused by gram-negative organisms.

   A variety of other conditions including thrombotic diseases, thrombocytopenia, chronic ulcerative colitis, chronic kidney diseases.
7. **Topically.** The corticosteroids can be used for the treatment of acute or chronic dermatoses, including atopic, seborrheic, some types of chronic eczematous dermatitis, and in infantile eczema, neurodermatitis, intertriginous psoriasis, and anogenital pruritus. Hydrocortisone has also been used effectively for the treatment of ulcerative colitis and other inflammatory conditions of the lower intestinal tract by rectal administration as suppositories or in aqueous suspension.

Contraindications   Corticosteroids are contraindicated in any situation where infection may be suspected as these drugs may mask infections. Also peptic ulcer, psychoses, acute glomerulonephritis, herpes simplex infections of the eye, vaccinia or varicella, the exanthematous diseases, Cushing's syndrome, active tuberculosis, myasthenia gravis.

Adrenoglucocorticoids should be used with caution in the presence of diabetes mellitus, hypertension, congestive heart failure, chronic nephritis, thrombophlebitis, osteoporosis, convulsive disorders, infectious diseases, diverticulitis, renal insufficiency, pregnancy.

Topical application in the treatment of eye disorders is contraindicated in dendritic keratitis, vaccinia, chickenpox, or other viral disease that may involve the conjunctiva or cornea. Also tuberculosis and fungal or acute purulent infections of the eye. Topical treatment of the ear is contraindicated in aural fungal infections and perforated eardrum. Topical use in dermatology contraindicated in tuberculosis of the skin, herpes simplex, vaccinia, varicella, and infectious conditions in the absence of anti-infective agents.

Untoward Reactions   Small physiological doses given as replacement therapy or short-term high dosage therapy during emergencies rarely cause side effects. Prolonged therapy may cause Cushing-like symptoms ("moon face") characterized by rounding of the face, excess fat on the face, neck, shoulders and abdomen; hirsutism; wasting of muscle tissue, especially the arms and legs; hyperglycemia, glycosuria (steroid diabetes); osteoporosis; spontaneous fractures; hypertension; edema; amenorrhea; changes in the skin and nails; ecchymoses; potassium depletion; alkalosis; mental disturbances, euphoria and manic-depressive states; obesity, increased appetite; peptic ulcer, epigastric distress; purpura; headache, and vertigo. Prolonged therapy with adrenocorticosteroids suppresses natural hormone production by the adrenal cortex and decreases urinary 17-hydroxycorticosteroids.

The glucocorticoids may cause linear growth suppression in children as well as a reversible pseudo-brain tumor syndrome characterized by headache, papilledema and oculomotor paralysis. Cataracts have also been reported in many patients after moderately high doses for more than 1 year.

They reduce inflammation (and therefore pain) in a diseased joint possibly inducing patients to overuse the joint.

Adrenocorticosteroids delay wound healing and tissue repair.

Eye Therapy

Application of corticosteroid preparations to the eye may reduce the aqueous outflow and increase ocular pressure thereby inducing or aggravating simple glaucoma. Ocular pressure therefore should be checked frequently in the elderly or in patients with glaucoma.

Stinging and burning may occur occasionally. Dendritic (herpes simplex) keratitis occasionally develops during adrenocorticoid therapy, in which case the drug must be discontinued.

Corneal perforation has occurred on occasion when the drugs were used for herpes zoster ophthalmicus or other disease that causes the cornea to thin.

Topical Use

Except when used over large areas, when the skin is broken, or with occlusive dressings, topically applied corticosteroids are not absorbed systemically in sufficiently large quantities to cause the untoward reactions noted in the previous paragraphs. Topically applied corticosteroids, however, may cause atrophy of the epidermis, drying of the skin, or atrophy of the dermal collagen. When used on the face, the agents may cause diffuse thinning and homogenization of the collagen, epidermal thinning, and striae formation. Topical corticosteroids should be used cautiously, or not at all, for infected lesions, and in that case, the use of occlusive dressings is contraindicated. Occasionally, topical corticosteroids may cause a sensitization reaction, which necessitates discontinuation of the drug.

Drug Interactions

Interactant	Interaction
Amphotericin B	Corticosteroids ↑ K depletion caused by amphotericin B
Antibiotics, broad spectrum	Concomitant use may result in emergence of resistant strains leading to severe infection

Drug Interactions (Continued)

Interactant	Interaction
Anticholinergics	Combination ↑ intraocular pressure; will aggravate glaucoma
Anticoagulants, oral	↓ Effect of anticoagulants by ↓ hypoprothrombinemia. Also ↑ risk of hemorrhage due to vascular effects of corticosteroids
Antidiabetic agents	Hyperglycemic effect of corticosteroids may necessitate an ↑ dose of antidiabetic agent
Barbiturates	↓ Effect of corticosteroids due to ↑ breakdown by liver
Contraceptives, oral	Estrogen ↑ anti-inflammatory effect of hydrocortisone by ↓ breakdown by liver
Estrogens	Estrogens ↑ anti-inflammatory effect of hydrocortisone by ↓ breakdown by liver
Ethacrynic acid (Edecrin)	Enhanced K loss due to K-losing properties of both drugs
Furosemide (Lasix)	Enhanced K loss due to K-losing properties of both drugs
Indomethacin (Indocin)	↑ Chance of GI ulceration
Phenytoin (Dilantin)	↓ Effect of corticosteroids due to ↑ breakdown by liver
Salicylates	Both are ulcerogenic. Also, corticosteroids may ↓ blood salicylate levels
Tetracyclines	Concomitant use may result in emergence of resistant strains leading to severe infection
Thiazide diuretics	Enhanced K loss due to K-losing properties of both drugs
Vitamin A	Topical vitamin A can reverse impaired wound healing in patients receiving corticosteroids

Laboratory Test Interferences

Alter electrolyte balance. ↑ Serum amylase, CO_2 content, and glucose. ↓ Serum uric acid.

Dosage

Dosage is highly individualized, according to both the condition being treated and to the response of the patient. Although the various adrenocorticosteroids are very similar in their actions, patients may respond better to one type of drug than to another. It is most important that therapy not be discontinued abruptly. Except for replacement therapy, treatment should always be aimed at the minimum effective dosage and shortest period of time. Long-term use often causes severe side effects. If corticosteroids are used for replacement therapy or high doses are used for prolonged periods of time, the dose must be *increased* if surgery is required.

For topical use, ointment, cream, lotion, solution, plastic tape, aerosol suspension and aerosol cream are selected, depending on dermatological condition to be treated.

Lotions are considered best for weeping eruptions, especially in areas subject to chafing (axilla, feet, and groin). Creams are suitable for most inflammations; ointments are preferred for dry scaly lesions.

Administration of Topical Corticosteroids

1. Cleanse area before application of medication.
2. Apply agent sparingly and rub gently into area.
3. Apply occlusive type dressing, as ordered, to promote hydration of stratum corneum and increase the absorption of the medication. Two methods are used to apply occlusive type dressing:
   a. Apply a heavy application of medication to cleansed area. Cover with a thin, pliable, nonflammable, plastic film which is then sealed to surrounding tissue with skin tape or held in place with gauze. Change the dressing every 3 to 4 days.
   b. Apply a light application of medication and cover with a damp cloth. Then cover with a thin pliable, nonflammable plastic film and seal to surrounding tissue with tape or hold in place with gauze. Change this dressing b.i.d.

Nursing Implications

1. Emphasize to the patient the need for regular medical supervision as dosage may have to be adjusted frequently.
2. Assist the patient in maintaining general hygiene with scrupulous cleanliness to avoid infection because antibody production is decreased by adrenocorticosteroids.
3. Check the patient for signs and symptoms of other diseases because adrenocorticosteroids mask the severity of most illnesses.
4. Weigh the patient before therapy is instituted and then daily under standard conditions. Anticipate that the patient will have a small weight gain due to increased appetite, but sudden increases are probably due to edema and must be reported. Edema occurs most frequently with cortisone or desoxycorticosterone acetate and less frequently with the new synthetic agents.
5. Monitor BP at least 2 times daily until the patient is stabilized on a maintenance dose. Report increases in BP.
6. Check the height and weight of children regularly because growth suppression is a hazard of adrenocorticosteroid administration.
7. Delay vaccination of patient on adrenocorticosteroid therapy because there is limited immune response during therapy with steroids.
8. Reassure parents of children who develop pseudo-brain tumor that these symptoms will disappear when therapy is discontinued.
9. Check the urine of patients with a history of diabetes before each meal and at bedtime because drug has a tendency to cause hyperglycemia and consequently glycosuria.
10. Check that patients on long-term therapy have blood tests periodically to determine glucose levels.
11. Check the patient's muscles for weakness and wasting (signs of negative nitrogen balance).
12. Warn patients to be particularly careful to avoid falls and other accidents because steroids may cause osteoporosis which makes the bones more susceptible to fractures.
13. Provide supportive measures and reassurance to patients who are having flare-ups explaining that symptoms are caused by forced reduction of drug dosage.
14. *Warn patients with arthritis not to overuse the now painless joint.*

Permanent joint damage may result from overuse because underlying pathology is still present though pain is relieved.

15. Advise patient to carry a card identifying the drug and dosage he/she is taking.

16. Explain to the patient the need for slowly withdrawing the drug when therapy is completed so that his/her own adrenal cortex will gradually be reactivated to take over the production of hormones.

17. Teach patient how to supplement diet with potassium-rich foods if indicated (e.g., citrus juices, bananas).

18. Teach the patient how to maintain a low-salt diet if ordered.

19. Anticipate that the patient's wounds will heal slowly because of the slow development of granulation tissue caused by steroid therapy.

20. Advise patients on long-term ophthalmic therapy to have frequent eye examinations as steroids may cause cataracts.

21. Observe for and report effects resembling Cushing's syndrome such as rounding of face, hirsutism, acne, muscular weakness, cervicothoracic hump, hypertension, osteoporosis, edema, amenorrhea, striae and thinning of skin and nails, ecchymosis, impaired glucose tolerance, negative nitrogen balance, alkalosis, and mental disturbances.

22. Advise the patient to report to physician any symptoms of gastric distress so that antacids, special diet, and possibly diagnostic x-rays may be ordered.

Topical Corticosteroids

23. Observe for local sensitivity reaction at site of application.

24. Withhold medication and report should sensitivity reaction be noted.

25. Observe closely for signs of infection because corticosteroids tend to mask infection.

26. Do not apply occlusive dressings when infection is present.

27. Monitor temperature of patient with large occlusive dressings q 4 hours, and remove dressing if temperature is elevated.

28. Observe patient for signs of systemic absorption of medication, such as edema and transient inhibition of pituitary—adrenal function.

BECLOMETHASONE DIPROPIONATE VANCERIL

Classification Adrenocorticosteroid, synthetic, glucocorticoid type.

Remarks Beclomethasone is suitable for inhalation therapy for bronchial asthma in patients who require chronic administration of glucocorticosteroids or those who are refractory to more conventional therapy. The drug is an effective topical anti-inflammatory acting on the bronchi and bronchioles. Beclomethasone is rapidly inactivated, and thus, the absorbed portion of the drug has few systemic effects. In glucocorticosteroid-dependent patients, beclomethasone often permits a decrease in the dosage of the systemic agent. Withdrawal of systemic corticosteroids must be carried out very gradually.

Note: If a patient is on systemic steroids, transfer to beclomethasone may be difficult, since recovery from impaired renal function may be slow.

Uses   Selected patients with bronchial asthma. Investigationally: hay fever, non-seasonal rhinitis, nasal polyps. Not suitable for rapid relief of bronchospasms or for relief of asthma that can be controlled by bronchodilators or other medication.

Contraindications   Status asthmaticus, acute episodes of asthma, hypersensitivity to drug or aerosol ingredients. Safe use in pregnancy, lactation, and children under 6 years of age not established.

Dosage   **PO (inhalation): usual,** 100 μg (2 inhalations) 3 to 4 times/day. **Severe:** 600–800 μg (12 to 16 inhalations/day). Up to maximum of 1 mg (20 inhalations) daily. When feasible, reduce to lowest effective dosage. **Pediatric 6–12 years: usual,** 50–100 μg (1 to 2 inhalations) 3 to 4 times/day, up to maximum of 500 μg (10 inhalations). *Investigational, hay fever,* **adults and children:** 50 μg (1 spray) in each nostril q.i.d. *Nonseasonal allergic rhinitis and nasal polyps,* **adults:** 50 μg (1 spray) in each nostril q.i.d.

In patients also receiving systemic glucocorticosteroids, beclomethasone should be started when condition of patient is relatively stable.

Administration   1. Follow these steps for administration of beclomethasone:
   a. Shake metal canister thoroughly immediately prior to use.
   b. Instruct patient to exhale as completely as possible.
   c. Place mouthpiece of inhaler into mouth and instruct patient to tighten lips around it.
   d. Instruct patient to inhale deeply through mouth while pressing metal canister down with forefinger.
   e. Instruct patient to hold breath for as long as possible.
   f. Remove mouthpiece.
   g. Instruct patient to exhale slowly.
2. A minimum of 60 seconds must elapse between inhalations.

Storage   To prevent explosion of contents under pressure, do not store or use near heat or open flame or throw in fire in incinerator. Keep secure from children.

Nursing Implications   1. Review with patient printed instructions included with inhaler and assess that he/she is using inhaler correctly.
2. Encourage drug compliance in patients not receiving systemic steroids, especially since improvement of respiratory function may not be apparent for 1 to 4 weeks.
3. Initiation of beclomethasone therapy in patients on systemic steroid therapy.
   a. Withdrawal of systemic steroids must be carried out *very* slowly as ordered by the doctor.

    b. Subjective signs of adrenal insufficiency, such as muscular pain, lassitude, and depression, must be reported to medical supervision even though respiratory function may have improved.

    c. Objective signs of adrenal insufficiency, such as hypotension and weight loss, must be assessed by nurse or doctor.

    d. Signs of adrenal insufficiency necessitate that systemic steroid dose be temporarily boosted and then be withdrawn more gradually.

    e. After withdrawal of systemic steroids, provide patient with a supply of oral glucocorticoids to be taken immediately if he/she is subjected to unusual stress or is experiencing an asthmatic attack. Physician must be called after steroids are taken.

4. Stress that inhaler should not be used for treatment of an asthmatic attack.

5. Caution against overuse of inhaler because more than 1 mg in adults or more than 500 μg in children may precipitate hypothalamic-pituitary axis depression, resulting in adrenal insufficiency.

6. Teach patient to be alert to localized fungal infection of mouth, which requires antifungal medication or possible discontinuation of drug.

7. Advise patients receiving bronchodilators by inhalation to use bronchodilator at least several minutes prior to use of beclomethasone to increase penetration of steroid and to reduce the potential toxicity from inhaled flurocarbon propellants of both inhalers.

8. Instruct patients to carry a card indicating his/her condition, diagnosis, treatment, and the possible need for systemic glucocorticoids, should he/she be exposed to unusual stress.

BETAMETHASONE CELESTONE

BETAMETHASONE ACETATE AND BETAMETHASONE SODIUM PHOSPHATE CELESTONE SOLUSPAN

BETAMETHASONE BENZOATE BENISONE, FLUROBATE, UTICORT

BETAMETHASONE DIPROPIONATE DIPROSONE

BETAMETHASONE SODIUM PHOSPHATE CELESTONE PHOSPHATE

BETAMETHASONE VALERATE VALISONE

Classification Adrenocorticosteroid, synthetic, glucocorticoid type.

General Statement   Causes low degree of sodium and water retention as well as potassium depletion. The injectible form contains both rapid acting and repository forms of betamethasone (mixture of betamethasone sodium phosphate and betamethasone acetate). Not recommended for replacement therapy in any acute or chronic adrenal cortical insufficiency because it does not have strong sodium-retaining effects.

Use   Anti-inflammatory, antiallergic.

Dosage   **PO: usual,** 1.2– 4.6 mg. **Extreme,** 0.6– 8.4 mg in divided doses. **IM:** 0.5– 9 mg daily depending on the specific disease. **Usual,** ½ to ⅓ the oral dose q 12 hr. *Intra-articular, intralesional:* 0.75– 9 mg depending on size of joint and condition.

Administration   Avoid injection into deltoid muscle because subcutaneous atrophy of tissue may occur.

Betamethasone dipropionate valerate and benzoate are used topically.

CORTICOTROPIN ACTH, ACTHAR, ADRENOCORTICOTROPIC HORMONE, CORTICOTROPIN

CORTICOTROPIN REPOSITORY CORTICOTROPIN GEL, CORTROPIN GEL, H.P. ACTHAR GEL

CORTICOTROPIN ZINC CORTROPHIN ZINC

Classification   Pituitary hormone.

General Statement   Corticotropin, or ACTH, is extracted from the anterior pituitary gland. The hormone stimulates the functional adrenal cortex to secrete its entire spectrum of hormones, including the corticosteroids.

The overall physiological effects of corticotropin are similar to those of cortisone. Since the latter is more easily obtainable, is more predictable, and has more prolonged activity, it is usually used for therapeutic purposes. ACTH is, however, very useful for the diagnosis of Addison's disease and other conditions in which the functionality of the adrenal cortex is to be determined.

Corticotropin cannot elicit a hormonal response from a nonfunctioning adrenal gland.

Uses   Diagnosis of adrenal insufficiency syndromes; severe myasthenia gravis. For same diseases as glucocorticosteroids, see p. 568.

Additional Contraindications   Cushing's syndrome, psychotic or psychopathic patients, active TB, active peptic ulcers. Use with caution in patients with diabetes and hypotension.

Additional Untoward Reactions
Acute allergic reactions.

In the treatment of myasthenia gravis, corticotropin may cause severe muscle weakness 2 to 3 days after initiation of therapy. Equipment for respiratory assistance must be on hand for such emergencies. Muscle strength recovers and improves 2 to 7 days after cessation of treatment, and improvement lasts for about 3 months.

Dosage
Highly individualized. **SC, IM or slow IV drip. Usual** (*aqueous solution*), **IM or SC:** 40 units in 3 divided doses. **IV:** 10–25 units of aqueous solution in 500 ml 5% dextrose injection over period of 8 hr. Infants and young children require larger dose per body weight than older children or adults.

Repository (gel or aqueous suspension with zinc hydroxide) IM or SC: 40 units q 24 to 72 hours. 12.5 units q.i.d. cause little metabolic disturbance; 25 units q.i.d. cause definite metabolic alterations.

As a general rule, patients are started on 10–12.5 units q.i.d. If no clinical effect is noted in 72 to 96 hours, dosage is increased by 5 units q few days to a final maximum of 25 units q.i.d.

Administration
Check label carefully for IV administration. **The label must say that the product is for intravenous use.**

IV administration should be slow, taking 8 hours.

Additional Nursing Implications
1. Before beginning IV administration of ACTH, check that patients with a known sensitivity to animal extracts have had sensitivity tests with the brand of corticotropin to be used.
2. Provide potassium intake during IV administration of ACTH either by foods as tolerated, or check with physician regarding administration of potassium by IV.
3. Observe and report exaggerated euphoria or nervousness and pronounced insomnia and depression as these are indications for reduction or stoppage of drug. Sedatives may be ordered as needed.

CORTISONE ACETATE COMPOUND E, CORTONE ACETATE

Classification
Adrenocorticosteroid, naturally occurring; glucocorticoid type.

Remarks
Equally effective when administered PO or IM. Action begins rapidly and is of shorter duration after PO administration. IM effective 24 to 48 hours. Single course of therapy should not exceed 6 weeks. Rest periods of 2 to 3 weeks are indicated between treatments.

Principal Uses
Primarily for replacement therapy in chronic cortical insufficiency. Also inflammatory or allergic disorders, but only for short-term use because the drug has a strong mineralocorticoid effect.

Dosage
PO or IM, initial *or during crisis:* 20–300 mg daily. Decrease gradually to lowest effective dose. *Anti-inflammatory:* 25–150 mg daily depending on severity of the disease. *Acute rheumatic fever:* 200 mg b.i.d. day 1,

thereafter 200 mg, daily. *Addison's disease* **Maintenance:** 10–25 mg daily and 4–6 gm sodium chloride.

DESONIDE TRIDESILON

Classification Adrenocorticosteroid for topical use.

Dosage Thin film of 0.05% ointment or cream is applied 2 to 3 times daily.

DESOXIMETASONE TOPICORT

Classification Adrenocorticosteroid for topical use.

Dosage Gently apply thin film of 0.25% cream b.i.d.

DESOXYCORTICOSTERONE ACETATE DOCA ACETATE, PERCORTEN ACETATE

DESOXYCORTICOSTERONE PIVALATE PERCORTEN PIVALATE

Classification Adrenocorticosteroid, naturally occurring; mineralocorticoid type.

General Statement Chiefly involved with electrolyte and water balance. It increases sodium and water retention and increases potassium excretion. Probably acts by altering the reabsorption patterns of the renal tubules. Desoxycorticosterone also decreases the concentration of sodium in sweat, saliva, and gastric juices. By restoring electrolyte balance and plasma volume to normal, the drug increases cardiac output, decreases nitrogen retention, increases fat and glucose absorption from the GI tract, and increases blood pressure.

Desoxycorticosterone does not affect protein or carbohydrate metabolism or skin pigmentation. It may have to be given in conjunction with a glucocorticoid.

Uses Primary and secondary adrenocortical insufficiency in Addison's disease and salt-losing adrenogenital syndrome.

Contraindication Use with caution in patients with hypertension.

Untoward Reactions Serious adverse effects may result from excessive dosage or prolonged treatment. These include increased blood volume, edema, increased blood pressure, enlargement of heart, headaches, arthralgia, ascending paralysis, and low potassium syndrome (sudden attacks of weakness, changes in ECG).

Dosage   **IM, Maintenance:** 1–5 mg daily. Also available as a long-acting suspension (25–100 mg IM, q 4 weeks); or as implantable pellets lasting 9–12 months. The latter are implanted surgically under asepsis.

Acute crisis: 10–15 mg b.i.d. for 1 or 2 days; supportive measures (whole adrenal cortical extract, cortisone or hydrocortisone, infusions of dextrose in isotonic sodium chloride solution, whole blood or plasma) may also be indicated.

Drug requirements and salt intake are inversely related. The higher the sodium intake, the lower are the requirements for the drug. Most patients need 3 mg of the drug when ingesting 3–6 gm of sodium chloride in addition to a normal diet. Potassium intake has no effect.

Administration   IM: use a 20-gauge needle and inject into upper outer quadrant of buttock.

DEXAMETHASONE DECADRON, DERONIL, DEXAMETH, DEXONE, HEXADROL, SK-DEXAMETHASONE. TOPICAL: AEROSEB-DEX, DECADERM, DECASPRAY, HEXADROL

Classification   Adrenocorticosteroid, synthetic; glucocorticoid type.

Remarks   Low degree of sodium and water retention. Diuresis may ensue when patients are transferred from other corticosteroids to dexamethasone. Not recommended for replacement therapy in adrenal cortical insufficiency.

Dosage   *Chronic diseases,* **PO: initial,** 0.75–9 mg daily. **Maintenance:** gradually reduce to minimum dose—0.5–3 mg daily. *Cerebral edema,* **adults:** *initially,* 10 mg **IV; then** 4 mg **IM** q 6 hr until maximum response noted. Switch to **PO** as soon as possible. **Children** 0.2 mg/kg/day in divided doses. **Topical:** Apply b.i.d.-t.i.d. *Acute life threatening crises, severe allergies:* 4–10 mg daily. *Leukemias, nephrotic syndrome:* 10–15 mg daily.

DEXAMETHASONE ACETATE DECADRON-LA, DECAMETH-LA, DEXACEN LA-8, DEXASONE-LA, L.A. DEZONE

Classification   Adrenocorticosteroid, synthetic, glucocorticoid type.

Remarks   This ester of dexamethasone is practically insoluble and provides the prolonged activity suitable for repository injections.

Dosage   **IM only:** 1–2 ml (8–16 mg) repeated at 1 to 3-week intervals. **Intraarticular and soft tissue injections:** 0.5–2 ml (4–16 mg) repeated at 1 to 3-week intervals. **Intralesional:** 0.1–0.2 ml (0.8–1.6 mg). Dose is expressed in terms of dexamethasone.

DEXAMETHASONE SODIUM PHOSPHATE DECADRON PHOSPHATE, DEKSONE, DEXASONE PHOSPHATE, DEXACEN-4, DEXON, DEZONE, HEXADROL PHOSPHATE, MAXIDEX OPHTHALMIC, SAVACORT-D, SOLUREX

Classification Adrenocorticosteroid, synthetic; glucocorticoid type.

Remarks In emergency situations when dexamethasone cannot be given PO. This drug is given IV or IM. Topical, ophthalmic, otic, intrasynovial, intra-articular, and intranasal use. Intrasynovial use is limited by the short duration of action of drug.

Aerosol preparation used for inhalation therapy in bronchial asthma.

Contraindications Acute infections, persistent positive sputum cultures of *Candida albicans*.

Dosage **IM, IV:** see *Dexamethasone*. **Intra-articular, intralesional, soft tissue:** 0.8–6 mg. **Intranasal, adults:** 2 sprays in each nostril 2 to 3 times/day; **children 6–12 years:** 1–2 sprays in each nostril b.i.d. depending on age. **Ophthalmic:** thin coating to area 3 to 4 times/day. **Oral inhalant, adults:** 3 inhalations (84 μg/activation) t.i.d.-q.i.d.; **children:** 2 inhalations t.i.d.-q.i.d. Dose may be gradually reduced.

Administration Do not use preparation containing lidocaine IV.

Additional Nursing Implication Spray only the number of times ordered for nasal spray.

FLUDROCORTISONE ACETATE FLORINEF ACETATE

Classification Adrenocorticosteroid, synthetic; mineralocorticoid type.

Remarks Produces marked sodium retention and inhibits excess adrenocortical secretion. Should not be used systemically for its anti-inflammatory effects. Supplementary potassium may be indicated.

Principal Uses Addison's disease and adrenal hyperplasia.

Dosage *Addison's disease,* **PO:** 0.1–0.3 mg daily to 0.1 mg 3 times/week. *Salt-losing adrenogenital syndrome:* 0.1–0.2 mg/day

FLUMETHASONE PIVALATE LOCORTEN

Classification Adrenocorticosteroid, synthetic.

Remark For *topical* application only.

Use Dermatoses.

Dosage   Apply 0.03% cream to affected area 3 to 4 times a day.

Administration   1. Rub gently into cleansed affected areas.
2. Add an additional film of cream when pliable plastic dressings are used.

FLUOCINOLONE ACETONIDE FLUONID, SYNALAR, SYNEMOL

Classification   Adrenocorticosteroid, synthetic.

Remark   For *topical* application.

Use   Dermatoses.

Dosage   Apply cream (0.01%, 0.025%, 0.2%), ointment (0.025%), or solution (0.01%) b.i.d.-t.i.d.

FLUOCINONIDE LIDEX, TOPSYN

Classification   Adrenocorticosteroid, synthetic.

Remark   For *topical* application.

Use   Dermatoses.

Dosage   Apply thin film of 0.05% cream, gel, or ointment 2 to 4 times a day.

Administration   Apply in small amounts by gently rubbing into cleansed affected area.

FLUOROMETHOLONE OXYLONE

Classification   Adrenocorticosteroid, synthetic.

Remark   Used only topically for susceptible skin diseases such as psoriasis and chronic neurodermatitis.

Dosage   Apply 0.025% cream 1 to 3 times daily as a thin film to cleansed affected area.

FLUPREDNISOLONE ALPHADROL

Classification   Adrenocorticosteroid, synthetic.

Remarks   Twice as potent an anti-inflammatory as prednisolone. Low sodium retaining activity. Not suitable as sole agent for treatment of Addison's disease.

Dosage   **PO,** *individualized. Rheumatoid arthritis:* **initial,** 2.25–18 mg daily for 3 to 7 days. **Maintenance:** 0.75–12 mg daily; **pediatric: initial,** 2.25–4.5 mg daily. **Maintenance:** 0.75–3 mg daily.

    Higher doses usually are given for *seasonal allergies, systemic lupus erythematosus, leukemia,* and *ulcerative colitis.* Drug usually is given in 4 divided doses, after meals and at bedtime.

FLURANDRENOLIDE CORDRAN

Classification   Adrenocorticosteroid, for topical use.

Remarks   Supplied as ointment, cream, lotion and tape.

Dosage   Apply prescribed strength, lotion (0.05%), cream (0.025% and 0.05%), or ointment (0.025% and 0.05%), 2 to 3 times daily. Tape (4 μg/sq cm), applied as occlusive dressing, is changed q 12 hr.

Administration/ Storage   Protect lotion from light, heat, and freezing.

HALCINONIDE HALOG

Classification   Adrenocorticosteroid, for topical use.

Dosage   Available as ointment (0.1%), cream (0.025%, 0.1%), or solution (0.1%). Apply 2 to 3 times daily.

Administration   Can be used in occlusive dressing during night (12 hours). Use without occlusion during day.

HYDROCORTISONE (CORTISOL) CORT-DOME, CORTENEMA, CORTEF, CORTRIL, HEB-CORT, HYDROCORTONE, OPTEF OPHTHALMIC, RECTOID, OTHERS

HYDROCORTISONE ACETATE BIOSONE, CORT-DOME ACETATE, CORTEF ACETATE, CORTRIL ACETATE, FERNISONE, HYDROCORTONE ACETATE, OTHERS

HYDROCORTISONE CYPIONATE CORTEF FLUID

HYDROCORTISONE SODIUM PHOSPHATE HYDROCORTONE PHOSPHATE

HYDROCORTISONE SODIUM SUCCINATE SOLU-CORTEF

HYDROCORTAMATE HYDROCHLORIDE ULCORT

Classification Adrenocorticosteroid, naturally occurring; glucocorticoid type.

Remarks On weight basis, more active, faster-acting, longer-lasting, and less irritating than cortisone.

Principal Uses Intra-articular. For IV administration for acute attack of adrenal insufficiency characterized by circulatory collapse, decrease in blood pressure, increase in pulse rate, and coma. Also status asthmaticus, allergic drug reactions, and collagen disease. Anti-inflammatory (short term only due to mineralocorticoid effect).

Dosage *Hydrocortisone. Chronic insufficiency,* **PO:** 10–20 mg as the base in 4 equally divided doses. *Other disease states:* 20–240 mg/day depending on disease. **IM, IV:** ⅓ to ½ oral dose q 12 hr. **Rectal:** 100 mg in retention enema. **Topical:** cream, apply t.i.d.-q.i.d. *Hydrocortisone acetate.* **Intra-lesional, intra-articular, soft tissue:** 5–50 mg. **Topical:** 0.25–2.5% solution or ointment. **Ointment:** apply t.i.d.-q.i.d. **Solution:** 1–2 gtts in conjunctival sac q 1 to 6 hr. *Hydrocortisone cypionate:* **Initial,** 20–500 mg. **Maintenance:** 10–260 mg. *Hydrocortisone sodium phosphate,* **IM, IV, SC:** see *Hydrocortisone. Hydrocortisone sodium succinate.* **IM, IV:** 50–300 mg. Higher doses have been used in cardiogenic or septic shock. *Hydrocortamate hydrochloride.* **Topical:** cream (0.1%) or lotion (0.5%).

Administration Check labels of parenteral hydrocortisone to verify route that can be used for a particular preparation because IM and IV are not necessarily interchangeable.

MEPREDNISONE BETAPAR

Classification Adrenocorticosteroid synthetic; glucocorticoid type.

Remarks Drug has minimal mineralocorticoid properties and is unsuitable as sole agent for adrenocorticosteroid replacement therapy.

Dosage **PO:** *individualized,* **initial,** 8–60 mg/day in 3 to 4 divided doses. When satisfactory response is attained, reduce to minimum effective dose; **pediatric,** *individualized:* based on age, condition to be treated, and response.

METHYLPREDNISOLONE MEDROL

METHYLPREDNISOLONE ACETATE DEPO-MEDROL, D-MED, DURA-METH, MEDRALONE, MEDROL ENPAK, MEPRED, METHYDROL, PRE-DEP, REP-PRED

METHYLPREDNISOLONE SODIUM SUCCINATE A-METHAPRED, SOLU-MEDROL

Classification   Adrenocorticosteroid, synthetic; glucocorticoid type.

Remarks   Low incidence of increased appetite, peptic ulcer, and psychic stimulation. Also low degree of sodium and water retention. May mask negative nitrogen balance. Methylprednisolone acetate has slower onset (12 to 24 hours) and longer duration (up to 1 week) than other soluble corticosteroid salts.

Uses   Anti-inflammatory, antiallergic, shock, ulcerative colitis. Methylprednisolone acetate is suitable for IM, intra-articular, and soft tissue injection. Methylprednisolone acetate is suitable for short-term emergency use and as retention enema for ulcerative colitis.

Dosage   *Highly individualized.*
   Methylprednisolone, **PO:** *Rheumatoid arthritis,* 6–16 mg daily. Decrease gradually when condition is under control. **Pediatric:** 6–10 mg daily. *Systemic lupus erythematosus,* **Acute:** 20–96 mg daily. **Maintenance:** 8–20 mg daily. *Acute rheumatic fever,* 1 mg/kg body weight daily. Drug is always given in 4 equally divided doses after meals and at bedtime. *Methylprednisolone acetate,* **not for IV use. IM:** *Adrenogenital syndrome:* 40 mg q 2 weeks; *rheumatoid arthritis:* 40–120 mg/week; *dermatologic lesions, dermatitis:* 40–120 mg/week; *asthma,* 80–120 mg. **Intra-articular, soft tissue and intralesional injection:** 10–80 mg. **Retention enema:** 40 mg 3 to 7 times/week for 2 or more weeks. **Topical, ointment:** 0.25–1% applied b.i.d.-q.i.d. *Methylprednisolone sodium succinate,* **IV, IM:** 4–48 mg depending on the disease; **pediatric:** not less than 0.5 mg/kg/day.

Administration   Solutions of methylprednisolone sodium succinate should be used within 48 hours after preparation.

PARAMETHASONE ACETATE HALDRONE

Classification   Adrenocorticosteroid, synthetic.

Remarks   Approximately two and one-half times as potent as prednisone. Rapid acting. Onset: 30 minutes; duration: 8 to 10 hours.

Dosage   **PO: initial,** 2–24 mg daily. **Maintenance:** 1.0–8 mg daily.

PREDNISOLONE DELTA-CORTEF, FERNISOLONE-P, METI-DERM, PREDNIS, PREDOXINE, STERANE, OTHERS

PREDNISOLONE ACETATE DURA-PRED, DELCORT-E, FERNISOLONE, KEY-PRED, METICORTELONE ACETATE, PREDCOR, SAVACORT, STERANE, OTHERS

PREDNISOLONE ACETATE AND PREDNISOLONE SODIUM PHOSPHATE DIPRED, DUA-PRED, DUO-PRED, JECTASONE, PANACORT R-P, PREDALONE R.P., SOLUJECT

PREDNISOLONE SODIUM PHOSPHATE HYDELTRASOL, KEY-PRED-SP, PSP-IV, SOL-PRED, OTHERS

PREDNISOLONE TEBUTATE HYDELTRA-T.B.A., METALONE-T.B.A., NOR-PRED T.B.A.

Classification   Adrenocorticosteroid, synthetic.

Remarks   Prednisolone is five times more potent than hydrocortisone and cortisone. Side effects are minimal except for GI distress.

Contraindication   Use with particular caution in diabetes.

Dosage   *Prednisolone,* **PO:** 5– 60 mg/day depending on disease being treated. **Topical:** 0.5% (cream or aerosol) applied b.i.d.-q.i.d. *Prednisolone acetate,* **IM: initial,** 4– 60 mg/day. **Not for IV use. Intralesional, intraarticular, soft tissue injection:** 5– 100 mg. **Topical:** 0.12%– 1% suspension, instill 1 to 2 gtts in conjunctival sac q 4 hr. *Prednisolone acetate and prednisolone sodium phosphate,* **IM only:** 10– 80 mg acetate and 5– 20 mg sodium phosphate q several days for 3 to 4 weeks. **Intraarticular, intrasynovial,** same as **IM.** *Prednisolone sodium phosphate,* **IM, IV:** 4– 60 mg/day. **Intralesional, intraarticular, soft-tissue injection:** 2– 30 mg. **Topical:** 0.125%– 1% solution, instill 1 to 2 gtts in conjunctival sac q 4 hr; 0.25% ointment, apply t.i.d.-q.i.d. *Prednisolone tebutate,* **intraarticular, intralesional, soft tissue injection:** 4– 30 mg.

Additional Nursing Implication   Ask the physician if drug should be administered with an antacid.

PREDNISONE DELTASONE, FERNISONE, LISACORT, METICORTEN, ORASONE, PARACORT, PREDNICEN-M, ROPRED, SERVASONE, SK-PREDNISONE, STERAPRED, OTHERS

Classification   Adrenocorticosteroid, synthetic.

Remarks   Drug is three to five times as active as cortisone or hydrocortisone. May cause moderate fluid retention. Is metabolized in liver to prednisolone which is the active form.

Dosage   *Highly individualized.* **PO (acute, severe conditions): initial,** 5– 60 mg daily, in 4 equally divided doses after meals and at bedtime. Decrease gradually by 5– 10 mg q 4 to 5 days to establish minimum maintenance dosage (5– 10 mg) or discontinue altogether until symptoms recur.

TRIAMCINOLONE ARISTOCORT, KENACORT, ROCINOLONE, SK-TRIAMCINOLONE, SPENCORT

TRIAMCINOLONE ACETONIDE ARISTOCORT, ARISTOCORT A, ARISTOGEL, ARISTODERM, CENOCORT A, KENALOG, TRAMACIN

TRIAMCINOLONE DIACETATE AMCORT, ARISTOCORT DIACETATE, CENOCORT FORTE, CINO-40, KENACORT DIACETATE, SPENCORT FORTIFIED, TRACILON, TRIACIN, TRIAM-FORTE, TRILONE, TRISTOJECT

TRIAMCINOLONE HEXACETONIDE ARISTOSPAN

Classification Adrenocorticosteroid, synthetic.

Remarks Somewhat more potent than prednisone. Onset of action: several hours. Duration: 1 or more weeks. Triamcinolone hexacetonide is restricted to the treatment of rheumatoid arthritis and osteoarthritis.

Additional Contraindications Use with special caution in patients with decreased renal function or renal disease.

Untoward Reactions Intra-articular, intrasynovial, or intrabursal administration may cause transient flushing, dizziness, local depigmentation, and rarely, local irritation. Exacerbation of symptoms has also been reported. A marked increase in swelling and pain and further restricted joint movement may indicate septic arthritis. Intradermal injection may cause local vesicular ulceration and persistent scarring.

Syncope and anaphylactoid reactions have been reported with triamcinolone regardless of route of administration.

Dosage *Highly individualized. Triamcinolone,* **PO: initial,** 8–60 mg/day depending on disease being treated. *Acute leukemias in* **children:** 1–2 mg/kg. *Triamcinolone acetonide,* **IM only (not for IV use).** *Usual:* 40 mg/week. A single **IM** dose 4 to 7 times the **PO** dose may control patient from 4 to 7 days to 3 to 4 weeks. **Intraarticular, intrabursal, tendon sheaths:** 2.5–15 mg. **Intradermal:** 1 mg/injection site. **Topical:** ointment or cream (0.025%–0.5%), **lotion** (0.025 and 0.1%); **gel or foam** (0.1%); **spray** (0.2 mg/3 second spray). Apply to area b.i.d.-q.i.d. *Triamcinolone diacetate,* **IM:** see *Acetonide.* **Intraarticular, intrasynovial:** 5–40 mg; **Intralesional, sublesional:** 5–48 mg (average limit/lesion usually 25 mg). *Triamcinolone hexacetonide,* **intraarticular:** 2–20 mg; **intralesional or sublesional:** up to 0.5 mg/square inch of affected area.

Additional Nursing Implications 1. Encourage the patient to ingest a liberal amount of protein as there is a tendency with this drug toward gradual weight loss associated with muscle wasting and weakening as well as a loss of appetite.

2. Offer encouragement and reassurance to patient to counteract drug-induced depression.
3. Warn the patient he/she may feel faint and tell him/her to lie down should this occur.

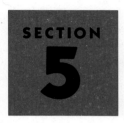

SECTION 5 estrogens, progestins, and oral contraceptives

Estrogens	Chlorotrianisene
	Dienestrol
	Diethylstilbestrol
	Diethylstilbestrol Diphosphate
	Estradiol
	Estradiol Cypionate
	Estradiol Valerate
	Estrogenic Substances
	Estrogenic Substances, Aqueous suspension

Estrogenic Substance in Oil
Estrogens, Combined, Aqueous or Oral
Estrogens Conjugated
Esterified Estrogens
Estrone Aqueous Suspension or in Oil
Estrone Piperazine Sulfate
Ethinyl Estradiol
Polyestradiol Phosphate

Progesterone and Progestins

Dydrogesterone
Ethynodiol Diacetate
Hydroxyprogesterone Caproate in Oil
Medroxyprogesterone Acetate
Megestrol Acetate

Norethindrone
Norethindrone Acetate
Norethynodrel
Norgestrel
Progesterone Aqueous or in Oil

Estrogen-Progestin Combinations

(Oral Contraceptives)
For trade names of various combinations, see Table 27.

ESTROGENS

General Statement

The estrogens are a group of natural female hormones first produced in large quantities during puberty. They are responsible for the development of primary and secondary female sex characteristics. From puberty on, estrogens are secreted primarily by the ovarian follicles during the early phase of the menstrual cycle. Their production decreases sharply at menopause, but small quantities continue to be produced. Men also produce some estrogens.

During each cycle, estrogens trigger the proliferative phase of the endometrium, affect the vaginal tract mucosa and breast tissue, and increase uterine tone. During adolescence, estrogens cause closure of the epiphyseal junction. Large doses inhibit the development of the long bones by causing premature closure and inhibiting endochondral bone formation. In adult women, they participate in bone maintenance by aiding the deposition of calcium in the protein matrix of bones. They increase elastic elements in the skin, tend to cause sodium and fluid retention, and have an anabolic effect by enhancing the turnover of dietary nitrogen and other elements into protein. Furthermore, they tend to keep plasma cholesterol at relatively low levels.

All natural estrogens, including estradiol, estrone, and estriol, are steroids. These compounds are either obtained from the urine of pregnant mares or are prepared synthetically. Nonsteroidal estrogens, including diethylstilbestrol, dienestrol, and chlorotrianisene, are always prepared synthetically.

Uses   Various estrogen-deficiency states, including menopausal syndrome (flushes, sweats, chills, paresthesia, muscle cramps, myalgia, and arthralgia). Stimulation of secondary sex characteristics at puberty (in primary amenorrhea resulting from delayed sexual maturation), postpartum suppression of lactation, in female hypogonadism, secondary amenorrhea, dysmenorrhea, kraurosis, pruritus vulvae, vaginitis in children, senile vaginitis and pruritus, inoperable cancer of the prostate and breast in males, prophylaxis in coronary atherosclerosis, hemostasis during uterine bleeding, replacement therapy after ovidectomy, symptomatic treatment of osteoporosis, and control dysfunctional uterine bleeding during menarche as well as in endometriosis. In combination with progesterone as oral contraceptive.

Contraindications   Cancerous or precancerous lesions of the breast (until 5 years past menopause) and of the genital tract. Administer with caution to patients with a history of thrombophlebitis, thromboembolism, asthma, epilepsy, migraine, cardiac failure, renal insufficiency, and diseases involving calcium or phosphorous metabolism, or a family history of mammary or genital tract cancer. Estrogen therapy may be contraindicated in patients with blood dyscrasias, hepatic disease, or thyroid dysfunction. Prolonged therapy is inadvisable in women who plan to become pregnant.

Estrogens also are contraindicated in patients who have not yet completed their bone growth.

Estrogens should be used with caution during pregnancy because they may masculinize the female fetus.

Untoward Reactions   Nausea and other GI disturbances, which usually disappear with usage. Also, headaches, malaise, irritability, depression, vertigo, breast engorgement and tenderness, paresthesia, lassitude, anxiety, insomnia. Purpura, hypersensitivity reactions, decreased glucose tolerance, edema due to salt and water retention, weight gain due to edema and nitrogen retention, leg cramps, porphyria cutanea tarda, chloasma, acne, leukorrhea, an increase in the size of preexisting uterine fibroid tumors, and hypercalcemia have been reported.

Long-term continuous estrogen therapy may produce endometrial hyperplasia and uterine bleeding. This may be prevented by cyclic administration of estrogens.

Intravaginal application of estrogens may induce a vaginal discharge.

Thrombophlebitis and pulmonary thromboembolism have been associated with the use of estrogens and oral contraceptives containing estrogen.

In males, estrogens may cause gynecomastia, loss of libido, arrest of spermatogenesis, and testicular atrophy.

Prolonged use of high doses may inhibit the function of the anterior pituitary.

Estrogen therapy affects many laboratory tests.

Drug Interactions

Interactant	*Interaction*
Anticoagulants, oral	↓ Anticoagulant response by ↑ activity of certain clotting factors
Anticonvulsants	Estrogen-induced fluid retention may precipitate seizures. Also, contraceptive steroids ↑ effect of anticonvulsants by ↓ breakdown in liver and ↓ plasma protein binding
Antidiabetic agents	Estrogens may impair glucose tolerance and thus change requirements for antidiabetic agent
Barbiturates	↓ Effect of estrogen by ↑ breakdown by liver
Corticosteroids	Estrogen ↑ anti-inflammatory effect of hydrocortisone by ↓ breakdown by liver
Meperidine (Demerol)	↑ Effect of meperidine due to ↓ breakdown by liver
Phenytoin (Dilantin)	See *Anticonvulsants*

Laboratory Test Interferences

Alter liver function tests and thyroid function tests. False + urine glucose test. BSP retention and serum glucose. ↓ Serum cholesterol and total serum lipids.

Dosage

PO, IM, SC, intravaginal, topical, or by implantation.

Most orally administered estrogens are metabolized rapidly and, with the exception of chlorotrianisene, must be administered daily.

Parenterally administered estrogens are released more slowly from their aqueous suspensions or oily solutions. Both types of preparations are suitable for treatment of estrogen deficiency states, requiring cyclic therapy.

Estrogens in pellet form can be implanted under the skin or in muscle tissue. This provides a fairly uniform release of estrogens for periods up to several months. This form of administration is suitable for long-term treatment of prostatic and mammary carcinoma.

Dosage of estrogens is highly individualized and is aimed at the minimal effective amount.

Cyclic therapy (3 weeks on, 1 week off) is usually recommended for women to avoid continuous stimulation of reproductive tissue.

To reduce postpartum breast engorgement, doses are administered during the first few days after delivery.

Nursing Implications

1. Emphasize to the patient that medical supervision is essential if she is on prolonged estrogen therapy.
2. Explain to the patient on cyclic therapy that she must take the medication for 3 weeks and then omit 1 week. She may then menstruate, but she will not become pregnant since she has not ovulated.
3. Instruct the patient to report unusual vaginal bleeding that may be caused by excessive amounts of estrogen.
4. Reassure the patient suffering from nausea that this usually disappears with the continuation of therapy. Nausea may be relieved by taking medication with meals or, if only one dose daily is administered, by taking medication at bedtime.
5. Observe for edema. Teach the patient how to check for presence of edema and to report.
6. Instruct the patient to weigh herself at least 2 times/week and to report sudden weight gain.
7. Observe for thrombophlebitis. Teach the patient how to check for phlebitis and to report if finding is positive.
8. Advise diabetic patients that estrogen may alter their glucose tolerance. Advise them to report positive urine tests promptly because dosage of antidiabetic medication may have to be adjusted.
9. Reassure male patients on estrogen therapy who may be developing feminine characteristics or suffering from impotence that these symptoms will disappear when the course of estrogen therapy has been completed.
10. Do not administer estrogen to mothers planning to breast-feed.
11. Teach the patient how to apply estrogen ointments locally and explain that there may be systemic reactions.
12. Teach the patient receiving intravaginal estrogen how to insert the suppository and instruct her to wear a perineal pad if vaginal discharge increases during treatment. Also advise the patient to store suppositories in the refrigerator.

CHLOROTRIANISENE TACE

Classification   Estrogen, synthetic, nonsteroidal.

Remarks   Chlorotrianisene has long-lasting effects after oral administration, which may be due to higher degree of storage in adipose tissue. The long duration of action of the drug makes it unsuitable for treatment of disorders that require cyclic therapy (menstrual disorders).

Use   Postpartum breast engorgement and prostatic cancer.

Dosage   **PO:** 12–25 mg daily for replacement therapy (cyclically for 21 days with oral progestin for last 5 days of therapy) or prostatic cancer. *Breast engorgement:* 72 mg b.i.d. for 2 days with first dose within 8 hr after delivery. *Atrophic vaginitis, kraurosis vulvae:* 12–25 mg daily given cyclically for 30 to 60 days.

DIENESTROL DV, ESTRAGUARD

Classification   Estrogen, synthetic, nonsteroidal.

Dosage   *Atrophic vaginitis* or *kraurosis vulvae,* **Cream,** 1–2 applicatorsful/day. **Suppository:** 1 daily, usually at night.

Storage   Protect from light.

DIETHYLSTILBESTROL DES, STILBESTROL

Classification   Estrogen, synthetic, nonsteroidal.

Remarks   Very potent nonsteroidal estrogen with long-lasting effect. This drug is not to be used during pregnancy because of the possibility of vaginal cancer in female offspring.

Contraindication   Pregnancy.

Dosage   **PO, IM, SC, Topical.** *Estrogen deficiency syndromes and vaginal conditions* **PO:** 0.2–0.5 mg up to 2 mg daily, give cyclically. *Palliative treatment of prostatic cancer,* **PO:** 1–3 mg daily with increases in advanced cases. *Postpartum breast engorgement,* **PO:** 5 mg 1 to 3 times/day for a total of 30 mg. *Mammary cancer (male),* **PO:** 15 mg daily. *Atrophic vaginitis or kraurosis vulvae:* 1 suppository daily, usually at bedtime.

DIETHYLSTILBESTROL DIPHOSPHATE STILPHOSTROL

Classification   Estrogen, synthetic, nonsteroidal.

Remarks   Potent, long-lasting nonsteroidal estrogen. This drug is not to be used during pregnancy because it may cause vaginal cancer in female offspring.

Dosage   *Palliative treatment of prostatic carcinoma,* **PO:** 50 mg t.i.d. up to 200 mg t.i.d.; **IV:** 500 mg on day 1 followed by 1 gm daily for 5 days. **Maintenance, IV:** 250–500 mg 1 to 2 times weekly.

ESTRADIOL ESTRACE, PROGYNON PELLETS

Classification   Estrogen, naturally derived, steroidal.

Remarks   Several forms of estradiol are available: estradiol, estradiol benzoate, estradiol cypionate, estradiol dipropionate, and estradiol valerate (see p. 592).

Many of the esters have a depot effect and are released slowly from the site of injection.

Uses Menopausal symptoms, functional uterine bleeding, atrophic and senile vaginitis, hypogenitalism, sexual infantilism, and amenorrhea or oligomenorrhea associated with hypogonadism.

Palliative treatment of inoperable prostatic and postmenopausal mammary cancer, postpartum breast engorgement, and occasionally as a pregnancy test.

Dosage *Individualized.* **IM:** *Menopause,* 1 mg/wk in divided doses for 2 to 3 weeks; **thereafter,** reduce dose to minimum needs. *Kraurosis vulvae:* 1–1.5 mg 1 or more times/week. *Prostatic cancer:* 1–5 mg 3 times/week. **SC:** 25 mg pellet for prostatic carcinoma. **PO,** *menstrual disorders, menopausal symptoms:* 1–2 mg daily. *Usual regimen,* 3 weeks on drug followed by 1 week off drug.

Storage Injectable solutions of the esters should be protected from light and stored at room temperature to prevent separation of crystals from oil solutions.

ESTRADIOL CYPIONATE DEPO-ESTRADIOL CYPIONATE, DEPOGEN, D-EST 5, DURAESTRIN, E-IONATE P.A., ESTRO-CYP, ESTROJECT-L.A., FEMOGEN-CYP, SPAN-F

Remark The drug is supplied in cottonseed oil.

Dosage **IM:** *Menopause,* 1–5 mg weekly for 2 to 3 weeks. *Kraurosis vulvae,* 5–10 mg. Repeat in 2 to 3 weeks.

ESTRADIOL VALERATE ARDEFEM, DELESTROGEN, DIOVAL, DURAGEN, ESTATE, ESTRATAB, ESTRAVAL PA, FEMOGEN LA, REP-ESTRA, SPAN-EST, VALERGEN

Remarks The drug is supplied dissolved in sesame oil. Often given in combination with progesterone.

Dosage **IM:** 5–20 mg q 3 to 4 weeks for *vasomotor symptoms, menopausal syndrome, replacement therapy. Prostatic carcinoma:* **maintenance,** 30 mg once q 1 to 2 weeks. *Postpartum breast engorgement,* 10–25 mg.

ESTROGENIC SUBSTANCES MENAGEN

ESTROGENIC SUBSTANCES, AQUEOUS SUSPENSION BESTRONE, CENTROGEN-20, ESTROLIN, ESTRONOL, FEMOGEN AQUEOUS, FORGEN AQUEOUS, KESTRIN AQUEOUS, WEHGEN

ESTROGENIC SUBSTANCE IN OIL FEMOGEN, GRAVIGEN, KESTRIN, URESTRIN

Classification   Estrogen, steroidal. These preparations contain a mixture of estrogens, mostly estrone.

Dosage   **IM,** *menopausal symptoms:* 0.1–0.5 mg 2 or 3 times/week. *Female hypogonadism, female castration, primary ovarian failure:* **initial,** 0.1–1 mg weekly as a single or divided dose. Dosage may be increased to 5 mg weekly. *Inoperable prostatic cancer:* 2–4 mg 2 to 3 times weekly. Response should become apparent within 3 months after initiation of therapy. **PO,** *menopausal symptoms:* 1–2 mg/day cyclically for 20 days/month. After symptoms are controlled, decrease dose to 1 mg or less/day. *Postpartum breast engorgement:* 4–6 mg/day for 6 to 7 days. *Prostatic carcinoma,* 2–3 mg/day indefinitely.

ESTROGENS, COMBINED, AQUEOUS DI-EST MODIFIED, DUOGEN-RP, EVAGEN, FEMSPAN, FOYGEN R-P, MER-ESTRONE, NEO-GENIC DA, SPANESTRIN P, THEELIN R-P, TRI-ES, TRI-ESTRIN

ESTROGENS, COMBINED, ORAL HORMONIN

Classification   Estrogen, steroidal.

Remarks   Combination of water soluble and water insoluble forms of estrone provides both rapid and prolonged estrogenic relief.

Use   Estrogenic deficiency states including atrophic vaginitis and kraurosis vulvae. Also, severe vasomotor symptoms.

Dosage   **Aqueous, IM only,** *individualized.* **Usual,** 0.25–1 ml 1 to 2 times/week. **Oral,** *cyclically for short-term use,* 1–2 tablets/day, of either strength tablet, depending on severity of symptoms.

ESTROGENS CONJUGATED CO-ESTRO, CONEST, ESTROATE, ESTROCON, ESTROPAN, FEMEST, FEM-H, KESTRIN, MENOGEN-1.25, MENOTAB, OVEST, PALOPAUSE, PREMARIN, SODESTRIN

ESTERIFIED ESTROGENS AMNESTROGEN, ESTABS, ESTRATAB, EVEX, GLYESTRIN, MENEST, SK-ESTROGENS, ZESTE

Classification   Estrogen, natural

Remarks   Mixture of sodium salts of sulfate esters of estrogenic substances: 50% to 65% estrone sodium sulfate and 20% to 35% equilin sodium sulfate. Isolated from urine of pregnant mares. Less potent than estrone.

Uses   Parenteral preparation: short-term emergency treatment of spontaneous capillary bleeding associated with surgery. Also, hemostasis
during dysfunctional uterine bleeding; oral preparation used for estrogen replacement therapy.

A cream for topical treatment of vaginal conditions is also available.

Dosage   **PO,** *menopausal syndrome, vasomotor symptoms, senile vaginitis, osteoporosis:* up to 1.25 mg daily. *Replacement therapy:* 1.25–7.5 mg daily;
give cyclically. *Mammary carcinoma:* 10 mg t.i.d. for 3 months. *Prostatic
carcinoma:* 1.25–2.5 mg t.i.d. *Postpartum breast engorgement:* 3.75 mg q
4 hr for 5 doses. **Cream:** 1–2 applicatorsful/day. **Suppository:** 1 daily,
usually at bedtime.

Storage   Injectable solutions are stable for 2 to 3 months at room temperature.
Solutions are incompatible with acids.

ESTRONE, AQUEOUS SUSPENSION OR IN OIL FOYGEN, GRAVIGEN AQUEOUS, THEELIN AQUEOUS, THEELIN IN OIL

ESTRONE PIPERAZINE SULFATE OGEN

Classification   Estrogen, steroidal, natural or synthetic.

Dosage   Individualized.

Estrone, **IM,** *menopausal symptoms,* 0.1–0.5 mg 1 or more times
weekly; *dysfunctional uterine bleeding,* 2–5 mg daily until bleeding
controlled; *prostatic cancer,* 2–4 mg 2 to 3 times weekly. **Topical:**
Nightly vaginal suppositories of 0.2 mg or topical application of cream,
several times daily if necessary.

Estrone piperazine sulfate, **PO,** *atrophic vaginitis and pruritus vulvae:*
0.625–5.0 mg daily; *menopausal symptoms:* 1.5 mg daily; *postpartum
breast engorgement:* 3.75 mg q 4 hr for 5 doses; *palliation of prostatic
cancer:* 3.5 mg t.i.d.; *dysfunctional uterine bleeding:* 3.75–7.5 mg daily
for several days followed by progestin for 1 week. *Intravaginally for
menopausal symptoms:* 1–2 applicatorsful/day.

ETHINYL ESTRADIOL ESTINYL, FEMINONE, ROLDIOL

Classification   Estrogen, steroidal, synthetic.

Remarks   The compound is a form of estradiol. It is effective orally and is a
component of many oral contraceptives.

Uses   Menopausal syndrome, hypogonadism, contraception, and hemostasis
in dysfunctional uterine bleeding.

Dosage **PO**, *menopausal syndrome:* **usual,** 1.25 mg/day. *Replacement therapy,* 1.25–7.5 mg/day for 3 weeks followed by rest period of 7 to 10 days; administer a progestin during last 5 days of therapy. *Mammary carcinoma:* 10 mg t.i.d. for at least 3 months. *Prostatic carcinoma:* 1.25–2.5 mg t.i.d. *Postpartum breast engorgement:* 3.75 mg q 4 hr for 5 doses or 1.25 mg q 4 hr for 5 days.

POLYESTRADIOL PHOSPHATE ESTRADURIN

Classification Estrogen, steroidal, natural or synthetic.

Remarks This compound is a form of estradiol. Only used for deep IM injection.

Principal Use Palliation of cancer of the prostate.

Dosage Administer 40–80 mg q 2 to 4 weeks.

Administration Injection is painful and may require concomitant administration of local anesthetic.

PROGESTERONE AND PROGESTINS

General Statement Progesterone is a natural female ovarian steroid hormone produced in large amounts during pregnancy. It is chiefly secreted by the corpus luteum during the second half of the menstrual cycle. During pregnancy, it is also produced by the placenta.

The hormone acts on the thick muscles of the uterus (myometrium) and on its lining (endometrium). It prepares the latter for the implantation of the fertilized ovum. Under the influence of progesterone, the estrogen-primed endometrium enters its "secretory phase," during which it thickens and secretes large quantities of mucus and glycogen. The myometrium relaxes under the effect of progesterone. During puberty, progesterone participates in the maturation of the female body, acting on the breasts and the vaginal mucosa.

Progesterone interacts, by feedback mechanism, with the hormones FSH and LH produced by the anterior pituitary. When progesterone and estrogen are high there is a decrease in the production of FSH and LH. This inhibits ovulation and accounts for the fact that progesterone is an effective contraceptive. Natural progesterone has to be injected, but a whole series of compounds with progesterone-type activity (collectively called progestins) can be taken orally. These substances are now routinely substituted for natural progesterone. Progesterone is essential for the maintenance of pregnancy.

Although progesterone stimulates the development of alveolar mammary tissue during pregnancy, it does not initiate lactation. On the contrary, it suppresses the lactogenic hormone, and lactation only starts postpartum when progesterone and estrogen levels have decreased.

Progesterone, like estrogen, can be used to relieve postpartum breast engorgement.

Uses Functional and dysfunctional uterine bleeding, primary and secondary amenorrhea, dysmenorrhea, premenstrual tension, endometriosis, infertility, toxemia of pregnancy, and afterpains. Contraception (alone or in combination with estrogens). Occasionally used for pregnancy tests. Responsiveness to progesterone in target organ depends on primary acting estrogen.

Contraindications Genital malignancies. Use with caution in case of asthma, epilepsy, and migraine.

Untoward Reactions Occasionally noted with short-term dosage, frequently observed with prolonged high dosage: spotting, irregular periods, nausea, and lethargy. Also, GI disturbances, edema, weight gain, thrombotic disease, headaches, dizziness, increase in body temperature, more severe menstrual irregularities, decreased libido, and jaundice. High dosage may cause masculinization of the female fetus.

Drug Interactions

Interactant	Interaction
Phenobarbital	↓ Effect of progesterone by ↑ breakdown by liver
Phenothiazines	↑ Effect of progesterone
Phenylbutazone	↓ Effect of progesterone

Dosage Progesterone must be administered parenterally. Other progestins can be administered PO and parenterally.

The usual schedule of administration for various conditions is as follows: *functional uterine bleeding, amenorrhea, infertility, dysmenorrhea, premenstrual tension and contraception:* days 5 through 25 of menstrual cycle. *Remark:* day 1 is the first day of menstrual flow.

Pregnancy test: **PO** for 3 to 5 days.

Nursing Implications
1. Inform the patient that GI distress may subside with use (after the first few cycles).
2. Caution the patient that she must report episodes of spotting or bleeding.
3. Observe the patient for thrombic disease (thrombophlebitis, pulmonary embolism, and cerebrovascular disease) and teach her how to diagnose symptoms that must be reported promptly.
4. Observe for edema. Instruct the patient to weigh herself at least 2 times/week and to report sudden weight gains.
5. Advise diabetic patients that progesterone may alter their glucose tolerance. Advise them to report positive urine tests promptly because dosage of antidiabetic medication may have to be adjusted.
6. Instruct the patient to note and report immediately early symptoms of ophthalmic pathology, such as headaches, dizziness, blurred vision, or partial loss of vision.

7. Inform family members that progestins may reactivate or worsen a psychic depression.
8. Observe the patient for yellowing of the sclera and instruct the patient to report any yellowish tinge to the sclera.
9. When administered to establish pregnancy, inform patient that in its absence she will menstruate 3 to 7 days after withdrawal.

DYDROGESTERONE DUPHASTON, GYNOREST

Classification   Progestational hormone, synthetic.

Remarks   Dydrogesterone has progestational activity without affecting basal body temperature, inhibiting ovulation, or suppressing menstruation. The compound is also devoid of estrogenic activity. Only effective after priming with estrogen.

Use   Menstrual abnormalities, infertility, and functional uterine bleeding.

Dosage   **PO,** *amenorrhea or dysmenorrhea:* 10–20 mg daily for 5 to 20 days.

ETHYNODIOL DIACETATE

Classification   Progestational hormone, synthetic.

Use   Only for oral contraception.

Dosage   See Table 27.

HYDROXYPROGESTERONE CAPROATE IN OIL CORLUTIN L.A., DELALUTIN, DURALUTIN, ESTRALUTIN, GESTEROL L.A., HYLUTIN, HYPROVAL P.A., HYPROXON, LUTATE, RELUTIN

Classification   Progestational hormone, synthetic.

Remarks   Hydroxyprogesterone caproate is relatively long acting (7 to 14 days) and is thus indicated when prolonged therapy is desired. The drug is devoid of androgenic effects. Priming with estrogen is necessary before response is noted.

Dosage   **IM,** *amenorrhea and other menstrual disorders:* 375 mg, anytime. *Cyclic therapy. Adenocarcinoma of uterine corpus (advanced):* 1–7 gm/week. *Test for endogenous estrogen production:* 250 mg, anytime.

Storage   1. Store at room temperature.
2. Wet syringe and needle may cause solution to become cloudy but does not affect potency.

MEDROXYPROGESTERONE ACETATE AMEN, DEPO-PROVERA, PROVERA

Classification Progestational hormone, synthetic.

Remarks Medroxyprogesterone acetate is devoid of estrogenic and androgenic activity. Medroxyprogesterone acetate is also available in depot form. Priming with estrogen is necessary before response is noted.

Dosage **PO,** *secondary amenorrhea, abnormal uterine bleeding with no organic pathology:* 5–10 mg daily for 5 to 10 days beginning on day 16 or 21 of menstrual cycle. *Pregnancy test:* 10 mg daily for 5 days. **IM,** *endometrial carcinoma:* **initial,** 400–1000 mg/week. **Maintenance:** 400 mg/month.

MEGESTROL ACETATE MEGACE

Classification Progestin, synthetic.

Remark The mechanism through which this compound has an antineoplastic effect is unknown.

Use Palliative treatment of endometrial or breast cancer.

Dosage **PO,** *breast cancer:* 40 mg q.i.d. *Endometrial carcinoma:* 40–320 mg/day in divided doses.

NORETHINDRONE NORLUTIN

NORETHINDRONE ACETATE NORLUTATE

Classification Progestational hormone, synthetic.

Remarks Norethindrone is twice as potent and norethindrone acetate is four times as potent as parenteral progesterone.

The compound has some estrogenic and androgenic properties and should not be used during pregnancy (masculinization of female fetus).

Norethindrone or norethindrone acetate, in combination with mestranol or ethinyl estradiol are widely used for oral contraception.

Dosage **PO,** *menstrual disorders, Norethindrone:* 5–20 mg daily; *Norethindrone acetate:* 2.5–10 mg daily. Start on day 5 of menstrual cycle and end on day 25. *Endometriosis, Norethindrone:* **initial,** 10 mg daily for 2 weeks. Increase by 5 mg/day q 2 weeks until 30 mg/day. *Norethindrone acetate:* ½ *norethindrone* dose using same regimen.

NORETHYNODREL

Classification Progestational hormone, synthetic.

Remarks   Slightly estrogenic. Estrogenization of breast-feeding infant may occur. Only used for oral contraception and menstrual abnormalities. May suppress lactation.

Dosage   See Table 27.

NORGESTREL

Classification   Progestin, synthetic.

Remark   This synthetic progestin suppresses ovulation primarily by inhibiting gonadotropin production.

Dosage   Drug is available in combination with ethinyl estradiol (Ovral); see Table 27.

PROGESTERONE AQUEOUS OR IN OIL AQUEOUS: GESTEROL, PROGELAN. IN OIL: GESTEROL, PROFAC-O, PROGELAN, LIPO-LUTIN

Classification   Progestational hormone, natural.

Remarks   Has minimal androgenic effect. IM injection of an oil solution acts more rapidly than SC injection of aqueous suspension. Pain and swelling at injection site are common.

Dosage   **IM,** *secondary amenorrhea,* 5–10 mg for 6 to 8 consecutive days. *Dysfunctional uterine bleeding:* 5–10 mg daily for 5 days.

ESTROGEN-PROGESTIN COMBINATIONS (ORAL CONTRACEPTIVES)

General Statement   Estrogen-progestin combinations, generally referred to as oral contraceptives, are now widely used. External supply of these hormones produces a state of pseudopregnancy in nongravid women.

In the combination regimen (combination of estrogen and progestin given for 20 or 21 days), estrogen suppresses ovulation by inhibiting release of the ovulation-triggering pituitary hormones (LH-FSH). The more prolonged progestin intake produces changes in the cervical mucus, alters the tubal transport of the ovum, and renders the endometrium less suitable for implantation of the blastocyst. These changes are believed to be detrimental to contraception.

Various mechanisms seem to operate in the case of contraception by the progestin-only preparations ("minipill"), including changes in the cervical mucus and alteration of the tubal transport of the ovum. This method of contraception is less reliable than combination therapy.

TABLE 27 COMBINATION ORAL CONTRACEPTIVE PREPARATIONS AVAILABLE IN U.S.

Name	Estrogen	Progestin
Brevicon (21 or 28 day)	Ethinyl estradiol (35 μg)	Norethindrone (0.5 mg)
Demulen (21 day)	Ethinyl estradiol (50 μg)	Ethynodiol diacetate (1 mg)
Demulen-28	Ethinyl estradiol (50 μg)	Ethynodiol diacetate (1 mg)
Enovid 5 mg (20 day)	Mestranol (75 μg)	Norethynodrel (5 mg)
Enovid 10 mg	Mestranol (150 μg)	Norethynodrel (9.85 mg)
Enovid-E (20 day)	Mestranol (100 μg)	Norethynodrel (2.5 mg)
Enovid-E 21	Mestranol (100 μg)	Norethynodrel (2.5 mg)
Loestrin 21 1.5/30	Ethinyl estradiol (30 μg)	Norethindrone acetate (1.5 mg)
Loestrin 21 1/20	Ethinyl estradiol (20 μg)	Norethindrone acetate (1 mg)
Loestrin-Fe 1.5/30 (28 day)	Ethinyl estradiol (30 μg)	Norethindrone acetate (1.5 mg)
Loestrin-Fe 1/20 (28 day)	Ethinyl estradiol (20 μg)	Norethindrone acetate (1.0 mg)
Lo/Ovral (21 or 28 day)	Ethinyl estradiol (30 μg)	Norgestrel (0.3 mg)
Modicon (21 or 28 day)	Ethinyl estradiol (30 μg)	Norethindrone (0.5 mg)
Norinyl-1 + 50 (21 day)	Mestranol (50 μg)	Norethindrone (1 mg)
Norinyl-1 + 50 (28 day)	Mestranol (50 μg)	Norethindrone (1 mg)
Norinyl-1 Fe 28	Mestranol (50 μg)	Norethindrone (1 mg)
Norinyl-1 + 80 (21 day)	Mestranol (80 μg)	Norethindrone (1 mg)
Norinyl-1 + 80 (28 day)	Mestranol (80 μg)	Norethindrone (1 mg)
Norinyl 2 mg (20 day)	Mestranol (100 μg)	Norethindrone (2 mg)
Norlestrin-21 1/50	Ethinyl estradiol (50 μg)	Norethindrone acetate (1 mg)
Norlestrin-28 1/50	Ethinyl estradiol (50 μg)	Norethindrone acetate (1 mg)
Norlestrin-Fe 1 mg	Ethinyl estradiol (50 μg)	Norethindrone acetate (1 mg)
Norlestrin-21, 2.5/50	Ethinyl estradiol (50 μg)	Norethindrone acetate (2.5 mg)
Norlestrin-Fe 2.5/50	Ethinyl estradiol (50 μg)	Norethindrone acetate (2.5 mg)
Ortho-Novum 1/50-21	Mestranol (50 μg)	Norethindrone (1 mg)
Ortho-Novum 1/50-28	Mestranol (50 μg)	Norethindrone (1 mg)
Ortho-Novum 1/80-21	Mestranol (80 μg)	Norethindrone (1 mg)
Ortho-Novum 1/80-28	Mestranol (80 μg)	Norethindrone (1 mg)
Ortho-Novum 2 mg (21 day)	Mestranol (100 μg)	Norethindrone (2 mg)
Ortho-Novum 10 mg (20 day)	Mestranol (60 μg)	Norethindrone (10 mg)
Ovcon-50	Ethinyl estradiol (50 μg)	Norethindrone (1 mg)
Ovcon-35	Ethinyl estradiol (35 μg)	Norethindrone (0.4 mg)
Ovulen (20 day)	Mestranol (100 μg)	Ethynodiol diacetate (1 mg)

TABLE 27   COMBINATION ORAL CONTRACEPTIVE PREPARATIONS AVAILABLE IN U.S. (*Continued*)

Name	Estrogen	Progestin
Ovulen-21	Mestranol (100 μg)	Ethynodiol diacetate (1 mg)
Ovulen-28	Mestranol (100 μg)	Ethynodiol diacetate (1 mg)
Ovral (21 day)	Ethinyl estradiol (50 μg)	Norgestrel (0.5 mg)
Ovral-28	Ethinyl estradiol (50 μg)	Norgestrel (0.5 mg)
Zorane 1/20	Ethinyl estradiol (20 μg)	Norethindrone acetate (1 mg)
Zorane 1.5/30 (28 day)	Ethinyl estradiol (30 μg)	Norethindrone acetate (1.5 mg)
Zorane 1/50 (28 day)	Ethinyl estradiol (50 μg)	Norethindrone acetate (1 mg)

Usual dosage: 1 tablet a day for 20 or 21 days. Sometimes an inert or iron-containing tablet is provided for the days during which no hormone-containing tablet is required (28 day).

Uses   Contraception, menstrual irregularity, menopause, acne, and hirsuitism.

Contraindications   History of cerebral vascular disease, thrombophlebitis, and/or pulmonary embolism, hypertension, ocular proptosis, partial or complete loss of vision, defects in visual field, diplopia, carcinomatous condition of the breast or genital tract, adolescents with incomplete epiphyseal closure, impaired hepatic function, undiagnosed genital bleeding. Use with caution in patients with asthma, epilepsy, migraine, diabetes, metabolic bone disease, renal or cardiac disease, and history of mental depression.

Untoward Reactions   The oral contraceptives have wide-ranging effects. These are particularly important since the drugs are given for long periods of time to healthy women.

Many authorities have voiced concern about the long-term safety of these agents.

The following side effects are noted in some patients: GI system: nausea (chief cause for discontinuation), vomiting, abdominal pain, diarrhea, constipation. Rarely jaundice. Cardiovascular system: possible thromboembolic disease, possible thrombophlebitis with or without pulmonary embolism. Possible hypertension, headache, migraine. Metabolism: edema, weight gain, folic acid deficiency resulting from malabsorption due to oral contraceptives. CNS: neuroophthalmic disorders, changes in mood. Reproductive system: increased cervical flow, breakthrough bleeding, altered menstrual pattern, tenderness and fullness of breasts, increase in size of fibroid tumors. Dermatologic manifestations: cholasma (melasma).

It is advisable to temporarily discontinue therapy after every 18 months continuous use.

Dosage   See Table 27, page 600 and Table 28, below.

Drug Interactions   See *Estrogens*, page 589, and *Progestins*, page 596.

Laboratory Test Interferences   Alter liver and thyroid function tests. ↓ Prothrombin time, 17-hydroxy-corticosteroids, 17-ketosteroids, and 17-ketogenic steroids. (Therapy with ovarian hormones should be discontinued 60 days prior to performance of laboratory tests.)

Administration   Take regularly with a meal or at bedtime.

Nursing Implications

1. Be aware that patients on combination therapy are susceptible to any of the untoward effects of estrogen and progesterone as noted in the *General Statement*. See *Nursing Implications* for estrogen and progesterone page 590 and page 596 respectively.
2. Be alert to patient's complaints of mood swings.
3. Withhold drug from lactating mothers until lactation is well established. An alternative method of contraception should be used during that period of time.
4. Teach patient
   a. That it is essential she be under medical supervision while taking oral contraceptives and that she must take the tablets as prescribed to prevent pregnancy.
   b. To take one missed tablet as soon as she remembers. If two consecutive tablets are missed, she should double the dosage for the next 2 days. She may then resume her regular schedule, but it is advisable for her to use additional contraceptive measures for the remainder of the cycle. If 3 tablets are missed, she should discontinue therapy and start a new course as indicated by the type of medication. Alternative contraceptive measures should be used when she is not taking tablets, and for 7 days after new course has been started.
   c. To discontinue therapy and consult her physician if she experiences symptoms of a thrombic disorder, such as pain in legs, pain in chest, respiratory distress, unexplained cough, severe headache, dizziness, or blurred vision.

TABLE 28 PROGESTIN-ONLY CONTRACEPTIVE PREPARATIONS AVAILABLE IN U.S.

Name	Manufacturer	Progestin
Micronor	Ortho	Norethindrone (0.35 mg)
Nor QD	Syntex	Norethindrone (0.35 mg)
Ovrette	Wyeth	Norgestrel (0.075 mg)

Dosage: 1 tablet daily every day of the year.

d. That oral contraceptives increase cervical mucus and susceptibility to vaginal infections which are more difficult to treat successfully.

e. To consult her physician for possible adjustment of dosage or a different combination if minor side effects such as nausea, edema, and skin eruptions persist after four cycles.

f. To report symptoms of eye pathology such as headaches, dizziness, blurred vision, or partial loss of sight.

g. To report missed menstruation. If 2 consecutive menstrual periods are missed, therapy should be discontinued until pregnancy is ruled out.

h. To have a yearly physical examination and a Pap smear.

i. Not to take tablets for longer than 18 months without consulting physician.

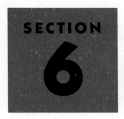

SECTION 6

ovarian stimulants

Chorionic Gonadotropin
Clomiphene Citrate

Menotropins

General Statement Ovarian stimulants are potent drugs to be used only in carefully selected patients. The fertility of the husband must be established prior to the treatment of the wife. A thorough clinical evaluation must also precede each new course of treatment.

CHORIONIC GONADOTROPIN ANDROID-HCG, ANTUITRIN S, A.P.L. SECULES, CHOREX, FOLLUTEIN, GLUKOR, GONADEX, LIBIGEN, PREGNYL

Classification Gonadotropic hormone.

General Statement Human chorionic gonadotropin (HCG) is extracted from the urine of pregnant women. The hormone, which is the basis of a very early and accurate pregnancy test, is produced by the trophoblasts of the fertilized ovum and by the placenta. The action of HCG resembles that of luteinizing hormone. In males, HCG stimulates androgen production by the testes, the development of secondary sex characteristics and testicular descent when no anatomical impediment is present. In women, HCG stimulates progesterone production by the corpus luteum and completes expulsion of the ovum from a mature follicle.

Uses   *Males:* Prepubertal cryptorchidism, hypogonadism due to pituitary insufficiency. *Females:* corpus luteum insufficiency, infertility (together with menotropins).

Contraindications   Precocious puberty, prostatic cancer or other androgen-dependent neoplasm, hypersensitivity to drug. Development of precocious puberty is cause for discontinuation of therapy. Since HCG increases androgen production, drug should be used with caution in patients in whom androgen-induced edema may be harmful (epilepsy, migraines, asthma, cardiac or renal diseases).

Untoward Reactions   Headache, irritability, restlessness, depression, fatigue, edema, precocious puberty, gynecomastia, pain at injection site.

Dosage   **IM only,** *Individualized, prepubertal cryptorchidism:* 1000–2000 USP units 3 times/week or 2500–5000 USP units 1 time/week, for maximum of 8 weeks. Treatment may be repeated after 10 weeks. *For cryptorchidism:* therapy is usually instituted between the age of 4 to 9 years. *Hypogonadism in males:* 500–1000 USP units 3 times/week for 3 weeks followed by same dose 2 times/week for 3 weeks. *Corpus luteum deficiency:* 500 USP units for 2 weeks starting on day 5 of menstrual cycle. Discontinue if bleeding occurs. Treatment may be repeated for 3 or 4 cycles. *Infertility:* 5,000–10,000 USP units 1 day after last dose of menotropins.

Administration/ Storage   Reconstituted solutions are stable for 1 to 3 months, depending on manufacturer, when stored at 2°–8° C (35.6°–46.4° F).

Nursing Implications
1. Teach patients to recognize and report edema.
2. Observe prepubescent male patient for appearance of secondary sex characteristics indicating sexual precocity that necessitates withdrawal of medication.
3. Arrange to have patient with cryptorchidism examined for testicular descent 1 time/week so as to evaluate response to therapy.
4. Withhold chorionic gonadotropin and report if bleeding occurs in female patients after 15th day of administration, if therapy is for corpus luteum deficiency.

CLOMIPHENE CITRATE CLOMID

Classification   Ovarian stimulant.

General Statement   Clomiphene induces ovulation in carefully selected anovulatory patients desiring pregnancy by increasing the release of gonadotropins. Patients usually respond (ovulate) after first course of therapy. Further treatment is inadvisable if pregnancy fails to occur after ovulatory responses.

Uses   Selected cases of female infertility. Investigational: Oligospermia.

Contraindications   Pregnancy, liver disease or history thereof, abnormal bleeding of undetermined origin. Ovarian cysts. The absence of neoplastic disease should be established before treatment is initiated. Therapy is ineffective in patients with ovarian or pituitary failure.

Untoward Reactions   Ovarian overstimulation. Ovarian enlargement (maximal a few days after discontinuation of therapy), flushing, abdominal-pelvic discomfort, bloating, nausea, vomiting, breast discomfort, blurred vision and other visual symptoms, and a variety of other complaints that occur rarely at recommended dosages.

Dosage   **PO,** *First course:* 50 mg daily for 5 days. *Second course:* same dosage. In absence of ovulation, dose may be increased to 100 mg/day for 5 days.

Therapy may be started any time in patients who had no recent uterine bleeding. Otherwise, on fifth day of cycle; after 30 days in patients who did not respond to previous course.

Note: Most patients will respond following the first course of therapy. Further therapy is not recommended if pregnancy does not result following 3 ovulatory responses.

Nursing Implications   Teach patient to:

a. Take basal body temperature and chart on graph.

b. Continue taking basal body temperature in AM and charting it to ascertain whether ovulation has occurred.

c. Discontinue drug and check with medical supervision if abdominal symptoms or pelvic pain occur because these indicate ovarian enlargement and/or ovarian cyst.

d. Discontinue drug and report to medical supervision should visual problems occur because retina may be affected and ophthalmologic examination may be required.

e. Avoid performing hazardous tasks involving body coordination or mental alertness because drug may cause light headedness, dizziness, or visual disturbances.

f. Discontinue medication and check with medical supervision if she suspects that she is pregnant, because drug may have teratogenic effect.

MENOTROPINS PERGONAL

Classification   Ovarian stimulant.

General Statement   Menotropins, extracted from the urine of post menopausal women, are a mixture of follicle stimulating hormone (FSH) and luteinizing hormone (LH). Treatment with menotropins usually only results in growth and maturation of ovarian follicles. Ovulation requires administration of human chorionic gonadotropin (HCG) the day after the last dose of menotropins has been administered.

Uses Infertility caused by secondary ovarian failure, primary or secondary amenorrhea (including galactorrhea), polycystic ovary syndrome, anovulatory cycles, oligomenorrhea.

Contraindications Pregnancy. Primary ovarian failure as indicated by high levels of urinary gonadotropins, ovarian cysts, intracranial lesions, including pituitary tumors. Thyroid or adrenal dysfunction. Absence of neoplastic disease should be established before treatment is initiated.

Untoward Reactions Ovarian overstimulation, hyperstimulation syndrome (maximal 7 to 10 days after discontinuation of drug), ovarian enlargement (20% of patients), ruptured ovarian cysts, hemoperitoneum, thromboembolism, multiple births (20%). Fever.

Dosage **IM,** *individualized;* **initial,** 75 IU of FSH and 75 IU of LH for 9 to 12 days, followed by 10,000 USP units of HCG on day after last dose of menotropins. *Subsequent courses:* same dosage schedule. In absence of ovulation, dose may be increased to 150 IU of FSH and 150 IU of LH for 9 to 12 days, followed by HCG as above for 2 or more courses. *Alternate regimen:* 500–700 IU FSH and LH in 3 equally divided doses on days 1, 4, and 8, followed by a single dose of 10,000 USP units of chorionic gonadotropin on day 10.

Administration Use reconstituted solution immediately. Discard unused portion.

Nursing Implications
1. *Withhold chorionic gonadotropin* and inform doctor if daily urinary estrogen excretion level is greater than 100 μg or daily estriol excretion is greater than 50 μg. These are signs of impending hyperstimulation syndrome.
2. Teach patient:
   a. That she must be examined at least every other day for signs of excessive ovarian stimulation during therapy and for 2 weeks thereafter.
   b. To collect 24 hr urine daily, which will be analyzed for estrogen. Provide her with a suitable container for collection.
   c. To deliver this sample to appropriate laboratory facility.
   d. To take basal body temperature and chart on graph.
   e. Signs and tests that indicate time of ovulation, such as increase in basal body temperature, and increase in the appearance and volume of cervical mucus, spinnbarkeit, and ferning of cervical mucus. Also explain significance of the urinary excretion of estriol as compared to untreated individual.
   f. That daily intercourse is advisable from the day before chorionic gonadotropin is administered and ovulation occurs.
   g. To abstain from intercourse in case of significant ovarian enlargement because this increases chance of rupturing ovarian cysts.
3. Should hyperstimulation syndrome occur:
   a. Explain to patient that hospitalization is necessary for close monitoring.
   b. Maintain intake and output and weigh daily to assist in monitor-

ing for hemoconcentration. Evaluate specific gravity of urine. Assess results of hematocrit and serum and urinary electrolytes.
c. Anticipate that sodium heparin will be ordered if hematocrit rises to critical levels.
d. Explain to patient the need for bed rest, fluid, and electrolyte replacement and the availability of analgesics if needed.

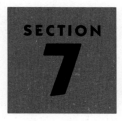

SECTION

7

abortifacients

Dinoprost Tromethamine	Sodium Chloride 20% Solution
Dinoprostone	Urea 40–50% Injection

General Statement

Several agents are used to induce abortions during the second trimester of pregnancy. These include the prostaglandins F_2 alpha and E_2 or highly concentrated solutions of sodium chloride (20%) or urea (40%–50%).

After administration, most of these agents induce evacuation of the uterus within a predictable number of hours. If uterine contractions fail to start or are not strong enough to expel the fetus, a second dose of the same abortifacient is administered. If this measure is again unsuccessful, the pregnancy must be terminated by another means, such as the administration of a different abortifacient, oxytocin, or surgery.

Second trimester abortions are usually carried out by a physician trained in amniocentesis and in a hospital in which intensive care and surgical facilities are available.

All abortifacients, except dinoprostone—which is a vaginal suppository—are administered intra-amniotically. Oxytocin is sometimes administered concurrently.

Administration

1. Have patient void before procedure to prevent injection of abortifacient into bladder.
2. Prepare abdomen with antiseptic solution.
3. Be prepared to assist while physician administers local anesthetic and inserts needle through abdominal wall (#14 gauge spinal needle with stylet) suitable for amniocentesis. One ml of amniotic fluid is withdrawn to check on position of needle.
4. If fluid withdrawn contains blood, needle must be repositioned. Otherwise, a teflon catheter is threaded beyond needle top; the needle is withdrawn and administration of abortifacient started.

5. An amount of amniotic fluid approximately equivalent to the volume of the abortifacient to be injected is removed through catheter.
6. The abortifacient is injected slowly, especially at first, to determine the sensitivity of the patient.
7. The catheter may be left in place for 24 to 48 hours to facilitate repeat administration of drug.
8. Be prepared to administer antibiotics prophylactically through catheter.
9. A small surgical dressing is applied to abdomen when catheter is withdrawn.

Nursing Implications

1. Provide emotional support to patient receiving an abortifacient because she is in great need of reassurance and acceptance and often lacks a good support system.
2. Explain abortion procedure, including administration of drug, labor, and delivery. Provide an opportunity for questions, and answer these appropriately.
3. Have antiemetics available to administer prior to procedure to minimize vomiting.
4. Remain close to patient and provide support as needed during administration of abortifacient.
5. Assess for onset of labor.
6. Monitor progress of labor, assessing frequency, length, and strength of contractions.
7. Monitor BP, temperature, pulse, and respiration to assess for hypertension, hemorrhage, dyspnea, bradycardia, and alterations in function of central nervous system.
8. Assess for nausea, vomiting, and diarrhea both to minimize discomfort and to prevent electrolyte imbalance.
9. If oxytocin is also administered, assess that contractions have ceased before initiating therapy. Utilize Y-tubing system in which one bottle contains IV solution and oxytocin, while the other contains only IV solution. In this manner, the drug can be discontinued but patency of the vein can be maintained when the switch to the drug-free infusion bottle is made. To prevent uterine rupture and cervical lacerations, discontinue oxytocin and notify doctor if contractions exceed 50 mm of Hg as measured on an electric monitor or last longer than 70 seconds without a period of complete relaxation of uterus in between contractions. Remain with patient receiving oxytocin for induction of labor.
10. Monitor patient during fourth stage of labor.
11. Assess patient for hemorrhage, fever, and signs of infection, which may indicate that placenta was retained after delivery of fetus.
12. Observe perineal area for trickle of blood from vagina which may be indicative of undetected cervical laceration.
13. Have RhoGam available for administration after delivery to unsensitized RH negative women.
14. *Teach Patient to*
    a. Observe for signs and symptoms of infection and hemorrhage.
    b. Avoid sex, tampons, or douches for 2 weeks postdelivery.

    c. Return for reexamination in 2 to 4 weeks.
    d. Recognize symptoms of depression, which are common after delivery.
    e. Wear a supporting bra, if lactation occurs after abortion.
    f. Use one of several suggested methods of contraception after postpartum examination if family planning is desired or medically indicated.

DINOPROST TROMETHAMINE PROSTIN F_2 ALPHA

Classification Abortifacient.

General Statement Prostaglandin F_2 alpha, the drug of choice, is administered intra-amniotically. By inducing uterine contractions similar to normal labor, it usually causes the fetus to be expelled in a matter of 20 to 48 hours. Drug facilitates dilation and softening of cervix. Dinoprost causes smooth muscle contraction and, thus, increases the motility of the GI tract which may be the cause of vomiting and/or diarrhea. The drug can also cause bronchospasms, vasoconstriction, and changes in blood pressure and heart rate.

Uses Late second trimester abortion (after week 16 of pregnancy).

Contraindications Hypersensitivity. Acute pelvic inflammatory disease. Use with caution in patients with history of asthma, glaucoma, hypertension, cardiovascular disease, or epilepsy.

Untoward Reactions Frequent: vomiting (50%), nausea (25%), diarrhea (20%). Also rarely: various pain reactions, bradycardia, substernal chest pain, headache, flushing, backache, bronchospasms, hypertension, hypotension, dizziness, syncope, breast pain. Also: cervical perforation, endometritis, diaphoresis, convulsions, paresthesias, dysuria, hematuria, polydipsia. *Note:* Dinoprost may induce an incomplete abortion and measures should be taken to insure complete abortion. Also, since dinoprost usually does not directly affect the fetal placental unit, it is possible that a live fetus may be born.

Dosage **Intra-amniotically:** 40 mg. An additional 10–40 mg may be administered after 24 hr following withdrawal of 1 ml of amniotic fluid, if abortion process has not started or is incomplete. If this still does not induce abortion, pregnancy must be terminated by other means.

Additional Administration 1. Inject first 5 mg at rate not exceeding 1 mg/minute while observing patient for hypersensitivity reactions and for vomiting, pain, or bronchoconstriction, signs that indicate that drug is not being administered into amniotic sac. If none of these untoward reactions occur, the remainder of the drug is administered over a period of 5 minutes.

2. Position patient for vaginal examination prior to each dose of drug to insure that intra-amniotic catheter has not prolapsed into vagina.

DINOPROSTONE PROSTIN E₂

Classification   Abortifacient.

General Statement   Dinoprostone is a prostaglandin that causes uterine contractions similar to normal labor. Uterine contractions usually begin 10 minutes after insertion, and the fetus is usually expelled in 12 to 14 hours. Abortions occur in about 90% of patients within 30 hours and are incomplete in 25% of the cases. Dinoprostone stimulates smooth muscles and increases the motility of the GI tract. Incomplete abortions must be completed by other means.

Intravenous infusion of dilute solutions of oxytocin are sometimes used concurrently to shorten the induction-to-labor time. Oxytocin can also be used when patient fails to abort within 48 hours of intra-amniotic dinoprostone administration.

Uses   Termination of pregnancy during second trimester, beyond twelfth week through the second trimester. Management of missed abortion and fetal death up to week 28. Benign hydatidiform mole.

Contraindications   Hypersensitivity to drug. Acute pelvic inflammatory disease. Use with caution for patients with history of asthma, epilepsy, hypo- or hypertension, cardiovascular, renal or hepatic disease, anemia, jaundice, diabetes, cervicitis, infected endocervical lesions, acute vaginitis.

Untoward Reactions   Vomiting (68%), diarrhea (40%), nausea (33%), transient mild fever (50%), headaches (10%), chills (10%), transient hypotension (10%). Also backache, joint inflammation, or pain, flushing or hot flashes, dizziness, vaginal pain, chest pain, dyspnea, endometritis, syncope or fainting, vaginitis, weakness, muscle cramps, nocturnal leg cramps, breast tenderness, blurred vision, coughing, rash, myalgia, stiff neck, dehydration, tremor, paresthesia, hearing impairment, urinary retention, pharyngitis, laryngitis, diaphoresis, eye pain, wheezing, cardiac arrhythmia, skin decoloration, vaginismus, tension. *Note:* Since dinoprostone does not directly affect the fetal placental unit, it is possible that a live fetus may be born.

Dosage   20 mg (1 vaginal suppository). Repeat if necessary q 3 to 5 hr until abortion occurs.

Administration
1. Insert high into vagina. A diaphragm may increase absorption.
2. Patient should remain supine for 10 minutes following insertion.
3. Times of administration of medication should be determined by patient tolerance and uterine contractability.
4. Store suppositories in freezer at 20° C (68° F).
5. Allow suppositories to warm to room temperature before removing foil wrapping and inserting.

Additional Nursing Implication   Sponge patient with water or alcohol and maintain hydration if patient has drug-induced fever.

SODIUM CHLORIDE 20% SOLUTION

Classification   Abortifacient.

General Statement   Instillation of 20% sodium chloride into the amniotic sac usually causes termination of pregnancy within 48 hours. Ninety-seven percent of patients abort within 72 hours. The abortion may be incomplete in 25–40% of all cases and then must be completed by other means.

Uses   Termination of pregnancy during second trimester (weeks 15 to 24).

Contraindications   Increased intra-amniotic pressure, as in actively contracting or hypertonic uterus. Suspected pelvic adhesions. Patients sensitive to sodium chloride overload (cardiovascular and renal disorders, hypertension and epilepsy), or suffering from blood disorders.

Untoward Reactions   Severe, life-threatening reactions (severe hypernatremia, cardiovascular shock, extensive hemolysis, necrosis of kidney, fever, flushing, edema, pulmonary embolism, pneumonia) have occurred when saline was inadvertently injected intravascularly. Other signs of intravascular injection include mental confusion, pelvic or abdominal pain, numbness of fingertips, tinnitus, salty taste or dry mouth.

Dosage   **Transabdominal intra-amniotic:** 45–250 ml of 20% sodium chloride solution. If labor has not begun within 48 hr after instillation, the patient should be reassessed by the physician.

Additional Administration
1. During instillation of saline pay close attention to complaints of patient (sensation of heat, thirst, severe headache, mental confusion, vague distress, lower back, pelvic or abdominal pain, tingling sensations, numbness of fingertips, a feeling of warmth about the lips and tongue, extreme nervousness or tinnitus) that may indicate that drug is not being instilled into amniotic sac. Be prepared to assist with 5% dextrose infusion and other supportive therapy to prevent hypernatremic shock.
2. Observe patient for 1 to 2 hr after instillation of hypertonic saline for untoward reactions and onset of labor.

Nursing Implications
1. Encourage patient to drink up to 2 liters of water on the day of the procedure to facilitate the excretion of salt.
2. Observe and report symptoms of hypernatremia following injection, such as thirst, rough dry tongue, flushed skin, elevated temperature, excitement, hypo– or hypertension, tachycardia, and numbness of finger tips.

3. Have available 5% Dextrose injection and IV administration set to use, should hypernatremia occur.

UREA 40%–50% INJECTION

Classification   Abortifacient.

General Statement   Hypertonic urea is sometimes used for inducing second trimester abortion. Oxytocin is often used concurrently. The mechanism is thought to involve the release of prostaglandins from cells, which are damaged by the concentrated urea. Average induction time of abortion is 18 to 30 hours, 80% of patients abort within 76 hours. In 30%–40% of patients, the uterine evacuation must be completed by surgical or other means.

Uses   Second trimester termination of pregnancy.

Contraindications   History of pelvic adhesions or pelvic surgery. Severely impaired renal function, frank liver failure, active intracranial bleeding, marked dehydration and major systemic disease.

Untoward Reactions   Nausea, vomiting, headaches, diarrhea, dehydration, myometrial necrosis, electrolyte depletion, including hyponatremia and hypokalemia. Also cervical laceration and perforation. Decrease in platelet count and level of fibrinogen. Accidental intravascular, intramyometrial, or intraperitoneal injection can lead to myometrial necrosis, dehydration, hyponatremia, hypokalemia or hyperkalemia.

Dosage   **Intra-amniotically:** 200–250 ml of 40%–50% urea solution (approximately 80 gm urea).

Additional Administration/ Storage

1. All amniotic fluid should be removed first to prevent sudden increases in intra-amniotic pressure.
2. Warm diluent in waterbath to 60°C (140°F) before mixing with urea. Administer at body temperature.
3. Urea solution should be used within a few hours after reconstitution, if stored at room temperature and within 48 hours, if stored at 2°–8°C (35.6–46.4°F).
4. Administer urea over period of 20 to 30 minutes.
5. Drug should be discontinued, if patient manifests symptoms of lower abdominal pain.

Additional Nursing Implications

1. Encourage fluids to prevent dehydration and to promote urea excretion.
2. Assess for muscle weakness and lethargy, signs of electrolyte imbalance.
3. Ascertain that blood chemistries are performed and results evaluated. Have IV fluids available to correct electrolyte imbalance.

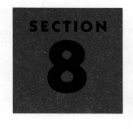
posterior pituitary hormones and related drugs

Posterior Pituitary Injection

Oxytocics	Ergonovine Maleate Methylergonovine Maleate	Oxytocin Oxytocin Citrate
Antidiuretic Hormone and Analogs	Desmopressin Acetate Lypressin	Vasopressin Injection Vasopressin Tannate Injection

The most important hormonal secretions of the posterior pituitary gland are the oxytocic hormone oxytocin and the antidiuretic hormone (ADH) vasopressin. Oxytocin acts on the smooth muscle of the uterus and alveoli of the breast. Vasopressin controls reabsorption of water from the glomerular filtrate and increases blood pressure by causing contraction of the vascular bed and increased peripheral resistance (pressor effect). Synthetic oxytocin and several oxytocic agents play a major role in obstetrics. Vasopressin and related substances are used for the treatment of diabetes insipidus, a disease characterized by loss of large volumes of dilute urine and dehydration.

Except for the posterior pituitary injection, which has oxytocic, vasopressor, and ADH activity, the drugs belonging to this group are used either for obstetric or antidiuretic purposes.

POSTERIOR PITUITARY INJECTION PITUITRIN, PITUITRIN-(S)

Classification   Posterior pituitary hormone.

General Statement   The natural extract of the posterior pituitary has oxytocic, vasopressor, and antidiuretic hormone properties. The rapid pressor effect of this drug may make its use hazardous. Most physicians now use more refined agents with specific oxytocic or antidiuretic properties.

Uses   Postoperative ileus, to stimulate expulsion of gas prior to pyelography, to achieve hemostasis in presence of esophageal varices, adjunct in the treatment of shock, diabetes insipidus, uterine stimulation after complete expulsion of placenta.

613

Contraindications Toxemia of pregnancy, cardiac disease, hypertension, epilepsy, advanced arteriosclerosis, first stage of labor. Use with great caution at any stage of delivery.

Untoward Reactions Common: facial pallor, increased GI motility, uterine cramps. Also tinnitus, anxiety, albuminuria, unconsciousness, eclamptic attacks, mydriasis, anaphylaxis, angioneurotic edema, urticaria.

Dosage **IM** (*preferred*) *and* **SC:** 5–20 units. *Postpartum hemorrhage:* 10 units.

Nursing Implications
1. Observe closely for allergic reaction following administration of medication and have emergency supportive medications and oxygen readily available.
2. Monitor BP closely for ½ hour following administration of medication because it reduces cardiac output and may diminish coronary blood flow.
3. Check with medical supervision whether additional medication is to be administered to prolong uterine contractions, because PPI is short acting.

OXYTOCICS

General Statement The uterus consists mainly of two types of tissues: (1) the *endometrium* or mucous membrane lining the inner surface whose function is governed chiefly by the ovarian hormones, and (2) the *myometrium*, a thick wall of smooth muscle heavily interlaced with blood vessels. The latter are necessary to supply the placenta and fetus with oxygen and nutrients.

An understanding of the different stages of labor is essential for the judicious use of drugs in obstetrics. Premature use of any agent might be harmful to mother and child.

Labor is divided into 3 stages. Stage I is characterized by the onset of strong regular contractions of the myometrium and complete dilatation of the cervix. Stage II begins with the complete dilatation of the cervix and ends with the delivery of the baby. Stage III begins after delivery, involves placental separation, and terminates with birth of the placenta.

Immediately after delivery, the smooth muscles of the uterus are completely relaxed (uterine atony), and during this time the patient may bleed heavily. This period of smooth muscle relaxation is followed by renewed contractions, which produce placental separation and also clamp shut the countless blood vessels exposed when the placenta separates from the uterus. The average amount of blood lost during this stage is 200–300 ml.

The drugs discussed in this section assist the uterus during the various stages of labor. The oxytocic drugs, like oxytocin and ergotamine, promote contraction.

Oxytocic agents are used occasionally to induce labor and to promote incomplete abortions.

As a rule, oxytocic agents are not used during the first or second stage of labor. The premature use of oxytocic agents may cause severe laceration and trauma to the mother (rupture of the uterus), and trauma—even death— to the infant.

Drug Interactions

Interactant	Interaction
Anesthetics, local	See vasoconstrictors
Cyclophosphamide	↑ Effect of oxytocics
Vasoconstrictors (anesthetics, etc.)	May have synergistic and additive effects with oxytocics. Concomitant use may result in severe, persistent hypertension and rupture of cerebral blood vessels

ERGONOVINE MALEATE ERGOTRATE MALEATE

Classification   Oxytocic agent.

Remarks   Natural alkaloid obtained from ergot (a fungus that grows on rye). The drug increases the rate, tone, and amplitude of uterine muscle contractions.

Uses   Prevention and treatment of postpartum and postabortal hemorrhage by producing firm uterine contractions and to decrease uterine bleeding. Occasionally used for migraine headaches.

Contraindications   Hypersensitivity to ergot. Usually, the drug should not be used before the placenta is delivered (third stage of labor). Induction of labor, threatened spontaneous abortion, uterine sepsis, obliterative vascular disease, hepatic or renal disease, during pregnancy, and cardiac disease.

Untoward Reactions   These occur rarely and include: nausea, vomiting, hypotension, bradycardia, allergic reactions, shock, rise in blood pressure, ergotism, drug gangrene, cerebrospinal symptoms, and spasms.

Dosage   **PO, IM, IV,** *Obstetrics* (any route): 0.2–0.4 mg 2 to 4 times daily for 2 days. Calcium-deficient patients may require 10–30 ml of a 10% solution of calcium gluconate prior to treatment with ergonovine maleate.
   Migraine, **PO:** 0.2–0.4 mg q hr until headache is relieved or until a total of 2 mg of the drug has been taken.

Administration/ Storage   Ampule must be stored in a cold place. If kept in the delivery room, it must be discarded after 60 days (loss of potency).

Nursing Implications
1. Check height, consistency, and location of fundus.
2. Check lochia.
3. Monitor vital signs for shock or hypertension after administration.
4. Have appropriate drugs available in case of hypertension.

5. Observe for severe cramping as this may suggest reduction in dose.
6. Check for early signs of accidental ergotism: nausea, vomiting, cramps, diarrhea, drowsiness, dizziness, headache and confusion, as drug is a derivative of lysergic acid. GI and CNS effects may occur before circulatory disturbances to hands and feet.

METHYLERGONOVINE MALEATE METHERGINE

Classification　Oxytocic agent.

Remarks　Synthetic substance whose structure and function closely resembles the natural alkaloid obtained from ergot. The drug promotes the rate, tone, and amplitude of uterine contractions. The intensity and duration of the effect produced somewhat exceeds that of ergonovine maleate. The onset of action is extremely rapid: 30 to 60 seconds after IV injection; 2 to 5 minutes after IM or PO administration.

Uses　Routine management of postpartum hemorrhage *after delivery of placenta* to hasten uterine involution. Should not be given routinely IV because of the possibility of inducing cerebral vascular accidents or hypertension.

Contraindications　Pregnancy. Should be given with caution in sepsis, obliterative vascular disease, impaired renal or hepatic function.

Untoward Reactions　Nausea, vomiting, transient hypotension or hypertension, bradycardia, headaches, dizziness, tinnitus, abdominal cramps, diaphoresis, temporary chest pain, and dyspnea.

Dosage　**PO, IM, or IV. PO:** 0.2 mg 3 to 4 times a day. **IM, IV:** 0.2 mg q 2 to 4 hr after delivery of placenta or during puerperium.

Administration/ Storage　Discolored ampules should be discarded. Drug should be protected from heat and light during storage.

Nursing Implications　See *Ergonovine Maleate*, page 615.

OXYTOCIN PITOCIN, SYNTOCINON

OXYTOCIN CITRATE PITOCIN CITRATE

Classification　Oxytocic agent.

Remarks　Synthetic compound identical with natural hormone isolated from posterior pituitary. Produces muscular contraction of uterus. Also stimulates flow (but not amount) of milk postpartum by contracting the smooth muscles of the myoepithelium. Oxytocin acts faster and for a shorter period of time than ergonovine. Onset: 3 to 7 minutes after IM; 1 minute after IV; and 30 minutes after buccal administration.

Uses Induction or stimulation of labor at term. Used to overcome true primary or secondary uterine inertia. Induction of labor with oxytocin is only indicated under certain *specific* conditions and is not usual because serious toxic effects can occur.

Oxytocin is indicated for the following:
1. Uterine inertia;
2. Induction of labor in cases of erythroblastosis fetalis, maternal diabetes mellitus, preeclampsia, and eclampsia;
3. Induction of labor after premature rupture of membranes in last month of pregnancy when labor fails to develop spontaneously within 12 hours;
4. Routine control of postpartum hemorrhage and uterine atony;
5. To hasten uterine involution;
6. To complete inevitable abortions after the 20th week of pregnancy.

Contraindications Hypersensitivity to drug, cephalopelvic disproportion, malpresentation of the fetus, undilated cervix, overdistention of the uterus, hypotonic uterine contractions, and history of caesarean section, or other uterine surgery. Also, predisposition to thromboplastin and amniotic fluid embolism (dead fetus, abruptio placentae), history of previous traumatic deliveries, or patients with four or more deliveries. Oxytocin should never be given IV undiluted or in high concentrations. Oxytocin citrate is contraindicated in severe toxemia, cardiovascular or renal disease. Do not administer PO to unconscious patients.

Untoward Reactions Mother: tetanic uterine contractions, rupture of the uterus, hypotension, tachycardia, and electrocardiographic changes after IV administration of concentrated solutions. Also, rarely, anxiety, dyspnea, precordial pain, edema, cyanosis, or reddening of the skin, and cardiovascular spasm. Water intoxication from prolonged IV infusion, maternal deaths due to hypertensive episodes, subarachnoid hemorrhage, or uterine rupture.

Fetus: death, premature ventricular contractions, bradycardia, tachycardia, hypoxia, intracranial hemorrhage due to overstimulation of the uterus during labor leads to uterine tetany with marked impairment of uteroplacental blood flow.

Remarks: hypersensitivity reactions occur rarely. When they do, they occur most often with natural oxytocin administered IM or in concentrated IV doses and least frequently after IV infusion or diluted doses. Accidental swallowing of buccal tablets is not harmful.

Oxytocin citrate (see also *Oxytocin*): nausea, vomiting, premature ventricular contractions, fetal cardiac arrhythmias, tetanic contractions of the uterus during induction of labor, and local vasoconstriction of the oral mucosa.

Dosage   **IM, SC, and IV** (*dilute solutions*), **intranasal.**

Induction of labor, **IV infusion:** *preferred*, using 10 units in 1000 ml isotonic saline or 5% dextrose. **Initial**, 0.001– 0.002 units/minute $^1/_{10}$–$^1/_5$ of a ml/min. Gradually increase by 0.001 units/minute (by 0.01 ml/min) until response (0.01–0.02 ml/min). *Postpartum*, **IM:** 3– 10 units, individual doses. *Postpartum bleeding:* 10– 40 units diluted in 1000 ml isotonic sodium chloride and given at rate to control bleeding. **IV.** *Oxytocin citrate*, **Buccal:** total usual dose to induce and complete labor: 1500– 2000 units usually given in increments of 200 units at 30-minute intervals. **Maximum total dose: 3000 units. Oxytocin, synthetic, Nasal:** 1 spray into one or both nostrils 2– 3 minutes before nursing or pumping breasts.

Administration
1. Use infusion pump when possible to regulate flow for induction or stimulation of labor.
2. Insert tablets into buccal space; alternate sides. Each tablet takes 30 minutes to dissolve.

Nursing Implications
1. A physician must always be in attendance when labor is being induced or stimulated with oxytocin.
2. Monitor closely: rate of flow of IV solution with oxytocin:
3. Closely monitor uterine contractions, fetal heart, and vital signs during induction of labor.
4. Report excessively long or strong contractions.
5. Report contractions above 50 mm Hg measured by electric monitor.
6. Observe patient for symptoms of water intoxication after prolonged administration of IV oxytocin. Check for urine output and edema.
7. If buccal membranes become dry, patients receiving buccal oxytocin citrate may rinse mouth with water before replacing tablets.

ANTIDIURETIC HORMONE AND ANALOGS

Vasopressin, the antidiuretic hormone, controls the reabsorption of water from the glomerular filtrate. Its deficiency causes diabetes insipidus or polyuria.

Patients suffering from a mild form of the disease can be treated by intranasal application of suitable substances (desmopressin, lypressin), whereas patients with severe disease may require systemic treatment with posterior pituitary injection, vasopressin, or vasopressin tannate.

Treatment requires individual dosage adjustment. Overdosage may cause fluid retention and hypernatremia. Another common adverse reaction is contraction of the smooth muscles of the intestine, uterus, and blood vessels. Animal proteins which may be present in the extracts of the pituitary glands may result in allergic reactions. Thus, synthetic preparations are preferred.

DESMOPRESSIN ACETATE DDAVP

Classification   Antidiuretic.

General Statement   This compound provides prolonged antidiuretic activity and is devoid of vasopressor and oxytocic side effects.

Uses   Central diabetes insipidus, temporary polyuria, and polydipsia associated with trauma to, or surgery of, the pituitary region.

Contraindications   Hypersensitivity to drug.

Untoward Reactions   Rare. High doses may cause dose-dependent transient headaches, nausea, nasal congestion, rhinitis, flushing, mild abdominal cramps and vulval pain. Side effects can be reduced by a reduction in dosage.

Dosage   **Intranasal only.** *Individualized, usual,* 0.1–0.4 ml/day as single or in 2 or 3 divided doses. Most patients require 0.2 ml/day in unequal doses adjusted to individual water metabolism pattern. **Pediatric 3 months– 12 years:** 0.05–0.3 ml/day as a single or divided dose; ¼ to ⅓ of patients can be controlled with one dose daily.

Administration/ Storage
1. Refrigerate DDAVP at 4° C (39.2° F).
2. Note carefully the three graduation marks on the soft flexible plastic nasal tube: 0.2, 0.1, and 0.05 ml. The 0.5 is not designated by number.
3. Cleanse and dry tube appropriately.
4. Measure dosage exactly because drug is very potent.

Nursing Implications
1. Anticipate that fluid intake should be restricted to avoid water intoxication, especially in the very young and the very old.
2. Anticipate that excessive fluid retention may be treated with a saluretic such as furosemide to induce diuresis.
3. Monitor duration of sleep and daily I & O because these parameters are used to estimate response.

LYPRESSIN DIAPID

Classification   Pituitary (antidiuretic) hormone.

General Statement   The drug is for topical (intranasal) use only. Particularly useful for treatment of patients with diabetes insipidus who are allergic or refractory to therapy with vasopressin of animal origin. See *Vasopressin.*

Uses   Diabetes insipidus of neurohypophyseal origin.

Contraindications   See *Vasopressin.*

Untoward Reactions   See *Vasopressin.* Also nasal congestion and irritation, rhinorrhea, heartburn. No allergic reactions have been noted.

Dosage   **Topical (intranasal), adults and children:** 1 (2 USP units) or more sprays 3 to 4 times daily. Four sprays in each nostril is maximum that can be absorbed at any one time. (Each spray contains approximately 7 μg lypressin.)

Administration
1. Encourage the patient to clear nasal passage before use.
2. Hold the bottle upright and insert the nozzle into the patient's nostril with the head in a vertical position.

Nursing Implications
1. Stress to patients or parents of patient not to increase the number of sprays at one time but rather to check with the physician if more frequent administration is needed. Usually the frequency of administration is increased rather than the number of sprays at one time.
2. Observe for dehydration by checking turgor of skin, condition of mucous membranes, and presence of thirst.

VASOPRESSIN INJECTION PITRESSIN

VASOPRESSIN TANNATE INJECTION PITRESSIN TANNATE

Classification   Pituitary (antidiuretic) hormone.

General Statement   The antidiuretic hormone ADH, more often referred to as vasopressin, is released from the anterior pituitary gland. The hormone regulates water conservation by promoting reabsorption of water by the distal portion of the renal tubules.

Insufficient output of ADH results in neurohypophyseal diabetes insipidus, characterized by the excretion of large quantities of normal but very dilute urine and excessive thirst. These symptoms result from primary (no organic lesion) or secondary (injury) malfunction of posterior pituitary. Vasopressin is effective in the treatment of the condition. It is ineffective when the diabetes insipidus is of renal origin (nephrogenic diabetes insipidus).

In addition to its diuretic properties, vasopressin also causes vasoconstriction (pressor effect) and increases the smooth muscular activity of the bladder, GI tract, and uterus.

Uses   Diabetes insipidus and relief of intestinal gaseous distention.

Contraindications   Vascular disease, especially when involving coronary arteries; angina pectoris. Chronic nephritis until reasonable blood nitrogen levels are attained. Caution in presence of asthma and epilepsy.

Untoward Reactions   Facial pallor, nausea, increases intestinal activity, such as belching, cramps and urge to defecate, uterine cramps, water intoxication, and hyponatremia (vomiting, headaches, confusion, lethargy, coma, convulsions). Large doses may cause increase in blood pressure and allergic reactions.

Drug Interactions

Interactant	Interaction
Acetaminophen (Tempra, Tylenol)	↑ Effect of vasopressin
Antidiabetics, oral	↑ Effect of vasopressin
Cyclophosphamide	↓ Effect of vasopressin

Dosage   *Vasopressin,* **SC, IM:** 5–10 units (0.25–0.5 ml) 3 to 4 times daily; **pediatric:** 2.5–10 units (0.125–0.5 ml) 3 to 4 times daily. *Vasopressin tannate,* **IM:** 1.5–5 units (0.3–1.0 ml) q 1 to 3 days; **pediatric:** 1.25–2.5 units (0.25–0.5 ml) q 1 to 3 days. **This preparation should never be given IV.**

Administration
1. **Never** administer vasopressin tannate in oil intravenously.
2. Shake vial of vasopressin tannate in oil before withdrawing dose.
3. Encourge patient to clear nasal passages well before insufflation.

Nursing Implications
1. Monitor intake and output to aid in evaluation of response to drug.
2. Observe for dehydration by checking turgor of skin, condition of mucous membranes, and thirst.
3. Observe for increased continence and decreased urinary frequency after drug is administered to improve bladder activity.
4. Assess for bowel sounds, passage of flatus, and resumption of bowel movements after drug is administered to improve peristalsis in the GI tract.
5. Monitor BP at least 2 times daily while the patient is on a regimen of vasopressin, and report untoward reactions, such as an excessive elevation of BP or lack of response to drug as characterized by lowering of blood pressure.

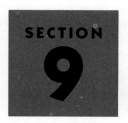

SECTION

9

growth hormone

SOMATOTROPIN ASELLACRIN, SOMATROPIN

Classification   Pituitary growth hormone.

General Statement   Somatotropin, a hormone, stimulates linear growth. Somatotropin is extracted from human pituitary glands. It is an anabolic agent stimulating intracellular transport of aminoacids and retention of nitrogen, phosphorus, and potassium. It stimulates both intestinal absorption and urinary excretion of calcium. The hormone inhibits intracellular glucose metabolism, and decreases the response to insulin. Other effects of this hormone include increased serum levels of phosphorus and alkaline phosphatase, increased synthesis of chondroitin sulfate and collagen, stimulation of intracellular lipolysis and fatty acid oxidation, and stimulation of urinary excretion of hydroxyproline.

Patients who fail to respond to somatotropin should be tested for somatotropin antibodies. During therapy the bone age should be monitored annually, especially in pubertal patients or those who receive concurrent thyroid hormone or androgen therapy.

Uses

Linear growth failure due to deficiency of pituitary growth hormone ascertained by failure of the latter to increase to above 5 to 7 ng/ml after administration of two of the following stimuli: hypoglycemia, arginine (IV), levodopa (PO), glucagon (IM).

Contraindications

Closed epiphyses. Use with caution in patients with diabetes or family history thereof, or intracranial lesions.

Untoward Reactions

Few. Antibodies to somatotropin, which interfere with treatment in 5% of the cases, pain at injection site. SC use may result in local lipoatrophy or lipodystrophy. These increase the likelihood of the production of antibodies to somatotropin.

Dosage

IM: 2 IU (1 ml) 3 times/week at minimum intervals of 48 hr. If growth rate is less than 2.5 cm during any 6-month period, dose may be doubled for the next 6 months.

Administration/ Storage

1. Administer IM.
2. Rotate injection site.
3. Unreconstituted vials may be stored at room temperature.
4. Store reconstituted vials in refrigerator and use within 1 month.
5. Reconstitute with bacteriostatic water for injection.

Nursing Implications

1. Measure height monthly.
2. Withhold drug and check with medical supervision if concomitant glucocorticoid therapy is ordered because steroids tend to inhibit response to somatotropin.
3. Check with medical supervision for frequency of glycosuria determinations.
4. Observe diabetic patients and those with family history thereof for symptoms of hyperglycemia and acidosis.

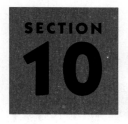

SECTION 10

androgens and anabolic agents

Dromostanolone Propionate
Ethylestrenol
Fluoxymesterone
Methandriol
Methandrostenolone
Methyltestosterone
Nandrolone Decanoate
Nandrolone Phenpropionate

Oxandrolone
Oxymetholone
Stanozolol
Testosterone
Testosterone Cypionate
Testosterone Enanthate
Testosterone Propionate

Miscellaneous Danazol

General Statement The principal male hormone manufactured by the interstitial cells of the testes is testosterone. Testosterone, its degradation products, and synthetic substitutes are collectively referred to as the androgens (from the Greek *andros,* man). Like the primary female hormones estrogen and progesterone, the production of testosterone is controlled by the gonadotropins, follicle-stimulating hormone (FSH), and the interstitial cell-stimulating hormone (ICSH), both of which are produced by the anterior pituitary.

At puberty, these gonadotropins initiate the production of testosterone, which in turn stimulates the development of primary sex organs and secondary sexual characteristics. Testosterone also stimulates bone and skeletal muscle growth, increases the retention of dietary protein nitrogen (anabolism), and slows down the breakdown of body tissues (catabolism). Androgens promote retention of sodium, potassium, nitrogen, and phosphorus and the excretion of calcium. Toward the end of puberty, testosterone hastens the conversion of cartilage into bone, thus terminating linear growth.

Treatment with testosterone and its congeners is complicated by the fact that the external supply of the hormone may depress secretion of the natural hormone through inhibitory effects on the pituitary. Too large a dose may cause permanent damage. Treatment is usually associated with a feeling of well being. In addition to testosterone and its various esters, several synthetic variants are available commercially.

Uses *Replacement therapy* when deficient endocrine function of the testes is present. Continued deficiency results in eunuchoidism. Such deficiency may become apparent when a body fails to mature sexually or later in life. Larger doses are required during puberty.

Sometimes treatment with testosterone is preceded by treatment with human chorionic gonadotropin (HCG) or ICSH. These pituitary

623

hormones may stimulate the testes to increase their production of testosterone.

Male climacteric, caused by the tapering off of natural hormone production. Therapeutic benefits in these patients are uncertain.

Cryptorchidism or undescended testes. *Oligospermia* or lack of viable motile sperm. *Menstrual disorders, premenstrual tension* often in combination with estrogens. *Antineoplastic,* carcinoma of the breast in females. *Osteoporosis,* senile, disuse. *Blood dyscrasias,* aplastic anemia, red cell aplasia, hemolytic anemias, myeloid metaplasia, lymphoma, leukemia, (androgens cause erythropoiesis). *Anabolism,* androgens that have been modified to minimize their sexual effects are usually used for this purpose. They are used as adjuncts in patients receiving corticosteroid therapy, to prevent osteoporosis, in patients convalescing from a wasting disease such as anemia, TB, or cancer to try and prevent loss of tissue and muscle, in severe disease states by promoting a positive nitrogen balance. Very rarely used for children with retarded growth (childhood dwarfism due to hypopituitarism mainly in males).

Contraindications   Prostatic or breast (males) carcinoma. Pregnancy (masculinization of female fetus). Use with caution in young boys who have not completed their growth (because of premature epiphyseal closure) or in patients with cardiac, renal or hepatic disorders (because of edema caused by androgen administration). Discontinue if hypercalcemia occurs.

Untoward Effects   Edema; retention of sodium, potassium, nitrogen, and phosphorus; cholestatic hepatitis (jaundice). (This condition is least pronounced with testosterone and its esters.) Creatinuria, steroid fever, gastrointestinal upsets, acne, priapism. In elderly males with Leydig cell failure, prostatic enlargement occurs.

In women: masculinization, acne, facial hair; voice becomes hoarse and deepens; increased libido. Symptoms subside with continued treatment. Hypercalcemia in patients with disseminated breast carcinoma. Baldness, excessive body hair, prominent musculature and veins, hypertrophy of the clitoris, menstrual cycle irregularity.

In children: serious disturbances of growth, bone (premature closure of the epiphyses), and precocious sexual development are possible.

Stomatitis, after buccal or sublingual administration.

Remarks: Diuretics are often used to control edema. Periodic tests for calcium, liver function, and cardiac function are indicated.

Drug Interactions

Interactant	Interaction
Anticoagulants, oral	Anabolic steroids ↑ effect of anticoagulants
Antidiabetic agents	Additive hypoglycemia
Barbiturates	↓ Effect of androgens due to ↑ breakdown by liver
Corticosteroids	↑ Chance of edema
Oxyphenbutazone (Tandearil)	Certain androgens ↑ effect of oxyphenbutazone
Phenylbutazone (Butazolidin)	Certain androgens ↑ effect of phenylbutazone

Laboratory Test Interference   Alter thyroid function tests. False + or ↑ BSP, alkaline phosphatase, bilirubin, cholesterol, and acid phosphatase (in women). Alteration of glucose tolerance tests.

Dosage   Androgens are given **PO, deep IM,** and by the **buccal** and **sublingual** route. See Table 29, page 626, for individual compounds.

Nursing Implications

1. Observe the patient closely for progression of disease during initial 6 to 8 weeks of therapy because this will necessitate withdrawal of drug.
2. Anticipate that the patient will be on the drug for at least 8 to 12 weeks before any conclusion can be drawn about its effectiveness. Be responsive to the patient's needs for emotional support during this trial period.
3. Provide a diet high in calories, proteins, vitamins, minerals, and other nutrients unless contraindicated.
4. Reassure female patients that growth of facial hair and development of acne are reversible once the drug is withdrawn.
5. Be alert to and report onset of permanent signs of virilization, such as deepening of the voice and clitoral enlargement.
6. Alert the physician to reports by female patients of increased libido. Such manifestations may require explanation and emotional support. Increased libido may be an early sign of serious toxicity.
7. Explain to patient that medication may cause menstrual cycle irregularities in premenopausal women and withdrawal bleeding in postmenopausal women.
8. Report priapism in male patients because this necessitates at least temporary withdrawal of drug.
9. Observe children closely for signs of premature puberty.
10. Observe for edema; weigh the patient at least 2 times/week. Check input and output.
11. Observe sclera, mucous membranes, and skin for signs of jaundice. Observe for pruritis which may occur before jaundice is noted.
12. Attempt to ascertain whether GI upset is due to medication.
13. In patients with high calcium levels the drug will have to be withdrawn and fluids administered to prevent renal calculi.

DANAZOL DANOCRINE

Classification   Androgen, synthetic.

General Statement   Danazol is a synthetic androgen that inhibits the release of the gonadotropins (follicle stimulating and luteinizing hormones) by the pituitary gland. In women, this arrests ovarian function, induces amenorrhea, and causes atrophy of normal and ectopic endometrial tissue. Ovulation and menstruation usually resume 60 to 90 days after drug is discontinued.

TABLE 29 ANDROGENS AND ANABOLIC AGENTS

Drug	Uses	Dosage	Remarks
Dromostanolone propionate (Drolban)	Antineoplastic; inoperable metastatic cancer of breast in women	**IM:** 100 mg 3 times weekly.	Observe for hypercalcemia. The regression produced by drug usually only lasts one year.
Ethylestrenol (Maxibolin)	Anabolic agent: to offset catabolic effects of corticosteroids and in certain forms of cancer, prolonged immobilization, retarded growth, osteoporosis, anemias	**PO, initial, adults:** 4–8 mg daily; **usual,** 4 mg daily. **Children under 12 years:** 1–3 mg daily.	Do not exceed 6 weeks therapy. Reinstitute if necessary after 4-week rest period. Fewer androgenic effects than methyltestosterone. However, these may be particularly marked in children. Drug may affect liver function; hence periodic liver function tests are indicated.
Fluoxymesterone (Halostestin, Ora-Testryl)	Androgen deficiency states in males (when hypogonadism starts in adult life); metastatic breast carcinoma in women; menopausal symptoms	*Hypogonadism, testicular hypofunction,* **PO:** 2–10 mg daily. *Inoperable mammary cancer:* 15–30 mg daily in divided doses. Give in 6-week courses interrupted by 3-week rest period. *Postpartum breast engorgement:* 2.5 mg at time of labor, 5–10 mg daily for 4 to 5 days.	Drug does not result in full sexual maturation in patients with prepuberal testicular function. Five times more potent than long-acting esters of testosterone or testosterone pellets when used as replacement therapy in males and androgen deficiency. GI disturbances more frequent than with other androgens.
Methandriol (Anabol, Andriol, Arbolic, Methabolic, Methydiol, Probolik, Steribolic)	Osteoporosis	**IM only:** 10–40 mg/day or 50–100 mg 1 to 2 times/week. **Pediatric:** 5–10 mg/day or less.	Observe children for evidence of androgenic effect of drug (which precludes increase in dosage) and report to medical supervisor.

626

| Methandrostenolone (Dianabol) | Anabolic effects: adjunct in chronic infections, corticosteroid therapy, negative nitrogen balance, osteoporosis | **PO: initial,** 5 mg daily. **Maintenance:** 2.5–5 mg. daily. **Intermittent therapy:** (6 weeks on, 3 weeks off) indicated for prolonged treatment. *Severe debilitation:* 10–20 mg daily for 3 weeks. | Low estrogenic, progestational, or corticoid effects. Patients with a history of hepatic dysfunction should have periodic liver function tests.

Additional Drug Interactions
Anticoagulants, oxyphenbutazone and phenylbutazone are potentiated by methandrostenolone. |
| Methyltestosterone (Android, Metandren, Oreton Methyl, Testred, Virilon) | Androgen deficiency states | *Androgen deficiency,* **PO:** 10–40 mg daily in divided doses. *Anabolic:* 10–20 mg daily. *Breast cancer in women:* 200 mg daily. *Postpartum breast engorgement:* 80 mg daily. **Sublingual or buccal:** ½ oral (tablet/capsule) dose. | Observe for jaundice. Less effective than long-acting esters of testosterone or of testosterone pellets. Ineffective in producing full sexual maturation in patients with prepuberal testicular failure; effective when hypogonadism begins in adult life.

Administration
1. Place linguet under the tongue or lower buccal pouch between gum and cheek
2. Eating, drinking, chewing or smoking must be avoided while linguet is in place because it may cause accidental swallowing, detrimental to absorption of hormone
3. Oral hygiene measures are suggested after absorption of linguet is completed

(Continued) |

TABLE 29   ANDROGENS AND ANABOLIC AGENTS (*Continued*)

Drug	Uses	Dosage	Remarks
Nandrolone decanoate (Anabolin LA, Androlone-D, Deca-Durabolin, Nandrolate)	Osteoporosis, anemias, debilitated states, metastatic breast cancer	**IM:** 50– 100 mg once a month for 4 months. **Children 2 to 13 years:** 25– 50 mg q 3 to 4 weeks.	A rest period of 6 to 8 weeks is suggested after 4 month course of therapy.
Nandrolone phenpropionate (Androlone, Anabolin I.M., Durabolin, Nandrolin, Spenbolic Improved)	Anabolic agent: growth retardation, osteoporosis, in corticosteroid therapy, inoperable mammary cancer in females	**IM, adults: initial,** 25– 50 mg 1 time/week, **then** 25 mg q 2 to 4 weeks. **Children 2 to 13 years:** 12.5– 25 mg q 2 to 4 weeks.	Children under 7 yr are particularly sensitive to the drug. Observe 1-month rest period after 3-month course of therapy.
Oxandrolone (Anavar)	Anabolic agent: reverses negative nitrogen balance, excess calcium and nitrogen excretion. Osteoporosis, and muscle wasting and tissue depletion. Suitable for patients recovering from surgery, infections, burns, severe traumatic injuries	**PO, adults:** 2.5 mg b.i.d. to q.i.d., **range:** 2.5– 20 mg daily. **Children under 12 years:** 0.25 mg/kg daily	Drug has low androgenic properties. Children may be particularly sensitive to the androgenic effects of oxandrolone. Therapy usually continued 2 to 4 weeks. Do not exceed 3 months.
Oxymetholone (Adroyd, Anadrol)	Same as oxandrolone	**PO,** *osteoporosis,* **adults only:** 2.5 mg t.i.d. up to 30 mg/day. *Anemias,* **adults or children:** 1– 5 mg/kg/day.	Do not exceed 30-day course in children or 90-days in any patient without a rest period.

Drug	Uses	Dosage	Remarks
Stanozolol (Winstrol)	Anabolic agent: preparation for elective surgery; postoperatively, in cancer patients, osteoporosis, burns, decubitus ulcers, and in conditions marked by negative nitrogen balance, muscle wasting and tissue depletion	**PO, adults:** 2 mg t.i.d. before or with meals or 2 mg daily in young women; **children up to 6 years:** 1 mg b.i.d.; **6–12 years:** up to 2 mg t.i.d.	May cause premature epiphyseal closure in children. Patients should be placed on high protein, high calorie diet. Periodic liver function studies required.
Testosterone (Andronaq, Android-T, Histerone, Malogen, Maltrone Aqueous, Oreton, Testaqua, Testoject) Testosterone Cypionate (Andro-Cyp, Depo-Testosterone, Depotest, Duratest, Jectatest-L.A., Malogen Cyp, Testoject) Testosterone Enanthate (Android-T, Andryl, Anthatest, Arderone, Delatestryl, Everone, Malogen L.A., Span-Test, Testate, Testo L.A., Testone L.A., Testostroval-P.A.) Testosterone Propionate (Malotrone-P)	Male sex hormone deficiency states, eunuchoidism, castration. Females: selected menstrual disorders, lactation suppression, advanced mammary cancer. Aplastic anemia, hypoplastic anemias	*Testosterone and testosterone propionate,* **IM only.** *Replacement therapy:* 10–25 mg 2 to 5 times/week; *postpartum breast engorgement:* 25–50 mg daily for 3 to 4 days; *breast cancer:* 100 mg 3 times/week. *Testosterone enanthate and cypionate,* **IM only.** *Replacement therapy:* 200–400 mg q 4 weeks; *oligospermia,* 100–200 mg q 4 to 6 weeks. **Pellets:** 2–67.5 mg pellets **SC** (lasts 3 to 5 months).	Natural hormone. Continue therapy for at least 2 months for satisfactory response and 5 months for objective response. Observe for priapism, virilization, hypercalcemia. Testosterone propionate is more effective than testosterone for parenteral injection because it is released more slowly. Priapism (persistent erection) may be a sign of overdosage. Drug is available in buccal tablets, as pellets for implantation and for intramuscular and subcutaneous injection. Action is short with intramuscular injection and very long when pellets are implanted subcutaneously. *Additional Drug Interactions* Chlorcyclizine and phenylbutazone inhibit testosterone.

629

Uses   Endometriosis amenable to hormonal management in patients who cannot tolerate other drug therapy or who have not responded to other drug therapy.

Contraindications   Undiagnosed genital bleeding, markedly impaired hepatic, renal and cardiac function, pregnancy and lactation.

Untoward Reactions   Weak symptoms of masculinization, such as mild hirsutism, decreased breast size, deepening of voice, oiliness of skin. Also acne, edema, weight gain, flushing, sweating, vaginitis, nervousness and emotional instability.

Dosage   **PO:** 400 mg b.i.d. for a period of 3 to 9 months. Begin therapy during menses, if possible.

Nursing Implications
1. Assure patient that hypoestrogenic side-effects usually disappear after drugs are discontinued.
2. Assess closely for signs of virilization, such as hirsutism, reduced breast size, deepening of voice, acne, increased oiliness of skin, weight gain, edema, and clitoral enlargement because some androgenic side effects may not be reversible and may necessitate change in dosage or discontinuation of drug.
3. Inform patient that ovulation will resume 60 to 90 days after drug is discontinued.
4. Observe patients with epilepsy, migraine, cardiac or renal dysfunction for edema because drug may cause fluid retention.

DIURETICS

Thiazides and Related Diuretics	Bendroflumethiazide	Hydroflumethiazide
	Benzthiazide	Methylchlothiazide
	Chlorothiazide	Metolazone
	Chlorothiazide Sodium	Polythiazide
	Chlorthalidone	Quinethazone
	Cyclothiazide	Trichlormethiazide
	Hydrochlorothiazide	
Carbonic Anhydrase Inhibitor Diuretics	Acetazolamide	Ethoxzolamide
	Acetazolamide Sodium	Methazolamide
	Dichlorphenamide	
Mercurial Diuretics	Mercaptomerin Sodium	Mersalyl with Theophylline
	Merethoxylline Procaine	
Osmotic Diuretics	Mannitol	
	Urea	
Xanthine	Theobromine Magnesium Oleate	
Miscellaneous Agents	Ethacrynate Sodium	Spironolactone
	Ethacrynic Acid	Triamterene
	Furosemide	

General Statement

The purpose of the diuretic drugs is to increase the urinary output of water and sodium. This corrects or prevents the retention of excessive fluid by various tissues (edema), which may be an important manifestation of many conditions (e.g., congestive heart failure, pregnancy, premenstrual tension).

The kidney is a complex organ with three main functions:
1. Elimination of waste materials and return of useful metabolites to the blood.
2. Maintenance of the acid-base balance.
3. Maintenance of an adequate electrolyte balance, which in turn governs the amount of fluid retained in the body.

Diuretic drugs can affect one or several of the processes involved in urine flow. The most important effects are:
1. Increase of the glomerular filtration rate.
2. Decrease the rate at which sodium is reabsorbed from the glomerular filtrate by the renal tubules.
3. Promotion of the excretion of sodium by the kidney.

Some of the commonly used diuretics, especially the thiazides, also have an antihypertensive effect.

Diuretic drugs can enhance the normal function of the kidney but cannot stimulate a failing kidney into action. According to their mode of action and chemical structure, the diuretics fall into the following classes: the thiazides (benzothiadiazides); the carbonic anhydrase inhibitors; the organic mercurial diuretics; osmotic diuretics; xanthine drugs; furosemide and ethacrynic acid; and potassium-sparing drugs.

Uses Edema, congestive heart failure, hypertension, pregnancy, and premenstrual tension.

Nursing Implications

1. Administer in the morning if drug is to be given daily so that the patient will have major diuretic effect before bedtime.
2. Explain to the patient that the drug may cause frequent urination in large amounts so that the patient may plan activities and not be alarmed by diuresis.
3. Have bedpan or commode readily available to assist the patient. Patients who are usually ambulatory may feel weak because of diuresis and may require bedpans. Use safety measures for patients affected by ataxia, confusion, or disorientation. Support ambulatory ataxic patients.
4. Weigh patient each morning under standard conditions, that is, after patient has voided and before patient has eaten or drunk fluids.
5. Maintain careful intake and output record of fluids. Report absence of or decrease in diuresis.
6. Examine the patient for edema: ambulatory patients may have edema of the lower extremities, whereas patients on bedrest are more likely to have edema of the sacral area. The abdomen may be measured with tape to evaluate ascites.
7. *Observe patients for signs of electrolyte imbalance:*
    a. *Hyponatremia* (low-salt syndrome)—characterized by muscle weakness, leg cramps, dryness of mouth, dizziness and GI disturbances.
    b. *Hypernatremia* (excessive sodium retention in relation to body water) characterized by CNS disturbances, such as confusion, loss of sensorium, stupor, and coma. Poor skin turgor or postural hypotention are not as prominent as when there are combined deficits of sodium and water.
    c. *Water intoxication* (caused by defective water diuresis)—characterized by lethargy, confusion, stupor and coma. Neuromuscular hyperexciteability with increased reflexes, muscular twitching, and convulsions may occur if water intoxication is acute.
    d. *Metabolic acidosis* —characterized by weakness, headache, malaise, abdominal pain, nausea, and vomiting. Hyperpnea occurs in severe metabolic acidosis. Signs of volume depletion, such as poor skin turgor, soft eyeballs, and a dry tongue, may be observed.
    e. *Metabolic alkalosis* —characterized by irritability, neuromuscular hyperexcitability and in severe cases, tetany.
    f. *Hypokalemia* (deficiency of potassium in blood)—characterized

by muscular weakness, failure of peristalsis, postural hypotension, respiratory embarrassment, and cardiac arrhythmias.

    g. *Hyperkalemia* (excess of potassium in blood)—characterized by early signs of irritability, nausea, intestinal colic and diarrhea; by later signs of weakness, flaccid paralysis, dyspnea, difficulty in speaking, and arrhythmias.

        Signs of electrolyte imbalance should be reported to the physician and physical safety for the patient should be provided.

8. Encourage patients for whom additional potassium intake is desirable to ingest foods high in potassium since this is preferable to potassium chloride tablets. Foods high in potassium are citrus, grape, cranberry, apple, pear, and apricot juices, bananas, meat, fish, fowl, cereals, and tea and cola beverages. Patients receiving diuretics and requiring potassium supplementation are encouraged to drink a large glass of orange juice daily unless it is contraindicated because of another preexisting condition such as diabetes or gastric ulcer.

9. Dilute liquid potassium preparations with fruit juice or milk to make them more palatable because they are bitter.

10. Observe patients on enteric-coated potassium tablets for abdominal pain, distention, or GI bleeding because such tablets can cause small bowel ulceration. Discontinue tablets if such symptoms appear.

11. Observe patients also receiving antihypertensive drugs for excessively low blood pressure, as diuretics potentiate antihypertensive agents. Caution patients to rise slowly from bed and to sit down or lie down should they feel dizzy or faint.

12. Check urine of diabetic patients and observe patients for signs of hyperglycemia since diuretics may precipitate symptoms of diabetes in latent or mild diabetic patients.

13. Check apical pulses of patients also receiving digitalis, as hyper- or hypokalemia associated with diuretic therapy may potentiate toxic effects of digitalis and precipitate cardiac arrhythmias.

14. Be alert to symptoms of sore throat, skin rash, or jaundice which are signs of blood dyscrasias due to drug hypersensitivity.

15. Extra cautious observation is advised for patients with a history of liver disease since electrolyte imbalance may cause stupor, coma, and death.

16. Note increased frequency of acute attacks of gout (pain in single joint) precipitated by diuretics in patients with history of the disease.

THIAZIDES AND RELATED DIURETICS

General Statement   The thiazides and related diuretics promote diuresis by decreasing the rate at which sodium and chloride are reabsorbed by the distal renal tubules of the kidney. By increasing the excretion of sodium and chloride, they force excretion of additional water. They also increase the excretion of potassium and, to a lesser extent, bicarbonate.

Sodium and chloride are excreted in approximately equal amounts.

The thiazides do not affect the glomerular filtration rate. Chemically, they are related to the sulfonamides. They do not have any antibiotic effects but may cause the same hypersensitivity reactions as the sulfonamides.

They also have an antihypertensive effect; the exact mechanism is unknown. This antihypertensive effect usually takes several days to become apparent.

The drugs potentiate several antihypertensive agents, especially the rauwolfia and veratrum alkaloids (see chapter 4, section 4).

The thiazides can be used for patients with some degree of kidney impairment. However, they must be used with caution because they can aggravate renal insufficiency.

To prevent low-salt syndrome, salt is usually not restricted for patients receiving thiazides.

The thiazides are powerful drugs and the nurse must be constantly on the lookout for the development of electrolyte imbalance, especially hypokalemia. Hypokalemia can cause cardiac arrhythmias as well as make the heart more sensitive to the toxic effects of digitalis.

The diuretic effects of most thiazides usually occur in approximately 2 hours. Peak excretion rates are attained after 4 to 6 hours. Total duration of action varies between 6 to 24 hours. Details are given in Table 30.

Patients resistant to one type of thiazide may respond to another.

Additional Uses Initiation and maintenance therapy of congestive heart failure; edematous renal conditions (nephrosis, nephritis); edema of pregnancy; premenstrual syndrome; adjunct in corticosteroid and other drug therapy that induces electrolyte and fluid retention; cirrhotic patients. The thiazides and related diuretics will not be active in cases of severe renal disease where glomerular filtration rate is severely reduced. Hypertension.

Contraindications Hypersensitivity to drug. Impaired renal function and advanced hepatic cirrhosis. Administer with caution to debilitated or elderly patients, or to those with a history of hepatic coma, or precoma, gout, diabetes mellitus, during pregnancy and lactation.

Drugs should not be used indiscriminately in patients with edema and toxemia of pregnancy even though they may be therapeutically useful because the thiazides may have adverse effects on newborn (thrombocytopenia and jaundice).

Thiazides and related diuretics may precipitate myocardial infarctions in elderly patients with advanced arteriosclerosis, especially if patient is also receiving therapy with other antihypertensive agents.

Patients with advanced heart failure, renal disease, or hepatic cirrhosis are most likely to develop hypokalemia.

Particular care must be exercised when thiazides are administered concomitantly with drugs that also cause potassium loss, such as digitalis, corticosteroids, and some estrogens.

TABLE 30 THIAZIDES AND RELATED DIURETICS

Drug	Dosage	Remarks
Bendroflumethiazide (Naturetin)	*Edema, hypertension,* **PO: initial,** 5 mg daily in AM, may be increased to 20 mg daily. **Maintenance:** 2.5–15 mg daily. **Pediatric, initial,** 0.1 mg/kg daily in 1 or 2 doses. **Maintenance:** 0.05–0.3 mg/kg daily in 1 or 2 doses.	Action lasts for about 24 hr. If administered every other day or 3–5 days/week, relatively low likelihood of causing electrolyte imbalance. When daily dose exceeds 20 mg, divided doses are recommended.
Benzthiazide (Aquapres, Aquascrip, Aquastat, Aquatag, Exna, Hydrex, Marazide, Proaqua, Urazide)	*Edema,* **PO: initial:** 50–200 mg daily. **Maintenance:** 50–150 mg daily. Divide dose when daily dose exceeds 100 mg. **Pediatric, all uses:** 1–4 mg/kg daily in 3 doses. *Hypertension:* **initial:** 50–200 mg; **maintenance:** according to patient response, up to 50 mg q.i.d.	Action begins within 2 hr; lasts 12–18 hr; peaks 4–6 hr.
Chlorothiazide (Diuril, Ro-Chlorozide) Chlorothiazide sodium (Diuril Sodium)	*Edema,* **PO:** 0.5–1 gm 1–2 times daily. **IV:** direct dissolve 500 mg in 18 ml isotonic solution b.i.d. Avoid extravasation of liquid into **SC** tissue. May be given **IV** in dextrose or NaCl solutions. *Hypertensive dose,* **PO only:** 250 mg b.i.d.– 500 mg t.i.d. **Pediatric:** 20 mg/kg daily in divided doses; infants under 6 months of age may require 30 mg/kg in 2 divided doses.	
Chlorthalidone (Hygroton)	*Edema,* **PO: initial,** 50–100 mg daily or 100 mg 3 times/week. **Maximum daily dose:** 200 mg. **Pediatric:** all uses, 2 mg/kg 3 times weekly. *Hypertension:* 25–50 mg as single daily dose up to 100 mg/day.	Give in AM with food. Has a more prolonged action than most thiazides (up to 72 hr). Particularly good for potentiating action and reducing dosage of other hypotensive agents.

(Continued)

TABLE 30   THIAZIDES AND RELATED DIURETICS (*Continued*)

Drug	Dosage	Remarks
Cyclothiazide (Anhydron)	*Edema,* **PO: initial,** 1–2 mg daily. **Maintenance:** 1–2 mg every 2 or 3 days. *Hypertension:* 2 mg 1–3 times/day. **Pediatric, all uses:** 0.02–0.04 mg/kg daily. **Maximum effective dose:** 8 mg. Divide dose if daily dosage exceeds 8 mg.	Prolonged duration of action (24 hr). Give in AM.
Hydrochlorothiazide (Chlorzide, Delco-Retic, Diaqua, Diucen-H, Diu-Scrip, Esidrex, Hydro-Chlor, Hydro-Diuril, Hydromal, Hydro-Z-25 & -50, Jen-Diril, Lexor, Loqua, Oretic, Tri-Zide, X-Aqua, Zide)	*Edema,* **PO:** 25–100 mg 1 to 2 times/day. 75–100 mg b.i.d. for severe edema. *Hypertension:* 50–100 mg once daily. **Pediatric:** 2–3 mg/kg daily divided into 2 doses.	Onset of action 2 hr; duration, 6–12 hr. Maximum at 4 hr. Divide daily dose larger than 100 mg. Give b.i.d. at 6–12 hr intervals.
Hydroflumethiazide (Diucardin, Saluron)	*Edema, hypertension,* **PO:** 50–200 mg daily. Single dose not to exceed 100 mg and daily dose not to exceed 200 mg. **Pediatric: all uses:** 1 mg/kg once daily.	Long-acting thiazide (18 to 24 hr).
Methylchlothiazide (Aquatensin, Enduron)	*Edema, hypertension,* **PO:** 2.5–10 mg daily initially. **Maintenance:** 2.5–5 mg once daily. **Pediatric, all uses:** 0.05–0.2 mg/kg daily.	Action may still be evident 24 hr after administration.
Metolazone (Diulo, Zaroxyolyn)	*Edema,* **PO:** 5–20 mg once daily. *Hypertension:* 2.5–5 mg once daily. Reduce all doses if possible when patient has stabilized.	Long-acting thiazide. Drug does not affect glomerular filtration rate. *Additional Contraindications* Pre-hepatic and hepatic coma. Do not use for children. *Additional Untoward Reactions* Bloating, palpitations, chest pain, chills.

TABLE 30   THIAZIDES AND RELATED DIURETICS (*Continued*)

Drug	Dosage	Remarks
Polythiazide (Renese)	*Edema, hypertension*, **PO:** 1–4 mg daily. Initial doses up to 12 mg daily in divided doses may be required. **Pediatric, all uses:** 0.02–0.08 mg/kg daily.	Very long acting (36 hr).
Quinethazone (Hydromox)	**PO:** 50–100 mg or more daily. For maintenance, adjust according to response	Sulfonamide that has same activity and side effects as thiazides. Long-acting. In addition to hypertension and renal insufficiency, used for edema associated with premenstrual tension and menopausal syndrome. May precipitate attacks of gout.
Trichlormethiazide (Aquazide, Aquex, Diurese, Kirkrinal, Metahydrin, Naqua, Spenzide)	*Edema;* **PO:** 1–4 mg daily, up to 16 mg may be required. *Hypertension:* 2–4 mg daily initial dose. **Maintenance:** 2–4 mg daily. **Pediatric, all uses:** 0.07 mg/kg daily.	Action prolonged for 24 hr or longer.

Untoward Reactions   Electrolyte imbalance: *hypokalemia* (most frequent) characterized by cardiac arrhythmias.

Hypokalemic alkalosis; hyponatremia (low-salt syndrome), characterized by weakness, lethargy, epigastric distress, nausea and vomiting. Hyperglycemia and aggravation of preexisting diabetes mellitus. Hyperuricemia which results in gout in susceptible individuals, renal colic, hematuria, crystalluria, increased blood ammonia. Hypotensive episodes during surgery. Blood dyscrasias. Allergic reactions. Hypersensitivity, photosensitivity, skin rash, necrotizing vasculitis of skin and kidney, allergic purpura. Also pancreatitis, jaundice and hepatic coma. Ulceration of small intestine if given with enteric coated potassium supplement.

Drug Interactions

Interactant	Interaction
Amphetamine	↑ Effect of amphetamine due to ↑ renal tubular reabsorption
Anticoagulants, oral	↓ Effect of anticoagulants by concentrating circulating clotting factors and ↑ clotting factor synthesis in liver

Drug Interactions (Continued)

Interactant	Interaction
Antidiabetic agents	Thiazides antagonize hypoglycemic effect of antidiabetic agents
Cholestyramine (Cuemid, Questran)	↓ Effect of thiazide due to ↓ absorption from GI tract
Corticosteroids	Enhanced K loss due to K-losing properties of both drugs
Diazoxide (Hyperstat)	Enhanced hypotensive effect. Also, ↑ hyperglycemic response
Digitalis glycosides	Thiazides produce ↑ K and Mg loss with ↑ chance of digitalis toxicity
Gallamine	↑ Muscle relaxation
Guanethidine (Ismelin)	Additive hypotensive effect
Lithium	Increased risk of lithium toxicity
Quinidine	↑ Effect of quinidine due to ↑ renal tubular reabsorption
Reserpine	Additive hypotensive effect
Tubocurarine	↑ Muscle relaxation
Vasopressors (sympathomimetics)	Thiazides ↓ responsiveness of arterioles to vasopressors

Laboratory Test Interference

Alter liver function tests, and electrolyte balance. False + or ↑ serum glucose (fasting), amylase.

Dosage

See Table 30. Drugs are preferentially given **PO,** but some preparations can be given parenterally. They are usually given in the morning so that peak effect occurs during the day.

Additional Nursing Implications

1. Anticipate that thiazide will be stopped at least 48 hours prior to surgery, because drug inhibits pressor effect of epinephrine.
2. Caution the patient not to ingest alcohol, since this causes severe hypotension with thiazides.
3. Warn the patient not to eat licorice when on thiazide therapy, because severe hypokalemia and paralysis may be precipitated.
4. Evaluate dietary potassium intake since potassium chloride supplement should only be given when dietary measures are inadequate. Liquid potassium preparations should be used since these do not produce ulcerations.

CARBONIC ANHYDRASE INHIBITOR DIURETICS

General Statement

This group of diuretics inhibits the enzyme carbonic anhydrase. The drugs promote the excretion of bicarbonate and sodium, which necessitates the extraction of additional fluid. There is also an increase in potassium excretion. The usefulness of the drugs is limited because they promote metabolic acidosis, which then inhibits their diuretic action. This difficulty is partially circumvented by giving the drugs on alternate days or alternating them with other diuretics, especially the mercurial diuretics. The latter tend to become less active because of their self-induced alkalosis. The carbonic anhydrase inhibitors are sulfonamides devoid of antibacterial activity. The carbonic anhydrase diuretics are, however, particularly useful in the treatment of glaucoma (reduction of intraocular pressure). The drugs have some antiepileptic activity.

Patients may respond to one carbonic anhydrase inhibitor and not to another. Failures in therapy may result from overdosage or too frequent use.

The drugs are mild, safe diuretics, not usually prescribed for the removal of large amounts of edema charcteristic of congestive heart failure. Carbonic anhydrase inhibitor diuretics may, however, play a role in maintenance programs and in milder forms of edema, associated with administration of corticosteroids or premenstrually. (For individual agents and dosages, see Table 31, p. 640.)

Additional Uses Edema due to chronic heart failure. More useful as adjunct to mercurial diuretics (potentiation or restoration of their effects) than when used alone. Decrease of intraocular pressure in glaucoma. Treatment of hyperkalemia due to incompatible blood transfusions, mild toxemia and edema of pregnancy, drug-induced edema, selected cases of emphysema and epilepsy, and edema of obesity.

Contraindications Idiopathic renal hyperchloremic acidosis, renal failure, hepatic insufficiency, and conditions associated with depressed sodium and potassium levels, such as Addison's disease and all other types of adrenal failure. Use with caution in the presence of mild acidosis, hepatic cirrhosis, advanced pulmonary disease, and pregnancy.

Untoward Reactions *Electrolyte imbalance:* Metabolic acidosis characterized by nausea, dizziness, numbness of fingers, toes, and lips, fatigue, drowsiness, headache, dry mouth, irritability, diarrhea, tinnitus, disorientation, dysuria, ataxia, and weight loss. *Hypersensitivity:* Like other sulfonamides, drug can cause blood dyscrasias, skin rashes, and fever. Also crystalluria and renal calculi.

Untoward reactions may be dose related and often are relieved by decrease in dosage. Alternate day therapy or rest periods allow kidney to recover.

Drug Interactions

Interactant	Interaction
Amphetamine	↑ Effect of amphetamine by ↑ renal tubular reabsorption
Antidepressants, tricyclic	↑ Effect of tricyclics by ↑ renal tubular reabsorption
Antidiabetic agents	Acetazolamide ↑ blood sugar in prediabetics and diabetics on oral hypoglycemics
Erythromycin	↑ Effect of erythromycin by ↑ renal tubular reabsorption
Lithium carbonate	↓ Effect of lithium by ↑ renal excretion

TABLE 31   CARBONIC ANHYDRASE INHIBITORS

Drug	Uses	Dosage	Remarks
Acetazolamide (Diamox, Rozolamide) Acetazolamide sodium (Diamox Parenteral)	Edema, epilepsy, mild toxemia of pregnancy, glaucoma, emphysema	*Edema*, **PO, IV, IM:** 250–375 mg daily or q other day in the AM. *Glaucoma:* 250 mg q 6 hr (range is 125 mg q 12 hr to 500 mg q 4 hr). **IV** route is preferred to **IM** because of alkalinity of solution.	1. Tolerance after prolonged administration may necessitate an increase in dosage. 2. Solutions diluted for IV injection can be stored at room temperature for 2 weeks, and in refrigerator for 4 weeks.
Dichlorphenamide (Daranid, Oratrol)	Glaucoma	**PO, priming dose, adults:** 100–200 mg followed by 100 mg q 12 hr until desired response manifested. **Maintenance, adults:** 25–50 mg 1 to 3 times/day.	Action noted in 1 hr. reaches a maximum in 2–4 and persists 6 hr.
Ethoxzolamide (Cardrase, Ethamide)	Edema, glaucoma, epilepsy, complications associated with blood transfusions (excess potassium)	*Edema*, **PO:** 62.5–125 mg in AM after breakfast either for 3 consecutive days or on alternate days. *Glaucoma:* 62.5–250 mg b.i.d.-q.i.d. *Epilepsy*, **maximum:** 750 mg daily with or without other anticonvulsant drugs.	1. Not suitable to initiate diuresis caused by severe congestive heart failure. 2. Action starts within 2 hr and lasts 8–12 hr.
Methazolamide (Neptazane)	Glaucoma	**PO:** 50–100 mg b.i.d. or t.i.d.	Maximum action 6 to 8 hr and lasts for 10 hr or more

Drug Interactions (Continued)	*Interactant*	*Interaction*
	Methenamine compounds	↓ Effect of methenamine compounds due to ↑ renal excretion
	Nitrofurantoin	↓ Effect of nitrofurantoin due to ↑ renal excretion
	Procainamide	↑ Effect of procainamide by ↑ renal tubular reabsorption
	Quinidine	↑ Effect of quinidine by ↑ renal tubular reabsorption

Administration Because of the self-inhibitory metabolic acidosis, the carbonic anhydrase drugs are usually administered during 3 consecutive days each week or every other day. Since kidney recovery does not play a role, intermittent administration is not necessary when drugs are used for glaucoma or epilepsy.

Additional Nursing Implication Caution the patient to maintain dosage and schedule prescribed by physician to maintain effectiveness of the drug and prevent metabolic acidosis.

Nursing Implications for Treatment of Glaucoma with Carbonic Anhydrase Inhibitors
1. Report if the patient complains of eye pain because drug may not be effective and intraocular pressure may be unrelieved or increasing.
2. Anticipate that carbonic anhydrase inhibitors should be administered at least once daily for treatment of glaucoma or epilepsy whereas in treatment of edema the drug is administered intermittently.

MERCURIAL DIURETICS

General Statement Mercurial diuretics promote diuresis by depressing the reabsorption of sodium and fixed anions in the renal tubules. The drugs may increase the excretion of potassium, although the effect is not as severe as with thiazides. During diuresis the urine contains about equal amounts of sodium and chloride.

Because they promote the excretion of chloride ions, the mercurial diuretics sometimes give rise to hypochloremic alkalosis.

The organic mercurial diuretics are rapidly excreted by the kidney. This minimizes the danger of mercury poisoning.

Diuresis usually sets in 1 to 2 hours after administration and reaches a maximum in 6 to 9 hours. Thus, drugs should be given in the morning. Diuresis is usually complete within 12 to 24 hours.

The response to the drug varies, but the average weight loss is about 2.5% of body weight.

Mercurial diuretics should be discontinued if diuresis is not observed within appropriate time.

Refractoriness to drug action results in the presence of low glomerular filtration rate or hypochloremic alkalosis. The latter might be caused by the mercurial diuretics.

Administration of xanthines may elevate low glomerular filtration rate.

Acidifying salts like ammonium chloride, potentiate the mercurial diuretics in the presence of alkalosis.

Additional Uses Principal: cardiac edema, cardiac asthma, decompensated patients with edematous distention of GI tract. Also chronic nephrosis, nephrotic stages of glomerulonephritis and ascites due to hepatic cirrhosis or portal obstruction.

Contraindications Absolute: hypersensitivity to drug (mercury ion), acute nephritis, ulcerative colitis, and malignant hypertension. Extreme caution must be exercised for other states of renal insufficiency and for patients with cardiac arrhythmias, those on digitalis, and after a recent myocardial infarction. Use extreme caution during pregnancy and lactation. IV administration should be reserved for extreme emergencies.

Untoward Reactions *Immediate fatal reactions* (very rare): precipitous fall in blood pressure, cardiac irregularities, cyanosis, dyspnea, and irregular, gasping respiration.

Immediate nonfatal reactions: flushing, pruritus, urticaria, dermatitis, and rarely, neutropenia, and agranulocytosis.

Systemic mercury poisoning: characterized by cardiac arrhythmias, ashen gray appearance of mouth and pharynx, gastric pain, vomiting, bloody diarrhea, stomatitis, foul breath, soreness of gums, and excessive salivation.

Other Untoward Effects *Electrolyte imbalance:* hypochloremic acidosis, hyponatremia, hypokalemia. Characterized by weakness, somnolence, muscle pain, shock, cardiac dysfunction. Dehydration. Acute urinary retention. Bone marrow depression. *Local reactions:* induration at injection site, thromboembolic disease. Hyperuricemia.

Drug Interactions

Interactant	*Interaction*
Antihypertensives	Additive antihypertensive effect
Corticosteroids	May lead to excessive potassium depletion
Digitalis	Mercurial diuretics potentiate toxic effects of digitalis because of potassium loss. Can lead to severe cardiac arrhythmias
Ethacrynic acid	↑ Effect of mercurial diuretics

Dosage See Table 32, p. 643. A test dose is often administered.

Administration
1. IM administration is preferred.
2. Administer IM deep into the muscle and massage well to minimize local irritation and pain.

3. Prior administration of 4–8 gm of an acid-producing diuretic such as ammonium chloride given in divided doses for 2 to 3 days before mercurial diuretic will potentiate diuresis.

Additional Nursing Implications

1. Anticipate that a sensitivity test dose of mercurial diuretics will be administered 24 hours prior to administration of full dose.
2. Observe urine for albumin, blood cells, and casts, which may indicate renal irritation.
3. Encourage good mouth care to prevent drug-induced stomatitis.
4. Examine rectum of patients receiving mercury suppositories for local irritation.
5. Monitor the patient's pulse after IV injection because ventricular arrhythmias may occur.
6. Be alert to symptoms of systemic mercury poisoning (see untoward reactions) and have dimercaprol available for treatment of toxicity.

TABLE 32 MERCURIAL DIURETICS

Drug	Dosage*	Remarks**
Mercaptomerin sodium (Thiomerin)	**SC** *preferred*, also **IM:** 0.5–2 ml daily (1 ml contains 125 mg). **IM** *preferred* for obese or debilitated patients.	Produces less local irritation than other mercurials (Check urine periodically: albumin, casts, blood). Use with caution in patients susceptible to arrhythmias. Store in refrigerator. Do not use turbid solutions. Inject beneath SC fat.
Merethoxylline procaine (Dicurin Procaine)	**SC or IM:** 0.5–2 ml daily.	Also contains procaine to reduce pain at site of injection. Rarely used. Do not administer to patients on sulfonamide therapy.
Mersalyl with theophylline (Foyuretic, Mercurasol, Mercutheolin, Mer-M, Mernephria, Mersalyn, Salyrgan-Theophyllin, Theo-Syl-R)	**IM, IV:** after *test dose* of 0.5 ml, 1.0 ml given the following day. *Usual dose:* 1–2 ml, 1 to 2 times/week. **Pediatric:** *test dose*, 0.2 ml; **then:** 0.5–1 ml on following day.	Each milliliter contains not less than 39.6% mercury in nonionizable form and 50 mg theophylline. Advisable to administer in the A.M. **Never administer SC.**

* In order to avoid large-scale toxic reactions, mercurial diuretics are initiated with small test dose (0.5 ml or less).
** Systemic acidosis potentiates diuresis. Treatment with mercurial diuretics often preceded by treatment for 2 to 3 days, with acid-producing diuretics (ammonium chloride or lysine hydrochloride).

OSMOTIC DIURETICS

General Statement Osmotic diuretics (mannitol and urea) increase the osmotic pressure of the glomerular filtrate inside the renal tubules. This decreases the amount of fluid and electrolytes that are reabsorbed by the tubules, thereby increasing the loss of fluid, chloride, sodium, and, to a lesser extent, potassium.

Osmotic diuretics retain their effectiveness even when the glomerular filtration rate is actually reduced, such as in hypovolemic shock, trauma, and dehydration. They are also effective when renal circulation is acutely compromised. Other diuretics lose their effectiveness under these circumstances.

The osmotic diuretics can prevent acute renal failure during prolonged surgery or trauma. They are also useful in decreasing abnormally high intracranial, cerebrospinal, and intraocular pressures.

Additional Uses Prevention of acute renal failure during or after extensive surgery. Selected cases of edema. Reduction or prevention of excess intracranial, cerebrospinal, or intraocular pressure during surgery, trauma, or disease. Prevention of renal failure associated with drug (secobarbital, imipramine, aspirin) or carbon tetrachloride intoxication. Acute episodes of glaucoma.

Contraindications Impaired renal or cardiac function, congestive heart failure, active intracranial bleeding, severe dehydration. Mannitol should not be used during pregnancy, in infants, or in children. Urea should not be injected IV into lower extremities of the elderly.

Untoward Reactions Nausea, vomiting, headaches, electrolyte imbalance, water intoxication, pulmonary edema, intraocular hemorrhages.

The transient expansion of blood volume may lead to circulatory overload and the possibility of pulmonary edema or of a cardiac crisis.

Additional Nursing Implications
1. Maintain strict intake and output. Measure output hourly and record.
2. Anticipate insertion of Foley catheter if patient is comatose, incontinent, or unable to void into a receptacle because therapy is based on very strict evaluation of intake and output.
3. Observe particularly for symptoms of water intoxication and for other types of electrolyte imbalance.
4. Observe at site of IV administration for edema due to extravasation into SC tissue and for thrombophlebitis due to local irritation of drug.
5. Monitor vital signs at least hourly while patient is being treated for acute episode.

MANNITOL D-MANNITOL, OSMITROL

Classification Diuretic, osmotic.

Remarks *Mannitol is not used for chronic edema.* A test dose is usually administered. Mannitol is usually discontinued when urine flow is greater than 100 ml/hour.

Untoward Reactions Nasal congestion, thirst, and mild angina-like chest pain. Local edema at injection site.

Drug Interaction May cause deafness when used in combination with kanamycin.

Dosage *Test dose,* **IV:** 200 mg/kg over period of 2 to 5 minutes. If urine flow corresponds to minimum of 40 ml/hr (as measured for 2 to 3 hr), the therapeutic dose can be given.

Individualized. **Always by IV infusion. Usual:** 50–100 gm/24 hrs. **Maximum,** for patients on mannitol, excreting less than 100 ml/hr, is 100 gm/24 hr.

Ophthalmology, neurosurgery (to reduce intraocular pressure): 1.5–2.0 gm/kg, as 20% solution over period of 30 to 60 minutes.

Diuresis during intoxication: 5% to 10% solution infused continuously as long as necessary up to maximum of 200 gm.

Additional Nursing Implications 1. Provide mouth care to relieve thirst and provide fluids if allowed.
2. Report chest pain.

UREA UREAPHIL

Classification Diuretic, osmotic.

Remarks Osmotic diuretic no longer used orally due to unpleasant taste, large doses required, and variable effectiveness by this route. See Abortifacients.

Contraindications See *Osmotic Diuretics,* p. 644.

Untoward Reactions Hypotension, acute psychosis, mental confusion, hyperthermia, nervousness, tachycardia, dehydration, syncope, pain, skin irritation, venous thrombosis, and phlebitis at injection site.

Drug Interactions

Interactant	Interaction
Anticoagulants	↑ Effect of anticoagulants
Lithium carbonate	↓ Lithium effect by ↑ renal excretion

Dosage **Slow IV infusion:** 1 gm/kg over 2 to 2½ hr. **Maximum in 24 hr:** 1.5 gm/kg or 120 gm in 24 hr. **Pediatric:** 0.1–1.5 gm/kg in 24 hr.

Administration Maximum IV administration rate: 4 mg/minute of a 30% solution to prevent increased hemolysis and increased capillary bleeding.

Additional Nursing Implications

1. Do not administer urea into lower extremities of elderly patients because drug has a fibrinolytic effect.
2. Observe patients with congestive heart failure closely, monitoring vital signs since increase in plasma volume by injection of the drug itself may precipitate pulmonary edema.
3. Observe for signs of personality change and report.
4. Provide close supervision and safety measures, such as side rails, because patient may be mentally confused and hypotensive.

XANTHINES

THEOBROMINE MAGNESIUM OLEATE ATHEMOL, ATHEMOL-N

General Statement

The diuretic effect of the xanthines has been known for a long time. Although the exact mechanism of action is not known, it is believed that the compounds increase cardiac function and act directly on the renal tubules, causing an increased excretion of sodium and chloride.

Potassium and urinary pH remain unaffected. Today the drugs are used infrequently.

Theophylline is by far the most potent diuretic of the xanthine group, although the only xanthine currently used is theobromine magnesium oleate.

Uses

Edema associated with congestive heart failure and acute pulmonary edema associated with elevated blood pressure. Arteriosclerosis and resultant peripheral vascular disorders. Xanthines are often used in combination with other diuretics. The drugs are also used in bronchial asthma (p. 484).

Contraindications

Angina pectoris and other conditions in which heart stimulation might be harmful. Peptic ulcer.

Untoward Reactions

GI disturbances (frequent): nausea, vomiting, diarrhea, abdominal cramps, and irritation of the gastric mucosa. CNS manifestations (disappear with usage): headaches, nervousness, insomnia, skin rash, palpitations, dizziness, light-headedness. Tolerance to drugs may develop; for maximum benefit drugs should be alternated with other agents.

Overdosage

Early signs: wakefulness, restlessness, irritability, alternating with drowsiness, tinnitus, extrasystoles, and anorexia. Late signs: fever, delirium, tonic extensor spasms, alternating with clonic convulsions, apathy, stupor, and coma. Increased vomiting. Vomitus may become tinged with blood, syrupy, or have the appearance of coffee grounds because of drug-induced acid stimulation of stomach.

The high acidity of vomitus may cause ulceration, esophageal perforation, and damage of mucosal membranes of lips and mouth. High blood pressure, cerebral edema, cardiovascular and respiratory collapse, shock cyanosis, and death may follow after 18 hours.

Children are especially susceptible to xanthines.

Treatment of Overdosage

Supportive sedatives for control of convulsions, parenteral fluids and electrolytes, and oxygen therapy if indicated.

Drug Interactions

Interactant	Interaction
Acidifying agents	↓ Effect of xanthines by ↑ renal excretion
Alkalinizing agents	↑ Effect of xanthines by ↓ renal excretion
Anticoagulants, oral	↓ Effect of anticoagulants by ↑ plasma pro-thrombin and Factor V
CNS stimulants	Concomitant use may result in excessive CNS stimulation

Dosage   **PO:** 200–400 mg t.i.d. After 6 weeks reduce to 200 mg t.i.d.

Administration   See *Adrenergic Sympathomimetic Agents*, p. 464.

Additional Nursing Implications

1. Report gastritis.
2. Reassure patient that a warm flush and pruritus, which may occur after administration of drug, are transient and harmless.
3. Also see *Adrenergic Sympathomimetic agents.*

MISCELLANEOUS AGENTS

ETHACRYNIC ACID EDECRIN

ETHACRYNATE SODIUM SODIUM EDECRIN

Classification   Diuretic.

General Statement

Ethacrynic acid inhibits the reabsorption of sodium and chloride by the renal tubule (mainly by acting on ascending loop of Henle). Large quantities of sodium and chloride and smaller amounts of potassium and bicarbonate ion are excreted during the diuresis.

The diuretic response to ethacrynic acid is not significantly depressed by changes in acid-base balance of the body as it is with mercurial diuretics. Ethacrynic acid renders the urine more acidic. Diuresis and electrolyte loss are more pronounced with ethacrynic acid than with the thiazide diuretics.

Onset of action is very rapid: 30 minutes after PO; 15 minutes after IV administration. It peaks at 2 hours after PO administration. Total duration: 2 hours after IV, 6 to 8 hours after PO administration.

Ethacrynic acid is often effective in patients refractory to other diuretics. It is preferably administered to hospitalized patients and used intermittently, especially since effectiveness of drug is reduced with continuous administration.

Additional Uses

Of value in patients resistant to less potent diuretics. Congestive heart failure, pulmonary edema, edema associated with nephrotic syndrome, ascites due to idiopathic edema, lymphedema, malignancy. Short-term use in pediatric patients with nephrotic syndrome or congenital heart disease.

Contraindications Anuria and severe renal damage. Patients with history of gout should be watched closely. To be used with caution in diabetic subjects and also in patients with hepatic cirrhosis. The latter are particularly prone to develop electrolyte imbalance.

Untoward Reactions Electrolyte imbalance (hypokalemia). The drug may also cause dehydration, reduction in blood volume, vascular complications, tetany, and metabolic alkalosis.

GI disturbances (frequent): anorexia, nausea, diarrhea, vomiting, acute pancreatitis, jaundice. Severe, watery diarrhea is an indication for permanent discontinuation of drug. GI bleeding, especially in patients on IV therapy or receiving heparin concomitantly.

CNS: tinnitus, hearing loss (permanent), vertigo, headache, blurred vision, apprehension, confusion, fatigue.

Hematologic: agranulocytosis, thrombocytopenia, neutropenia.

Other side effects: skin rashes, abnormal liver function tests in seriously ill patients, fever, chills, hematuria.

Ethacrynic acid increases uric acid levels and may precipitate attacks of gout. The drug may also produce changes in glucose metabolism (hyperglycemia and glycosuria).

Drug Interactions

Interactant	Interaction
Alcohol	↑ Orthostatic hypotension

Aminoglycoside antibiotics
  Gentamicin
  Kanamycin
  Neomycin
  Streptomycin
	Additive ototoxicity and nephrotoxicity

Anticoagulants, oral	↑ Effect of anticoagulants by ↓ plasma protein binding
Antidiabetic agents	Ethacrynic acid antagonizes hypoglycemic effect of antidiabetics
Barbiturates	↑ Orthostatic hypotension
Cephaloridine	↑ Risk of ototoxicity and nephrotoxicity
Corticosteroids	Enhanced K loss due to K-losing properties of both drugs
Digitalis glycosides	Ethacrynic acid produces excess K and Mg loss with ↑ chance of digitalis toxicity
Furosemide (Lasix)	Combination may result in hypokalemia, tachycardia, deafness, hypotension. **Do not use together.**
Lithium	↑ Risk of lithium toxicity due to ↓ renal clearance
Narcotics	↑ Orthostatic hypotension

Dosage   *Ethacrynic acid* is administered **PO;** *sodium ethacrynate* is given **IV.** Because of local pain or irritation, **the drug should not be given SC or IM.** *Individualized* according to response. **Typical PO regime:** *day 1:* 50 mg; *day 2:* 50 mg b.i.d; *day 3:* 100 mg AM, 50–100 mg PM. **Maximum daily dose:** 400 mg. Drug is always given after meals.

     Pediatric: initial, 25 mg given AM. May be increased by 25 mg daily. After desired response, dose may be reduced to minimum maintenance dose.

     IV, adult: initial, 50 mg or 0.5 mg/kg, injected slowly. Usually one dose is sufficient to initiate diuresis, but dose may be repeated at other injection site.

Administration/ Storage   Reconstitute sodium ethacrynate according to directions on vial. Do not use hazy or opalescent solutions, and do not administer simultaneously with whole blood or its derivatives. Use dilutions within 24 hours.

Additional Nursing Implications

1. Observe the patient for excessive diuresis (>2 pounds daily) because electrolyte imbalance is more likely to occur at higher rates of diuresis. Drug may have to be discontinued until homeostasis is achieved.
2. Consult with physician regarding need for supplementary potassium.
3. Observe patients having rapid excessive diuresis for pain in calves, pelvic area, or in chest because rapid hemoconcentration may cause thromboembolic effects.
4. Observe for GI effects that may necessitate discontinuation of drug. Severe diarrhea mandates permanent discontinuation of ethacrynic acid.
5. Check stools for blood.
6. Observe urine for hematuria.
7. Observe the patient for vestibular disturbances and do not administer IV concomitantly with another ototoxic agent.

FUROSEMIDE LASIX

Classification   Diuretic.

General Statement   Furosemide inhibits the reabsorption of sodium and chloride in the ascending loop of Henle, resulting in the excretion of sodium, chloride and, to a lesser degree, potassium and bicarbonate ions. The resulting urine is more acid. Diuretic action is independent of changes in patients' acid-base balance.

     The diuretic has a rapid onset of action: 1 hour after PO and IM administration; 5 minutes after IV administration. After PO or IM administration, action peaks after 1 to 2 hours and lasts 4 to 8 hours. Peak of activity after IV administration is 30 minutes, duration 2 hours.

     Furosemide has a slight antihypertensive effect.

     The drug may be effective for patients resistant to thiazides, and those with reduced glomerular filtration rates. Furosemide can be used in conjunction with spironolactone, triamterene, and other diuretics *except* ethacrynic acid. **Never use with ethacrynic acid.**

Additional Uses   Edema associated with coronary heart failure, nephrotic syndrome, hepatic cirrhosis, ascites, and hypertension. IV for acute pulmonary edema, and severe hypercalcemia. Drug should be given intermittently (2 to 4 days per week) followed by rest period.

Contraindications   Anuria, hypersensitivity to drug, severe renal disease associated with azotemia and oliguria, hepatic coma associated with electrolyte depletion, pregnancy, and pediatric patients.

Untoward Reactions   Also see *Untoward Reactions* for *Thiazides* p. 637.
This powerful agent is prone to cause electrolyte depletion, including hypokalemia, severe dehydration, gout, and metabolic alkalosis. Various types of dermatitis, blurred vision, postural hypotension, nausea, vomiting and diarrhea, weakness, fatigue, light-headedness, dizziness, muscle cramps, thirst, urinary bladder spasms, and urinary frequency have occasionally been reported.
Caution: Since drug is extremely powerful, patient should be in hospital when therapy is initiated and should continue under close medical supervision.
Because this drug is resistant to the effects of pressor amines and potentiates the effects of muscle relaxants, it is recommended that oral drug be discontinued one week before surgery and IV drug two days prior to surgery.

Drug Interactions

Interactant	Interaction

Aminoglycoside Antibiotics
  Gentamicin
  Kanamycin
  Neomycin
  Streptomycin
	Additive ototoxicity and nephrotoxicity

Anticoagulants	↑ Effect of anticoagulant due to ↓ plasma protein binding
Antidiabetic Agents	Furosemide antagonizes hypoglycemic effect of antidiabetics
Cephalosporins	↑ Renal toxicity of cephalosporins
Corticosteroids	Enhanced K loss due to K-depleting properties of both drugs
Digitalis glycosides	Furosemide produces excess K and Mg loss with ↑ chance of digitalis toxicity
Ethacrynic Acid (Edecrin)	Combination may result in hypokalemia, tachycardia, deafness, hypotension. **Do Not Use Together.**
Lithium	↓ Renal clearance of lithium leading to ↑ risk of toxicity

Drug Interactions (Continued)

Interactant	Interaction
MAO inhibitors Pargyline (Eutonyl) Tranylcypromine (Parnate)	Combination may result in severe hypotension with possibility of shock
Salicylates	↑ Risk of salicylate toxicity due to ↓ renal excretion
Skeletal Muscle Relaxants Succinylcholine Tubocurarine	Furosemide ↑ effect of skeletal muscle relaxants

Dosage

Edema, **PO: initial,** 40–80 mg daily. For resistant cases, dosage can be increased by 40 mg q 6 to 8 hr until desired diuretic response is attained. *Hypertension,* **PO:** 40 mg b.i.d. Drug can also be given **IV or IM,** if necessary. *Acute pulmonary edema,* **IV:** 40 mg, an additional 20 mg can be given every 1 to 2 hr. *Emergency (hypertensive crisis):* 100–200 mg **(IV or IM)** over period of 1 to 2 minutes. *Hypercalcemia,* **IV:** 80–100 mg q 1 to 2 hr until serum calcium levels are normal; **then PO:** 120 mg. **Infants/children, PO:** 2 mg/kg as single dose; can increase by 1–2 mg/kg up to maximum of 6 mg/kg. **IV, IM:** 1 mg/kg.

Administration/ Storage

1. Discoloration by light does not affect potency.
2. Store in light-resistant container.

Additional Nursing Implications

1. Monitor BP closely when drug is administered for hypertension, especially initially.
2. Observe patients having rapid diuresis for dehydration and circulatory collapse. Monitor BP and pulse.
3. Observe the patient for ototoxicity, when patient has renal impairment or is receiving other ototoxic drugs.
4. Be alert to signs of vascular thrombosis and embolism, particularly in the elderly.
5. Assure the patient that pain after IM injection is transient and will pass.
6. Caution patients to consult with their physician before taking aspirin because salicylate intoxication occurs at lower level because of competitive renal excretory sites.

SPIRONOLACTONE ALDACTONE

Classification

Diuretic, potassium-sparing.

General Statement

Spironolactone is a steroid compound that antagonizes (blocks) the sodium-retaining effects of the hormone aldosterone. More sodium, and more fluid, are thus eliminated from the body. Drug prevents excessive excretion of potassium.

    Onset of diuresis with spironolactone is gradual. Urine output increases over a period of 3 days. Diuresis reaches a maximum on day 3 and declines thereafter. Effect persists for 2 to 3 days. Spironolactone also has an antihypertensive effect.

Additional Uses Edema due to congestive heart failure, cirrhosis of the liver, nephrotic syndrome, idiopathic edema, primary hyperaldosteronism, and essential hypertension. Frequently used as adjunct with potassium-losing diuretics when it is important to avoid hypokalemia.

Contraindications Acute renal insufficiency, progressive renal failure, hyperkalemia, and anuria. Patients receiving potassium supplements.

Untoward Reactions Electrolyte imbalance, hyperkalemia, hyponatremia (characterized by dryness of the mouth, lethargy, and thirst), and slight acidosis. Also drowsiness; headaches; mental confusion; GI disturbances, including diarrhea; cutaneous eruptions; drug fever; ataxia; gynecomastia; and mild androgenic effects, including hirsutism, irregular menses, and deepening of voice. Prolonged use may cause increase in aldosterone. Most of these reactions are rare and reversible.

Drug Interactions

Interactant	Interaction
Anticoagulants, oral	Inhibited by spironolactone
Antihypertensives	Potentiation of hypotensive effect of both agents. Reduce dosage, especially of ganglionic blockers by one-half
Digitalis	The potassium-conserving effect of spironolactone may decrease effectiveness of digitalis. Though severe consequences have occurred in patients with impaired kidney function, drugs are often given concomitantly. Monitor closely
Diuretics, other	Often administered concurrently because of potassium-sparing effect of spironolactone. Severe hyponatremia may occur. Monitor closely
Norepinephrine	↓ Responsiveness to norepinephrine.
Potassium salts	Since spironolactone conserves potassium excessively, hyperkalemia may result. Rarely used together
Salicylates	Large doses may ↓ effects of spironolactone
Triamterene	Hazardous hyperkalemia may result from combination

Dosage **PO, adult:** 100 mg daily in divided doses. Treatment should be maintained for at least 5 days. Adjust dosage according to response. **Usual maximum maintenance:** 200 mg daily. **Pediatric:** 1.7–3.3 mg/kg daily in 4 divided doses.

Administration Protect drug from light.

Additional Nursing Implications
1. Anticipate that supplemental potassium will be avoided in therapy with patient on spironolactone because drug is potassium sparing.
2. Warn patients on large doses experiencing drowsiness and ataxia against driving a car or operating dangerous machinery.

3. Observe the patient for tolerance to drug which may be characterized by edema and reduced urine output.
4. Observe patients with a history of liver disease for stupor and coma.

TRIAMTERENE DYRENIUM

Classification   Diuretic, potassium-sparing.

General Statement   Triamterene acts directly on tubular transport of electrolytes by promoting the excretion of approximately equal amounts of sodium and chloride. A corresponding volume of fluid is also excreted. Unlike many other diuretics, it does not increase the excretion of potassium and may even decrease it. It increases urinary pH by promoting excretion of bicarbonate ion. Triamterene is of most value when it is combined with other diuretics.

Diuresis starts 2 hours after administration, but the maximum effect of the drug may only be reached after several days usage. This makes the drug unsuitable for initiation of therapy in patients with severe congestive heart failure.

Withdraw drug slowly as an excessive excretion of potassium may occur with abrupt withdrawal. Patients with hepatic cirrhosis and ascites are more susceptible to hypokalemia.

Lab work to check BUN, creatinine, and serum electrolytes should be done periodically.

Additional Uses   Congestive heart failure, idiopathic edema, edema associated with hepatic cirrhosis, nephrotic syndrome, steroid therapy, late pregnancy, and secondary hyperaldosteronism. Hypertension (in combination with a thiazide).

Contraindications   Hypersensitivity to drug, severe renal insufficiency, and severe hepatic disease. Pregnancy.

Untoward Reactions   Electrolyte imbalance, including hyponatremia, hyper- and hypokalemia, and increases in serum uric acid levels, especially in patients predisposed to gout. GI distress: nausea, vomiting, and diarrhea. Dizziness, drowsiness, hypotension, weakness, muscular cramps, dry mouth, headache, blood dyscrasias, photosensitivity, and hypersensitivity have occasionally been reported.

Drug Interactions

Interactant	Interaction
Antidiabetics, oral	Triamterene antagonizes hypoglycemic effect of antidiabetics
Antihypertensives	Potentiated by triamterene
Digitalis	Inhibited by triamterene
Spironolactone	Should not be used concomitantly

Dosage   *Edema*, **initial;** 100 mg 1 to 2 times daily after meals; **maximum daily dose:** 300 mg. **Maintenance:** 100 mg q other day.

Hypertension (usually given in combination with a thiazide): 100 mg b.i.d. after meals.

Triamterene dosage usually reduced by one half when other diuretic is added to regimen.

Administration   Minimize nausea by giving drug after meals.

Additional Nursing Implications

1. Observe for hyperkalemia, an indication for withdrawal of drug, since cardiac irregularities may result.
2. Anticipate that supplemental potassium will be avoided during treatment with triamterene because drug is potassium-sparing.
3. Observe for signs of fever, sore throat, and rash—signs of blood dyscrasias.
4. Observe for signs of uremia characterized by lethargy, headache, drowsiness, vomiting, restlessness, mental wandering, and foul breath.

CHAPTER 9

ELECTROLYTE, CALORIC AND WATER BALANCE

Electrolytes	Magnesium Sulfate Potassium Salts	Sodium Chloride
Caloric Agents	Carbohydrates: Dextrose Fructose Invert Sugar	Other: Crystalline Amino Acid Infusion Essential Amino Acid Injection Protein Hydrolysate Intravenous Fat Emulsion

SUMMARY TABLE OF ELECTROLYTES, CARBOHYDRATES, AND PROTEIN SOLUTIONS

Acidifying Agent	Ammonium Chloride	
Alkalinizing Agents	Sodium Bicarbonate Sodium Lactate	Tromethamine
Potassium Removing Resin	Sodium Polystyrene Sulfonate	

General Statement

Water, electrolytes, and nutrients are used as adjuncts in the management of a great variety of disorders and conditions. Since there is a close link between fluid volume and electrolyte balance, these two subjects will be discussed together.

The electrolyte concentration of the body varies within extremely narrow limits (see Appendix 1). Any major deviation from normal quickly results in physiological changes manifested by dehydration, fluid retention, and disturbance of the acid-base balance. Severe illness (chronic or acute), shock, trauma, poisoning, burns and certain medications often affect the fluid and electrolyte balance of the body. The administration of suitable replacements to prevent or correct disequilibration of the fluid and electrolyte balance is an important aspect of patient care.

Fluid and electrolytes can be supplied orally, subcutaneously (rare) or intravenously. The oral route should be chosen whenever possible. Parenteral therapy should be discontinued at the earliest point feasible.

Numerous single and multiple electrolyte replacement solutions with or without carbohydrates are commercially available.

Drugs are often added to parenterally administered solutions, and the nurse must be aware of possible interactions and incompatibilities. Unless specifically instructed to do otherwise, it is advisable to add only one drug at a time to the intravenous assembly.

Fluid balance can also be manipulated with diuretics. These are discussed in Chapter 8. Calcium, an electrolyte, is discussed in Chapter

7, Section 3. Blood volume expanders are discussed in Chapter 3, Section 3.

Detailed information on the major electrolytes, and caloric agents is presented in the following chapter. Table 33, page 666 presents information on these agents and commonly used mixtures in summary form.

Please note that the dosage of IV solutions is highly individualized especially for infants, children, elderly, or debilitated patients and those suffering from cardiovascular diseases.

MAGNESIUM SULFATE

Classification   Electrolyte.

General Statement   Magnesium is an important cation present in the extracellular fluid at a concentration of 1.5–2.5 mEq/liter. It is also present extracellularly, especially in muscle tissue and in bone. Magnesium is believed to play a major role in nerve impulse transmission.

Hypomagnesemia is characterized by neurological symptoms, such as muscle irritation, clonic twitching, tremors, and tetany. Hypomagnesemia is often accompanied by hypocalcemia and hypokalemia. *Hypermagnesemia* is characterized by central nervous system depression.

Uses   Replacement therapy in magnesium deficiency. Adjunct in TPN.

Contraindications   Use with caution in patients with renal disease because magnesium is removed from the body solely by the kidneys; in the presence of heart block or myocardial damage.

Untoward Reactions   Magnesium intoxication, vasodilation. Low doses cause flushing and sweating; higher doses cause a sharp decrease in blood pressure and respiratory paralysis.

Dosage   *Hypomagnesemia,* **mild, IM:** 1 gm q 6 hr 4 times total (or total of 32.5 mEq/24 hr). **Severe, IM:** up to 2 mEq/kg over 4 hr or, **IV:** 5 gm (40 mEq) in Dextrose 5% by **slow** infusion over period of 3 hr. *Hyperalimentation,* **adults:** 8–24 mEq/day; **infants:** 2–10 mEq/day.

Treatment of Magnesium Intoxication   a. Use artificial ventilation immediately.
b. Have 5–10 mEq of calcium (e.g., 10–20 ml of 10% calcium gluconate) readily available for IV injection.

Administration   1. IM: deep injection of 50% concentrate is appropriate for adults. A 20% solution should be used for children. IV: dilute as specified by manufacturer.
2. Administer slowly and cautiously at a rate not exceeding 1.5 ml of a 10% concentrate/minute.

Nursing Implications

1. Withhold drug and check with doctor prior to administration if
   a. Patellar reflexes are absent.
   b. Respirations are below 16/minute.
   c. Urinary output was less than 100 ml during past 4 hours.
   d. There is flushing, sweating, hypotension, or hypothermia, early signs of hypermagnesemia.
   e. There is a previous history of heart block or myocardial damage.
2. Do not administer magnesium sulfate for 2 hours preceding delivery of baby.
3. Monitor newborn for neurological and respiratory depression if mother received continuous IV therapy with magnesium sulfate during 24 hours preceding delivery.
4. Be prepared to assist with emergency treatment of magnesium intoxication. Have available equipment for artificial ventilation and calcium gluconate IV.

POTASSIUM SALTS

Classification   Electrolyte.

General Statement   Potassium is the major cation of the body's intracellular fluid. It is essential for the maintenance of important physiological processes, including cardiac, smooth, and skeletal muscle function, acid-base balance, gastric secretions, renal function, tissue synthesis, and carbohydrate metabolism. Symptoms of hypokalemia include weakness, cardiac arrhythmias, fatigue and in severe cases flaccid paralysis and inability to concentrate urine.

The usual adult daily requirement of potassium is 40–80 mg. In adults, the normal plasma concentration of potassium ranges from 3.5 to 5 mEq/liter. Concentrations up to 5.6 mEq/liter are normal in children.

Both hypokalemia and hyperkalemia, if uncorrected, can be fatal; thus, potassium must always be administered very cautiously.

Potassium is readily and rapidly absorbed from the gastrointestinal tract. Though a number of salts can be used to supply the potassium cation, potassium chloride is the agent of choice since hypochloremia frequently accompanies potassium deficiency. Dietary measures (bananas, orange juice) can often prevent and even correct potassium deficiencies.

Potassium is excreted by the kidney and is partially reabsorbed from the glomerular filtrate.

Uses   Correction of potassium deficiency caused by vomiting, diarrhea, excess loss of gastrointestinal fluids, hyperadrenalism, malnutrition, debilitation, prolonged negative nitrogen balance, dialysis, metabolic alkalosis, diabetic acidosis, certain renal conditions, cardiac arrhythmias, cardiotonic glycoside toxicity, and myasthenia gravis (experimentally).

Long-term electrolyte replacement regimen or total parenteral nutrition with potassium-free solutions. Correction of potassium deficiency possibly caused by certain drugs, including many diuretics, adrenal corticosteroids, testosterone or corticotropin.

Prophylaxis after major surgery when urine flow has been reestablished.

Contraindications

Severe renal function impairment, postoperatively before urine flow has been reestablished. Crush syndrome, Addison's disease, hyperkalemia, acute dehydration. Administer with caution in the presence of cardiac disease and in patients receiving potassium-sparing drugs.

Untoward Reactions

Hyperkalemia, characterized by electrocardiographic changes (tall peaked T-waves, depression of the S-T segment, disappearance of the P-waves, and widening and slurring of the QRS segment).

Clinically, hyperkalemia is characterized by paresthesia of the extremities, listlessness, mental confusion, weakness or heaviness of the legs, cold skin, grey pallor, peripheral collapse with fall in blood pressure, cardiac arrhythmias. Death results from cardiac depression, arrhythmias, or cardiac arrest.

Nausea, vomiting, diarrhea, abdominal discomfort.

Small-bowel ulcerations may result from administration of enteric-coated potassium chloride tablets.

Dosage

Highly individualized. Oral administration is preferred because the slow absorption from the GI tract prevents sudden, large increases in plasma potassium levels. Dosage is usually expressed as mEq/liter of potassium. The acetate, bicarbonate, chloride, citrate and gluconate salts are usually administered orally. The chloride, acetate, and phosphate may be administered by **slow IV** infusion. *Prophylaxis:* 20 mEq/day; *correction of hypokalemia:* 40–100 mEq/day or more. Infants may require 2–3 mEq/kg.

PO: administer dosage in 2 to 4 doses daily. Correct hypokalemia slowly over period of 3 to 7 days to avoid hyperkalemia.

For patients with potassium levels greater than 2.5 mEq/liter, administer no more than 200 mEq in 24 hr at a maximum rate of 10 mEq/hr.

For patients with potassium levels less than 2.0 mEq/liter and marked electrocardiographic changes or paralysis: administer up to 400 mEq in 24 hr at a maximum rate of 40 mEq/hr.

For patients with accompanying metabolic acidosis, an alkalinizing potassium salt (potassium bicarbonate, potassium citrate, or potassium acetate) should be selected.

Treatment of Overdosage

(Plasma potassium levels greater than 6.5 mEq/liter.) All measures must be monitored by electrocardiogram. Measures consist of actions taken to shift potassium ions from plasma into cells by

1. **Sodium Bicarbonate:** IV infusion of 40–160 mEq over period of 5 minutes. May be repeated after 10 to 15 minutes if ECG abnormalities persist.

2. **Dextrose:** IV infusion of 300–500 ml of 10%–25% injection over period of 1 hour. Insulin is sometimes added to dextrose (5–10 units per 20 gm of dextrose) or given separately.
3. **Calcium gluconate—or other calcium salt:** (only for patients not on digitalis or other cardiotonic glycosides): IV infusion of 0.5–1 gm (5–10 ml of a 10% solution) over period of 2 minutes. Dosage may be repeated after 1 to 2 minutes if ECG remains abnormal.

When ECG is approximately normal, the excess potassium should be removed from body by administration of polystyrene sulfonate, hemo- or peritoneal dialysis (patients with renal insufficiency) or other means.

Administration   PO:

1. Dilute or dissolve liquid potassium in fruit or vegetable juice if not already in flavored base.
2. Chill to increase palatability.
3. Instruct patients to swallow enteric-coated tablets and not dissolve them in their mouths.
4. Administer dilute liquid solutions of potassium rather than tablets to patients with esophageal compression.

Parenteral:

1. Administer very slowly as ordered for individual patient by the doctor.
2. Administer only in a dilute solution and do not exceed 20 mEq of potassium/hour.
3. Ensure uniform distribution of potassium by inverting container during addition of potassium solution and then by agitating container. Squeezing the plastic container will not prevent potassium chloride from settling to the bottom.
4. Check site of administration frequently for pain and redness because drug is extremely irritating.

Nursing Implications

1. Discontinue ingestion of potassium-rich foods and oral potassium medication when parenteral potassium administration is initiated.
2. Withhold oral potassium medication if abdominal pain, distention, or GI bleeding occurs.
3. Be alert to symptoms of hypokalemia, such as weakness, cardiac arrhythmias, and fatigue, that indicate a low intracellular potassium level even though the serum potassium level is within normal limits.
4. Assess that urinary flow is adequate before starting administration of potassium because impaired renal function can lead to hyperkalemia.
5. Withhold potassium medication from patients with oliguria, anuria, or azotinuria, chronic adrenal insufficiency, or extensive tissue breakdown as in burns.
6. Do not administer potassium medication to patients receiving potassium-sparing diuretics, such as spironolactone or triamterene.

7. Monitor ECG when patient is on parenteral potassium for signs of hyperkalemia as noted in *Untoward Reactions.*
8. Monitor serum potassium while patient is receiving parenteral potassium. (Norm: 3.6– 5.5 mEq/L).
9. Assess for signs of hyperkalemia, such as listlessness, mental confusion, weakness or heaviness of legs, flaccid paralysis, cold skin, grey pallor, hypotension, cardiac arrhythmias, and heart block.
10. Be prepared to assist with emergency treatment of hyperkalemia. Have available sodium bicarbonate, calcium gluconate, and regular insulin for parenteral use.
11. Teach patient: a) the relationship of potassium to other medication regimen to improve compliance, b) symptoms of hypokalemia and hyperkalemia, need to report these, and, c) to ingest potassium-rich food, such as citrus juices, bananas, apricots, raisins, and nuts, after parenteral potassium is discontinued.

SODIUM CHLORIDE

Classification Electrolyte.

General Statement Sodium is the major cation of the body's extracellular fluid. It plays a crucial role in maintaining the fluid and electrolyte balance. Excess retention of sodium results in overhydration (edema, hypervolemia), which is often treated with diuretics. Abnormally low levels of sodium result in dehydration. Normally, the plasma contains 136 to 145 mEq sodium and 98 to 106 mEq chloride/liter. The average daily requirement of salt is approximately 5 gm.

Hyponatremia is characterized by abdominal and muscle cramps, fatigue, headaches, vertigo, decrease in blood pressure, muscle weakness and poor skin turgor.

Hypernatremia is characterized by CNS dysfunction, confusion, neuromuscular excitation, edema, elevated temperature and blood pressure, seizures and coma. Sodium chloride and increased water intake is usually used to correct all types of dehydration.

Uses Sodium and fluid replacement, heat prostration, cramps.

Contraindications Congestive heart failure, severely impaired renal function. Administer with caution to patients with cardiovascular, cirrhotic, renal disease, in presence of hyperproteinemia, and in patients receiving corticosteroids or corticotropin.

Untoward Reactions Hypernatremia, postoperative intolerance of sodium chloride characterized by cellular dehydration, asthenia, disorientation, anorexia, nausea, oliguria, and increased BUN levels.

Dosage **PO:** *individualized* as required. Commonly used solution contains 3– 4 gm NaCl and 1.5– 3 gm sodium bicarbonate/liter. *Heat cramps:* 1 gm

NaCl with q glass of water. **IV:** *individualized* as required. *Hypotonic* (0.11–0.45% NaCl) solutions are used when fluid losses exceed electrolyte depletion. *Isotonic* (0.9% NaCl providing approximately physiological concentrations of sodium and chloride ions). *Hypertonic* (3% or 5%) when sodium loss exceeds fluid loss.

Administration   Hypertonic injections of NaCl must be given slowly and cautiously in a volume not to exceed 100 ml/hr. Plasma electrolyte levels should be determined before additional sodium chloride is given.

Nursing Implications
1. Assess patient for signs of hypernatremia, such as flushed skin, elevated temperature, rough dry tongue, edema, hypertension or hypotension, tachycardia, urine specific gravity above 1.02 and serum sodium above 146 mEq/liter.
2. Interrupt IV and report condition of patient to doctor should these signs occur.

CARBOHYDRATES

Classification   Caloric agents.

General Statement   The simplest and most easily absorbed caloric agents are dextrose (D-glucose) and fructose, or an equimolar mixture of the two—invert sugar. Fructose and dextrose are monosaccharides. They can replace and supplement orally absorbed food and water. They decrease excess ketone formation, spare body proteins and electrolytes.

One liter of a 10% solution of any of the above provides 340–380 calories. Five percent solutions are approximately isotonic. Both 5% and 10% solutions are used to correct dehydration and supply calories. More concentrated solutions also have a diuretic effect. *Remark:* Solutions without NaCl should not be used as diluents for blood.

Contraindications   Do not use concentrated (hypertonic) solutions in the presence of intracranial or intraspinal hemorrhages or delirium tremens in dehydrated patients.

Administration
1. The amount of fluid to be received in a specific time is to be ordered by the doctor. The amount is highly individualized, especially in children.
2. Administer concentrated solution into large, central vein to prevent irritation.

Nursing Implications
1. Iso-osmolar (isotonic) parenteral therapy:
   Assess for signs of cerebral edema manifested by slow pulse rate, high blood pressure, and headaches. *Reduce* rate of flow markedly should these symptoms occur and report to doctor.
2. Hyperosmolar (hypertonic) parenteral therapy:
   a. Assess for signs of dehydration manifested by rapid pulse rate, low BP, and restlessness. *Reduce* rate of flow markedly should these symptoms occur, and report to doctor.

b. Determine that hyperosmolar solution does not run faster than 3–4 ml/minute to prevent further electrolyte imbalance and local irritation.

c. Assess site of infusion for redness and pain since hyperosmolar solutions can cause sclerosis and thrombophlebitis.

d. Anticipate that a 5% dextrose solution will be administered following abrupt withdrawal of hypertonic dextrose solution to prevent hypoglycemia.

DEXTROSE (D-GLUCOSE)

Classification   Caloric agent, carbohydrate.

Remarks   Most widely used carbohydrate.

Uses   To supply calories and water when non-electrolytic fluid and caloric replacement are necessary. Also, to spare proteins and minimize loss of electrolytes. Toxemia of pregnancy, renal failure (use 20% solution), diabetic acidosis (use 2.5% dextrose and 0.45% NaCl), reduction of cerebrospinal fluid pressure and to maintain blood volume (use 50% solution). To correct insulin reaction (hypoglycemia), use 50% solution.

Additional Contraindications   Hyperglycemia.

Untoward Reactions   Hyperglycemia and glycosuria (with rapid administration of hypertonic solution), thrombosis (concentrated solutions), or phlebitis.

Dosage   *Individualized, usual,* **IV:** 1–3 liters of 5%–10% solution daily. *Diuretic:* 500–1000 ml of 20% solution; 50–100 ml of 50% solution when indicated.

Administration   Maximum rate of administration to avoid hyperglycemia: 0.5 gm/kg/hr.

FRUCTOSE LEVULOSE

Classification   Caloric agent, carbohydrate.

Remarks   More rapidly metabolized and converted to glycogen than dextrose. When necessary can be administered more quickly than dextrose (100 gm in 1 hour). Suitable for diabetic patients because it does not require insulin to be metabolized.

Uses   To supply calories, water, to spare body proteins and electrolytes.

Contraindications   Acute hypoglycemia (use dextrose instead), hereditary fructose intolerance.

Untoward Reactions   In infants, rapid administration has caused an increase in pulse and respiratory rate and liver size, accompanied by a decrease in blood pH and CO_2.

Dosage   **IV:** *individualized,* **usual,** 1– 3 liters of 10% solution. **Infants:** 100– 1,000 ml of 10% solution; **children:** 200– 2,000 ml of 10% solution. Each 10 ml of solution contain approximately 1 gm of fructose.

Administration   IV only. Unless otherwise instructed, administer slowly, especially in children (rate should not exceed 1 gm/kg/hour).

INVERT SUGAR TRAVERT

Classification   Caloric agent, carbohydrate.

Remarks   Equimolar mixture of dextrose and fructose; the combination is more rapidly utilized than dextrose alone. A 5% solution is sometimes administered together with amino acids.

Dosage   *Individualized.* **IV: usual,** 1– 3 liters of 10% solution.

Administration   The rate is determined by the reaction of patient.

CRYSTALLINE AMINO ACID INFUSION AMINOSYN, FREAMINE II, TRAVASOL, VEINAMINE

ESSENTIAL AMINO ACID INJECTION NEPHRAMINE

PROTEIN HYDROLYSATE AMIGEN, AMINOSOL, C.P.H., TRAVAMIN

Classification   Nutritional agent.

General Statement   Seriously or chronically ill patients often need intravenous administration of nutritional supplements. One of the limitations of parenteral nutrition is that the average patient can only handle 2500– 3000 ml of fluid daily. Moreover, in order to minimize injury to the blood vessels, solutions administered via the peripheral veins must be isotonic. This requirement limits the number of calories that can be administered via that route (usually up to 200 cal/liter).

Infusion through the large subclavian vein (central parenteral administration) permits the administration of more concentrated (hypertonic) solutions. At first, these consisted mostly of hypertonic glucose solutions. Today, these simple carbohydrate solutions are supplemented by protein hydrolysates or mixtures of essential amino acids, which supply the body with the amino acids (nitrogen) essential for tissue formation and repair.

Three types of preparations are available today.

1. *Protein Hydrolysates:* prepared from protein (casein or fibrin) which is degraded into its constituent amino acids and low molecular weight peptides. The nitrogen from the peptides is not as easily assimilated by the body as the nitrogen from free amino acids. These preparations contain both essential and non-essential amino acids as well as electrolytes. These solutions are especially likely to cause allergic reactions.
2. *Essential Amino Acid Injection:* A mixture of essential amino acids often with electrolytes, minerals and vitamins. The preparation is administered with dextrose.
3. *Crystalline Amino Acid Infusions* contain both essential and non-essential amino acids in crystalline form, as well as electrolytes.

Total parenteral nutrition (TPN) regimens also provide the carbohydrates, whose calories are essential for the proper utilization of the amino acids, electrolytes, and vitamins. TPN regimens have a nitrogen-sparing effect and promote a positive nitrogen balance and protein synthesis.

The proper administration of TPN products requires a thorough knowledge of the nutritional needs of the patients, as well as of their fluid and electrolyte balance. Patients receiving TPN must be frequently evaluated by means of complete clinical laboratory tests. Malfunction of a major metabolic pathway or organ system (impaired kidney function, congestive heart failure) may rapidly result in major complications.

The concentrated sugar solutions may result in hyperglycemia if given too fast, and insulin must be added.

Patients on TPN must be monitored closely.

Initially blood glucose levels are measured every 6 to 12 hours, and electrolytes daily. During routine administration, blood glucose and electrolytes are measured 2 to 3 times a week. Acid-base balance, liver and kidney function, calcium, magnesium, blood ammonia, serum proteins, formed elements of blood, vitamin levels, and lipids are also monitored.

The success of TPN is gauged by weight gain and positive nitrogen balance. Adults should gain approximately 340 gm/day, infants 2–35 gm/day.

Uses　Pre- and postoperative support, fistulas of the GI tract, inflammatory bowel disease, cancer, burns, starvation, renal, cardiac and liver failure, psychosis. *Pediatrics:* neonatal surgery, chronic intractable diarrhea; investigational: low birth weight. Supplemental as protein-sparing nutrition.

Contraindications　Hypersensitivity to any component. Severe uncorrected acid-base imbalance, decreased circulating blood volume, anuria, oliguria, severe liver disease.

Untoward Reactions　Allergic reactions. Headache, dizziness, chills, nausea, vomiting, flushing of skin with sensation of warmth (these effects can be minimized by using slow infusion). Hyperglycemia, glycosuria, osmotic diuresis, dehydration (using hyperosmolar preparations), sepsis (3%–7% in institutions practicing aseptic techniques, higher in others). Electrolyte and fluid imbalance, fever, hypersensitivity reactions, pneumothorax, hemothorax. Also, metabolic acidosis, hyperammonemia (especially with essential amino acid injection), hypophosphatemia, alkalosis, hypo- and hypervitaminosis, elevated hepatic enzymes, phlebitis (along vein used for infusion), thrombosis. *Pediatric patients:* bone demineralization.

Dosage

Daily need: protein 0.9 gm/kg; **infants and children:** 1.4–2.2 gm/kg; **debilitated adults:** 1–1.5 gm/kg; **debilitated children:** 2–3 gm/kg. Nitrogen is only assimilated when adequate proteins are given at same time. *Calorie (carbohydrate)/nitrogen ratio:* 100–200 non-protein calories per gm of nitrogen to achieve positive nitrogen balance. The commercial solutions are available in different strengths. TPN should be initiated slowly. **For adults:** 1 liter on day one; 2 liters on day 2; up to 3 liters on day 3. The therapy should be terminated by infusing decreasing concentrations of dextrose over a period of at least 24 hr, to avoid rebound hypoglycemia.

Administration/ Storage

1. Solutions should be prepared in the pharmacy.
2. Store prepared solutions at 4° C (39.2° F).
3. Use prepared solutions within 24 hours.

Nursing Implication

See *Nursing Implications* for *Central Parenteral Administration* in Section 1, p. 15.

Additional Nursing Implications

1. Observe for allergic reaction to protein hydrolysate characterized by pruritus, urticaria, and wheals. Report positive observations to doctor.
2. Report blood sugar determinations over 200 mg/100 ml indicating need for insulin to be added to TPN.
3. Report fractional urine determinations of 3^+–4^+ indicating need for insulin to be added to TPN.
4. Discontinue TPN if blood sugar exceeds 1000 mg/100 ml and substitute a hypo-osmolar solution to prevent neurological dysfunction and coma.

INTRAVENOUS FAT EMULSION INTRALIPID 10%

Classification

Nutritional agent.

General Statement

The product contains soybean oil (10%), egg yolk phospholipids (1.2%), glycerin (2.25%), and water for injection. It provides 1.1 cal/ml. Since it is isotonic, it can be administered into a peripheral vein. The fat emulsion provides essential fatty acids (e.g., linoleic, oleic, palmitic) that may be necessary to maintain normal cellular membrane function. The preparation increases heat production, oxygen consumption, and decreases the respiratory quotient (ratio of CO_2/O_2; normal: 0.77–0.90).

TABLE 33 PARENTERAL ELECTROLYTE, CARBOHYDRATE, OR PROTEIN SOLUTIONS

Preparation	Information on Content	Use	Other Information
Alcohol in Dextrose Infusion	5% or 10% alcohol & 5% dextrose in water for IV infusion only.	Increase caloric intake.	Alcohol intoxication may occur if infused too rapidly. Contraindicated in conditions where alcohol should not be used.
Ammonium Chloride	2.14%; 21.4% & 26.7% —both to be diluted before IV infusion. Also can be given by hypodermoclysis.	Chloride loss due to vomiting, gastric suction, gastric fistula drainage. To acidify urine; overuse of mercurial diuretics.	May also be necessary to replace potassium. Excessive doses may cause metabolic acidosis. Due to severe pain, SC use is not recommended. Dose: 10 ml of the 2.14% soln/kg for alkalotic adults and infants.
Combined Electrolyte Solutions (Ringer's Injection, Lactated Ringer's Inj., Ionosol D-CM, Plasma-Lyte Inj., Acetated Ringer's Inj., Plasma-Lyte 56, Isolyte S, Isolyte E, Normosol R, Plasma-Lyte 148, Polyonic R 148, Polysal)	These products contain varying amounts of Na^+, K^+, Ca^{++}, Mg^{++}, Cl^-. Some contain lactate, acetate, and/or gluconate.	Electrolyte replacement.	
Crystalline Amino Acid Infusions (Aminosyn 5%, 7%, 10%, 3.5% M; Freamine II, Travasol 5.5%, 8.5%; 3.5% Travasol M w/Electrolyte 45; Veinamine)	These products contain varying amounts of protein, essential and non-essential amino acids, and electrolytes. Percent refers to the protein concentration.	Total parenteral (central) nutrition/hyperalimentation (all products can be used except Aminosyn 3.5 M & 3.5% Travasol M w/Electrolyte 45). Supplemental parenteral (peripheral) nutrition (Veinamine diluted with D-5-W or D-10-W is used).	Complete familiarity with amino acid injection therapy is essential because there are many possible cautions with their use.

Solution	Concentration	Use	Comments
Dextrose (in water) (D-2½-W, D-5-W, D-10-W, D-20-W, D-40-W, D-50-W, D-60-W, D-70-W)	2½%, 5%, 10% by IV infusion	Protein-sparing (peripheral) nutrition (Aminosyn 3.5 M, 3.5% M w/Electrolyte 45 are used; Aminosyn 5% & Travasol 5.5% or 8.5% can be used if diluted with fluids and electrolytes).	Prolonged IV infusion of 5% dextrose may cause phlebitis. If hypertonic solutions are administered too rapidly, hyperglycemia, glycosuria, and hyperosmolarity may result. Thrombosis may result if hypertonic solutions are given in peripheral veins. Concentrated solutions should not be used if intracranial or intraspinal hemorrhage is present or in delirium tremens in dehydrated individuals.
	2½%, 5%, 10% by IV infusion	Peripheral infusion to provide calories when non-electrolyte fluid is needed.	
	20%, 50% (hypertonic)	Needed calories in minimal volume of water; 50% used in hyperinsulinemia or insulin shock.	
	40%, 50%, 60%, 70%	Concentrated source of calories for central IV infusion when mixed with other solutions.	
Dextrose-Electrolyte Solutions.		All are for electrolyte and caloric replacement.	
a) Dextrose in NaCl	2½%–10% dextrose in 0.11%–0.9% NaCl		
b) KCl in Dextrose	0.075%–0.3% KCl in 5% dextrose		
c) KCl in Dextrose and NaCl	20–40 mEq KCl in 5% dextrose & 0.45% NaCl; 0.075%–0.3% KCl in 5% dextrose & either 0.2% or 0.45% NaCl		
d) Dextrose in Lactated Ringer's	2½%–10% dextrose in Lactated Ringer's		
e) Dextrose in Acetated Ringer's	5%–10% dextrose in Acetated Ringer's		
f) Many other products			
Dextrose & Electrolyte Solutions w/Vitamins	Most contain various B vitamins in 5% dextrose; in addition, some contain 0.9% NaCl	Replacement of vitamins electrolytes, and calories.	

(Continued)

667

TABLE 33 PARENTERAL ELECTROLYTE, CARBOHYDRATE, OR PROTEIN SOLUTIONS (*Continued*)

Preparation	Information on Content	Use	Other Information
Essential Amino Acid Injection (Nephramine)	Mixture of essential amino acids administered with hypertonic dextrose	For total parenteral nutrition (hyperalimentation). For reversible renal decompensation. Hypertonic solutions of essential amino acids and dextrose may be administered via central venous catheter.	Hyperglycemia may result. May need to supplement K, P, and Mg. Fluid balance must be monitored in renal failure patients. Use with special caution in low birth-weight infants. Dose: 250–500 ml containing about 1.5–3 gm nitrogen in 13–26 gm essential amino acids/day. Usually 250 ml is mixed with 500 ml 70% dextrose.
Fructose (Levulose)	10% fructose in water	Used in place of solns. containing glucose or invert sugar for fluid replacement and increased calories. To be used only for IV infusion.	Contraindicated for acute hypoglycemia. Use in infants may result in increases in pulse and respiratory rates and liver size as well as decreases in blood pH and CO_2. Rates of 2.0 gm/kg/hour have resulted in metabolic acidosis in infants (do not give more than 1 gm/kg/hour to either infants or adults).
Fructose-Electrolyte Solutions	These products contain 5%–15% fructose with varying amounts of Na^+, K^+, Mg^{++}, Cl^-, phosphate, lactate, and/or acetate.	Replacement therapy.	
Invert Sugar (Travert)	5% or 10%. Contains equal parts of dextrose and fructose.	Non-electrolyte and caloric replacement.	Fructose increases the utilization of dextrose. See information on dextrose and fructose.

Invert Sugar-Electrolyte Solutions	These products contain 5%–10% invert sugar with varying amounts of Na^+, K^+, Mg^{++}, Ca^{++}, Cl^-, phosphate and/or lactate.	Replacement of electrolytes and calories.	
IV Fat Emulsion (Intralipid 10%)	10% soybean oil, 1.2% egg yolk phospholipids, 2.25% glycerin in water for injection. The major fatty acids present are linolenic, linoleic, oleic, and palmitic acids.	Caloric and essential fatty acid source in patients requiring parenteral nutrition for more than 5 days. In essential fatty acid deficits. Used as part of a total parenteral (IV) nutrition program.	Do not mix with electrolyte or other nutrient solutions and no additives can be placed in container. If there is oiling out of the emulsion, do not use. Use with caution with severe liver damage, anemia or blood coagulation disorders, and pulmonary embolism. Many possible adverse reactions.
Magnesium Sulfate	10%, 12.5%, 25%, and 50% solutions	Hypocalcemia and magnesium deficiency esp. if tetany present. In total parenteral nutrition to prevent hypomagnesemia. Can be used both IV or IM.	Use with caution in kidney impairment. Be aware of possible magnesium intoxication (respiratory paralysis and sharp drop in blood pressure). Onset of intoxication can be detected by absence of patellar reflex.
Phosphate (Potassium or Sodium)	Potassium phosphate provides 3 mM PO_4 and 4.4 mEq K/ml; Sodium phosphate provides 3 mM PO_4 and 4 mEq Na/ml.	To prevent or correct hypophosphatemia. As an additive to large volume IV fluids.	K phosphate contraindicated in hyperkalemia and Na phosphate contraindicated in hypernatremia. Must be diluted before use and to avoid intoxication, must be infused slowly. Phosphate intoxication results in a decrease in serum Ca and hypocalcemic tetany may be manifested. Note usual precautions in administering Na or K.

(Continued)

TABLE 33 PARENTERAL ELECTROLYTE, CARBOHYDRATE, OR PROTEIN SOLUTIONS (*Continued*)

Preparation	Information on Content	Use	Other Information
Phosphate-Carbonate Buffer (BUFF)	Full strength provides 72 mg Na biphosphate & 69 mg Na carbonate in 10 ml (equivalent to 2 mEq Na, 1 mEq PO_4, and 1 mEq carbonate)	Additive to adjust pH of acidic IV solns. to physiological range.	Must be diluted before use. Add to IV solution immediately before use.
Potassium Salts Potassium Acetate Potassium Chloride	40 or 50 mEq/20 ml 10–90 mEq in various volumes	Both used for moderate to severe potassium deficit due to: malnutrition, loss of GI fluids, diabetic acidosis, metabolic alkalosis, hyperadrenocorticism, primary aldosteronism, healing phase of scalds or burns; cardiac arrhythmias esp. if due to digitalis glycosides.	Contraindicated in conditions resulting in increased serum K levels or decreased renal excretion. Infuse slowly to avoid potassium intoxication. Hypokalemia with metabolic acidosis should be treated with alkalinizing K salt. Be sure kidney function is normal. Dilute before use and only use IV.
Protein Hydrolysates (Amigen 5%, 10%; Aminosol 5%; C.P.H. 5%; Travamin 5%, 10%)	Solution of amino acids or low molecular weight peptides from hydrolysis of casein or fibrin; also contains electrolytes. Percent refers to the protein concentration.	Central venous hyperalimentation	See Crystalline Amino Acid Infusion
Protein Products— See *Crystalline Amino Acid Infusions, Essential Amino Acid Injection,* or *Protein Hydrolysates*			
Ringer's Injection, Lactated (Hartman's Soln.)	Contains mixture of electrolytes approximating that of blood plasma: Na, 130 mEq/l; K, 4 mEq/l; Ca, 2.7 mEq/l; Cl, 109.7 mEq/l; lactate, 28 mEq/l.	Dehydration accompanied by mild acidosis	Dose is individualized. Patient must be assessed for signs of electrolyte imbalance.
Ringer's Solution	Contains electrolytes at levels approximating blood plasma: Na, 147 mEq/l; K, 4 mEq/l; Ca, 5 mEq/l; Cl, 155.5 mEq/l.	Replacement of electrolytes and fluid	Ringer's Solution is less likely to induce edema than isotonic saline. Dose is individualized. Patient must be assessed for signs of electrolyte imbalance.

Sodium Acetate	40 mEq/20 ml (equivalent to 2 mEq Na and 2 mEq acetate/ml).	Source of hydrogen acceptors in acidotic states; hyponatremia.	
Sodium Bicarbonate	4, 4.2, 5, 7.5, 8.4% solutions equivalent to 480, 500, 595, 892, 1000 mEq/liter respectively	Metabolic acidosis; to alkalinize the urine to hasten excretion in certain drug intoxications; severe diarrhea	Contraindicated in Cl loss due to vomiting or continuous GI suction and in diuretics producing hypochloremic alkalosis. Be aware of contraindications and warnings with use of sodium. Rapid injection of hypertonic solns. in children under 2 yrs may produce hypernatremia, decrease in CSF pressure, and possible intracranial hemorrhage. Precipitation or haze may result from sod. bicarbonate-calcium mixtures. Alkalosis may result from overdose.
Sodium Chloride Intravenous Infusions	0.45%, 0.9%, 3%, 5% NaCl	The 0.45% and 0.9% solns. are used for fluid and/or NaCl loss; the 3 or 5% solns. are used for hyponatremia and hypochloremia	Contraindicated in congestive heart failure or severe renal impairment and in edema with sodium retention. Administer with caution to patients with decompensated cardiovascular, cirrhotic, or nephrotic disease and in patients receiving corticosteroids. To avoid pulmonary edema, administer 3% or 5% solution slowly. Monitor plasma electrolytes.
Injection for Admixtures	50, 60, 100, 120 mEq	Electrolyte replacement	
Diluents	0.9% Injection; Bacteriostatic Injection	For dilution of other substances to be infused.	
Sodium Lactate	The 1/6 molar injection contains 167 mEq/l each of Na and lactate. Also available as 50 mEq and 120 mEq preps.	Alkalinizing agent. Metabolic acidosis.	

(Continued)

671

TABLE 33 PARENTERAL ELECTROLYTE, CARBOHYDRATE, OR PROTEIN SOLUTIONS (*Continued*)

Preparation	Information on Content	Use	Other Information
Sodium, Potassium, Ammonium Chlorides	Contains Na, 63 mEq/l; K, 17 mEq/l., NH₄, 70 mEq/l.; and Cl, 150 mEq/l.	Gastric fluid replacement.	Give only to patients with adequate renal function. Can be given SC or IV. Ascertain urinary output before starting as K content is high. Assess patient for clinical signs of electrolyte imbalance.
Tromethamine (Tham, Tham-E)	Contains 18 gm tromethamine (150 mEq)/500 ml. Tham-E contains Na, 30 mEq/l.; K, 5 mEq/l.; and Cl, 35 mEq/l and tromethamine.	Acts as a proton acceptor in acidotic states; used especially in cardiac bypass surgery and cardiac arrest.	Contraindicated in anuria and uremia. Large doses may depress ventilation. Exercise care to prevent perivascular infiltration. Overdosage may cause hypoglycemia. Do not administer for longer than 1 day except in life-threatening situations. Administer by slow IV infusion. Monitor blood values and urinary output during use.

Use Source of calories and essential fatty acids for prolonged parenteral nutrition (longer than 5 days). Fatty acid deficiency.

Contraindications Disturbances of fat metabolism (e.g., lipoid nephrosis, pathological hyperlipemia).

Untoward Reactions Sepsis, vein irritation, thrombophlebitis. Less frequently: allergic reactions, cyanosis, hyperlipemia, hypercoagulability, various GI and neurological symptoms. Delayed untoward reactions: splenomegaly, hepatomegaly, thrombocytopenia, leukopenia, disturbances in liver function tests, and overloading syndrome.

Dosage **IV,** as part of total parenteral nutrition regimen. **Maximum:** 2.5 gm/kg/day. **Pediatric maximum:** 4 gm/kg/day. The product should not exceed 60% of daily caloric intake. *Fatty acid deficiency:* 8% to 10% of caloric intake.

Administration/ Storage
1. Discard if oiling out occurs before administration.
2. May be given parenterally or centrally using a separate line, though it can be administered into same peripheral vein as carbohydrate-amino acid solutions using a Y-connection located near infusion site. Flow rate of each solution should be controlled separately by infusion pump. Do not use filters.
3. Do not mix with electrolytes, drugs, vitamins, or other nutrient solutions.
4. Start infusion slowly. **Adults:** 1 ml/min for first 15–30 minutes; **pediatric:** 0.1 ml/minute for first 10–15 minutes. If no untoward reaction occurs, increase rate to give **Adults:** 500 ml in 4 hours; **pediatric:** 1 gm/kg in 4 hours.
5. Give only 500 ml on day 1 (adults). If patient has no adverse reaction, dosage can be increased on subsequent days.
6. Store in refrigerator at 4°–8°C (39.2°–46.4°F).

Nursing Implications Observe patient closely for first 10 to 15 minutes of administration for allergic reaction to medication.

ACIDIFYING AGENTS

AMMONIUM CHLORIDE

Classification Urinary acidifying agent, electrolyte.

General Statement The ammonium ion is metabolized to urea liberating hydrogen ions that acidify the urine. Ammonium chloride also induces diuresis. The salt is rapidly absorbed from the GI tract. Prolonged administration, especially in patients with impaired kidney function, may cause severe metabolic acidosis. The full effect of the drug only becomes apparent after several days.

Uses Systemic acidifier used for the prevention or correction of metabolic alkalosis due to chloride ion loss caused by vomiting, gastric fistula drainage, gastric suction, excessive alkalinizing medication, or over-use of mercurial diuretics. To induce diuresis in premenstrual tension and Ménière's syndrome. Adjunct in the treatment of urinary calculi, lead poisoning, and bromism.

Contraindications Marked renal and hepatic impairment. Lack of accurate blood chemistry determinations.

Untoward Reactions Metabolic acidosis, sodium and potassium depletion, skin rash, headaches, hyperventilation, bradycardia, progressive drowsiness, mental confusion, phases of excitement alternating with coma, calcium deficiency, tetany, hyperglycemia, glycosuria, twitching, convulsions, hyperreflexia, EEG abnormalities. PO: also severe GI irritation (nausea, vomiting, anorexia, diarrhea).

Drug Interactions

Interactant	Interaction
Aminosalicylic acid	↑ Chance of aminosalicylic acid crystalluria
Amphetamine	↓ Effect of amphetamine by ↓ renal tubular reabsorption
Antidepressants, tricyclic	↓ Effect of tricyclics by ↓ renal tubular reabsorption
Salicylates	↑ Effect of salicylates by ↑ renal tubular reabsorption

Dosage **PO:** 4–12 gm daily in divided doses q 2 to 4 hr; **pediatric:** 75 mg/kg daily in 4 divided doses. Drug is more effective as diuretic when rest periods of a few days are part of regimen (i.e., 3 days on, 2 days off). *Premenstrual tension:* 1.5 gm b.i.d. for 4 to 5 days, premenstrually.

IV (*metabolic alkalosis*): *Highly individualized* and based on blood chemistry determinations (CO_2 combining power or chloride ion deficit). Always start with minimal dosage. **Usual, adults and children:** 10 ml/kg of 2.14% solution at a rate of 0.9–1.3 ml/minute up to 2 ml/minute.

Has also been administered by hypodermoclysis in infants and young children into the midlateral aspect of thigh because this area is less sensitive than frontal aspect of thigh.

Administration
1. PO: To minimize GI effects, give after meals or as enteric-coated tablets.
2. Administer liquid with acid juices, raspberry, or cherry syrup to mask saline taste.
3. Do not administer with milk or any other alkaline solution, because these are incompatible with ammonium chloride.
4. Parenteral: Carbon dioxide combining power and serum electrolytes should be monitored prior to and periodically during IV infusion so as to avoid serious acidosis.

Nursing Implications
1. Have on hand sodium bicarbonate or sodium lactate for treatment of electrolyte loss or acidosis.
2. Anticipate administration of potassium supplements if hypokalemia occurs.
3. Assess for untoward reactions.
4. Do not administer to patients with a history of liver impairment.
5. Anticipate intermittent administration of drug to maintain diuresis.
6. Discontinue administration at site of hypodermoclysis if pain occurs.

ALKALINIZING AGENTS

SODIUM BICARBONATE NEUT

Classification   Alkalinizing agent. See also page 709, *Drugs for the Treatment of Common Medical Conditions.*

Remarks   Sodium bicarbonate neutralizes hydrochloric acid by forming sodium chloride and carbon dioxide (1 gm of sodium bicarbonate neutralizes 12 mEq of acid).

Uses   As adjunct in sulfonamide therapy, treatment of metabolic acidosis, antacid, increases excretion of drugs by alkalinizing the urine, severe diarrhea.

Contraindications   Renal disease, congestive heart failure, patients on restricted sodium diet. Pyloric obstruction. Use with extreme caution for patients losing chloride through vomiting or continuous GI suction and in those in whom diuretics reduce hypochloremic alkalosis.

Untoward Reactions   Systemic alkalosis characterized by dizziness, abdominal cramps, thirst, anorexia, nausea, vomiting, diminished breathing, convulsions.

Drug Interactions

Interactant	*Interaction*
Amphetamine	↑ Effect of amphetamine by ↑ renal tubular reabsorption
Antidepressants, tricyclic	↑ Effect of tricyclics by ↑ renal tubular reabsorption
Erythromycin	↑ Effect of erythromycin in urine due to ↑ alkalinity of urine
Lithium carbonate	Excretion of Li is proportional to amount of sodium ingested. If patient on sodium-free diet, may develop Li toxicity since less Li is excreted
Methenamine compounds	↓ Effect of methenamine due to ↑ alkalinity of urine
Nitrofurantoin	↓ Effect of nitrofurantoin due to ↑ alkalinity of urine

Drug	*Interactant*	*Interaction*
Interactions		
(Continued)	Procainamide	↑ Effect of procainamide due to ↓ excretion by kidney
	Quinidine	↑ Effect of quinidine by ↑ renal tubular reabsorption
	Tetracyclines	↓ Effect of tetracyclines due to ↓ absorption from GI tract

Dosage   **PO** (*adjunct to sulfonamide therapy*): **initial,** 4 gm. **Maintenance:** 2 gm q 4 hr. *Metabolic acidosis:* Gastric lavage with 3%–5% solution; leave about 100 ml in stomach of patient. **IV:** *individualized,* 1.5% isotonic solution contains 15 gm of sodium bicarbonate/L (or 178 mEq of sodium and 178 mEq of bicarbonate).
   Cardiac arrest, **adults, IV:** 200–300 mEq bicarbonate as a 7.5%–8.4% solution.
      Infants up to 2 years, IV: 8 mEq/kg/day as a 4.2% solution.

Administration
1. Hypertonic solutions must be administered by the physician.
2. Isotonic solutions should be administered slowly as ordered as too rapid administration may result in death due to cellular acidity. Check rate of flow frequently.

Nursing Implications
1. Observe acidotic patients being treated with sodium bicarbonate for relief of dyspnea and hyperpnea and report because the drug must be discontinued when these conditions are relieved.
2. Observe acidotic patients being treated with sodium bicarbonate for edema since this may necessitate a change to potassium bicarbonate.

SODIUM LACTATE

Classification   Systemic alkalinizing agent.

General Statement   Sodium lactate is an effective acid-neutralizing agent because it removes hydrogen ions. It is converted in the liver to glycogen which is easily degraded to carbon dioxide and water. Sodium lactate also supplies sodium ions. Sodium bicarbonate is usually preferred as an alkalinizing agent.

Uses   Metabolic acidosis due to sodium deficiency resulting from vomiting, starvation, uncontrolled diabetes mellitus, acute infections or renal failure. Adjunct in sulfonamide therapy (alkalinization of urine).

Contraindications   Respiratory alkalosis, acidosis, accompanying congenital heart disease with persistent cyanosis.

Untoward Reactions   Metabolic acidosis (from overtreatment).

Dosage **IV.** *Highly individualized* and based on blood level of sodium ion. The following formula can be used to estimate correct dose:

$$\text{Dose in ml of 1.5 M sodium lactate (167 mEq/liter each of sodium and lactate ions)} = \frac{(60 - \text{plasma CO}_2) \times}{(0.8 \text{ body weight in pounds})}$$

Administration Administration rate should not exceed 300 ml/hour (60 drops/minute) of 1/6 M solution.

Nursing Implications Assess patient by observing clinical signs and laboratory results for electrolyte balance.

TROMETHAMINE THAM

Classification Systemic alkalinizing agent.

General Statement Tromethamine is an organic buffering substance that actively binds hydrogen ions, decreasing and correcting acidosis. It also increases urine flow, urinary pH, excretion of CO_2, and electrolytes. 75% of the drug is eliminated within 8 hours.

Uses Prevention and correction of systemic acidosis, especially that accompanying cardiac-bypass surgery and cardiac arrest.

Contraindications Uremia and anuria, pregnancy. Administer with caution to patients with renal disorders.

Untoward Reactions Transient decrease of blood glucose, respiratory depression, hyperkalemia, extravasation. Tests on blood pH, pCO_2, bicarbonate, glucose, electrolytes should be determined before, during, and after administration of tromethamine.

Dosage **IV:** Minimum amount to correct acid-base imbalance. The amount of tromethamine can be estimated using the following formula:

$$\text{ml of 0.3 M tromethamine solution required} = \text{body weight (kg)} \times \text{base deficit (mEq/liter)} \times 1.1$$

Acidosis in cardiac bypass surgery: 500 ml (150 mEq). Severe cases may require 1000 ml. *Acidosis in cardiac arrest* (given at the same time as other standard procedures are being applied): 3.5–6.0 ml/kg in a peripheral vein.

Administration 1. Concentration of solution administered *must not* exceed 0.3 M.
2. Prepare a 0.3 M solution of tromethamine by adding 1000 ml of sterile water for injection to 36 gm of lyophilized tromethamine.
3. Infuse slowly.
4. Administer into the largest antecubital vein through a large needle or indwelling catheter and elevate limb.

5. For treatment of cardiac arrest, the drug may be injected into the ventricular cavity if the chest is open. If the chest is not open, the drug may be injected into a large peripheral vein.
6. Do not administer longer than 1 day unless acute life-threatening situation exists.
7. Discontinue administration *immediately*, if extravasation occurs. The treatment for extravasation is administration of 1% procaine hydrochloride with hyaluronidase to reduce venospasm and dilute drug in local tissues. Phentolamine mesylate (Regitine) has been used for local infiltration for its adrenergic blocking properties. If necessary, a nerve block of the autonomic fibers may be done.

Nursing Implications

1. Assess for respiratory depression.
2. Have mechanical equipment for mechanical ventilation readily available.
3. Assess for weakness, moist pale skin, tremors, and a full bounding pulse, symptoms of hypoglycemia following rapid or high dosage of drug.
4. Ascertain that blood chemistries are done before, during, and after administration of drug and monitor results.
5. Assess for nausea, diarrhea, tachycardia (later bradycardia), oliguria, weakness, numbness or tingling, symptoms of hyperkalemia, more likely to occur in patients with impaired renal function.

POTASSIUM REMOVING RESIN

SODIUM POLYSTYRENE SULFONATE KAYEXALATE

Classification Ion exchange resin (potassium).

General Statement Sodium polystyrene sulfonate is a resin that exchanges sodium ions for potassium ions. The exchange primarily takes place in the large intestine. Treatment with the resin is not very quantitative. Too much or too little potassium, and to a lesser extent, calcium and magnesium may be removed. Thus, the patient's electrolytes must be monitored very carefully to avoid hyperkalemia or hypokalemia, hypocalcemia, or hypomagnesemia. Sorbitol is often administered concurrently to prevent constipation.

The therapy with sodium polystyrene sulfonate is governed by serum potassium levels, which must be determined daily. Discontinue therapy when potassium levels have reached 4–5 m Eq/liter.

Serum calcium determinations should be performed when therapy exceeds 3 days.

Uses Adjunct in treatment of hyperkalemia due to acute renal shutdown.

Contraindications Use with caution for patients sensitive to sodium overload (cardiovascular diseases) or for those receiving digitalis preparations since the action of these agents is potentiated by hypokalemia.

Untoward Reactions Fecal impaction, constipation, sodium retention, edema, hypokalemia, hypocalcemia, hypomagnesemia. GI effects: anorexia, nausea, vomiting, diarrhea. Overhydration, pulmonary edema.

Drug Interactions

Interactant	Interaction
Aluminum hydroxide	↑ Chance of intestinal obstruction
Aluminum or magnesium-containing antacids or laxatives	Systemic alkalosis and ↓ effect of exchange resin

Dosage **PO (preferred):** 15 gm suspended in 150–200 ml water 1 to 4 times daily (1 gm of resin contains 4.1 mEq sodium) Sorbitol: 10–20 ml of 70% solution q 2 hr initially, **then** so adjusted that 2 diarrheal stools are produced daily. *High retention enema:* 30 gm suspended in 100–200 ml of 1% methylcellulose solution, 10% dextrose, or 25% sorbital solution.

Administration/ Storage
1. Give resin suspended in a small amount of water or syrup (3–4 ml/gm resin). If necessary, resin can be administered through a nasogastric tube, either as aqueous suspension, mixed with dextrose, or as a peanut or olive oil emulsion.
2. Rectal administration:
   a. First administer cleansing enema.
   b. To administer medication insert soft large-size rubber tube (French 28) into rectum for distance of 20 cm until well into sigmoid colon and tape in place.
   c. Suspend resin into 100 ml or less of vehicle (see *Dosage*) at body temperature. Administer by gravity while stirring suspension.
   d. Flush suspension that remains in container with 50–100 ml fluid, clamp tube, and leave in place.
   e. Elevate hips—or ask patient to assume knee-chest position (for a short time)—if there is back leakage.
   f. Enema should be kept in colon as long as possible (3 to 4 hours).
   g. Resin is removed by colonic irrigation with 2 quarts of a *non-sodium* containing solution warmed to body temperature. Returns are drained constantly through a Y-tube.
3. Use freshly prepared solutions within 24 hours. Do not heat resin.

Nursing Implications
1. Assess for clinical signs of electrolyte imbalance related to magnesium, calcium, sodium, and potassium, and monitor blood chemistries.
2. Monitor intake and output.
3. Report increased urinary output because this may be an indication of increased potassium excretions, and the use of sodium polystyrene sulfonate may be contraindicated.
4. Encourage patient to retain medication rectally for several hours.

CHAPTER 10
HISTAMINES/ ANTIHISTAMINES

Azatadine Maleate
Bromodiphenhydramine Hydrochloride
Brompheniramine Maleate
Carbinoxamine Maleate
Chlorpheniramine Maleate
Clemastine Fumarate
Cyclizine Hydrochloride
Cyclizine Lactate
Cyproheptadine Hydrochloride
Dexchlorpheniramine Maleate
Dimenhydrinate
Dimethindene Maleate

Diphenhydramine Hydrochloride
Diphenylpyraline Hydrochloride
Doxylamine Succinate
Meclizine Hydrochloride
Methdilazine Hydrochloride
Promethazine Hydrochloride
Pyrilamine Maleate
Trimeprazine Tartrate
Tripelennamine Citrate
Tripelennamine Hydrochloride
Triprolidine Hydrochloride

General Statement

Antihistamines antagonize the action of histamine, which plays a crucial role in allergic reactions. Histamine is found stored in almost every type of tissue in the body. It is released from the tissue into the vascular system on the action of certain stimuli; that is, tissue injury, antigen-antibody reactions (allergic reactions), and extreme cold. When released into the vascular system, histamine has the following effects:

1. Dilation and increased permeability of the small arterioles, capillaries, and precapillaries, which result in increased permeability to fluid. This causes a fall of blood pressure in humans. The outflow of fluid into the subcutaneous spaces results in edema. The local edema in the nasal mucosa caused by histamine is responsible for the nasal congestion associated with allergies. It may also cause laryngeal edema.
2. Histamine contracts some smooth muscles such as those in the bronchioles; the resulting bronchoconstriction is believed to account for the role histamine plays in bronchial asthma. Histamine also causes the uterus to contract.
3. Histamine stimulates acid secretion in the stomach. It is used diagnostically to stimulate the gastric glands to test gastric function. It also increases bronchial, intestinal, and mild salivary secretions.
4. Histamine dilates cerebral vessels, and small doses can cause an intense headache.
5. Histamine causes pain and itch because it stimulates the sensory nerve endings.

Several histamine-induced reactions (anaphylactic shock) and severe attacks of asthma are treated with epinephrine, which produces effects diametrically opposed to the action of histamine or corticosteroids which alter the response of the patient to asthma-inducing agents. Less severe reactions can often be controlled by antihistamines.

Histamine phosphate is used for the diagnosis of pheochromocytoma and achlorhydria.

ANTIHISTAMINES

The group of drugs commonly referred to as antihistamines are used to antagonize the action of histamine on peripheral structures; they therefore completely or wholly prevent increased capillary permeability leading to edema, itching, and smooth muscle contraction, which may lead to bronchospasms. Antihistamines do not prevent histamine release from tissues.

Some antihistamines resemble histamine from a chemical point of view. These agents fall into several categories and seem to act by competing for receptor sites of the cells involved in initiating the allergic response.

The antihistamines do not control all of the untoward effects of histamine. Even though they usually prevent edema formation and itching associated with allergic reactions, they are ineffective in controlling hypotension and increased gastric secretion. The antihistamines are not effective against allergic reactions that are not caused by histamine release.

The antihistamines also have a CNS depressant effect. Although mostly annoying (drowsiness), the effect is sometimes used therapeutically in the treatment of parkinsonism and insomnia. Many of the antihistamines also abolish motion sickness, nausea, and vertigo and are used for this purpose.

There are many antihistamines on the market. They are very similar in their overall actions and will be treated as a group.

The duration of action of most antihistamines is 4 to 6 hours for a single dose, although most piperazines have a longer duration of action. Many antihistamines are also available as timed-released preparations.

The antihistamines can be subdivided chemically as follows. The most outstanding characteristics of each subgroup are listed; the group to which individual drugs belong is given in Table 34.

1. **Ethylenediamine Derivatives.** The CNS depressant effect of this group of drugs is weak and thus they cause less drowsiness than other antihistamines. They frequently cause GI distress. Tripelennamine (Pyribenzamine) belongs to this group.
2. **Ethanolamine Derivatives.** Group most likely to cause CNS depression (drowsiness). Low incidence of GI side effects. Also effective as antiemetics. Diphenhydramine (Benadryl) belongs to this group.
3. **Alkylamines.** Members of this group are among the most useful antihistamines. They are effective at relatively low dosage and are most suitable agents for daytime use. They can cause both CNS stimulation and depression (paradoxical excitation and drowsiness). Individual response to agents is variable. Chlorpheniramine maleate (ChlorTrimeton) is a member of this group.

4. **Phenothiazines** (see also *Phenothiazines*, Chapter 5, Section 8). Mostly used for their CNS depressant effect. Promethazine hydrochloride (Phenergan) is a member of this group.

5. **Piperazines.** Members of this group have prolonged antihistaminic activity, with a comparatively low incidence of drowsiness. However, their CNS depressant effect affects the alertness of the patient sufficiently to make the operation of dangerous machinery (driving) hazardous.

6. **Miscellaneous Agents.**

Uses   Symptomatic relief of allergic symptoms caused by histamine release. Nasal congestion accompanying allergic rhinitis, hay fever, and the common cold.

Symptomatic treatment of allergic dermatoses, drug-induced allergic skin reactions, atopic dermatitis, contact dermatitis, pruritus ani, vulvae, and insect bites.

Angioneurotic edema, blood transfusion reaction, Ménière's disease, and serum sickness.

Topical application may relieve vernal (seasonal) conjunctivitis and hypersensitivity to ophthalmic medications.

Allergic reactions to other drugs may respond to antihistamines.

Topical or local anesthetic during certain diagnostic procedures.

The CNS-depressant effect of certain of the drugs has proven helpful in the treatment of parkinsonism and drug-induced extrapyramidal reactions. They decrease rigidity and improve speech and voluntary movements.

The antifungistatic activity of certain members of the group has been used for the treatment of tinea pedia (athlete's foot).

Contraindications   Hypersensitivity to the drug, narrow-angle glaucoma, prostatic hypertrophy, stenosing peptic ulcer, and pyloroduodenal or bladder neck obstruction.

Pregnancy, or possibility thereof (some agents), lactation, premature or newborn infants. Administer with caution to patients with convulsive disorders.

Untoward Reactions   CNS depression: sedation ranging from mild drowsiness to deep sleep. Dizziness, lassitude, disturbed coordination, muscular weakness.

Paradoxical excitation (especially in children) including: restlessness, insomnia, tremors, euphoria, nervousness, delirium, palpitations, and even convulsions.

Antihistamines can precipitate epileptiform seizures in patients with focal lesions.

GI effects: epigastric distress, dryness of mouth, anorexia, nausea, vomiting, and diarrhea or constipation.

Miscellaneous effects: allergic hypersensitivity reactions, including skin rashes and photosensitization. These occur most frequently after topical administration.

Also xerostomia, dysuria, impotence, vertigo, visual disturbances, tinnitus, tightness of the chest, sweating, hypotension or hypertension, tachycardia, personality changes, headache, faintness, and paresthesia.

TABLE 34 COMMON ANTIHISTAMINES

Drug	Type	Dosage	Remarks
Azatadine maleate (Optimine)	5	**PO:** 1–2 mg b.i.d. Use lower dosage in elderly	Has prolonged action. Used for allergic rhinitis and chronic urticaria. Should not be used in patients with asthma or children under 12 years of age, pregnancy, lactation.
Bromodiphenhydramine HCl (Ambodryl)	2	**PO, adult:** 25 mg t.i.d. up to 150 mg daily.	
Brompheniramine maleate (Bromatane, Dimetane, Puretane, Spentane, Symptom 3, Veltane)	3	**PO, adults:** 4–8 mg t.i.d.-q.i.d. or 8–12 mg of sustained release b.i.d.; **pediatric, infants–6 years:** 0.5 mg/kg daily or 15 mg/m²/day in divided doses; **6 years and above:** ½ adult dose. **IM, IV, SC, adult:** 10 mg q 6 to 12 hr. **maximum:** 40 mg daily; **children under 12 years:** 0.5 mg/kg/day or 15 mg/m²/day in divided doses.	Can be given parenterally. Causes mild drowsiness. Do not use solution containing preservatives for IV injection.
Carbinoxamine maleate (Clistin)	2	**Adult:** 4 mg, 3 to 4 times/day, *long-acting:* 8–12 mg q 6–12 hours; **pediatric:** 2 to 4 mg t.i.d.-q.i.d.	Low incidence of side effects; causes drowsiness, dizziness, dryness of mouth, and GI distress.
Chlorpheniramine maleate (Ahbid, Allerbid, Allerid O.D., Alermine, Allermine, Antagonate, Chlo-Amine, Chloramate, Chlor-Hab, Chlor-Mal, Chlorophen, Chlorspan, Chlortab, Chlor-Trimeton, Ciramine, Histaspan, Histex, Histrey, Kloromin, Phenetron, Ru-Hist, T. D. Alermine, Pyranistan, Teldrin, Trymegen)	3	**PO, adults:** 2–4 mg t.i.d.-q.i.d.; **pediatric:** 1–2 mg t.i.d.-q.i.d. **Sustained Release:** 8–12 mg at bedtime or q 8 to 10 hr during day; **pediatric 6–12 years:** 8 mg during day or at bedtime. **SC, IM, IV** (see *Remarks*): 10–20 mg; dose may be increased to 40 mg in 24 hr; **pediatric, SC:** 0.35 mg/kg/day in 4 divided doses.	Low incidence of side effects; drowsiness. The drug can be administered parenterally as prophylaxis to drug reactions or blood transfusion. Only preparation *without* preservative may be given IV. If drugs are compatible, chlorpheniramine may be administered in same syringe. Chlorpheniramine for injection *without* preservative may be added directly to blood transfusion. Not recommended for children under 6 years of age.

Drug		Dosage	Comments
Clemastine Fumarate (Tavist)	5	**PO:** 2.68 mg 1 to 3 times/day. Not to exceed 8.04 mg/day. *Long-acting:* **initial,** 1.34 mg b.i.d. Not to exceed 8.04 mg/day.	Do not use in children under 12 years of age. Frequently causes drowsiness.
Cyclizine hydrochloride (Marezine Hydrochloride) Cyclizine lactate (Marezine Lactate)	5	**PO:** 50 mg t.i.d.-q.i.d. up to maximum of 200 mg daily; **pediatric 6–10 years:** ½ adult dose (24 hr). **IM:** 50 mg t.i.d.-q.i.d. or as required; **pediatric 6–10 years:** 1 mg/kg t.i.d. (24 hr).	Contraindicated in pregnancy. May cause drowsiness, dizziness, hyperirritability. Used widely as an antiemetic.
Cyproheptadine hydrochloride (Cyprodine, Periactin)	5	**PO:** 4–20 mg daily. Not to exceed 0.5 mg/kg daily; **pediatric (use for maximum of 6 months) 2–6 years:** 2 mg t.i.d. not to exceed 12 mg daily; **6–14 years:** 4 mg t.i.d. Not to exceed 16 mg daily	Contraindicated in glaucoma and urinary retention. Particularly indicated for treatment of pruritic dermatoses, angioedema, migraine. Resembles phenothiazines. May cause drowsiness, dryness of mouth.
Dexchlorpheniramine maleate (Polaramine)	3	**PO:** 2 mg t.i.d.-q.i.d. **Sustained release:** 4–6 mg b.i.d. **Pediatric under 12 years:** ½ adult dose; **infants:** ¼ adult dose. (Do not use sustained release)	May cause mild drowsiness.
Dimenhydrinate (Dimenest, Dimentabs, Dramamine, Reidamine, others)	2	**PO:** 50–100 mg q 4 hr; **pediatric 8–12 years:** 25–50 mg t.i.d. **Rectal:** 100 mg 1 to 2 times/day. **IM, IV:** 50 mg.	Widely used against motion sickness; may cause drowsiness. May mask ototoxicity due to aminoglycoside antibiotics (Gentamicin, Kanamycin, Neomycin, Streptomycin)
Dimethindene maleate (Forhistal Maleate, Triten)	3	**PO, adults and children over 6 years:** 2.5 mg 1 to 2 times daily.	Particularly useful in pruritus (allergic and nonallergic). May cause drowsiness, various GI manifestations, dry mouth, urinary frequency.
Diphenhydramine hydrochloride (Benachlor, Benadryl, Bendylate, Benahist, Benaject, Benylin, Diphen, Diphen-Ex, Diphenallin, Diphenadril, Eladryl, Fenylhist, Habdryl, Hydrexin, Nordryl, Phen-Amin, SK-Diphenhydramine, Tusstat, Valdrene, Wehdryl)	2	**PO, adults, usual,** 25–50 mg t.i.d.-q.i.d. **IV and IM:** 10–50 mg up to maximum single dose of 100 mg. **Maximum daily dose:** 400 mg. **Pediatric: IV, IM:** 5 mg/kg or 150 mg/m² /day divided into 4 doses during 24-hour period up to maximum of 300 mg/day. **PO:** 12.5–25 mg t.i.d. or 5 mg/kg/day.	Can be given parenterally (avoid SC) and topically. Also used for motion sickness and emotionally disturbed children. Protect from light. Drowsiness decreases with usage. May affect blood pressure when given parenterally.

(Continued)

685

TABLE 34 COMMON ANTIHISTAMINES (*Continued*)

Drug	Type	Dosage	Remarks
Diphenylpyraline hydrochloride (Diafen, Hispril)	6	**PO adults and children 6–12 years:** 2 mg t.i.d.-q.i.d.; **sustained release:** 5 mg 1 to 2 times/day; **under 6 years:** 1–2 mg 1 to 2 times daily. Do not exceed 4 mg daily or use sustained release form.	Low incidence of side effects; drowsiness, headaches, dizziness, dry mouth.
Doxylamine succinate (Decapryn)	2	PO: 12.5–25 mg q 4 to 6 hr; **pediatric 6–12 years:** 6.25–12.5 mg q 4 to 6 hr.	High degree of sedation.
Meclizine hydrochloride (Antivert, Bonine, Wehvert)	5	PO, *motion sickness:* 25–50 mg daily. *Vertigo:* 25–100 mg daily in divided doses.	Mostly used for motion sickness. May cause drowsiness, dry mouth, blurred vision
Methdilazine hydrochloride (Tacaryl Hydrochloride)	4	PO: 8 mg b.i.d.-q.i.d.; **Pediatric, infants:** 2 mg b.i.d.; **over 3 years:** 4 mg b.i.d.	Indicated for allergic and nonallergic pruritus. Tablet must be chewed properly. May cause drowsiness. See also *Phenothiazines.*
Promethazine hydrochloride (Fellowzine, Ganphen, Historest, K-Phen, Phenazine, Pentazine, Phencen, Phenergan, Phenoject, Promethamead, Prorex, Protha-	4	**PO:** 12.5 mg in AM or when necessary, and 25 mg at bedtime. Can be given as suppository (25 mg) or parenterally. **IM or IV:** 12.5–25 mg; can be repeated after 2 hrs if necessary. **Pediatric:** 0.13 mg/kg in	Very potent antihistamines with prolonged action. Also used as sedative and for motion sickness. Severe drowsiness. Also see *Phenothiazines.* Because of high

zine, Provigan, Quadnite, Remsed, V-Gan-50, Zipan)		AM and when necessary; 0.5 mg/kg at bedtime.	incidence of side effects, use cautiously in ambulatory patients.
Pyrilamine maleate (Allertoc, Zem-Histine)	1	**PO, adults: 25–100 mg b.i.d.-q.i.d.; pediatric 6–12 years: 12.5–25 mg q.i.d.**	
Trimeprazine tartrate (Temaril)	4	**PO:** 2.5 mg q.i.d.; **pediatric younger than 3 years:** 1.25 mg t.i.d.; **maximum:** 5 mg daily; **3–12 years:** 2.5 mg q.i.d.; **maximum:** 10 mg daily. Do not give timed-release capsule to children younger than 7 years of age.	Symptomatic relief of acute and chronic pruritus. Also see *Phenothiazines*. May cause drowsiness (decreasing with usage), dizziness, dry mouth.
Tripelennamine citrate (PBZ Citrate) Tripelennamine hydrochloride (PBZ Hydrochloride, PBZ-SR)	1	Dose based on HCl salt. **PO, adult: 25–50 mg q 4 to 6 hours; pediatric: 5 mg/kg/day or 150 mg/m²/day in divided doses. Maximum daily dose:** 300 mg. **Sustained Release, adults:** 100 mg in AM and PM; **children over 5 years:** 50 mg in AM and PM.	Citrate more palatable than hydrochloride. Low incidence of side effects: moderate sedation, mild GI distress, paradoxical excitation, hyperirritability.
Triprolidine hydrochloride (Actidil)	3	**PO, adults:** 2.5 mg b.i.d.-t.i.d.; **pediatric 4 months–2 years:** 0.3 mg t.i.d.-q.i.d.; **2–4 years:** 0.6 mg t.i.d.-q.i.d.; **4–6 years:** 0.9 mg t.i.d.-q.i.d. **Up to 6 years:** use syrup only; **6–12 years:** ½ adult dose.	Rapid onset; low incidence of side effects. May cause drowsiness, dizziness, GI distress, paradoxical excitation, hyperirritability.

Blood dyscrasias have been reported very infrequently.

Prolonged topical application of antihistamines is not recommended because the sensitized skin of allergic-type patients may be further sensitized by continuous application of such agents (rebound effect).

Topical preparations should not be applied to denuded or weeping areas.

Antihistamines should be discontinued prior to skin testing procedures.

Acute Toxicity   Antihistamines have a wide therapeutic range. Overdosage can nevertheless be fatal. Children are particularly susceptible. Overdosage can cause both CNS overstimulation and depression. The overstimulation is characterized by hallucinations, incoordination, and tonic-clonic convulsions. Fixed, dilated pupils, flushing, and fever are common in children. Cerebral edema, deepening coma and respiratory collapse occur usually within 2 to 18 hours.

Overdosage in adults usually starts with severe CNS depression. Treatment of overdosage is symptomatic and supportive. Respiratory stimulants given during depression may only hasten the onset of convulsions. A short-acting depressant, such as sodium thiopental (Pentothal) may be used IV to treat convulsions.

Dosage   **Usually PO.** See Table 34, p. 684. Parenteral administration is seldom used because of irritating nature of drugs.

Topical usage is also limited because antihistamines often cause hypersensitivity reactions. When given for motion sickness, antihistamines are usually given 30 to 60 minutes before anticipated travel.

Drug Interactions

Interactant	Interaction
Alcohol, ethyl	See *CNS Depressants*
Antidepressants, tricyclic	Additive anticholinergic side effects
CNS depressants	Potentiation or addition of CNS depressant effects. Concomitant use may lead to drowsiness, lethargy, stupor, respiratory depression, coma, and possibly death
Antianxiety agents	
Barbiturates	
Narcotics	
Phenothiazines	
Sedative-hypnotics	
Methotrimeprazine (Levoprome)	See *CNS Depressants*
Monoamine Oxidase Inhibitors	Intensification and prolongation of anticholinergic side effects.

Administration   1. Inject IM preparations deep into the muscle because preparations tend to be irritating to tissue.
2. Decrease GI side effects by administering with meals or with milk.

Nursing Implications

1. Caution the patient against driving a car or operating other machinery until response to medication (drowsiness) has worn off. Sedative effect may disappear spontaneously after several days administration.
2. Use side rails for patients sedated with antihistamines.
3. Assist patients experiencing dizziness, lassitude, or weakness.
4. Advise the patient to report side effects to physician, who may change dose or order another antihistamine which may have less side effects for this particular patient. The patient should not discontinue medication without consulting physician.
5. Advise the patient to consult with physician before taking any depressants because antihistamines tend to potentiate other CNS depresants.
6. Caution the patient to store antihistamines out of the reach of children because large doses may be fatal.

11 VITAMINS

Vitamin A	Vitamin A	
Vitamin B Complex	Calcium Pantothenate Cyanocobalamin Cyanocobalamin Crystalline Folic Acid Leucovorin Calcium Hydroxocobalamin	Nicotinamide Nicotinic Acid Pyridoxine Hydrochloride Riboflavin Thiamine Hydrochloride
Vitamin C	Ascorbate Calcium Ascorbate Sodium	Ascorbic Acid
Vitamin D	Vitamin D	Calcitrol
Vitamin E	Vitamin E	
Vitamin K	Menadiol Sodium Diphosphate Menadione	Phytonadione

General Statement

Vitamins are essential for the normal metabolic functioning of the body. A normal diet usually provides enough vitamins for a healthy individual. However, there are some situations and disease states, such as malabsorption syndromes or blood dyscrasias, in which supplemental vitamins may be of value.

The minimum daily requirement (MDR) for most vitamins has been determined, and is often used as a standard. The abbreviations RDDA and RDA (recommended daily dietary allowance) are also often used on the labels of vitamin preparations. There is no advantage in giving patients excessive amounts of vitamins. Vitamins are also usually prescribed during pregnancy and for children during maximum periods of growth.

Vitamins are divided into fat-soluble (A, D, E, K) and water-soluble (B, C) vitamins.

In addition to vitamins listed in this section the body also requires small amounts of certain minerals such as iodine, magnesium, iron, calcium, phosphorus, copper, zinc, manganese.

Nursing Implications

1. Encourage patients to eat a nutritionally sound diet.
2. Be prepared to discuss the composition of a nutritious diet and foods that may be substituted on low cost diets, as well as how a diet may be adapted to meet a patient's particular physiologic and cultural needs. (See Table 35 for foods high in specific vitamins and minerals.)
3. Discuss how to read labels of vitamin preparations to ascertain that the recommended daily allowance is met and explain that such

TABLE 35   VITAMINS AND RELATED SUBSTANCES, FUNCTION, U.S. RDA FOR ADULTS AND FOOD SOURCE

Substance*	Needed For	Good Food Sources	Usual Therapeutic Dose
Vitamin A 4000–5000 I.U.	Helps to form and maintain healthy function of eyes, skin, hair, teeth, gums, various glands, and mucous membranes. It is also involved in fat metabolism. *Deficiency symptoms:* night blindness, hyperkeratosis of skin, xerophthalmia.	Whole milk, eggs, green leafy vegetables (e.g., spinach, kale, broccoli, turnip greens, brussel sprouts).	Up to 100,000 units/day
Vitamin B₁ (thiamine) 1.0–1.5 mg	Helps get energy from food by promoting proper metabolism of sugars. *Deficiency symptoms:* beriberi, peripheral neuritis, cardiac disease.	Milk, chicken, fish, red meat, liver, whole grain bread, green leafy vegetables.	5–30 mg/day
Vitamin B₂ (riboflavin) 1.1–1.8 mg	Functions in the body's use of carbohydrates, proteins and fats, particularly to release energy to cells. *Deficiency symptoms:* cheilosis, angular stomatitis, dermatitis, photophobia.	Milk, eggs, red meat, liver, whole grain, enriched bread, green leafy vegetables.	10–30 mg/day
Vitamin B₆ (pyridoxine) 1.6–2.0 mg	Has many important roles in protein metabolism. It also aids in the formation of red blood cells and proper function of the nervous system, including brain cells. *Deficiency symptoms:* seborrhea-like skin lesions; nerve inflammations, anemias, epileptiform convulsions in infants.	Green leafy vegetables, red meat, whole grains, green beans.	25–100 mg/day
Vitamin B₁₂ (cobalamin) 3.0 µg	Helps to build vital genetic material (nucleic acids) for cell nuclei, and to form red blood cells. Essential for normal function of all body cells, including brain and other nerve cells as well as tissues that make red cells. *Deficiency symptoms:* pernicious anemia	Milk, fish (salt water), red meat, liver, oysters, kidneys.	1–2 µg/day
Folic acid 0.4 mg	Assists in the formation of certain body proteins and genetic materials for the cell nucleus, and in the formation of red blood cells. *Deficiency symptoms:* macrocytic anemia (nutritional).	Green leafy vegetables, liver.	.1–15 mg/day

692

Vitamin	Function	Sources	Dosage
Pantothenic acid 10.0 mg	A key substance in body metabolism involved in changing carbohydrates, fats, and proteins into molecular forms needed by the body. Also required for formation of certain hormones and nerve regulating substances. *Deficiency symptoms* (rare): Fatigue, malaise, headache, sleep disturbance, cramps.	Eggs, green leafy vegetables, nuts, liver, kidneys.	Not known
Niacin (niacinamide) 13–20 mg	Present in all body tissues and is involved in energy-producing reactions in cells. *Deficiency symptom:* pellagra.	Eggs, red meat, liver, whole grain, whole grain enriched bread.	100–1000 USP units/day
Biotin 0.30 mg	It is involved in the formation of certain fatty acids and the production of energy from the metabolism of glucose. It is essential for the working of many chemical systems in the body.	Eggs, green leafy vegetables, string beans, kidneys, liver.	
Vitamin C 45 mg	To help form and keep bones, teeth and blood vessels healthy. It is also important in the formation of collagen, a protein that helps support body structures such as skin, bone and tendon. *Deficiency symptom:* scurvy (hemorrhages, loose teeth, gingivitis)	Potatoes, green leafy vegetables, lemons, tomatoes, oranges, green peppers, strawberries, cantaloupes.	100–1000 mg/day
Vitamin D (including D_2 and D_3) 400 I.U.	For strong teeth and bones. To help the body use calcium and phosphorus properly. *Deficiency symptoms:* infantile rickets, infantile tetany, osteomalacia	Milk, egg yolks, tuna, salmon, cod liver oil.	400–1600 USP units/day
Vitamin E (tocopherol) 12–15 I.U.	To help normal red blood cells, muscle and other tissues. Protects fat in the body's tissue from abnormal breakdown. *Deficiency symptoms:* abnormal fat deposits, creatinuria, macrocytic anemia (when associated with protein deficiency).	Vegetable oil, whole grains.	Not established
Vitamin K (need in human nutrition established but levels have not yet been determined)	For normal blood clotting. *Deficiency symptoms:* hemorrhages, prolonged clotting time.	Green leafy vegetables	See drug entry

(Continued)

TABLE 35 VITAMINS AND RELATED SUBSTANCES, FUNCTION, U.S. RDA FOR ADULTS AND FOOD SOURCE
(Continued)

Substance*	Needed For	Good Food Sources	Usual Therapeutic Dose
Iron 10–18 mg	An essential part of hemoglobin, the protein substance which enables red cells to carry oxygen throughout the body. It is also part of certain important enzymes.	Red meat, egg yolk, liver, green vegetables (e.g., spinach, kale, broccoli, chard, turnip greens, brussel sprouts).	
Calcium 800–1200 mg	To help build strong bones and teeth. Also required for activity of nerve and muscle cells, including the heart, and for normal blood clotting	Milk, egg yolk, tuna, salmon, cheese.	
Phosphorus 800–1200 mg	Essential in building and maintaining strong teeth and bones, in quick release of energy, in muscle contraction, and in nerve function	Milk, fish, meat, whole grain.	
Iodine 100–150 μg	Forms an integral part of hormones produced by the thyroid gland, which is involved in the regulation of cell metabolism.	Seafoods (shrimp, oysters, fish) and iodized salt.	
Copper 2.0 mg	Is present in many organs, including the brain, liver, heart and kidneys. It occurs as part of important proteins, including certain enzymes involved in brain and red cell function. Also needed for making red blood cells.	Kidneys, nuts, raisins, chocolate, mushrooms.	
Magnesium 300–400 mg	Is an important constituent of all soft tissues and bones. It helps trigger many vital enzyme reactions in humans.	Broccoli, whole grain enriched bread, meat.	
Zinc 15 μg; Fluorine, Cobalt, Chromium, Selenium, Manganese, Molybdenum	Zinc considered essential every day for normal skeletal growth and tissue repair. Fluorine makes the teeth harder. Cobalt is an integral part of the vitamin B_{12} molecule. The others are needed in a wide variety of body functions.	Whole grains, broccoli, liver, meat, strawberries, oranges.	

* Values given are *Recommended Daily Allowances* for individuals over 11 years of age. National Academy of Sciences, 1974.

vitamins are usually satisfactory for supplementation, unless the physician orders larger doses of a vitamin.

4. Warn patients against overdosing themselves with vitamins.
5. Observe patients, particularly the young and the elderly, for symptoms of vitamin deficiencies, such as an inflamed tongue or cracks at the corner of the mouth and refer them to medical supervision. (See Table 35 for deficiency symptoms.)
6. Advise patients to store vitamins in a cool place in a light-resistant container to minimize loss of potency.
7. Advise patients not to take mineral oil at the same time that they ingest fat-soluble vitamins such as A, D, E, and K because the vitamins will be dissolved in the oil and not be absorbed by the body.
8. Caution patients on anticoagulant therapy not to take vitamin preparations containing vitamin K.

VITAMIN A ACON, ALPHALIN, AQUASOL A, DISPATABS, VI-DOM-A

Classification Fat-soluble vitamin.

General Statement Vitamin A deficiency can lead to night blindness, xerophthalmia, and, if prolonged, blindness. Vitamin A, as such, is only found in animal sources but the body can manufacture vitamin A from carotene. Excess vitamin A can lead to hypervitaminosis A (see *Untoward Reactions*), which is treated by withdrawal of the vitamin.

Uses Vitamin A deficiency and prophylaxis during periods of high requirement, such as infancy, pregnancy, and lactation. Supplements may also be required in patients with steatorrhea, severe biliary obstruction, cirrhosis of the liver, total gastrectomy and xerophthalmia, nyctalopis, certain hyperkeratoses of the skin, and lowered resistance to infection.

Untoward Reactions Hypervitaminosis A, characterized by pseudotumor cerebri, irritability, miosis, anorexia, loss of hair, dry skin, pruritus, tender extremities, hepatomegaly and spleenomegaly, roentgenographic evidence of elevation of the periosteum of the long bones, high serum vitamin A levels, increased serum lipids, hypoplastic anemia, leukopenia, clubbing of the fingers and advanced skeletal development.

Drug Interactions

Interactant	Interaction
Corticosteroids	Impairment of wound healing in patients receiving topical Vitamin A. Systemic Vitamin A may inhibit anti-inflammatory effect of systemic corticosteroids.
Oral contraceptives	Results in significant ↑ plasma Vitamin A

Dosage **PO, adults,** *severe deficiency:* 100,000 USP units daily for 3 days followed by 50,000 USP units daily for 2 weeks. **Follow-up:** 10,000–20,000 USP units daily for 2 months. **IM:** 100,000 I.U. daily for 3 days, followed by 50,000 I.U. daily for 2 weeks.

Children 1–8 years: 17,500– 35,000 I.U. daily for 10 days, **infants:** 7,500– 15,000 I.U. daily for 10 days.

VITAMIN B COMPLEX

General Statement
This large, assorted group of vitamins is usually considered together because all members are water soluble and all can be obtained from the same sources, such as yeast and liver. Since the individual vitamins have completely different functions, they shall be considered separately.

Drug Interaction
Anticoagulants (oral) may interact with B complex vitamins and cause hemorrhage.

CALCIUM PANTOTHENATE (VITAMIN B₅) PANTHOLIN

Classification
Vitamin B complex.

General Statement
This compound can replace pantothenic acid, an essential nutrient that participates in the metabolism of sugars, fats, and proteins (Krebs cycle).

Pantothenic acid deficiency in animals is characterized by neurological symptoms, keratitis, dermatitis, a fatty liver, and necrotic lesions of the adrenal cortex. Pantothenic acid deficiency in humans has never been diagnosed.

Uses
Although specific indications are absent, the drug has been used for the treatment of peripheral neuritis, muscular cramps, during pregnancy, for delirium tremens, systemic lupus erythematosus, and acute cataract disorders.

Contraindication
Hemophilia.

Untoward Reaction
Allergic symptoms have occurred occasionally.

Dosage
PO: 10 mg/day for approximate daily allowance; 20– 100 mg/day for experimental purposes.

CYANOCOBALAMIN (VITAMIN B₁₂) KAYBOVITE, RHODAVITE

CYANOCOBALAMIN CRYSTALLINE (VITAMIN B₁₂) BERUBIGEN, BETALIN 12, COBAVITE, COBEX 1000, CRYSTI-12, DODEX, HYDROXO-12, KAYBOVITE 1000, REDISOL, RUBESOL 1000, RUBRAMIN PC, RUVITE 1000, SYTOBEX, VI-TWELL

General Statement
Cyanocobalamin (Vitamin B₁₂) is a cobalt-containing substance produced by certain microorganisms, such as *Streptomyces griseus*. The vitamin can also be isolated from liver.

The action of cyanocobalamin is identical to that of the antianemic factor of liver.

This vitamin is essential for hematopoiesis, cell reproduction, nucleoprotein and myelin synthesis.

Products containing less than 500 μg vitamin B_{12} are not to be used for the treatment of pernicious anemia.

Uses
Pernicious anemia, tropical and nontropical sprue, nutritional macrocytic anemia due to vitamin B_{12} deficiency, certain types of megaloblastic anemia of infancy. Vitamin B_{12} is particularly suitable for the treatment of patients allergic to liver extract. Vitamin B_{12} sometimes provides quick relief in conditions associated with severe pain such as tic douloureux, and with certain forms of neuritis (alcoholic, diabetic, etc.) *Note:* Folic acid is not a substitute for vitamin B_{12} although concurrent folic acid therapy may be required.

Untoward Reaction
Hypersensitivity reactions probably caused by impurities.

Drug Interactions

Interactant	Interaction
Aminosalicyclic acid	↓ Vitamin B_{12} absorption
Chloramphenicol	Chloramphenicol ↓ response to vitamin B_{12} therapy
Neomycin	Neomycin ↓ response to vitamin B_{12} therapy

Dosage
Cyanocobalamin, **PO, adults,** *nutritional vitamin B_{12} deficiency:* 25 μg daily. *Cyanocobalamin Crystalline, vitamin B_{12} deficiency,* **PO:** 1,000 μg/day. *Patients with normal intestinal absorption:* 15 μg/day. **IM:** 30 μg/day for 5 to 10 days; **then** 100–200 μg/month **IM** or **SC** until remission is complete. Higher doses may be necessary in the presence of neurologic or infectious disease, or hyperthyroidism. *Schilling test:* 1000 μg **IM** (flusing dose).

Administration
Stable for 1 year in isotonic sodium chloride solution if kept sterile.

FOLIC ACID FOLVITE

LEUCOVORIN CALCIUM

Classification
Vitamin B complex.

General Statement
Folic acid is required for nucleoprotein synthesis (DNA) and the maintenance of normal levels of mature red cells (erythropoiesis). The vitamin is readily available in a great variety of foods, including liver, kidney, and leafy vegetables.

Uses
Megaloblastic and macrocytic anemia resulting from folic acid deficiency; nutritional macrocytic anemia, megaloblastic anemias of

pregnancy, infancy and childhood, and megaloblastic anemia associated with primary liver disease, intestinal obstruction, anastomoses, or sprue. Supplemental folic acid may also be required by patients on renal dialysis or receiving drugs that interfere with folic acid metabolism, such as methotrexate, phenytoin, and barbiturates.

Folic acid is sometimes administered in conjunction with vitamin B_{12} for the treatment of refractory or aplastic anemia.

Contraindication Administer with caution to patients with undiagnosed anemias, since improvement of blood picture may mask neurological complications of pernicious anemia.

Untoward Reactions Allergic responses, characterized by erythema, skin rash, itching, general malaise, respiratory difficulties, and bronchospasms have been observed occasionally.

High dosages (15 mg daily for 1 month or more) may cause GI distress (anorexia, nausea, abdominal distention, flatulence, and bad taste in mouth), altered sleep patterns, difficulty in concentration, irritability, overactivity, excitement, mental depression, confusion, and impaired judgment. Pernicious anemia may be obscured with doses of folic acid of 1 mg or more daily.

Drug Interaction *Folic acid* decreases phenytoin blood levels due to increased breakdown by liver.

Dosage *Folic acid,* **PO, usual,** 0.25–1 mg daily. **Maintenance (per day), infants:** 0.1 mg; **children 4 years and less:** 0.3 mg; **adults and children over 4 years:** 0.4 mg; **pregnancy or lactation:** 0.8 mg. The dose may need to be increased in alcoholics, and patients with hemolytic anemia, chronic infections, or anticonvulsant therapy.

Folic acid can be administered by deep **IM, SC, or IV** injection if **PO administration** is not feasible or malabsorption syndrome is suspected. *Leucovorin Calcium.* **IM,** 1 mg/day.

Administration/ Storage Store folic acid solutions in a cold place.

HYDROXOCOBALAMIN ALPHA REDISOL, ALPHA-RUVITE, CRYSTI-12 GEL, NEO-BETALIN 12, RUBESOL-LA 1000, SYTOBEX-H

Classification Vitamin B complex.

General Statement This compound can be converted to cyanocobalamin by the body and has the same therapeutic function as cyanocobalamin.

Hydroxocobalamin is absorbed more slowly from the injection site and its action is thought to be more prolonged.

Uses Same as cyanocobalamin.

Untoward Reactions   Pain at injection site, transient diarrhea; rarely allergic reaction.

Dosage   *Hydroxocobalamin Crystalline*, **IM only:** 30 μg/day for 5 to 10 days; **then,** 100 μg/month. Concurrent folic acid therapy may be required.

NICOTINOMIDE NIACINOMIDE

NICOTINIC ACID DIACIN, NIAC, NIACIN, NICALEX, NICO-400, NICOBID, NICOCAP, NICOLAR, NICOTINEX, TEGA-SPAN, TINIC, VASOTHERM, WAMPOCAP

Classification   Vitamin B complex.

General Statement   Nicotinic acid and nicotinamide are water-soluble, heat-resistant vitamins. They are prepared synthetically. They are specific for the treatment and prophylaxis of pellagra but do not alleviate the polyneuritis and cheilosis that frequently accompany the disease. Nicotinic acid also has vasodilating effects which may produce mild flushing, itching, and burning. Nicotinamide does not produce such side effects and is preferred when large doses or parenteral administration is required.

Uses   *Nicotinic acid:* pellagra or prophylaxis thereof. Headaches. Adjunct in treatment of vascular spasms, peripheral arteriosclerosis, angina pectoris, Raynaud's disease, varicose and decubital ulcers and other conditions associated with impaired blood and poor peripheral circulation. Hyperlipidemia.
    Nicotinamide: pellagra and prophylaxis thereof.

Drug Interaction

Interactant	*Interaction*
Sympathetic Blocking Agents	↑ Vasodilatory effect → postural hypotension.

Dosage   *Vitamin source,* **PO:** 0.5–3.0 gm/day in divided doses with or following meals. **SC, IM, IV:** *usual,* 300–500 mg/day (range 0.1–3.0 gm/day). *Hyperlipidemia,* **PO:** 1.5–6.0 gm/day in 3–4 doses.

Nursing Implications   1. Explain to patients that flushing is a frequent side effect.
2. Advise patients who feel weak and dizzy after taking niacin to lie down until they are feeling recovered and then to inform physician.

PYRIDOXINE HYDROCHLORIDE (VITAMIN B$_6$) BEESIX, HEXA-BETALIN, HEXACREST, HEXAVIBEX, PYROXINE

Classification   Vitamin B complex.

| General Statement | Pyridoxine hydrochloride is a water-soluble, heat resistant vitamin. It is destroyed by light. It is prepared synthetically. Its role in the body is not clearly understood, although it seems to be required for the metabolism of amino acids. |

General Statement — Pyridoxine hydrochloride is a water-soluble, heat resistant vitamin. It is destroyed by light. It is prepared synthetically. Its role in the body is not clearly understood, although it seems to be required for the metabolism of amino acids.

Uses — Irradiation sickness. Prophylaxis of isoniazid-induced peripheral neuritis. Infants with epileptiform convulsions. Hypochromic anemias due to familial pyridoxine deficiency, some cases of hypochromic or megaloblastic anemias.

Drug Interactions

Interactant	Interaction
Chloramphenicol	B_6 may prevent chloramphenicol-induced optic neuritis
Levodopa	Pyridoxine reverses levodopa-induced improvement in Parkinson's syndrome. Pyridoxine and vitamin preparations containing pyridoxine should be avoided in patients receiving levodopa

Dosage — *Dietary deficiency,* **PO, IM, IV:** 10–20 mg daily for 3 weeks; **then,** 2–5 mg/day for several weeks. *Adjunct in the administration of isoniazid:* 100 mg/day for 3 weeks; **then** 50 mg/day. *Vitamin B_6 dependency syndrome:* **initial,** up to 600 mg/day; **then** 50 mg/day for life.

RIBOFLAVIN (VITAMIN B₂)

Classification — Vitamin B complex.

General Statement — Riboflavin is a water-soluble, heat-resistant substance. It is sensitive to light. Riboflavin deficiency is characterized by characteristic lesions of the tongue, lips and face, photophobia, itching, burning and keratosis of the eyes. Riboflavin deficiency often accompanies pellagra.

Uses — Riboflavin deficiency. Adjunct, with niacin, in the treatment of pellagra.

Drug Interactions

Interactant	Interaction
Chloramphenicol	Riboflavin may counteract bone marrow depression and optic neuritis due to chloramphenicol
Tetracyclines	Antibiotic activity ↓ by riboflavin

Dosage — **PO, adults and children over 12 years of age:** 5–50 mg daily depending on severity of disease.

THIAMINE HYDROCHLORIDE (VITAMIN B₁) BETALIN S

Classification — Vitamin B complex.

Remarks   Water-soluble vitamin, stable in acid solution. The vitamin is decomposed in neutral or acid solutions.

Uses   Thiamine deficiency states and associated neurological and cardiovascular symptoms. Prophylaxis and treatment of beriberi. Alcoholic neuritis, neuritis of pellagra, and neuritis of pregnancy. To correct anorexia due to thiamine insufficiency.

Untoward Reaction   Parenteral administration of large doses may produce anaphylactic shock.

Drug Interaction   Since Vitamin B$_1$ is unstable in neutral or alkaline solutions, the vitamin should not be used with substances as citrates, barbiturates, or carbonates which yield alkaline solutions.

Dosage   **PO:** 5– 100 mg/day with meals. **IM** (*for beriberi*): 10– 20 mg t.i.d. for 2 weeks; **then, PO:** 5– 10 mg/day for 1 month. **IV** route used for beriberi with myocardial failure.

Additional Nursing Implication   Be prepared with epinephrine to treat anaphylactic shock should it occur after a large parenteral dose of thiamine.

VITAMIN C

ASCORBATE CALCIUM CALSCORBATE

ASCORBATE SODIUM CENOLATE, C-JECT, CEVITA, LIQUI-CEE

ASCORBIC ACID ASCOR, ASCORBAJEN, ASCORBICAP, BEST-C, CEBID, CECON, CEMILL, CETANE TIMED, CEVALIN, CEVI-BID, CE-VI-SOL, CEVITA, CHEW-CEE, C-LONG, FLAVORCEE, PROLONG 'C', SARO-C, TETA C-SYRUP-500, VITACEE, VITERRA C

Classification   Vitamin C.

General Statement   Vitamin C (ascorbic acid) is a specific antiscorbutic, antiscurvy substance. The vitamin is unstable and easily destroyed by air, light, and heat. Vitamin C is essential to the maintenance of the connective and supporting tissue of the body.

Vitamin C deficiency leads to scurvy, which is characterized by changes in the fibrous tissues, the matrix of dentine, bone, cartilage, and the vascular endothelium.

The stores of vitamin C in the body are depleted very rapidly and patients on IV feeding may develop ascorbic acid deficiency. This may cause a delay in healing in patients who have undergone surgery. Due to an increased rate of oxidation during infectious diseases, the daily requirements of vitamin C rise.

Uses Treatment of scurvy and prophylaxis thereof. Vitamin C supplementation is indicated for burn victims, debilitated patients, and as an adjunct in iron therapy and in patients on prolonged IV feedings.

Drug Interactions

Interactant	Interaction
Aminosalicylic acid	↑ Chance of aminosalicylic acid crystalluria
Amphetamine	↓ Effect of amphetamine by ↓ renal tubular reabsorption
Antidepressants, tricyclic	↓ Effect of tricyclics by ↓ renal tubular reabsorption
Digitalis	Calcium ascorbate may cause cardiac arrhythmias in patients receiving digitalis
Salicylates	↑ Effect of salicylates by ↑ renal tubular reabsorption
Sulfonamides	↑ Chance of crystallization of sulfonamides in urine

Dosage **PO,** *therapeutic:* 100–200 mg daily. *Prophylaxis:* 50 mg daily. **Pediatric, infants,** *therapeutic:* 30–50 mg daily. *Prophylaxis:* 10 mg daily. **IM, IV:** 200 mg/day up to 1–2 gm/day in severe deficiency. *Aid for burn patients:* 200–500 mg/day. *Pre-surgical in gastrectomy patients:* 1 gm/day 4 to 7 days before surgery.

Administration
1. Sodium ascorbate can be administered IM or IV.
2. Calcium ascorbate should never be injected SC. IM injection may cause tissue necrosis in infants.

VITAMIN D

CALCIFEROL, DELTALIN, DRISDOL, GELTABS

Classification Vitamin D.

General Statement Two compounds, cholecalciferol (vitamin D_3) and ergocalciferol (vitamin D_2) have vitamin D or antirachitic properties.

In addition, humans can convert many sterol compounds to vitamin D when exposed to sunlight (ultraviolet irradiation).

Fish liver oils and irradiated milk are an excellent source of vitamin D.

Vitamin D deficiency is characterized by inadequate absorption of calcium and phosphate. During periods of active growth, vitamin D deficiency may lead to rickets. In the adult, vitamin D deficiency may lead to osteomalacia (adult rickets).

Uses   Infantile rickets or prophylaxis thereof, spasmophilia and osteomalacia (adult rickets), hypoparathyroidism, infantile tetany.
Prophylaxis: Adjunct in diseases that may lead to vitamin D deficiency: diarrhea, steatorrhea, biliary obstruction, and other abnormalities of the GI tract that may interfere with absorption.

Untoward   Excess doses of vitamin D (150,000–300,000 units daily) over prolonged
Reactions   periods of time may lead to hypervitaminosis D. This condition may result in a mobilization of calcium from bone tissue, which in turn may lead to osteoporosis and pathological calcification of the soft tissues such as the kidney.
Early symptoms of hypervitaminosis D are anorexia, nausea, vomiting, diarrhea, bloody stools, polyuria, muscular weakness, lassitude and headaches.
Patients on prolonged, high-dosage vitamin D therapy should have regular Sulkowitch tests for urinary excretion of calcium.

Drug
Interactions

Interactant	*Interaction*
Mineral Oil	↓ Absorption of fat-soluble vitamins
Thiazide Diuretics	In hypoparathyroidism → hypercalcemia

Dosage   *Usual requirement:* 400 units daily; 800 units daily may be required during pregnancy and lactation. *Vitamin D resistant rickets,* **PO,** 12,000–500,000 units/day. *Osteomalacia,* **PO:** 10,000–50,000 units/day. *Familial hypophosphatemia:* 40,000–160,000 units/day. *Renal tubular reabsorption deficits:* 50,000–500,000 units daily. *Acute parathyroid tetany:* **initial,** 50,000–100,000 units/day. **Maintenance,** 25,000–100,000 units daily.

Nursing   Observe urine for cloudiness and red color—indications of toxicity
Implications when massive doses are used.

CALCITROL ROCALTROL

Classification   Vitamin D.

General   Calcitrol is the most active form of vitamin D_3. It stimulates intestinal
Statement   calcium transport as well as having an action on bone, the kidneys, and parathyroid gland. It is rapidly absorbed from the intestine and its effect lasts from 3 to 5 days.

Use   Hypocalcemia in patients on chronic renal dialysis.

Contraindications Hypercalcemia. Vitamin D toxicity. *Note:* Serum phosphate levels should also be controlled in patients undergoing dialysis. This may be accomplished by aluminum carbonate or hydroxide gels.

Untoward Reactions

Overdosage of vitamin D is potentially dangerous (See *Vitamin D*). Early signs of toxicity include hypercalcemia, fall in serum alkaline phosphatase, GI disturbances (nausea, vomiting, metallic taste, constipation, dry mouth), weakness, headache, and muscle and bone pain.

Drug Interactions

Interactant	Interaction
Cholestyramine	↓ Absorption of calcitrol from intestine
Digitalis	↑ Chance of cardiac arrhythmias due to hypercalcemia
Mg-containing Antacids	↑ Chance of hypermagnesemia

Treatment of Overdose

Immediate discontinuation of calcitrol therapy, institution of a low calcium diet, and withdrawal of any calcium supplements. In acute accidental overdosage, induction of emesis or gastric lavage is beneficial if the overdose is discovered within a short time; also, administration of mineral oil may increase fecal excretion of the drug.

Dosage

Highly individualized. Effectiveness of drug depends on adequate daily intake of calcium; thus, calcium supplements may be necessary. **PO:** Usual, **initial,** 0.25 µg/day. May be increased by 0.25 µg/day at 2 to 4 week intervals only after serum calcium levels determined. **Maintenance,** *hemodialysis patients:* 0.5–1.0 µg/day.

Nursing Implications

Teach patient and/or family to:

1. Have blood and urine tests performed periodically as ordered to evaluate calcium, magnesium, phosphorus, and alkaline phosphatase levels.
2. Avoid magnesium-containing antacids.
3. Withhold drug and report to medical supervision if weakness, nausea, vomiting, dry mouth, constipation, muscle pain, bone pain, or a metallic taste (early symptoms of vitamin D intoxication) occur.
4. Take medication in dosage prescribed since the dosage for each patient is highly individualized.
5. Adhere to diet and calcium supplementation recommended.
6. Avoid non-prescription medications unless prescribed by medical supervision.

VITAMIN E

VITAMIN E (TOCOPHEROL, TOCOPHEROL ACETATE) AQUASOL E, D-ALPHA-E, E-FEROL, EPROLIN, EPSILAN-M, HY-E-PLEX, KELL-E, LETHOPHEROL, MAXI-E, PRO-COTE E, TOCOPHER-CAPS, TOCOPHER-400, TOCOPHER-PLUS, TOKOLS, VITERRA E

Classification   Vitamin E.

General Statement Vitamin E refers to a group of fat-soluble substances including alpha-, beta-, gamma, and delta-tocopherol. The exact physiological function of vitamin E is difficult to ascertain. Deficiency symptoms have been studied mainly in animals.

The usefulness of the vitamin for therapeutic purposes is questionable. However, it is consumed in large amounts by food faddists.

Uses Vitamin E deficiency (only established use), macrocytic megaloblastic anemia in children, hemolytic anemia in premature infants.

Contraindications None known.

Untoward Reactions Large doses over prolonged periods may cause skeletal muscle weakness, disturbances of reproductive functions, and GI upset.

Drug Interaction Vitamin E decreases the response to iron therapy.

Dosage **Usual,** RDA, **children 4–6 years:** 9 IU; **adult males:** 15 IU; **adult females:** 12 IU. **Pregnancy or lactation:** 15 IU. *Note:* potencies of products differ widely; thus the dosage should be based on International Units.

VITAMIN K

Classification Vitamin K.

General Statement Vitamin K is essential for the biosynthesis of prothrombin and other blood clotting factors by the liver. The chief manifestation of vitamin K deficiency is an increase in bleeding tendency. This is demonstrated by ecchymoses, epistaxis, hematuria, GI bleeding, postoperative and intracranial hemorrhage.

Vitamin K is available as a water-soluble (some salts of menadione) and fat-soluble (phytonadione) preparation.

Uses Primary and drug-induced hypoprothrombinemia, especially that caused by anticoagulants of the coumarin and phenindione type. Vitamin K cannot reverse the anticoagulant activity of heparin.

Large doses of salicylates, quinine, barbiturates, and therapy with agents that suppress the intestinal flora (antibiotics and sulfonamides) may also cause vitamin K deficiency.

Vitamin K malabsorption syndromes. Adjunct during whole blood transfusions. Preoperatively to prevent the danger of hemorrhages in surgical patients who may require anticoagulant therapy.

Prophylaxis of hypoprothrombinemia of the newborn.

Certain forms of liver disease. Hemorrhagic states associated with obstructive jaundice, celiac disease, ulcerative colitis, sprue, and GI fistulas.

Contraindications Severe liver disease. Use with caution in neonates.

MENADIOL SODIUM BISULFATE HYKINONE

MENADIOL SODIUM DIPHOSPHATE (K₄) KAPPADIONE, SYNKAYVITE

MENADIONE (K₃)

General Statement

The pharmacologic action of these compounds is identical. Menadione sodium diphosphate is water soluble and is directly absorbed from the GI tract, even in the absence of bile. Menadione is oil soluble. To be effective, it requires the presence of bile (nonobstructed bile duct) or concomitant administration of bile salts.

Use

Vitamin K deficiency, primary or drug-induced. (For details see vitamin K, p. 705.)

Contraindications

Severe liver disease. Use with caution in neonates.

Untoward Reactions

Occasional skin rash, nausea, and diarrhea. The drug may cause hyperbilirubinemia and fatal kernicterus in neonates.

Drug Interactions

Interactant	Interaction
Antibiotics	Antibiotics may inhibit the body's production of vitamin K and may lead to bleeding. Vitamin K supplements should be given
Anticoagulants, oral	Vitamin K antagonizes anticoagulant effect
Cholestyramine	↓ Effect of vitamin K by ↓ absorption from GI tract

Dosage

Menadione, **PO, IM:** 2–10 mg/day. Not for use in infants. In presence of bile obstruction, bile salts (300 mg ox bile/mg menadione) should be administered when menadione is given PO.

Menadiol sodium bisulfite (about ½ as potent as menadione), **SC, IM, IV:** 2.5–5 mg/day. In severe deficiency use larger doses. *Obstructive jaundice or other conditions interfering with vitamin absorption:* 5–10 mg/day.

Menadiol sodium diphosphate (about ½ as potent as menadione) **PO, SC, IM, IV,** *hemorrhagic states,* **adults:** 5–15 mg or more daily; **children,** 5–10 mg daily. *Anticoagulant overdosage,* **IM:** 75 mg, repeated if necessary. *Hemorrhagic disease of newborn:* 6–12 mg given parenterally to mother during labor or 3 mg to infant immediately following delivery.

Nursing Implication

Check dosage for infants very carefully because overdosage may result in irreversible brain damage.

PHYTONADIONE (VITAMIN K₁) AQUA-MEPHYTON, KONAKION, MEPHYTON

Classification Vitamin K.

General Statement Phytonadione is identical with neutral vitamin K. The compound is rapidly destroyed upon exposure to light.

Phytonadione is rapid acting (onset: IV administration, 15 minutes; PO administration, 6 to 10 hours), and is the agent of choice in presence of threatened or ongoing hemorrhage. Bleeding is usually controlled within 12 to 24 hours.

Remarks Heparin may be used to correct overdosage of phytonadione.

Uses See *General Statement* on vitamin K, page 705.

Contraindications Some forms of hepatic disease. In some cases of liver diseases, phytonadione may actually increase prothrombin time.

Untoward Reactions Phytonadione should only be used in cases of abnormal (prolonged) prothrombin time. Frequent determinations of prothrombin time are indicated during therapy.

IV administration may cause severe reactions leading to death. May be transient flushing of the face, sweating, a sense of constriction of the chest, and weakness. Cramplike pain, weak and rapid pulse, convulsive movements, chills and fever, hypotension, cyanosis, or hemoglobinuria have been reported occasionally. Shock, cardiac, and respiratory failure may be observed.

Hyperbilirubinemia and severe hemolytic anemia have been observed in infants following administration of large doses of phytonadione.

Dosage **PO, IM, IV, SC. IV** administration is reserved for emergency situations; rate of **IV** administration should not exceed 1 mg/min. **IM and SC** administration are indicated for patients unsuitable for **PO** therapy.

Anticoagulant-induced hypoprothrombinemia: (1) In the absence of bleeding, **PO, IM, or SC:** 2.5–10 mg or more (up to 25 mg). Repeated after 12 to 48 hr if prothrombin time has not reached normal levels (2) In the presence of hemorrhage or threatened hemorrhage, **IV:** 10–50 mg; **children:** 5–10 mg. *Preoperatively to offset effects of anticoagulant therapy,* **PO, IM, SC** (given 24 hr before surgery): 5–25 mg; **IV** (12 hr before surgery): 10–25 mg or more. *Prophylaxis of hemorrhagic disease of the newborn,* **IM, to mother:** 1–5 mg 12 to 24 hr prior to delivery; **IM, to newborn:** 0.5–1 mg. *Acute hemorrhagic disease of newborn,* **IV:** 1 mg or **IM:** 2 mg for several days.

Administration/ Storage 1. Store injectable emulsion or colloidal solutions in cool, 5°–15° C (41°–59° F), dark place.
2. Do not freeze.

3. Protect vitamin K from light. IV should be completed within 2 to 3 hours.
4. Do not administer faster than 10 mg/minute by IV.
5. Mix emulsion only with water or 5% D/W.
6. Mix colloidal solution with 5% D/W, isotonic sodium chloride injection, or dextrose and sodium chloride injection.

Nursing Implications

1. Check that prothrombin times are being done while the patient is on therapy and have therapy evaluated.
2. Observe patient, during parenteral administration, for sweating, transient flushing of face, a sense of constriction of chest, weakness, tachycardia, hypotension which may progress to shock, cardiac arrest, and respiratory failure.

DRUGS FOR TREATMENT OF COMMON MEDICAL CONDITIONS

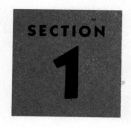

antitussives and expectorants

Narcotic Antitussive	Codeine	
Nonnarcotic Antitussives	Benzonatate Chlophedianol Hydrochloride Dextromethorphan Hydrobromide	Levopropoxyphene Napsylate Noscapine
Expectorants	Acetylcysteine Guaifenesin	Terpin Hydrate Elixir Tyloxapol

General Statement The cough is a useful protective reflex mechanism through which the body attempts to clear the respiratory tract of excess mucus or foreign particles. Coughing may accompany respiratory disease. In such cases, it will usually clear up by itself within a few days. It may also indicate an underlying organic disease whose cause should be ascertained. Coughing, however, can and sometimes should be treated symptomatically. There are two common types of cough: productive (cough accompanied by expectoration of mucus and phlegm) and nonproductive (dry cough).

Antitussive agents can be divided into narcotic and nonnarcotic products. Such agents depress a cough by depressing the activity of the cough center in the brain or by a local action.

NARCOTIC ANTITUSSIVE

CODEINE

See *Narcotic Analgesics*, page 357.

NONNARCOTIC ANTITUSSIVES

General Statement The drugs belonging to this category depress the cough reflex by a variety of mechanisms. All of them are more effective in the treatment of nonproductive cough than in cough associated with copious sputum. Many of the agents have local anesthetic properties. They do not produce dependence.

Contraindication Antitussive medication should be avoided during the first trimester of pregnancy unless otherwise decided by a physician.

Nursing Implications

1. Advise the patient to take antitussive as prescribed and to discard remaining medication after course of therapy because medication for cough should be taken under medical supervision.
2. Acquaint the patient with side effects of drugs.
3. Stress to women of childbearing age that antitussives are, for the most part, contraindicated in pregnancy.
4. Report if the patient continues to sound congested or is unable to bring up phlegm.
5. Advise the patient not to eat or drink fluids for at least 15 minutes after he/she has taken a cough syrup that has a demulcent effect.
6. Provide supportive nursing care measures, such as offering and encouraging increased fluid intake, positioning the patient in a sitting position, splinting an incision during coughing, and providing soothing warm liquids to reduce mucosal irritation.

BENZONATATE TESSALON

Classification Nonnarcotic antitussive.

Remarks Benzonatate is as effective as codeine. PO, onset, 30 minutes; duration: 2 to 8 hours.

Uses Respiratory conditions including pneumonia and bronchitis; chronic conditions including emphysema, tuberculosis, and pulmonary tumors; bronchial asthma. Adjunct in surgery when cough should be suppressed.

Untoward Reactions Nasal congestion, chills, skin rash, GI upset, dizziness, and drowsiness. Rarely, hypersensitivity. Parenteral administration may cause temporary increase in blood pressure.

Dosage **PO:** 100 mg t.i.d. or more (up to 600 mg daily). **Pediatric under 10 years:** 50 mg t.i.d.-q.i.d.

CHLOPHEDIANOL HYDROCHLORIDE Ulo

Classification Nonnarcotic antitussive.

Remarks This drug depresses the cough reflex selectively. It has an antihistaminic effect.

Uses Symptomatic treatment of nonproductive cough and bronchial asthma.

Untoward Reactions CNS stimulation includes excitation, hyperirritability, nightmares, and hallucinations, which are relieved by withdrawal of drug. Should be used cautiously when given concomitantly with CNS stimulants or depressants.

Dosage   **Adults and children over 12 years:** 25 mg t.i.d.-q.i.d.; **pediatric 2–6 years:** 12.5 mg t.i.d.-q.i.d.; **6–12 years:** 12.5–25 mg t.i.d.-q.i.d. **Do not give to children under 2 years.**

DEXTROMETHORPHAN HYDROBROMIDE BENYLIN DM COUGH, CHLOROSEPTIC-DM, CONGESPIRIN, FORMULA 44, HOLD 4-HOUR, ROMILAR, PERTUSSIN 8 HOUR, SPEC-T, STOP-KOFF, SUCRETS, SYMPTOM 1

Classification   Nonnarcotic antitussive.

Remarks   Dextromethorphan is about equal to codeine in its antitussive activity. Onset of action, 15 to 30 minutes; duration, 3 to 6 hours. It produces little CNS depression. Common ingredient of nonprescription cough medication; does not produce physical dependence.

Use   Symptomatic relief of nonproductive chronic cough.

Drug Interaction   Contraindicated with monoamine oxidase inhibitors.

Dosage   **PO:** 10–20 mg q 4 hr or 30 mg q 6 to 8 hr. **Pediatric 2–6 years:** ¼ adult dose; **6–12 years:** ½ adult dose.

LEVOPROPOXYPHENE NAPSYLATE NOVRAD NAPSYLATE

Classification   Nonnarcotic antitussive.

Remarks   Levopropoxyphene has a local anesthetic action. It does not interfere with expectoration and does not affect respiratory tract fluid.

Use   Symptomatic treatment of nonproductive cough.

Untoward Reactions   Nausea, skin rash, urticaria, drowsiness, jitteriness, dizziness.

Dosage   **PO:** 100 mg q 4 hr up to a maximum of 600 mg/day. **Pediatric,** approximately 0.5 mg/lb q 4 hr; **25 pounds:** 75 mg; **50 pounds:** 150 mg; **75–100 pounds:** 200 mg.

NOSCAPINE TUSSCAPINE

Classification   Nonnarcotic antitussive.

Remark   This alkaloid is said to be as effective as codeine.

Use   Symptomatic treatment of nonproductive cough.

Untoward Reactions   Slight drowsiness and occasional nausea. Allergic reactions, including acute vasomotor rhinitis and conjunctivitis.

Dosage **PO:** 15–30 mg t.i.d.-q.i.d. not to exceed 120 mg/day; **pediatric 6 to 12 years:** 15 mg t.i.d.-q.i.d. not to exceed 60 mg/day.

EXPECTORANTS

ACETYLCYSTEINE MUCOMYST

Classification Expectorant.

General Statement Acetylcysteine reduces the viscosity of purulent and nonpurulent pulmonary secretions and permits their expectoration, or removal by mechanical means.

Acetylcysteine is incompatible with antibiotics and should be administered separately.

Uses Adjunct in the treatment of acute and chronic bronchitis, emphysema, and other bronchopulmonary disorders.

Routine care of patients with tracheostomy, pulmonary complications after thoracic or cardiovascular surgery, or in post-traumatic chest conditions.

Pulmonary complications of cystic fibrosis. Diagnostic bronchial studies.

Contraindications Sensitivity to drug. Use with caution in patients with asthma and in the elderly.

Untoward Reactions Acetylcysteine increases the incidence of bronchospasm in patients with asthma. The drug may also increase the amount of liquified bronchial secretions, which must be removed by suction if cough is inadequate. Other side effects include stomatitis, hemoptysis, nausea, and rhinorrhea.

Dosage Administer 10% or 20% solution by nebulization, direct application, or direct intratracheal instillation.

Nebulization into face mask: 1–10 ml of 20% solution or 2–10 ml of 10% solution 3 to 4 times daily. *Closed tent or croupette:* 300 ml of 10% or 20% solution per treatment. *Direct instillation into tracheostomy:* 1–2 ml of 10%–20% solution every 1 to 4 hr. *Diagnostic procedures:* 2 to 3 doses of 1–2 ml of 20% or 2–4 ml of 10% solution by nebulization or intratracheal instillation.

Administration/ Storage
1. Use nonreactive plastic, glass, or stainless steel equipment for administration.
2. Administer via face mask, face tent, oxygen tent, head tent, or by positive pressure breathing machine as indicated.
3. Administer with compressed air for nebulization. Hand nebulizers are contraindicated.
4. After prolonged nebulization, dilute the last fourth of the medication

with sterile water for injection to prevent concentration of medication.

5. Note that the solution may develop a light purple color that does not affect the action of the medication.

6. Closed bottles are stable for 2 years when stored at 20°C. Open bottles should be stored at 2°–8°C and should be used within 96 hours.

Nursing Implications

1. Observe asthmatics particularly for bronchial spasm demonstrated by wheezing and increased congestion.

2. Have available bronchodilators such as isoproterenol for aerosol inhalation should bronchospasm occur.

3. Provide mechanical suction to remove secretions if patient is unable to cough up secretions and have endotrachial tube available.

4. Advise the patient that the nauseous odor that may be perceived on the initiation of treatment will soon not be noticeable.

5. Wash the patient's face after nebulization, as medication may cause stickiness.

GUAIFENESIN (GLYCERYL GUAIACOLATE) GLYCOTUSS, GLYTUSS, HYTUSS, PROCO, ROBITUSSIN, 2/G, OTHERS

Classification　Expectorant, local.

General Statement　Guaifenesin increases the fluid of the respiratory tract. This reduces the viscosity of respiratory secretions and facilitates their expectoration. The drug is more effective than ammonium chloride or terpin hydrate for the treatment of tubercular cough but less effective than the iodides for the treatment of bronchical asthma.

Guaifenesin is an active ingredient of many nonprescription cough preparations.

Use　Symptomatic treatment of productive cough.

Untoward Reactions　At very high levels: GI upset and emesis.

Drug Interaction　Inhibition of platelet adhesiveness by guaifenesin may result in bleeding tendencies.

Dosage　**PO:** 200–400 mg q 4 hr up to 800 mg daily; **pediatric:** 50–100 mg 3 to 4 times daily as required.

TERPIN HYDRATE ELIXIR

TERPIN HYDRATE AND CODEINE ELIXIR

Classification　Expectorant, local.

General Statement	Terpin hydrate is alleged to decrease the excessive bronchial secretion, liquify sputum, and facilitate expectoration. Terpin hydrate is often combined with codeine, a narcotic, which specifically depresses the cough reflex. Terpin hydrate elixir contains about 43% alcohol, and Terpin hydrate and codeine elixir contains 10 mg codeine per 5 ml and is subject to federal narcotic regulations.
Use	Symptomatic treatment of cough.
Contraindications	Peptic ulcer and severe diabetes mellitus. Also see *Codeine*, page 357.
Untoward Reactions	See *Codeine*, page 357.
Dosage	*Terpin hydrate elixir*, **PO:** 5–10 ml every 3 to 4 hr as needed. *Terpin hydrate and codeine elixir*, **PO:** 5 ml 3 to 4 times daily.
Nursing Implications	Warn the patient that excessive use of drug may lead to oversedation and prolonged use may lead to dependence.

TYLOXAPOL ALEVAIRE

Classification	Mucolytic, expectorant.
General Statement	Tyloxapol has detergent-like properties. It reduces the viscosity of purulent and nonpurulent pulmonary secretions. It also decreases the force with which these cling to various surfaces in the lungs, facilitating expectoration by natural processes.
Uses	Adjunct in the treatment of bronchopulmonary diseases characterized by excessive or thickened excretions, or conditions in which the normal processes of elimination are suppressed, such as bronchiectasis, lung abscess, intrathoracic surgery. As a vehicle for antibiotics and other medications in diseases, such as pertussis, croup, laryngitis, bronchiolitis, poliomyelitis, bronchial asthma, pneumonia, and tracheotomy.
Contraindications	Sensitivity to drug.
Untoward Reactions	Tyloxapol increases the incidence of bronchospasms in patients with asthma.
Dosage	500 ml of undiluted prepared solution (0.125% tyloxapol, 2% sodium bicarbonate, 5% glycerol) administered over period of 12 to 24 hours. *Ambulatory patients:* oral nasal nebulizer, 10–20 ml.

Administration	1. Tyloxapol may be administered via:
	   a. a clean nebulizer attached to an air compressor or oxygen source.
	   b. a face mask.
	   c. an open topped or closed cooled tent.

2. For continuous administration, adjust rate of flow according to needs, with 500 ml of solution to last for 12 to 24 hours.
3. For intermittent administration, nebulize 30 to 90 minutes t.i.d. or q.i.d. using a smaller nebulizer, such as the De Vilbiss #640.
4. Do not use hand-bulb technique because of amount of solution is too large.
5. When used as a vehicle for other medications, administer in amount of tyloxapol ordered (usually 60 ml).

Nursing Implications

1. Anticipate that effect of expectorant may not be demonstrated for several days or more of continuous therapy.
2. Report if patient complains of irritation because this is caused by the alkaline pH of medication and tissue damage may result.
3. Be alert to occurrence of nausea and report because it may interfere with patient's nutritional status and ability to maintain liquid intake.
4. Observe solution of tyloxapol for contamination because it tends to support bacterial growth. Autoclave contaminated solutions or discard.

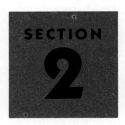

SECTION 2

gastrointestinal drugs

Gastric Antacids and Adsorbents

Aluminum Hydroxide Gel
Aluminum Hydroxide Gel, Dried
Aluminum Phosphate Gel
Basic Aluminum Carbonate Gel
Calcium Carbonate Precipitated
Dihydroxyaluminum Aminoacetate
Dihydroxyaluminum Sodium Carbonate

Magaldrate
Magnesia Magma
Magnesium Carbonate
Magnesium Oxide
Magnesium Trisilicate
Sodium Bicarbonate

Miscellaneous   Cimetidine   Dexpanthenol

General Statement

Acute and chronic gastrointestinal disturbances are among the most common medical conditions requiring treatment. The drugs specifically used to treat GI disturbances are listed in this section. Other drugs used for the treatment of GI disturbances, such as the cholinergic and anticholinergic agents or the opiates, are discussed elsewhere.

GASTRIC ANTACIDS AND ADSORBENTS

General Statement

Hydrochloric acid, secreted as part of the gastric juices, is necessary for digestion. In particular, it maintains the stomach at the low pH (1–2) necessary for the optimum activity of the digestive enzyme pepsin.

Under certain circumstances, people become sensitive to their own gastric juice. Adverse reactions vary from an unpleasant burning sensation (heartburn) to life-threatening peptic or duodenal ulcers.

The initial cause for ulceration is as yet unknown. It is believed that peptic ulcers are caused by a decrease in the resistance of stomach tissue to hydrochloric acid, whereas duodenal ulcers are associated with an increase in the secretion of acid by the parietal cells.

Various drugs and dietary measures are used for the treatment of hyperacidity states and ulcers; use of antacids is an important part of this regimen. Drugs used as antacids are simple chemicals that work by (1) neutralizing the acid directly; (2) buffering the acid; or (3) adsorbing the acid.

Most of the antacids used today form products that are not absorbed systemically. Some, like sodium bicarbonate, form products that affect the pH of the body fluids and electrolyte balance. By eliminating excess acid, the antacids provide relief from pain and promote healing.

Some antacids also coat the naked ulcer to protect it, as much as possible, from further contact with the acid content of the stomach.

Antacids containing magnesium have a laxative effect. Those that contain aluminum or calcium have a constipating effect. This is why patients are often given alternating doses of a laxative and a constipating antacid. Antacids with such different side effects are sometimes combined in a single preparation.

The antacids have few untoward reactions. Excessive blood levels of magnesium may cause CNS depression. This is why magnesium-containing antacids should be given cautiously to patients with impaired renal function.

Nursing Implications

1. Carefully observe patients on antacid therapy for constipation if they are on medication containing calcium or aluminum. Encourage extra fluids unless contraindicated and consult with physician when laxatives or enemas seem indicated.
2. Carefully observe patients on antacid therapy for diarrhea if they are on medication containing magnesium. Report diarrhea to physician because change of medication or alternation with an aluminum- or calcium-containing antacid may be indicated.
3. Encourage patients on antacid therapy to take medication with the amount of water or milk prescribed because liquid acts as a vehicle transporting the medication to the stomach where the action is desired.
4. Administer laxative or cathartic dose at bedtime as medication takes about 8 hours to be effective and the effect should not interfere with the patient's rest.

ALUMINUM HYDROXIDE GEL AMPHOJEL, NO-CO-GEL

ALUMINUM HYDROXIDE GEL, DRIED ALU-CAP, ALU-TAB, AMPHOJEL TABLETS, DIALUME

Classification	Antacid.
General Statement	A nonsystemic antacid that works by neutralization. The drug has a mildly demulcent action and is slightly constipating. Aluminum hydroxide and phosphorus form insoluble phosphates that are eliminated in the feces. This yields a relatively phosphorus-free urine and prevents phosphate stone formation in individuals prone to them. One gram of aluminum hydroxide gel neutralizes 25 mEq of acid.
Uses	Adjunct in the treatment of gastric and duodenal ulcer. Management of phosphate stone formation in kidneys, ureters, and bladder.
Contraindications	Sensitivity to aluminum. Peptic ulcer associated with pancreatic deficiency, diarrhea, or low phosphorus diet. Aluminum hydroxide preparations contain sodium and thus should not be administered to patients on a low sodium diet.
Untoward Reactions	Lowering of serum phosphate level, phosphorus deficiency, constipation, and intestinal obstruction.
Drug Interactions	Aluminum hydroxide gel inhibits the absorption of tetracyclines, barbiturates, digoxin, phenytoin, warfarin, quinidine, and anticholinergics decreasing their effect.
Dosage	*Gel*, **PO:** 5–10 ml q 2 to 4 hr (more effective than the tablet) or tablets containing 300 mg or 600 mg q.i.d. with water (tablets should be chewed before swallowing). *Urinary calculi:* 40 ml after meals and at bedtime; 300-mg tablet corresponds to approximately 5 ml gel.
Administration	1. Administer gel in a half glass of water. 2. Teach the patient to chew tablets before swallowing them and to take them with milk or water. 3. For administration by stomach tube, dilute commercial solution 2 or 3 times with water. Administer this at a rate of 15–20 gtt per minute. Total daily dose is approximately 1.5 liters of the diluted suspension.
Additional Nursing Implications	1. Check that urine specimen is collected at least once a month to determine urinary phosphate when drug is given in management of phosphatic urinary calculi. 2. Check that patient is on a low phosphorus diet of 1.3 gm of phosphorus, 700 mg of calcium, 13 gm of nitrogen, and 2500 cal when patient is being treated for phosphatic urinary calculi.

ALUMINUM PHOSPHATE GEL PHOSPHALJEL

Classification   Antacid.

General Statement   Aluminum phosphate has antacid, astringent, and demulcent properties similar to aluminum hydroxide gel but with only half the neutralizing power. The drug does not interfere with phosphate metabolism and is thus preferred for patients who cannot maintain a high phosphorus diet. Also preferred in the presence of diarrhea or pancreatic juice deficiency.

Uses   Antacid; peptic ulcer.

Contraindication   Sensitivity to aluminum.

Untoward Reactions   Intestinal obstruction and constipation.

Dosage   **PO:** 15–30 ml undiluted q 2 hr between meals and at bedtime, alone or with milk or water.

BASIC ALUMINUM CARBONATE GEL BASALJEL

Uses   Hyperacidity. With low phosphorus diet to prevent phosphate urinary stones by reducing urinary phosphate levels.

Contraindications   Sensitivity to aluminum.

Untoward Reaction   Constipation.

Dosage   *Antacid:* 1–2 tablets or capsules or 1–2 teaspoons of suspension. *Extra strength suspension:* ½–1 teaspoon. *Urinary calculi:* 2–6 capsules or tablets or 1–2 tablespoons suspension 1 hr after meals and at bedtime. *Extra strength suspension:* 1–3 teaspoons.

CALCIUM CARBONATE PRECIPITATED AMITONE, ALKA-2, DICARBOSIL, EQUILET, MALLAMINT, P.H. TABLETS, TRIALKA, TUMS

Classification   Antacid.

Remarks   Nonsystemic antacid regarded by some as the antacid of choice. It has a rapid onset of action, high neutralizing capacity (1 gm neutralizes about 21 mEq acid), and its activity is relatively prolonged. Since calcium carbonate is constipating, it is often alternated or even mixed with magnesium salts.

Uses   Antacid; peptic ulcer.

Untoward Reactions   Constipation, eructation, flatulence, hypercalcemia with occasional metastatic calcifications, alkalosis, azotemia, renal dysfunction, GI hemorrhage, and rebound hyperacidity.

Dosage   **PO:** *individualized usual dose*, 1–4 gm 4 or more times daily with water. *Severe symptoms;* 2–4 gm q hr. Tablets should be chewed before swallowing.

DIHYDROXYALUMINUM AMINOACETATE ROBALATE

General Statement   Nonsystemic antacid with adsorbent and protective properties similar to aluminum hydroxide but reported to act more rapidly. Dihydroxyaluminum aminoacetate has more neutralizing capacity than aluminum hydroxide but the liquid aluminum hydroxide preparation is more effective.

    Often alternated with magnesium salts to counteract constipating effect.

Uses   Peptic ulcer. Antacid for hyperacidity, gastritis, enteritis, pyrosis, and diarrhea.

Contraindication   Sensitivity to aluminum.

Untoward Reaction   Constipation.

Dosage   **PO:** 0.5–1 gm after meals and at bedtime; 1–2 gm q 2 to 4 hr may be required to alleviate severe discomfort.

DIHYDROXYALUMINUM SODIUM CARBONATE ROLAIDS

See *Dihydroxyaluminum Aminoacetate.*

Dosage   1 or 2 tablets chewed as required.

MAGALDRATE RIOPAN

Classification   Antacid.

Remarks   Chemical combination of aluminum hydroxide and magnesium hydroxide. This compound is an effective nonsystemic antacid. It buffers (pH 3.0–5.5) without causing alkalosis.

Use   Antacid.

Contraindications Sensitivity to aluminum. Use with caution in patients with impaired renal function.

Untoward Reactions Mild constipation and hypermagnesia.

Dosage **PO: tablets or suspension,** 400–800 mg q.i.d. between meals and at bedtime. Frequency of administration may have to be increased initially to every hour to control severe symptoms.

MAGNESIUM CARBONATE

Classification Antacid.

Remarks Nonsystemic antacid with high neutralizing capacity (1.0 gm neutralizes 20 mEq of acid). During neutralization, carbon dioxide forms in the stomach. To counteract catharsis, magnesium carbonate is often alternated with aluminum hydroxide (see also p. 718).

Uses Antacid, laxative.

Contraindication Use with caution in patients with renal impairment.

Untoward Reactions Diarrhea, abdominal pain, nausea, vomiting, and magnesium intoxication.

Drug Interaction Tetracyclines are inhibited by magnesium salts.

Dosage **PO,** *antacid:* 0.5–2 gm between meals with water (tablets should be chewed before swallowing). *Cathartic:* 8.0 gm.

Administration Give with one-half glass of water.

MAGNESIUM HYDROXIDE MILK OF MAGNESIA, MINT-O-MAG

Classification Antacid, cathartic.

General Statement Depending on dosage, drug simply acts as an antacid or as a laxative. Neutralizes hydrochloric acid. Does not produce alkalosis and has a demulcent effect. One milliliter neutralizes 2.7 mEq of acid.
     Often alternated with aluminum hydroxide to counteract cathartic effect.

Uses Antacid, laxative.

Untoward Reactions Diarrhea, abdominal pain, nausea, vomiting.

Drug Interactions	Interactant	Interaction
	Procainamide	Procainamide ↑ muscle relaxation produced by Mg salts

	Skeletal muscle relaxants (surgical)
	    Succinylcholine
	    Tubocurarine
		↑ Muscle relaxation

	Tetracyclines	↓ Effect of tetracyclines due to ↓ absorption from GI tract

Dosage **PO:** *antacid*, 5– 10 ml q.i.d.; *laxative*, **adult:**15– 30 ml in the morning or evening. **Children:** 2.5– 5 ml with water. *Milk of magnesia/aluminum hydroxide combination:*5– 30 ml q 2 to 4 hr.

Administration
1. Give suspension with water. Administer combined magnesia magma and aluminum hydroxide gel with one-half glass of water.
2. Provide a slice of orange or orange juice after administration as a laxative to minimize the unpleasant aftertaste.
3. Administer laxative dose at bedtime as medication takes about 8 hours to be effective and thereby will not interfere with patient's rest.

MAGNESIUM OXIDE MAOX, MAG-OX 400, OXABID, PAR-MAG, URO-MAG

Classification Antacid, cathartic.

General Statement Nonsystemic antacid, slower acting than sodium bicarbonate, with more prolonged activity. The compound has a rather high neutralizing capacity (1.0 gm neutralizes 50 mEq acid).

In order to reduce the cathartic effect of the drug, the compound can be alternated with calcium salts. For example: sodium bicarbonate and calcium carbonate powder (Sippy Powder No. 1) is alternated with sodium bicarbonate and magnesium oxide powder (Sippy Powder No. 2).

Uses Antacid, cathartic.

Contraindication Poor renal function.

Untoward Reactions Abdominal pain, nausea, diarrhea. May cause CNS depression in patients with poor renal function.

Drug Interactions Tetracyclines are inhibited by magnesium salts.

Dosage **PO,** *antacid:* 0.25– 1 gm with water or milk as required. *Cathartic:* 4 gm. *Sippy Powder No. 1 or Sippy Powder No. 2:* 1.3 gm as required.

Administration Administer antacid with water or milk.

Additional Nursing Implications Explain to patients why Sippy Powder No. 1 and 2 are alternated.

MAGNESIUM TRISILICATE

Classification Antacid

Remarks Nonsystemic antacid with marked adsorbent and protective properties and a relatively long action (1.0 gm neutralizes 50 mEq acid). The drug protects the crater of the ulcer. Like all magnesium salts, it has a mild laxative effect and is often used in combination with aluminum hydroxide.

Use Antacid.

Contraindication Use with caution in patients with renal disease.

Untoward Reactions Abdominal pain, nausea, diarrhea, and magnesium intoxication.

Drug Interactions Tetracyclines are inhibited by magnesium salts.

Dosage **PO:** 0.5–1 gm q.i.d. Tablets should be chewed before swallowing. Combined with aluminum hydroxide: 5–30 ml in one-half glass of water every 2 to 4 hr.

Administration
1. Instruct the patient to chew tablets before swallowing and then drink 60 ml of water.
2. Administer combination of magnesium trisilicate with aluminum hydroxide in 120 ml of water.

SODIUM BICARBONATE SODA MINT

Classification Antacid, systemic alkalizer.

General Statement Systemic antacid that neutralizes hydrochloric acid by forming sodium chloride and carbon dioxide (1 gm of sodium bicarbonate neutralizes 12 mEq of acid). Provides temporary relief of peptic ulcer pain and of discomfort associated with indigestion. The drug has a short duration of action and alkalinizes urine. Although it is widely used by the general public, it is rarely prescribed as an antacid by the physician because of its high sodium content and because it may cause alkalosis. The drug also often causes rebound acid secretions. For more details see *Electrolytes Section*, chapter 9, p. 671 and 675.

Uses   As an adjunct in sulfonamide therapy (prevents crystal deposition in renal tubules by alkalinizing urine); for the treatment of acidosis. Antacid.

Contraindications   Renal disease, congestive heart failure, patients on restricted sodium diet, pyloric obstruction. Use with caution in patients with edema and cirrhosis. Do not use as an antidote for strong mineral acids because carbon dioxide is formed, which may cause discomfort and even perforation.

Untoward Reactions   "Acid rebound" (increased acid secretion by the stomach), gastric distention, alkalosis (characterized by dizziness, abdominal cramps, thirst, anorexia, nausea, vomiting, diminished breathing, convulsions). Sodium bicarbonate leaves the stomach readily and its neutralizing action is therefore short-lived. This may cause an increased secretion of acid (rebound effect). Furthermore, sodium bicarbonate is absorbed into the bloodstream where it may cause systemic alkalosis.

Drug Interactions   See Sodium Bicarbonate, *Electrolytes* Section, p. 675.

Dosage   *Adjunct to sulfonamide therapy:* **initial,** 4 gm. **Maintenance:** 2 gm q 4 hr. *Metabolic acidosis:* Gastric lavage with 3% to 5% solution and leave about 100 ml in stomach of patient. *Antacid:* 0.3–2 gm as necessary.

   IV, *Metabolic acidosis: individualized,* 1.5% solution contains 15 gm of sodium bicarbonate per liter (178 mEq of sodium and 178 mEq of bicarbonate). This is an isotonic solution.

Administration   1. Hypertonic solutions must be administered by the physician.
2. Isotonic solutions should be administered slowly as ordered as too rapid administration may result in death due to cellular acidity. Check rate of flow frequently.

Nursing Implications   1. Observe acidotic patients being treated with sodium bicarbonate for relief of dyspnea and hyperpnea and report as the drug must be discontinued when these conditions are relieved.
2. Observe acidotic patients being treated with sodium bicarbonate for edema as this may necessitate a change to potassium bicarbonate.
3. Caution the general public not to take sodium bicarbonate routinely for gastric distress but rather to consult a physician instead. Excessive use of the drug may cause a rebound effect with increased acid secretion or systemic alkalosis and formation of phosphate crystals in the kidney.

MISCELLANEOUS

CIMETIDINE TAGAMET

Classification   Histamine H_2 receptor blocking agent.

**General
Statement** A recently developed drug—cimetidine—decreases the acidity of the stomach by blocking the action of histamine, a substance involved in triggering gastric acid secretion. Cimetidine blocks the action of histamine by competitively occupying the histamine (H_2) receptors in the gastric mucosa. This, in turn, inhibits the release of gastric (hydrochloric) acid. The onset of action of cimetidine is rapid (within 1 hour) and suppresses postprandial, daytime and nighttime gastric acid secretion. It is *not* an anticholinergic agent.

Uses Short-term (up to 8 weeks) treatment of duodenal ulcers. Management of gastric acid hypersecretory states (Zollinger-Ellison syndrome).
Investigationally: for osteoarthritis patients intolerant to aspirin and for patients with renal failure.

Contraindications Pregnancy, children under 12, nursing mothers.

**Untoward
Reactions** Rare. Mild and transient diarrhea, muscle pain, dizziness and rash, mild gynecomastia. Small increases in plasma creatinine and serum transaminase.

**Drug
Interactions**

Interactant	Interaction
Antacids	↑ Absorption of cimetidine in some patients
Wafarin	Potentiation of anticoagulant effect (↑ prothrombin time)

Dosage **PO:** *Duodenal ulcers:* 300 mg q.i.d. with meals and at bedtime, for a period of 4 to 6 weeks. Administer with antacids. Dosage may be increased to 2400 mg/day in patients with hypersecretory conditions.
IV (rare): *hypersecretory conditions, intractable ulcers:* 300 mg q 6 hr. *Renal failure,* **PO or IV:** 300 mg q 8 to 12 hr.

Administration 1. For IV injection or infusion. Dilute as specified by manufacturer and inject over period of 1–2 minutes, or infuse intermittently.
2. Administer oral medication with meals and at bedtime.

**Nursing
Implication** Advise patient to continue taking medication as ordered for 4 to 6 weeks until healing has been observed by endoscopic examination.

DEXPANTHENOL ILOPAN

Classification Smooth muscle stimulant.

**General
Statement** Dexpanthenol, a precursor of Coenzyme A, stimulates the smooth muscles of the GI tract. Satisfactory response is unlikely in the presence of hypokalemia.

Uses Prophylactic after major abdominal surgery to minimize development of paralytic ileus abdominal distention. Retention of flatus or delay in resumption of normal intestinal motility. Paralytic ileus.

Contraindication   Hemophilia.

Drug Interactions

Interactant	Interaction
Antibiotics ⎫ Barbiturates ⎬ Narcotics ⎭	Allergic reactions of unknown cause

Dosage   **IM:** *prophylaxis or postoperative abdominal distention:* 250–500 mg. Repeat once after 2 hr; **then** q 6 hr until danger of distention has passed. *Paralytic ileus:* 500 mg. **IM:** repeat after 2 hr, **then** q 4 to 6 hr. Continue above regimens until all danger of distention has passed (usually for a period of 48 to 72 hr or longer).

Dexpanthenol can be administered by IV drip when mixed with 5% dextrose or lactated Ringer's solution.

Administration
1. Delay administration of dexpanthenol for 12 hours after administration of neostigmine or similar drug, or for 1 hour after administration of succinylcholine.
2. Do not administer full strength solution into vein.

Nursing Implications
1. Listen for bowel sounds to evaluate the effectiveness of dexpanthenol.
2. Ask patients whether they are passing flatus, an indication of peristaltic activity.
3. Assess the patient for hypokalemia manifested by apathy, muscle weakness, atonia, cardiac arrhythmias, and impaired respirations, and report to medical supervision as dexpanthenol is not effective if the patient is in a hypokalemic state.

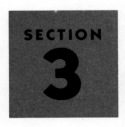

SECTION 3

cathartics (laxatives)

Stimulant Cathartics
Bisacodyl
Bisacodyl Tannex Enema
Cascara Sagrada
Castor Oil
Castor Oil, Emulsified
Danthron
Glycerin Suppositories
Phenolphthalein
Senna
Sennosides A and B, Calcium Salts

Saline Cathartics
Fleet Enema
Magnesium Carbonate
Magnesium Citrate
Magnesium Hydroxide
Magnesium Oxide
Magnesium Sulfate (Epsom Salt)
Phospho-Soda
Potassium Phosphate
Potassium Sodium Tartrate
Sodium Phosphate
Sodium Phosphate Effervescent
Sodium Sulfate

Bulk-Forming Cathartics	Methylcellulose	Psyllium Hydrophilic Muciloid
	Sodium Carboxymethylcellulose	
Emollient Cathartics	Dioctyl Calcium Sulfosuccinate	Mineral Oil
	Dioctyl Sodium Sulfosuccinate	Poloxamer 188

General Statement

Difficult or infrequent passage of stools (constipation) is a symptom of many conditions ranging from purely organic causes (obstruction, megacolon) to common functional disorders. Patients confined to bed may often develop constipation. Constipation may also be of psychological origin. The underlying cause of constipation should be elucidated by a physician, especially since a marked change in bowel habits may be a symptom of a pathological condition.

The cathartics discussed in this section are effective because they act locally either by specifically stimulating the smooth muscles of the bowel or by changing the bulk or consistency of the stools. The cathartics can be divided into four categories: (1) *stimulant cathartics:* substances that chemically stimulate the smooth muscles of the bowel so as to increase contractions: (2) *saline cathartics:* substances that increase the bulk of the stools by retaining water; (3) *bulk-forming cathartics:* nondigestable substances that pass through the stomach and then increase the bulk of the stools; and (4) *emollient laxatives:* agents that soften hardened feces and facilitate their passage through the lower intestine.

Today cathartics are prescribed less frequently for chronic constipation than in the past. In fact, continued use of laxatives has been held responsible for some cases of chronic constipation and other intestinal disorders because the patient may start to depend on the psychological effect and physical stimulus of the drug rather than on his own natural reflexes. Prevention of constipation should include adequate fluid intake and diet as well as daily exercise.

Uses

Cathartics are indicated for the following conditions: anorectal lesions like hemorrhoids; for diagnostic procedures and in conjunction with surgery or anthelmintic therapy; and in cases of chemical poisoning.

Contraindications

Severe abdominal pain that *might* be caused by appendicitis, enteritis, ulcerative colitis, diverticulitis, intestinal obstruction. The administration of cathartics in such cases might cause rupture of the abdomen or intestinal hemorrhage.

Untoward Reactions

Dehydration, disturbance of the electrolyte balance, and chronic constipation.

Drug Interactions

Interactant	Interaction
Anticoagulants, oral	↓ Absorption of vitamin K from GI tract induced by cathartics may ↑ effects of anticoagulants and result in bleeding
Digitalis	Cathartics may ↓ absorption of digitalis
Tetracyclines	↓ Effect of tetracyclines due to ↓ absorption from GI tract

Nursing Implications

1. Advise the patient that a daily bowel movement is not essential and that one or two bowel movements may be missed without harm to health.
2. Advise the patient that rather than relying on cathartics, it would be far better to include more fluids and bulk in the diet and more exercise in daily activity, if such are not contraindicated. Explain that regular use of cathartics can lead to chronic constipation.
3. Promote better bowel function without the use of cathartics by either assisting the patient to the bathroom or by providing a commode at the bedside and ensuring privacy.
4. Advise patients who have abdominal pain or a sudden change in bowel habits to go for medical supervision rather than self-medicating with cathartics.
5. Administer cathartics at a temperature and in or with a substance that makes it more palatable.
6. Administer a cathartic at a time when it will not interfere with the patient's digestion and absorption of nutrients.
7. Note the length of time it takes for the prescribed cathartic to take effect and administer it in such a manner that the time of its action will not interfere with the patient's rest.
8. Keep a record of patient's bowel function and response to cathartics so that they will be given only as needed.
9. Check directions carefully and administer accordingly when cathartics are ordered to prepare the patient for diagnostic studies. Explain how the drug will affect him/her and stress the importance of procedure for accurate diagnostic study.

STIMULANT CATHARTICS

BISACODYL BICOL, BISCOLAX, BON-O-LAX, CO DYLAX, DULCOLAX, LAXADAN SUPULES, ROLAX, SK-BISACODYL, THERALAX, TULAX, VACTROL

Classification   Cathartic, stimulant.

General Statement   Bisacodyl is a local chemical stimulant that acts by increasing the contraction of the muscles of the colon. Bisacodyl is not absorbed systemically and can be administered orally or as a rectal suppository. It is not contraindicated in pregnancy or in the presence of cardiovascular, renal, or hepatic disease.

It produces a gentle bowel movement and soft, formed stools.

It usually acts within 6 to 8 hours after PO administration and 15 to 60 minutes after rectal administration.

Uses   Cleansing of colon preoperatively and postoperatively and for diagnostic procedures (radiology, barium enemas, proctoscopy), colostomies, and chronic constipation.

Contraindications   Acute surgical abdomen or acute abdominal pain.

Untoward Reactions Mild abdominal cramps. Suppositories may cause burning sensation.

Dosage **PO:** 10–15 mg at bedtime or before breakfast; **pediatric over 6 years:** 5 mg. **Rectal, adults and children over 2 years:** 10 mg; **infants:** 5 mg.

Administration/ Storage

Bisacodyl Tablets

1. Administer at bedtime for effectiveness in morning.
2. Otherwise administer before breakfast so that drug will not interfere with the patient's rest at night but rather will be effective within 6 hours.
3. Advise patient that he/she must swallow tablets whole and not chew them or crush them. Children who cannot swallow pills will be unable to take medication PO.
4. Refrigerate bisacodyl tablets at a temperature not exceeding 30° C (86° F).
5. Anticipate for surgery, radiography, or sigmoidoscopy preparation that the drug should be given orally the night before and by rectal suppository in AM.

Bisacodyl Suppositories

1. Administer at a time least likely to interfere with patient's rest.
2. Anticipate that the suppository will be effective in 15 minutes to 2 hours and provide for adequate toileting facilities.

Nursing Implication Advise the patient not to take tablets within 1 hour of ingesting milk or antacid.

BISACODYL TANNEX ENEMACLYSODRAST

Classification Cathartic, stimulant.

General Statement Bisacodyl tannate is a complex of bisocodyl (see preceding drug) and tannic acid. The tannic acid increases the solubility of the bisacodyl.

Solutions of bisacodyl tannate are stable. Bisocodyl, however, is often mixed with barium sulfate for diagnostic studies. These mixed solutions should be used immediately after preparation.

Bisacodyl tannate is only used rectally. The astringent effects of the tannic acid decrease the mucous secretions of the lining of the large intestine. The tannic acid is also said to improve the adherence of the contrast medium to the sides of the bowel.

Uses Cleansing enema prior to radiologic examination of colon; for sigmoidoscopic and proctoscopic procedures.

Contraindications Extensive ulcerations of colon, children younger than 10 years of age, and pregnancy.

Untoward Reaction If absorbed, tannic acid may be hepatotoxic.

Dosage/ Administration	1. Prepare bisacodyl tannex equivalent to 1.5 mg of bisacodyl and 2.5 gm of tannic acid (one packet of commercially available product) in 1 liter of lukewarm water for administration.
	2. For use as radiopaque enema adjuvant: 1 to 2 packets.
	3. For use as a colonic cleansing enema: 3 packets.
	4. No more than 4 packets should be used within 72 hours.
	5. Anticipate that for radiologic examination or sigmoidoscopic or proctoscopic procedures, the patient will be placed on a residue-free diet 1 day before examination and 30–60 ml castor oil will be ordered for administration 16 hours before the examination. A cleansing enema of bisacodyl tannex may be administered on the day of the exam and may be repeated as necessary.

CASCARA SAGRADA CAS-EVAC, BILEO-SECRIN, FLUID EXTRACT CASCARA SAGRADA, FLUID EXTRACT CASCARA SAGRADA AROMATIC

Classification Cathartic, stimulant.

General Statement The compound is the dried bark of the *Rhamnus purshiana* tree. It stimulates the contractions of the colon without affecting the small intestine. It produces a soft stool within 8 to 12 hours.

Cascara sagrada is available as a fluid extract and as a less effective but better-tasting aromatic, debittered fluid extract. The substance may enter the milk of a nursing mother.

Use Constipation.

Dosage **PO,** *fluid extract:* 1 ml; *aromatic fluid extract:* 5 ml; *tablets:* 325 mg. **Cas-Evac:** 1.25–2.5 ml b.i.d. or 2.5–5.0 ml at bedtime.

Nursing Implication Advise the patient that cascara may cause his/her urine to appear yellow-brown or reddish.

CASTOR OIL

EMULSIFIED CASTOR OIL ALPHAMUL, NELOID

Classification Cathartic, stimulant.

Remarks This cathartic is obtained from the seeds of *Ricinus communis*. It increases peristalsis. The drug produces prompt and complete evacuation of the bowel within approximately 6 hours.

Use Prompt evacuation of bowel.

Contraindications Pregnancy, menstruation, abdominal pain, and intestinal obstruction.

Untoward Reactions Severe diarrhea, abdominal pain, dehydration, and changes in electrolyte balance, including hyperkalemia, acidosis, or alkalosis.

Dosage *Castor oil:* 15–60 ml prior to diagnostic procedures; **infants:** 1–5 ml; **children over 2 years:** 5–15 ml. *Castor oil emulsified,* **PO:** 15–60 ml; **infants less than 2 years:** 1.25–7.5 ml; **children over 2 years:** 5–30 ml. Dose depends on strength of preparation.

Nursing Implications
1. The more palatable oil-in-water emulsion aromatized with flavoring agents is preferred.
2. Disguise taste of plain castor oil with a glass of orange juice.

DANTHRON ANAVAC, DANAVAC, DORBANE, MODANE, WESLAX

Classification Cathartic, stimulant.

Remarks Danthron stimulates peristalsis in the large intestine. The onset of the drug is slow (12 hours after ingestion).

 The drug is often combined with a fecal moistening agent such as dioctyl sodium sulfosuccinate.

Use Constipation.

Contraindications Pregnancy, lactation, nausea, vomiting, or abdominal pain.

Untoward Reactions Severe diarrhea, hyperkalemia, and dehydration.

Dosage **PO:** 37.5–150 mg with evening meal; 300 mg may be required occasionally.

Nursing Implication Inform patient that danthron may cause urine to appear pink or red in color.

GLYCERIN SUPPOSITORIES

Classification Cathartic, stimulant.

Remarks Used as suppository to promote defecation by irritating rectal mucosa.

Contraindications Should not be used in the presence of anal fissures, fistulas, ulcerative hemorrhoids, or proctitis.

Dosage One adult or infant-size suppository inserted as needed. Habitual use may result in mucous membrane irritation.

Administration/ Storage Store in tight container in refrigerator below 25° C (77° F).

PHENOLPHTHALEIN ALOPHEN, ESPOTABS, EVAC-U-GEN, EVAC-U-LAX, EX-LAX, FEEN-A-MINT, PHENOLAX, PRULET

Classification Cathartic, stimulant.

Remarks The drug primarily acts on the large intestine. It produces a semifluid stool in 6 to 8 hours with little or no colic. The residual effect of drug may persist for 3 to 4 days. Phenolphthalein is a component of many over-the-counter laxatives.

Use Simple constipation.

Untoward Reactions Hypersensitivity reactions: dermatitis, pruritus; rarely, nonthrombocytopenia purpura.

Dosage **PO: usual,** 60 mg. Doses up to 200 mg are commonly used. Usually taken at bedtime.

Nursing Implications Teach patient and/or parent:

1. That phenolphthalein imparts red color to alkaline stools or urine.
2. To store medication out of children's reach so it will not be ingested as "candy."
3. To stress to children that Ex-Lax is a medication and not candy.

SENNA BLACK DRAUGHT, CASAFRU, SENOKOT, SENOLAX, X-PREP

SENNOSIDES A AND B, CALCIUM SALTS GLYSENNID

Classification Cathartic, stimulant.

General Statement Senna is prepared from the dried leaf or fruit of the *Cassia acutifolia* or *Cassia angustifolia* tree. The powder is comparable to cascara.
 It increases peristalsis of the large intestine and colon. The effect appears 6 to 10 hours after administration.

Uses Constipation, preoperative and prediagnostic procedures involving the GI tract.

Contraindications Irritable colon, nausea, vomiting, abdominal pain, and appendicitis or possibility thereof. Administer with caution to nursing mothers.

Untoward Reactions Abdominal pain, colic, and diarrhea.

Dosage *Senna.* **PO:** 2 tablets. **Rectal suppositories** (652 mg of standard senna concentrate): 1 at bedtime. Pregnant women and children should receive one-half of the standard dose. *Granules:* ½–1 teaspoon. *Syrup,* **adults:** 1–3 teaspoons (depending on the preparation) at bedtime.

Sennosides A and B: 12–24 mg at bedtime; **children 6 to 10 years:** 12 mg at bedtime.

Nursing Implications

Teach patient:

1. That gripping pain is a symptom of overdosage. Drug must be omitted when this occurs and patient should check with physician.
2. The drug imparts a yellowish-brown color to acid urine and a reddish color to alkaline urine.

SALINE CATHARTICS

General Statement

Saline laxatives increase the bulk of the stools by attracting and holding large amounts of fluids. The increased bulk results in the mechanical stimulation of peristalsis. The saline cathartics should be administered with sufficient fluid so as not to cause dehydration of the patient.

The saline cathartics, which include magnesium sulfate, milk of magnesia (see antacids), magnesium citrate, sodium phosphate, sodium sulfate, potassium sodium tartrate, and potassium phosphate are very similar in activity, differing mostly with respect to palatability, cost, and efficiency.

There is always some systemic absorption of the saline cathartics. This presents a problem in the case of magnesium ions, which may cause magnesium intoxication when given to patients with poor renal function. Magnesium intoxication is characterized by drowsiness, dizziness, and other signs of CNS depression. Thirst may be an early sign of magnesium intoxication.

The action of saline cathartics is fast (1 to 2 hours), and they are suitable for rapidly cleaning the entire intestinal tract. They are particularly suitable for the collection of stool specimens and in case of intestinal poisoning. See Table 36, page 734, for individual agents.

BULK-FORMING CATHARTICS

Bulk-forming cathartics increase the bulk of the feces and stimulate peristalsis by mechanical means.

METHYLCELLULOSE COLOGEL, HYDROLOSE

SODIUM CARBOXYMETHYLCELLULOSE CMC, CELLULOSE GUM

Classification   Cathartic, bulk-forming.

TABLE 36 SALINE CATHARTICS

Drug	Use*	Dosage	Remarks
Fleet enema	Catharsis, constipation	4 oz (rectal only). **Children: 2 oz (rectally).**	Contains 16 gm sodium biphosphate and 6 gm sodium phosphate/100 ml.
Magnesium carbonate (see p. 721)			
Magnesium citrate	Catharsis, constipation	**PO:** 200–300 ml (100 ml contain 1.75 gm of magnesium oxide).	Observe for magnesium intoxication. Do not give in case of poor renal function. *Administration* Store preferably in refrigerator to improve taste. *Nursing Implications* 1. Remain with patient and encourage drinking the entire solution at once. 2. Provide a cold solution of medication for this makes it taste best. 3. Observe for signs of magnesium toxicity. (For characteristics, see p. 656 and 733).
Magnesium hydroxide (see p. 721)			
Magnesium oxide (see p. 722)			

Drug	Uses	Dosage	Administration/Remarks
Magnesium sulfate (Epsom Salt)	Catharsis, constipation. Occasionally as CNS depressant, preoperatively. Also, 25%–50% solution used as compress or soak for relief of inflammatory conditions.	PO: 15 gm. Effective 1 to 2 hr.	*Administration* Dissolve in glassful of ice water or other fluid to lessen the disagreeable taste.
Phospho-soda (Fleet)	Catharsis, constipation	PO: 10–20 ml in ½ glass cold water.	Contains 18 gm sodium phosphate and 48 gm sodium biphosphate/100 ml.
Potassium phosphate	Catharsis, constipation	PO: 4 gm.	Similar to sodium phosphate.
Potassium sodium tartrate (Rochelle salt)	Catharsis, constipation	PO: 10 gm.	*Administration* Administer before breakfast dissolved in a glassful of warm water. Relatively pleasant tasting.
Sodium phosphate	Catharsis, constipation	PO: 4 gm. Exsiccated sodium phosphate: 2 gm.	Relatively pleasant tasting. Somewhat less effective than magnesium or sodium sulfate. Available as flavored solution.
Sodium phosphate effervescent	Catharsis, constipation	PO: 10 gm Sodium phosphate solution: 5–10 ml.	*Administration* Administer before breakfast dissolved in a glassful of warm water. Pleasant tasting. Also contains sodium bicarbonate, tartaric, and citric acids. Dry powder liberates carbon dioxide upon addition of water.
Sodium sulfate (Glauber's Sulfate)	Catharsis, constipation	PO: 15 gm.	Very vile tasting. As effective as magnesium sulfate.

*All saline cathartics are used, when appropriate, prior to GI surgery or diagnostic procedures.

General Statement　These indigestible fibers form a colloidal, bulky gelatinous mass on contact with water. The fibers pass through the stomach and increase the bulk of the feces; this stimulates peristalsis. The drug is usually effective within 12 to 24 hours.

Several nonprescription laxatives contain methylcellulose. Both compounds have antacid properties.

Uses　Chronic constipation, colostomy, weight control, and as antacid.

Contraindications　Intestinal obstruction, ulceration, and severe abdominal pain.

Untoward Reactions　Diarrhea, nausea, vomiting, and esophageal obstruction resulting from chewing of tablets.

Dosage　**PO,** *Methylcellulose:* 1–1.5 gm 2 to 4 times daily; *Sodium carboxymethylcellulose:* 1.5 gm 2 to 4 times daily; **pediatric:** 500 mg 2 to 3 times daily.

Administration
1. Warn the patient to swallow tablets whole and not to chew them because this may cause esophageal obstruction.
2. Follow each dose with a glass of water or milk to prevent impaction.

PSYLLIUM HYDROPHILIC MUCILOID EFFERSYLLIUM, HYDROCIL PLAIN, KONSYL, L.A. FORMULA, LAXAMEAD, METAMUCIL, MODANE BULK, MUCILOSE, MUCILLIUM, REGACILIUM, SIBLIN, SYLLACT

Classification　Cathartic, bulk-forming.

General Statement　This drug is obtained from the fruit of various species of plantago. These preparations may also contain dextrose, sodium bicarbonate, monobasic potassium phosphate, citric acid, and benzyl benzoate.

The powder forms a gelatinous mass with water which adds bulk to the stools and stimulates peristalsis. It also has a demulcent effect on an inflamed intestinal mucosa.

Contraindications　Severe abdominal pain, or intestinal obstruction.

Dosage　**PO:** 4–7 gm 1 to 3 times daily. Pediatric dose proportionately smaller.

Administration
1. Thoroughly mix each dose in a glass of cool water or other liquid.
2. Follow with an additional glass of liquid.
3. Do not give routinely because it may cause dependency.

EMOLLIENT CATHARTICS

General Statement　As their name implies, these laxatives promote defecation by softening the feces. These agents are useful when it is desirable to keep the feces soft or when straining at stool is undesirable.

In addition to mineral oil (liquid petrolatum), which is seldom used today, this group of laxatives include several surface-active agents that lower the surface tension of the feces and promote their penetration by water and fat. This increases the softness of the fecal mass.

Except for mineral oil, the compounds are not absorbed systemically and do not seem to interfere with the absorption of nutrients.

Uses   Constipation associated with dry, hard stools, megacolon, bedridden patients, and cardiovascular and other diseases in which straining at stool should be avoided. After rectal surgery, especially hemorrhoidectomy.

DIOCTYL CALCIUM SULFOSUCCINATE SURFAK

DIOCTYL SODIUM SULFOSUCCINATE AFKO-LUBE, BU-LAX, COLACE, COLOCTYL, COMFOLAX, DILAX, DIOMEDICONE, DIOSUCCIN, DIOSUX, DISONATE, DOCTATE, DOSS, DOXINATE, D-S-S, DUOSOL, LAXINATE, MODANE SOFT, MOLATOC, PARLAX, PROVILAX, REGUL-AIDS, REGUTOL, REVAC, SOFTEZE, SOFTON, STULEX

Classification   Cathartic, emollient.

Remarks   These substances are surface-active laxatives. They should not be given concomitantly with mineral oil because surface-active agents may promote absorption of oil. May cause diarrhea.

Use   To lessen strain of defecation in persons with hernia or cardiovascular diseases, megacolon, or bedridden patients.

Contraindications   Nausea, vomiting, abdominal pain, and intestinal obstruction.

Dosage for All Agents   **PO: adults and children over 12 years:** 50–240 mg daily; **pediatric under 3 years:** 10–40 mg daily; **3 to 6 years:** 20–60 mg daily; **6 to 12 years:** 40–120 mg daily.

Administration: Dioctyl Sodium Sulfosuccinate   Administer oral solutions with milk or fruit juices to help mask bitter taste.

MINERAL OIL AGORAL PLAIN, FLEET OIL RETENTION ENEMA, KONDREMUL PLAIN, NEO-CULTOL, PETROGALAR PLAIN

Classification   Cathartic, emollient.

General Statement   This mixture of liquid hydrocarbons obtained from petroleum softens the stools and lubricates the GI tract. It coats the feces and thus prevents dehydration. It is effective 6 to 8 hours after administration.

Small amounts of mineral oil are absorbed systemically. Because the preparation coats the intestinal mucosa and thus prevents the normal absorption of vitamins A, D, and K, and other nutrients, care must be taken not to administer with foods or meals. Mineral oil can also be given as an enema to soften feces. The preparation is also available as an emulsion.

Uses Constipation, to avoid straining under certain conditions, such as rectal surgery, hemorrhoidectomy, and certain cardiovascular conditions.

Contraindications Nausea, vomiting, abdominal pain, or intestinal obstruction.

Untoward Reactions Regular use may produce nutritional (vitamins A, D, K) deficiency or lipid pneumonia. Regular use during pregnancy may decrease vitamin K absorption sufficiently to cause hypoprothrombinemia in the newborn.

Drug Interactions

Interactant	Interaction
Anticoagulants, oral	↑ Hypoprothrombinemia by ↓ absorption of vitamin K from GI tract. Also, mineral oil could ↓ absorption of anticoagulant from GI tract
Sulfonamides	↓ Effect of nonabsorbable sulfonamide in GI tract

Dosage **PO:** 15–30 ml at bedtime, **children:** 5–15 ml at bedtime. **Rectal, adults:** 90–120 ml; **children 2 years and older:** 30–60 ml.

Administration
1. Do not administer with food because oil may delay digestion and prevent absorption of vitamins.
2. Do not administer with vitamin preparation since again the medication will interfere with the absorption, especially of vitamins A, D, and K.
3. Administer at bedtime and, unless contraindicated, follow with orange juice or give patient a piece of orange to suck on. The emulsion is pleasant tasting and does not require orange to make it palatable.
4. Store in refrigerator to make medication more palatable.
5. Administer mineral oil to the elderly, debilitated, and to children slowly and carefully to prevent aspiration which may result in lipid pneumonia. Check with physician whether other relief for condition might be utilized if there seems to be a danger of aspiration.
6. For an oil retention enema, administer slowly via catheter. Follow 20 minutes later with cleansing enema as ordered.

Nursing Implications
1. Since mineral oil may cause hypoprothrombinemia in the newborn, warn pregnant women not to take medication to relieve constipation but rather to check her medical supervision for suitable medication.
2. Check perianal area of patients taking more than 30 ml of mineral oil because they are prone to leakage of feces through anal sphincter and

thus need more frequent cleansing and a perianal pad to prevent soiling of clothes and bedding.

POLOXAMER 188 POLYKOL

Classification	Cathartic, emollient.
Remarks	Surface active agent with emulsifying and wetting properties similar to dioctyl sodium sulfosuccinate. This physiologically inert substance permits water and fats to penetrate stools so that they are softer.
Uses	To decrease straining of defecation in presence of hernia or cardiovascular disease. Also megacolon and for bedridden patients with constipation.
Dosage	**PO:** 250 mg b.i.d.-t.i.d. for not more than five days; **pediatric 6 to 12 years:** 250–500 mg daily.
Administration	Administer as a single or divided dose which may be reduced after several days of therapy.

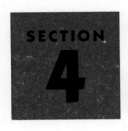

SECTION

4 antidiarrheal agents

Systemic Agents	Diphenoxylate Diphenoxylate Hydrochloride with Atropine	Loperamide Hydrochloride Paregoric
Local Agents	Bismuth Subcarbonate Charcoal, Activated Cholestyramine Resin Donnagel Donnagel PG	Kaolin with Pectin Mixture Kaopectate Lactobacillus Cultures Parepectolin

General Statement   Diarrhea accompanies many different disorders and the treating physician should attempt to elucidate the underlying cause of its manifestations. When diarrhea is caused by an infectious organism, the physician may prescribe a specific antibiotic or chemotherapeutic agent to eradicate the causative agent.

Often diarrhea is a self-limiting natural defense reaction by means of which the body rids itself of a toxic or irritating substance. Dehydration and disturbance of the electrolyte balance can be a major complication of diarrhea. Symptomatic antidiarrheal therapy can prevent extreme dehydration.

Most antidiarrheal agents are used for symptomatic relief. Anticholinergic drugs (p. 506), which reduce the excessive motility of the intestine, are also effective constipating agents.

Antidiarrheal agents fall into two categories: those that act locally on the intestine and its content and those that act systemically.

SYSTEMIC AGENTS

DIPHENOXYLATE

DIPHENOXYLATE HYDROCHLORIDE WITH ATROPINE
COLONIL, LOFENE, LOFLO, LOMO-PLUS, LOMOTIL, LONOX, LO-TROL, RO-DIPHEN-ATRO

Classification   Antidiarrheal agent, systemic.

General Statement   Diphenoxylate is a systemic constipating agent chemically related to the narcotic analgesic drug meperidine (Demerol). Diphenoxylate inhibits GI motility and has a constipating effect. The more widely used preparation (Lomotil) contains small amounts of atropine sulfate. This is thought to prevent the overusage of diphenoxylate, which might lead to dependence.

Uses   Symptomatic treatment of chronic and functional diarrhea. Also, diarrhea associated with gastroenteritis, irritable bowel, regional enteritis, malabsorption syndrome, ulcerative colitis, acute infections, food poisoning, postgastrectomy, and for drug-induced diarrhea. Therapeutic results for control of acute diarrhea are inconsistent. Also used in the control of intestinal passage time in patients with ileostomies and colostomies.

Contraindications   Cirrhosis, advanced liver disease, or glaucoma.

Untoward Reactions   Nausea, vomiting, abdominal cramps, drowsiness, dizziness, pruritus, skin rash, restlessness, and insomnia. Headache, tachycardia, numbness of the extremities, blurred vision, dryness of mouth, swelling of the gums, euphoria, depression, weakness, and general malaise occur rarely.

Drug Interactions

Interactant	Interaction
Barbiturates	CNS depressant effects of barbiturates may be potentiated by diphenoxylate
Monoamine Oxidase Inhibitors	↑ Chance of hypertensive crisis
Narcotics	↑ Effect of narcotics

Overdosage   Overdosage is characterized by flushing, lethargy, coma, hypotonic reflexes, nystagmus, pinpoint pupils, tachycardia and respiratory depression.

Treatment: Gastric lavage and assisted respiration.

IV administration of a narcotic antagonist, see page 365. Administration may be repeated after 10 to 15 minutes. Observe patient and readminister antagonist if respiratory depression returns.

Dosage   **PO: initial,** 5 mg t.i.d.-q.i.d., **children:** 0.3–0.4 mg/kg/day in divided doses. Contraindicated in children under 2 years of age. Also see below.

Pediatric	Total daily dose*
2– 5 years	6 mg
5– 8 years	8 mg
8– 12 years	10 mg

* Based on 4 ml per teaspoonful or 2.00 mg of diphenoxylate.

Each tablet or 5 ml of liquid preparation contains 2.5 mg diphenoxylate hydrochloride and 25 μg of atropine sulfate. Dosage should be maintained at initial levels until symptoms are under control; then reduce to maintenance levels.

Additional Nursing Implications
1. Observe patients on combination of Lomotil and barbiturates or other narcotics closely for potentiation of CNS depression.
2. Observe patients with liver disease who are receiving Lomotil for signs of impending coma such as minor mental aberrations and motor disturbances, untidiness, drowsiness, night wandering, faraway look in eye, and a coarse or "flapping" tremor of the hands.
3. Caution patients to follow exactly the recommended dosage schedule.
4. Store out of reach of children since accidental overdosage may result in fatality.
5. Have Narcan readily available in case of overdosage.

LOPERAMIDE HYDROCHLORIDE IMODIUM

Classification   Antidiarrheal agent, systemic.

General Statement   Loperamide is a piperidine derivative that slows intestinal motility by acting on the nerve end receptors embedded in the intestinal wall. The prolonged retention of the feces in the intestine results in reducing volume of the stools, increases viscosity, and decreases fluid and electrolyte loss. The drug is reported to be more effective than diphenoxylate.

Uses   Symptomatic relief of acute, non-specific diarrhea, chronic diarrhea associated with inflammatory bowel disease, reduction of volume discharged from ileostomies.

Contraindications   Discontinue drug promptly if abdominal distention develops in patients with acute ulcerative colitis. Safe use in pregnancy and children under twelve years of age not established. In conditions where pregnancy is to be avoided.

Untoward Reactions   Abdominal pain, distention or discomfort, constipation, drowsiness, dizziness, fatigue, dry mouth, nausea, vomiting, rash, and epigastric distress. (All these may be caused by the diarrheal syndrome.)

Dosage   **PO,** *acute diarrhea:* **initial,** 4 mg, followed by 2 mg after each unformed stool up to maximum of 16 mg/day. *Chronic diarrhea:* 4–8 mg/day as a single or divided dose. **Pediatric:** 80–240 μg/kg/day in 2 to 3 divided doses.

In acute diarrhea discontinue drug after 48 hr if ineffective. In chronic diarrhea discontinue if 16 mg daily for 10 days is ineffective.

PAREGORIC CAMPHORATED OPIUM TINCTURE

Classification   Antidiarrheal agent, systemic.

General Statement   The active principle of the mixture is opium (0.04% morphine). The preparation also contains benzoic acid, camphor, and anise oil.

Morphine increases the muscular tone of the intestinal tract, decreases digestive secretions, and inhibits normal peristalsis. The slowed passage of the feces through the intestines promotes dessication, which is a function of the time the feces spend in the intestine.

Uses   Acute diarrhea. Mild narcotic physical dependence in infants born to addicted mothers.

Contraindications   See *Morphine,* page 360. Do not use in patients with diarrhea caused by poisoning until toxic substance has been eliminated.

Untoward Reactions   See *Morphine,* p. 360.

Drug Interactions   See *Narcotic Analgesics,* p. 352.

Dosage   Preparation contains 0.04% morphine. **PO:** 5–10 ml 1 to 4 times daily (4 ml contain 1.6 mg of morphine). **Pediatric:** 0.25–0.5 ml/kg after each loose stool. **Infants** (*withdrawal symptoms*): 0.5–0.6 ml 4 to 6 times daily until withdrawal symptoms are relieved. Reduce dosage to 2 to 4 times a week over period of 10 days.

Nursing Implications   1. Adhere to the regimen prescribed by the physician.
2. Once diarrhea has abated, check with the physician for further instructions. Continued use of the drug may result in excessive constipation.
3. Read the order, the medicine card, and the label of the bottle care-

fully to ensure that correct medication is being administered. This is extremely important because opium tincture contains 25 times more morphine than paregoric.

4. Give paregoric with water to insure that it will reach stomach. Mixture of paregoric and water will have milky appearance.
5. Observe patients on prolonged use of drug for signs of physical dependence. Even though paregoric contains relatively little morphine its long-term use may lead to dependence.
6. Preparations containing paregoric are subject to the Controlled Substances Act.
7. Store in light-resistant container.
8. Have Narcan on hand in case of overdosage.

LOCAL AGENTS

General Statement
These are only moderately successful in the treatment of diarrhea, and their mode of action is not completely understood. The local agents consist of inert, nonabsorbable material, such as kaolin, charcoal, or bismuth. The individual particles of these preparations have large surface areas that are believed to adsorb fluid and toxic substances.

Some locally acting antidiarrheal agents, such as kaolin and pectin, have demulcent properties that can protect the irritated, inflamed walls of the intestine. Many nonprescription antidiarrheal preparations consist of a mixture of several locally acting agents. See Table 37, p. 744.

Contraindications
The locally acting antidiarrheal agents are not absorbed systemically and there are no known contraindications.

Untoward Reactions
Prolonged use may result in constipation or interfere with the proper absorption of nutrients.

Nursing Implications
1. Maintain a daily record indicating the frequency, character, and number of stools.
2. Analyze the stool record to evaluate the patient's response to medication.
3. Be alert to increased diarrhea or development of constipation, because either may require dosage adjustment.
4. Advise the patient to follow regimen prescribed by his/her physician because this is essential for control of diarrhea. Highly spiced foods and foods high in fat should be eliminated from the diet of patients suffering from diarrhea.
5. Caution parents of infants and young children under 5 years of age to consult a doctor rather than to administer antidiarrheal medications on their own because children are more susceptible to the consequences of severe fluid and electrolyte depletion.
6. Advise the patient to stop taking medication once diarrhea is controlled or constipation will result.
7. Advise patient at home to consult his/her physician should several doses of medication prove ineffective in controlling diarrhea.

TABLE 37 LOCALLY ACTING ANTIDIARRHEAL AGENTS

Drug	Main Use	Dosage	Remarks
Bismuth subcarbonate	Symptomatic treatment of diarrhea, gastritis, enteritis, dysentery, ulcerative colitis, ulceration of bowel. Adjuvent in treatment of amebiasis	**PO:** 0.5–4 gm, q 2 to 4 hr as capsule or as a powder suspended in water or milk with camphorated opium tincture (paregoric).	Also has some antacid and demulcent properties. Preferred to bismuth subnitrate.
Charcoal, activated	Emergency treatment of drug poisoning, dyspepsia, diarrhea, flatulence, dysentery	1–8 gm. In emergency, dosage may be approximated by stirring activated charcoal in water to consistency of thick soup.	Most valuable single agent for emergency treatment of certain cases of drug poisoning (mercuric chloride, strychnine, phenobarbital). Also, part of universal antidote.
Cholestyramine resin (Cuemid, Questran)	See *Hypocholesterolemics*, p. 288.		
Donnagel	Symptomatic treatment of diarrhea	**Initial,** 30 ml, **then** 15–30 ml after each BM. **Infants weighing 10 lbs:** 2.5 ml; **20 lbs:** 5 ml; **30 lbs and over:** 5–10 ml after each BM.	Mixture of kaolin, pectin and 3 anticholinergics (atropine, scopolamine, hyoscyamine). For contraindications, etc. see individual agents.

Drug	Use	Dosage	Remarks
Donnagel PG	Same as above plus opium		
Kaolin with pectin mixture	Symptomatic relief of diarrhea	**PO; adults:** 60– 120 ml; **children over 12 years:** 60 ml; **6–12 years:** 30– 60 ml; **3 to 6 years:** 15– 30 ml.	Kaolin is a clay consisting of aluminum silicate, mainly effective in small intestine
Kaopectate (Kalpec, Kao-Con, Paocin, Pargel)	Symptomatic relief of diarrhea	60– 120 ml repeated as necessary. **Pediatric:** half adult dose.	Mixtures of kaolin (20%) and pectin (1%) are popular and freely available. Kaolin-pectin ↓ effect of lincomycin due to ↓ absorption from GI tract.
Lactobacillus cultures (Bactid, Lactinex)	Treatment of side effects of diarrhea.	*Bactid:* two 100 mg capsules 2–4 times/day. *Lactinex:* 4 tablets or 1 packet (1 gm) 3–4 times/day with food, milk, or juice.	These bacterial cultures apparently help restore the normal intestinal flora after use of antimicrobial drugs and suppress emergence of some pathogenic staphylococci and candida.
Parepectolin	Antidiarrheal	**PO, adults:**15– 30 ml; **pediatric:** 2.5– 10 ml. Dose given after evacuation up to a maximum of 4 doses in 12 hr.	Mixture contains pectin, kaolin, and opium. See Kaolin with Pectin mixture.

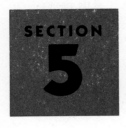

SECTION 5

emetics/antiemetics

Emetics	Apomorphine Hydrochloride
Antiemetics	Benzquinamide Hydrochloride
	Buclizine Hydrochloride
	Cyclizine Hydrochloride
	Dimenhydrinate
	Diphenhydramine Hydrochloride
	Diphenidol Hydrochloride
	Hydroxyzine
	Meclizine

Ipecac Syrup

Phosphorated Carbohydrate Solution
Prochlorperazine
Prochlorperazine Edisylate
Prochlorperazine Maleate
Scopolamine Hydrobromide
Thiethylperazine Maleate
Trimethobenzamide Hydrochloride

EMETICS

General Statement Emetics are used in case of acute poisoning to induce vomiting when it is desirable to empty the stomach promptly and completely after ingestion of toxic materials.

Vomiting can be elicited either by direct action on the chemoreceptor trigger zone (CTZ) in the medulla, or by indirect stimulation of the GI tract. Some agents act in both ways.

Nursing Implications
1. Do not administer an emetic if patient is comatose or semiconscious, has taken a convulsant poison, such as strychnine, or has ingested a corrosive substance like a strong acid or caustic, or petroleum distillates like kerosene.
2. Have on hand the following for the treatment of poison ingestion: gastric lavage equipment, oxygen, positive pressure apparatus, emergency drugs, and intravenous equipment and fluids.
3. Position the patient on side after administration of emetic to prevent aspiration when patient vomits.
4. Have available 200–300 ml of water at time of administration as emetics are usually administered with water.

APOMORPHINE HYDROCHLORIDE

Remarks Apomorphine is a synthetic derivative of morphine. It produces emesis by stimulating the CTZ. Vomiting occurs within 5 to 15 minutes.

The drug is not effective when administered PO since it may result in excessive CNS depression. **Do not give second dose.**

Use Oral poisoning.

Contraindications   Shock, drug-induced CNS depression, ingestion of corrosive substances, petroleum distillates, and lye and for patients sensitive to morphine.

Dosage   **SC:** 5– 10 mg; **pediatric:** 0.066 mg/kg. **Do not repeat.**

Administration/ Storage
1. Do not use solutions with emerald green hue indicating that drug has disintegrated.
2. Store solution in the dark in a closed container.

Additional Nursing Implications
1. Patient should drink 200– 300 ml water immediately before injection.
2. Observe for respiratory distress for at least 1 hour after administration of apomorphine as it may depress the respiratory center.
3. Chart apomorphine given in Narcotic Book in compliance with the Controlled Substances Act.

IPECAC SYRUP

General Statement   Ipecac is an alkaloid extracted from Brazil root. The active principle acts both locally on the gastric mucosa and centrally on the CTZ. Vomiting occurs within 15 to 60 minutes in 90% of all patients.

Ipecac is also used as an expectorant and for croup to make cough more productive. The drug does not act as quickly as apomorphine, but a second dose may be given. **Ipecac syrup must not be confused with ipecac fluid extract which is 14 times as strong.**

Uses   Oral poisoning, nauseating expectorant.

Contraindications   With corrosives or in individuals who are unconscious, semicomatose, severely inebriated or in shock.

Activated charcoal should not be given simultaneously with ipecac syrup as charcoal adsorbs ipecac and will nullify the effect.

Dosage   **PO,** *Emetic, Syrup,* **adults and children over 1 year:** 15 ml; **children less than 1 year:** 5– 10 ml. Administration should be followed by 200– 300 ml water for adults and 100– 200 ml water for children. May be repeated once if vomiting does not occur in 20 min.

Administration   Check label of medication closely so that the syrup and the fluid extract are not confused.

ANTIEMETICS

General Statement   Nausea and vomiting can be caused by a great variety of conditions, such as infections, drugs, radiation, motion, organic disease, or psychological factors. The underlying cause for the symptoms must be elicited before emesis is corrected.

The act of vomiting is complex. The vomiting center in the medulla responds to stimulation from many peripheral areas as well as to stimuli from the CNS itself, chemoreceptor trigger zone (CTZ), vestibular apparatus of the ear, and the cerebral cortex.

The selection of an antiemetic depends on the cause of the symptoms as well as on the manner in which the vomiting is triggered.

Many drugs used for other conditions, such as the antihistamines, phenothiazines, barbiturates and scopolamine, have antiemetic properties and can be so used. (For details see appropriate sections.) These agents often have serious side-effects (mostly CNS depression) that make their routine use undesirable. Several miscellaneous antiemetics are treated here.

Drug Interaction   Because of their antiemetic and antinauseant activity, the antiemetics may mask overdosage caused by other drugs.

Nursing Implications
1. Observe the patient closely for other untoward symptoms besides nausea since antiemetic may mask signs of overdosage of other drugs or pathology, such as increased intracranial pressure or intestinal obstruction.
2. Caution the patient against driving or performing hazardous tasks until his/her individual response to the drug has been evaluated. Antiemetics tend to cause drowsiness and dizziness.

BENZQUINAMIDE HYDROCHLORIDE EMETE-CON

Classification   Antiemetic.

General Statement   Benzquinamide hydrochloride is an antiemetic presently used only during anesthesia and surgery. The drug is a benzoquinoline derivative whose antiemetic activity is attributed to its depressant effect on the chemoreceptor trigger zone. Onset of action is rapid (15 minutes after parenteral administration) and the effect lasts for 3 to 4 hours.

Uses   Prevention and treatment of nausea during anesthesia and surgery.

Contraindications   Hypersensitivity to drug. Pregnancy; children under 12 years of age. IV for cardiac patients.

Untoward Reactions   Drowsiness. Also, insomnia, restlessness, headache, excitement, nervousness, dry mouth, shivering, sweating, hiccups, flushing, salivation, blurred vision have been reported. Various effects on cardiovascular system (hypertension, hypotension, dizziness, arrhythmias) have been reported especially after IV administration. Also various GI effects.

Drug Interaction   Use lower dose of benzquinamide in patients receiving epinephrinelike drugs or pressor agents.

Dosage   **IM:** 50 mg or 0.5– 1 mg/kg. May be repeated after 1 hr, **then** q 3 to 4 hr. **IV:** 25 mg or 0.2–0.4 mg/kg. Inject slowly (½ to 1 minute); switch to **IM** after one **IV** dose.

Administration/ Storage
1. Reconstituted solution stable for 14 days at room temperature.
2. Store solution and unreconstituted powder in light-resistant containers.
3. For prophylaxis give 15 minutes prior to when patient is expected to regain consciousness from anesthesia.

BUCLIZINE HCL

Classification   Antiemetic, antihistamine.

General Statement   Piperazine-type antihistamine used primarily to suppress nausea and vomiting through an action on the CNS.

Uses   Nausea, vomiting, dizziness of motion sickness, Meniere's syndrome, labyrinthitis.

Contraindications   Hypersensitivity to drug, pregnancy. Safe use in children not established.

Untoward Reactions   Drowsiness, dryness of mouth, headache, nervousness.

Drug Interactions   See *Antihistamines*, page 688.

Dosage   **PO: usual,** 50 mg alleviates nausea and prevents motion sickness. May be repeated after 4 to 6 hr. *Severe nausea:* up to 150 mg. **Maintenance:** 50 mg b.i.d.

Administration
1. Take 30 minutes before departure.
2. Tablet can be chewed, swallowed whole, or dissolved in mouth.

CYCLIZINE HYDROCHLORIDE MAREZINE
See *Antihistamines*, page 685.

Antiemetic Dosage   **PO:** 50 mg t.i.d.-q.i.d. Not to exceed 200 mg/day. **IM:** 50 mg t.i.d.-q.i.d. **PO, pediatric 6–10 years:** ½ the adult dose.

DIMENHYDRINATE DRAMAMINE, DIMENEST, REIDAMINE, OTHERS
See *Antihistamines*, page 685.

Dosage   **PO, Rectal, IM, IV:** 50–100 mg t.i.d.-q.i.d.; **pediatric 8 to 12 years (except IV):** 5 mg/kg daily in 4 divided doses, up to maximum of 150 mg daily. No **IV** dosage has been established for children.

DIPHENHYDRAMINE HYDROCHLORIDE BAX, BENADRYL, FENYLHIST, ROHYDRA, VALDRENE

See *Antihistamines*, Table 34, p. 685.

DIPHENIDOL HYDROCHLORIDE VONTROL HYDROCHLORIDE

Classification   Antiemetic.

Remarks   The drug seems to have a depressant action on labyrinth excitability. Like the phenothiazines, it may also depress the CTZ or vomiting center.

Uses   Nausea and vomiting associated with infectious diseases, malignancies, radiation sickness, general anesthesia, motion sickness, labyrinthitis, and Meniere's disease. The drug is effective 30 to 45 minutes after PO and 15 minutes after parenteral administration. It is effective for 3 to 6 hours.

Contraindications   Hypersensitivity to drug, anuria, pregnancy, infants under 6 months or weighing less than 25 pounds. Administer with caution to patients with glaucoma, pyloric stenosis, pylorospasm, obstructive lesions of GI and urinary tract, and sinus tachycardia.

Untoward Reactions   Drowsiness, dry mouth, nausea, indigestion, blurred vision, dizziness, skin rash, malaise, headache, weakness, heartburn, nervousness, and urticaria. Discontinue drug at once in case of hallucinations, disorientation, or confusion.

Dosage   **PO:** 25–50 mg q 4 hr. **IM** (*acute symptoms*): 20–40 mg. May be repeated once after 1 hr, and q 4 hr thereafter. **IV or IV infusion:** 20 mg (maximum of 2 doses by this route and only for adult, hospitalized patients). **Maximum adult dosage:** 300 mg. **Pediatric, PO:** 0.88 mg/kg up to maximum of 5.5 mg/kg in 24 hr. **IM:** 0.44 mg/kg up to maximum of 3.3 mg/kg in 24 hr. Use only 1 week if there is serious vestibular disease requiring treatment.

Additional Nursing Implications   1. Observe the patient, especially within first 3 days of starting drug for possible hallucinations, disorientation, or confusion. Reassure the patient that these symptoms decrease 3 days after drug is stopped.
2. Be prepared to monitor BP in adults after parenteral administration and in children after postoperative administration.
3. Monitor intake and output and report oliguria as this interferes with excretion of the drug.

4. Stress to the patient the necessity for hospitalization or close medical supervision when drug is used.
5. Be prepared in case of overdosage to assist with gastric lavage, monitor BP and respiration, and to supply supportive measures such as oxygen or mechanical respiration.

HYDROXYZINE ATARAX, VISTARIL

See *Antianxiety Agents*, Chapter 5, Section 7.

MECLIZINE ANTIVERT, BONINE, WEHVERT, OTHERS

See *Antihistamines*, page 686.

Antiemetic Dosage   **PO:** 25–50 mg daily; **pediatric:** dosage not established. *Vertigo:* 25–100 mg daily.

PHOSPHORATED CARBOHYDRATE SOLUTION EMETROL, NAUSETROL

Classification   Antiemetic.

General Statement   These low cost, mint-flavored syrups are concentrated carbohydrate solutions with phosphoric acid. They are claimed to relieve nausea and vomiting by a direct action on the GI tract wall.

Uses   Symptomatic relief of nausea and vomiting due to a variety of causes, including vomiting due to psychogenic factors, morning sickness, motion sickness, nausea or vomiting due to drug therapy, and regurgitation in infants.

Contraindications   Diabetes.

Dosage   **Adults:** 15–30 ml; **infants and children:** 5–10 ml. Dose may be repeated.

Administration
1. *Do Not* dilute.
2. Do not allow liquids PO for 15 minutes after administration.
3. In case of nausea, repeat at 15-minute intervals until condition is under control.
4. Regurgitating infants: 5 to 10 minutes before each feeding; refractory cases: 30–45 ml ½ hr before feeding.
5. Morning sickness: On arising and q 3 hr thereafter or when nausea threatens.

Nursing Implications
1. Do not administer this concentrated carbohydrate solution to a diabetic.
2. Anticipate that this emetic will not cause toxicity, side effects, or mask symptoms of organic disease.

PROCHLORPERAZINE COMPAZINE

PROCHLORPERAZINE EDISYLATE COMPAZINE EDISYLATE

PROCHLORPERAZINE MALEATE COMPAZINE MALEATE

See *Phenothiazines*, page 377.

Uses   Postoperative nausea and vomiting, radiation sickness, vomiting due to toxins.

Dosage   **PO:** 5– 10 mg 3 to 4 times daily. *Timed release:* 15 mg on arising, or 10 mg q 12 hr. **Rectal:** 25 mg b.i.d. **IM:** 5– 10 mg q 3 to 4 hr. *Postoperatively and postpartum control of vomiting:* 10– 30 mg. **Pediatric, PO and Rectal:** 0.4 mg/kg daily in 3 to 4 divided doses. **IM:** 0.13 mg/kg is usually sufficient to control vomiting.

SCOPOLAMINE HYDROBROMIDE

See *Anticholinergics*, Chapter 6, Section 5.

THIETHYLPERAZINE MALEATE TORECAN MALEATE

Classification   Antiemetic.

Remarks   Phenothiazine derivative acting on CTZ zone. For details, see *Phenothiazines*, page 368.

Uses   Control of nausea and vomiting of various origins.

Contraindications   Severe CNS depression, comatose states, pregnancy, children under 12 years of age. Administer with caution to patients with liver or kidney disease. The drug, when administered PO, is effective in 30 minutes; the effect lasts 4 hours.

Untoward Reactions   Drowsiness, dryness of mouth and nose, restlessness, hypotension, extrapyramidal complications.

Dosage   **PO, Rectal, IM:** 10– 30 mg 1 to 3 times daily. Do not use **IV.** Dosage for children not established.

Administration   Administer by deep IM injection.

Additional Nursing Implications

Review *General Statement* and *Nursing Implications* for phenothiazines, pages 368 and 373.

1. Do not administer to a patient with depressed respiratory rate, to patients in a comatose state, or to those performing hazardous tasks.
2. Observe the patient for postural hypotension manifested by weakness, dizziness, and faintness. Monitor BP.
3. Have available levarterenol and phenylephrine should hypotension occur because epinephrine is contraindicated.
4. Observe and report extrapyramidal symptoms, such as torticollis, dysphagia, random movements of the eyes, or convulsions.
5. Have available caffeine sodium benzoate and Benadryl IV for relief of extrapyramidal symptoms.

TRIMETHOBENZAMIDE HYDROCHLORIDE TIGAN

Classification

Antiemetic.

General Statement

An antiemetic related to antihistamines but with weak antihistaminic properties. Believed to depress CTZ of medulla. The drug is less effective than phenothiazines but has fewer side effects. Not suitable as sole agent for severe emesis. Onset of action after PO or IM administration: 10–40 minutes. Duration: 3 to 4 hours. Can be given rectally.

Uses

Emesis during surgery, radiation-induced nausea and vomiting; pregnancy.

Contraindications

Hypersensitivity to drug, and when suppositories are used, to benzocaine. Do not use suppositories for neonates; do not use IM in children.

Untoward Reactions

Few. Occasionally parkinson-like symptoms, hypersensitivity, rarely adverse CNS manifestations, blood dyscrasias, jaundice. After IM administration: pain at injection site.

Dosage

PO: 250 mg b.i.d.-q.i.d. **Rectal and IM:** 200 mg t.i.d.-q.i.d. **Pediatric:** 30–90 pounds, **PO and rectal:** 100–200 mg. t.i.d.-q.i.d.; **under 30 pounds, rectal,** 100 mg t.i.d.-q.i.d.

Administration

Inject drug IM deeply into the upper outer quadrant and be careful to avoid escape of fluid from needle so as to minimize local reaction.

Additional Nursing Implications

1. Do not administer suppositories to patients allergic to benzocaine or similar local anesthetics.
2. Observe for skin reaction which is the first sign of hypersensitivity to drug.
3. Check with the patient whether there is any local reaction to suppositories.

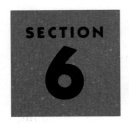

SECTION 6

digestants

Dehydrocholic Acid
Sodium Dehydrocholate Injection
Glutamic Acid Hydrochloride
Hydrochloric Acid, Diluted

Ketocholanic Acids
Ox Bile Extract (Bile Salts)
Pancreatin
Pancrelipase

General Statement Digestants are agents that replace or supplement one of the many enzymes or other chemical substances that participate in the digestion of food. They are rarely indicated for therapeutic reasons but may be required for elderly patients or those suffering from certain deficiency diseases of the GI tract. They may also be required after GI surgery.

Commonly used digestants include hydrochloric acid, bile salts, and the enzymes produced by the stomach and glands associated with digestion.

Nonprescription preparations also contain many of the same ingredients as prescription drugs; however, these are usually present at levels too low to be effective.

DEHYDROCHOLIC ACID CHOLAN DH, DECHOLIN, HEPAHYDRIN, NEOCHOLAN

SODIUM DEHYDROCHOLATE INJECTION DECHOLIN SODIUM

Classification Digestant.

General Statement This drug is a modified derivative of the bile acids. Dehydrocholic acid is believed to increase the flow of bile and facilitate evacuation of the gallbladder. The drug may increase the absorption of fats.

In allergic or asthmatic patients, IV administration of sodium dehydrocholic acid should be preceded by a skin test.

Uses Flushing action after surgery of the biliary tract to promote drainage of an infected common bile duct as well as chronic and recurring cholangitis. Promotion of fat absorption in cirrhosis and steatorrhea (excessive fat in stools which makes them large, bulky, and foul smelling). Sodium dehydrocholate injection is used for diagnostic purposes to determine circulation time.

Contraindications Complete obstruction of the biliary tract, acute hepatitis, asthma. Use with caution in patients with a history of asthma and allergies.

Untoward Reactions	Systemic administration: anaphylactoid reaction, nausea, vomiting, diarrhea, abdominal pain, headache, tachycardia, hypotension, faintness, dyspnea, sweating, chills, fever, erythema, pruritus, and urticaria.
Dosage	*Dehydrocholic acid*, **PO**: 250–500 mg b.i.d.-t.i.d. after meals for 4 to 6 weeks. Discontinue drug if no improvement is noted after 4 to 6 weeks. *Sodium dyhydrocholate injection*, **IV**: 20% solution, *day 1:* 5–10 ml; *days 2 to 3:* 10 ml. Replace by **PO** medication as soon as possible. **Diagnosis—circulation time:** 3–5 ml.
Nursing Implications (Dehydrocholic Acid)	1. Check that skin test was done on patients with a history of allergy or asthma prior to injection of dehydrocholic acid. 2. Have epinephrine available in case of allergic response to IV administration of drug. 3. Observe after IV injection for extravasation into the perivascular tissue because pain, redness and swelling may occur. Report and apply warm compresses should extravasation occur. 4. Instruct patient who will be taking medication at home to consult the physician if pain persists or if severe nausea and pain develop. 5. Be prepared to assist the physician in determining circulation time, defined as the time it takes from injection of the drug into the cubital vein until the patient perceives a bitter taste that passes from the base of the tongue to its tip. The range of normal values is 8 to 16 seconds.

GLUTAMIC ACID HYDROCHLORIDE ACIDULIN

Classification	Digestant.
Remarks	On contact with water this compound releases hydrochloric acid, which acidifies the stomach. Thus, the drug has the same effect as hydrochloric acid but is easier to administer because it comes in capsule form. Is also combined with pepsin.
Uses	Hypochlorhydria, achlorhydria, as an adjunct in pernicious anemia or gastric cancer.
Contraindications	Hyperacidity and peptic ulcer.
Untoward Reaction	An overdose may result in systemic acidosis.
Dosage	**PO**: 340–1000 mg t.i.d. before meals. (Each capsule contains the equivalent of 0.6 ml of diluted hydrochloric acid.)
Nursing Implications	1. Advise the patient to keep capsules dry before ingesting. 2. Have on hand sodium bicarbonate or sodium lactate or other alkaline solution to treat overdosage.

HYDROCHLORIC ACID, DILUTED

Classification Digestant.

Remarks Diluted hydrochloric acid (10% w/v) is used to supplement or replace that which occurs naturally in the stomach.

Uses Hypochlorhydria, hydrochloric acid deficiency often occurring in the elderly (is frequently associated with pernicious anemia or gastric cancer).

Contraindications Hyperacidity and peptic ulcer.

Untoward Reactions Prolonged administration may disturb electrolyte balance (depletion of sodium bicarbonate) and increase the levels of sodium chloride.

Dosage Administer 2–8 ml of a 10% solution copiously diluted. Dilute each milliliter with at least 25 ml of water.

Nursing Implications
1. Tell the patient to sip medication with meal.
2. Instruct the patient to sip medication through a straw to protect tooth enamel (do not use a metal straw).
3. Advise the patient to use an alkaline mouth wash if he/she is still finishing the hydrochloric acid solution after the meal.

KETOCHOLANIC ACIDS KETOCHOL

Classification Digestant.

Remarks One mg of ketocholanic acid derived from beef bile corresponds to one mg of dehydrochloric acid.

Uses Laxative.

Dosage **PO:** 250–500 mg t.i.d. with meals.

Nursing Implications
1. Advise patient to increase intake of fluids and roughage in diet and include exercise (unless contraindicated) to prevent constipation rather than relying on ketocholanic acids—which may result in drug dependency.
2. Observe patient whose bile is draining away from the GI tract or who is on long-term therapy for signs of nutritional deficiency precipitated by inadequate digestion and absorption of nutrients. Bile salts may be necessary to prevent or alleviate nutritional deficiency. Also see *Nursing Implications 1 to 4 of Dehydrochloric Acid*, p. 755.

OX BILE EXTRACT BILE SALTS, BILRON

Classification Digestant.

Remarks	Natural dried extract of ox bile containing a minimum of 45% cholic acid.
Uses	Bile deficiency states. Partial biliary obstruction, steatorrhea. To increase the secretion of bile by the liver and promote absorption of fats and fat-soluble vitamins. Laxative.
Contraindications	Complete mechanical biliary obstruction. Use with caution in patients with obstructive jaundice.
Untoward Reactions	Nausea, vomiting, and diarrhea.
Dosage	Administer 300–500 mg with water b.i.d.-t.i.d. after meals.
Administration	Caution the patient not to chew tablets because they are bitter.

PANCREATIN ELZYME 303, PANTERIC, VIOKASE

Classification	Digestant.
Remarks	This mixture of enzymes (mainly lipase, amylase, and trypsin) is obtained from hog pancreas. It promotes the digestion of food.
Uses	Pancreatic deficiency diseases. Invalids with poor digestion. Sometimes used to predigest food.
Contraindications	Give with caution to patients sensitive to hog protein.
Dosage	Administer 0.325–1.0 gm with meals.
Administration	1. Advise patient to swallow and not chew tablets. 2. Do not administer granules alone as the enzymes would be destroyed. 3. Sprinkle granules on food or add to milk or water for those unable to swallow capsules. 4. Do not give with hot foods.
Nursing Implications	1. Check that the patient maintains diet ordered. 2. Observe for constipation and anorexia indicating overdosage.

PANCRELIPASE COTAZYM, ILOZYME, KU-ZYME-HP

Classification	Digestant.
Remarks	Enzyme concentrate obtained from hog pancreas. The preparation contains high concentrations of digestive enzymes, especially lipase. The product is more effective than pancreatin.

Uses   Replacement therapy in symptomatic relief of malabsorption syndromes caused by pancreatic deficiency of organic origin as in cystic fibrosis of pancreas, cancer of the pancreas, and chronic inflammation of the pancreas.

Contraindication   Give with caution to patients hypersensitive to hog protein.

Dosage   **PO** dosage should be calculated according to fat content of diet. Approximately 300 mg/17 gm dietary fat. Usually the dose is 1–3 tablets or capsules at each meal or 1 with each snack. The dose of powder is 1–2 packets before meals or snacks.

Administration   Pediatric: for young children the content of the capsule can be sprinkled on food. After several weeks of use, dosage should be adjusted according to therapeutic results.

Nursing Implication   Check that patient maintains prescribed diet.

HEAVY METAL ANTAGONISTS

Calcium Disodium Edetate
Deferoxamine Mesylate
Dimercaprol

Disodium Edetate
Penicillamine

General Statement
Heavy metals are toxic because they tie up reaction sites and thus inactivate key biological substances, such as enzymes. This leads to poisoning and often to death.

Heavy metal antagonists have the ability to bind the metal ions as a nonpoisonous, complex "chelate" compound that is eliminated without toxic reaction by the kidneys. The word "chelate" comes from the Greek and means "claw." A chelating compound holds a metal ion like a claw, removing it from circulation.

Heavy metal poisoning occurs as a consequence of overdosage with certain drugs (i.e., gold compounds for the treatment of rheumatoid arthritis, iron for the treatment of anemia, mercurial diuretics) or because of accidental ingestion of such widespread substances as lead-containing paint, lead tetraethyl, arsenic-containing weed-killers, and pesticides.

CALCIUM DISODIUM EDETATE CALCIUM DISODIUM VERSENATE, CALCIUM EDTA

Classification
Heavy metal antagonist.

General Statement
Calcium disodium edetate displaces lead and cadmium from biological molecules and body tissues. It is used primarily for lead poisoning, but also for zinc, copper, chromium, manganese and nickel. It is ineffective in mercury or arsenic poisoning. It also combines with free heavy metal ions in the extra-cellular fluid. The resulting, inactive chelate is eliminated by the kidneys.

After institution of IV therapy, peak of lead excretion occurs within 24 to 48 hours. Lead encephalopathy is sometimes treated with both calcium disodium edetate and BAL, injected in separate deep IM sites.

Uses
Acute lead poisoning and lead encephalopathy; diagnosis of lead poisoning. Effective in reducing the incidence of residual neurologic damage. Chronic lead poisoning when accompanied by accidental overdosage of PO or parenteral iron, cadmium poisoning, and porphyria.

759

Contraindication   Use with extreme caution in the presence of renal disease.

Untoward Reactions   Few side effects are noted when drug is administered at prescribed dosage levels. The greatest danger is kidney damage and kidney failure that may occur when drug is given at too high dosage.

Other side effects include: malaise, fatigue, excessive thirst, numbness and tingling, followed by sudden fever and shaking chills, myalgia, arthralgia, headache, GI disturbances, and transitory allergic manifestations. Thrombophlebitis.

Prolonged administration may cause kidney damage, transient bone marrow depression, GI disturbances, and mucotaneous lesions.

Dosage   One gram of calcium disodium edetate removes about 3–5 mg lead. Dosage is determined by lead titer of blood (60 μg/100 ml of whole blood or 100 μg/liter of 24-hr urine specimen indicative of lead poisoning). The drug is usually administered IV.

IV, adults: 50 mg/kg/day. **Maximum total dose:** 550 mg/kg/course. **Maximum duration of course:** 2 weeks. Course may be repeated once after a rest period of 2 weeks. **IM:** Route of choice for children. Dose should not exceed 0.5 gm/30 pounds b.i.d. (about 75 mg/kg/day). **PO** (rare): 4 gm daily in divided doses; **pediatric:** 60 mg/kg. Course may be repeated after a rest period of 2 weeks for oral administration. Not advisable to give more than two courses of therapy. *Diagnosis:* 3 doses of 25 mg/kg given at 8-hr intervals. In case of lead poisoning urinary excretion of lead increases to 500 μg lead/24-hr urine sample.

Administration   IV: Dilute 5 ml ampul to 250 to 500 ml with suitable diluent. Administer to asymptomatic adults over a period of 1 hour minimum b.i.d. and to symptomatic adults over a period of 2 hours minimum. Drug may be given for up to 5 days. Administration then may be resumed after a rest period of 2 days. IM (preferred in children): Inject with procaine (1 ml of 1% procaine solution for each ml of concentrated calcium disodium edetate or equivalent amount of crystalline procaine) to reduce pain at injection site.

Nursing Implications

1. Check that patient has urine flow before initiating therapy with EDTA.
2. Provide large amounts of milk orally to facilitate removal of lead salts from the gut if lead has been ingested. Enemas are also administered to hasten removal of lead.
3. Check that x-ray is taken before initiation of EDTA therapy to ascertain that all lead has been removed from gut.
4. Monitor intake and output.
5. Unless contraindicated, encourage fluid intake to facilitate excretion of lead.
6. Avoid contact of EDTA with contaminated skin of patient, because contact increases systemic absorption.
7. Check that daily urinalysis is done to determine proteinuria,

hematuria, and renal cells. Should these occur, withhold drug, report to doctor.

8. Discontinue medication if anuria occurs to prevent high tissue levels of drug.
9. Check that tests for BUN are done periodically to detect renal damage.
10. Monitor pulse regularly because medication may cause cardiac arrhythmias.
11. Check that serum lead levels are performed periodically to evaluate drug response. Children with lead levels above 40 μg/100 ml of blood require treatment.

DEFEROXAMINE MESYLATE DESFERAL MESYLATE

Classification Heavy metal antagonist.

Remarks Deferoxamine is a complex organic molecule that reacts with iron. The resulting chelate is excreted by the kidneys.

Uses Adjunct in the treatment of iron intoxication. Also used for iron storage diseases (investigational use) and thalassemia.

Contraindications Severe renal disease, anuria. Use with caution for patients with pyelonephritis.

Untoward Reactions Hypotension, tachycardia, skin rashes, GI irritation, shock. All these symptoms are more common after IV administration.

Long-term therapy may cause allergic-type reactions (pruritus, rash, anaphylactoid reactions), blurring of vision, abdominal discomfort, diarrhea, leg cramps, tachycardia, fever, and cataracts.

Dosage **IV infusion** can be used in emergencies such as cardiovascular collapse. 1 gm at a rate not to exceed 15 mg/kg/hr; follow by 0.5 gm q 4 hr for 2 doses; **then** same as **IM.**

IM, *preferred:* **initial,** 1 gm; **then** 500 mg at 4-hr intervals for 2 doses. Subsequent 500 mg doses may be given if necessary q 4 hr to 12 hr up to total of 6 gm/24 hr.

Administration
1. Dissolve deferoxamine mesylate by adding 2 ml of sterile water to each ampule.
2. For IV administration use physiological saline, or Ringer's Lactate and administer *slowly* at a rate not exceeding 15 mg/kg/hour.
3. Discard dissolved drug if not used within 2 weeks.
4. Do not administer by SC route as induration may occur.

Nursing Implications
1. Be prepared to assist with induction of emesis, gastric lavage, suction, maintenance of airway, administration of IV fluid and blood, and provision of oxygen and vasopressors to prevent or treat shock due to iron intoxication, and/or acidosis.

2. Observe patients in shock (BP and pulse) for improvement and report. The physician may wish to transfer to IM administration as soon as patient is out of shock.
3. Have epinephrine readily available for allergic type reactions.
4. Anticipate that pain and induration at the site of administration may occur.
5. Inform patient that drug may give urine a reddish color.
6. Observe patients with a history of pyelonephritis for pain and hematuria caused by deferoxamine inducing an exacerbation of the disease.

DIMERCAPROL BAL IN OIL

Classification   Heavy metal antagonist.

General Statement   This compound was developed as an antidote to the arsenic-containing war gas Lewisite. It forms a chelate with a number of heavy metal ions, including arsenic, mercury, and gold. The resulting chelate is eliminated by the kidneys. To be effective the drug must be administered promptly after poisoning is noted.

Uses   Acute arsenic, mercury and gold poisoning, resulting from overdosage with mercurial diuretics, arsenicals, gold salts, accidental ingestion of mercury, arsenic, or gold-containing salts. Wilson's disease.

Contraindications   Iron, cadmium, or selenium poisoning. Hepatic insufficiency. Use with caution in the presence of renal insufficiency.

Untoward Reactions   At recommended dosage levels there are few side effects. Doses of 5 or more mg/kg may cause transient nausea, vomiting, headache, lacrimation, salivation, a burning sensation of lips, mouth, throat, eye extremities, generalized muscular pain, constriction of chest, and hypertension.
Children may also develop fever. At very high doses dimercaprol may cause coma or convulsions and metabolic acidosis.
Drug must be discontinued if renal insufficiency develops.

Drug Interactions

Interactant	Interaction
Cadmium salts ⎫ Iron salts ⎪ Selenium salts ⎬ Uranium salts ⎭	Dimercaprol may increase toxicity of these heavy metal salts

Dosage   **IM,** *mild arsenic and gold poisoning:* 2.5 mg/kg q.i.d. for days 1 and 2; b.i.d. on day 3; once daily for 10 days thereafter or until recovery is complete. *Severe arsenic or gold poisoning:* 3 mg/kg q 4 hrs for days 1 and 2; q.i.d. on day 3; b.i.d. for 10 days. *Mercury poisoning:* **initial,** 5 mg/kg, **then** 2.5 mg/kg 1 or 2 times daily for 10 days. *Acute lead encephalopathy:* 4 mg/kg alone initially; **then** q 4 hr in combination with EDTA administered in a separate site.

Administration
1. Check with physician whether a local anesthetic may be given with IM injection to minimize pain at injection site.
2. Inject IM deeply into muscle and massage after injection.

Nursing Implications
1. Reassure the patient that untoward GI and CNS effects will pass within 30 to 90 minutes.
2. Monitor the patient's BP, pulse, and temperature to help evaluate reaction to drug.
3. Have ephedrine or an antihistamine available for either premedication or for later use if the patient should have an untoward reaction.
4. Anticipate that the medication should have an unpleasant garliclike odor.
5. Be careful when preparing medication or administering medication not to allow fluid to come in contact with skin as it may cause a skin reaction.

DISODIUM EDETATE DISODIUM VERSENATE, ENDRATE DISODIUM

Classification
Heavy metal antagonist.

Remarks
Although disodium edetate has the same properties as calcium disodium edetate, it is not recommended for use as a heavy metal antagonist because it may cause hypocalcemia. It is used, however, for the emergency treatment of hypercalcemia; kidney function, blood pressure, and electrolytes should be monitored during therapy.

Uses
Emergency treatment of hypercalcemia and pathologic calcification. Experimentally in the management of atherosclerosis and intermittent claudication. Digitalis toxicity.

Contraindications
Use with caution in patients with clinical or subclinical hypokalemia.

Untoward Reactions
Pain at infusion site, thrombophlebitis, chills, fever, back pain, hypotension, muscle cramps, vomiting, urinary frequency, skin eruptions, anorexia, nausea, and diarrhea. Rapid injection may produce hypocalcemic tetany and convulsions, respiratory arrest, and severe arrhythmias.

Dosage
IV: Individualized and depending on degree of hypercalcemia. **Recommended maximum dose, adult:** 50 mg/kg up to a total of 3 gm daily for a period of 5 days, followed by a rest period of 2 days. Course may be repeated, if necessary, to a total of 15 doses. **Children:** 40 mg/kg up to a maximum of 70 mg/kg/day.

Administration
1. Check label on vial carefully that drug is disodium edetate and not calcium disodium edetate.
2. Dilute medication in 500 ml of 5% dextrose solution or isotonic saline solution as ordered.

3. Infuse slowly over 3 to 4 hours.
4. Do not extend the recommended dose, concentration, or rate of administration.

Nursing Implications

1. Record which vein is used for site of administration as repeated use of the same vein is likely to result in thrombophlebitis. Greater dilution of the solution and slower administration reduces the incidence of thrombophlebitis if the same vein must be used.
2. Administer with the patient in Fowler's position according to the patient's comfort.
3. Monitor BP during infusion as a transitory hypotension may occur, which would necessitate lowering the patient until hypotension has passed and blood pressure stabilized.
4. Be alert to a generalized systemic reaction that may occur from 4 to 8 hours after infusion of the drug and usually subsides within 12 hours. Report such a reaction and provide supportive care for fever, chills, back pain, vomiting, muscle cramps, or urinary urgency should they occur.
5. Warn diabetic patients that drug may cause hypoglycemia and that physician should be consulted whether to reduce insulin or increase food intake should patient feel hypoglycemic or urine test be negative for sugar.

PENICILLAMINE CUPRIMINE

General Statement

Penicillamine is a degradation product of penicillin. It is devoid of antibiotic activity. Penicillamine combines with copper, iron, mercury, and lead. The resulting biologically inactive chelate is readily excreted by the kidneys.

Patients should be closely watched during initiation of therapy. Urinalysis, CBC, and hemoglobin determinations should be performed regularly. Body temperature must be checked nightly.

Use

Copper toxicity. For use in rheumatoid arthritis, Wilson's disease, and cystinuria see p. 429. For all details except dosage for heavy metal intoxication see p. 429.

Dosage

Dosage is usually calculated on the basis of the urinary excretion of copper; 1 gm penicillamine promotes excretion of 2 mg copper.

PO: Usual Initial, adults and older children: 250 mg q.i.d. Dosage may have to be increased to 4 gm daily. A further increase does not produce additional excretion. **Pediatric, infants over 6 months:** 250 mg daily.

Patient should also receive sulfurated potash (40 mg) or a cation exchange resin such as Carbo-Resin (15–20 gm) with each meal.

For Administration and Nursing Implications see p. 430.

MISCELLANEOUS AGENTS

Adenosine Phosphate
Azathioprine
Beta-Carotene
Bromocriptine Mesylate
Cromolyn Sodium
Disulfiram
Guanidine Hydrochloride
Hyaluronidase

Lactulose
Morrhuate Sodium
Pigmenting Agents—Psoralens
  Methoxsalen
  Trioxsalen
Pralidoxine Chloride
Sodium Tetradecyl Sulfate
Streptokinase-Streptodornase

ADENOSINE PHOSPHATE ADENOCREST, ADENOSINE 5-MONOPHOSPHATE, AMP, COBALASINE, MUSCLE ADENYLIC ACID, MY-B-DEN

Classification Miscellaneous.

General Statement The adenosine phosphates are essential to the energy economy of muscle tissue. The therapeutic effects of adenosine phosphate in reducing tissue edema and inflammation are believed to result from increasing levels of adenosine triphosphate (ATP) or from its vasodilator effect.

Uses Adjunct in treatment of varicose vein ulcers and chronic thrombophlebitis (pre- and post-operatively). Tenosynovitis, intractable pruritus, and multiple sclerosis.

Contraindications Use with caution in patients with history of asthma, myocardial infarction, or cerebral hemorrhage.

Untoward Reactions Local reaction at injection site. Slight flushing, dizziness, diuresis, palpitations, headaches, diarrhea, rash. May increase symptoms of bursitis or tendonitis.

Dosage **IM** (*as sodium salt in repository gelatin vehicle*): 20–100 mg/day for 3 to 4 days, followed by single dose q other day or 3 times/week. After initial response, reduce to 20 mg 1 to 2 times/week. *Aqueous solution* (*sodium salt*): 20 mg 1 to 3 times/day or once/hr for 5 doses on each of first 3 days. Reduce to 20 mg/day as needed. *Alternate dosage regimen:* 100 mg/day as single dose, followed by 100 mg on alternate days as needed. **Sublingual** (*as acid*) **to supplement IM administration:** 20 mg q hr for 5–7 doses for 4 to 7 days. **Thereafter,** 40–100 mg/day.

Administration Instruct patients taking sublingual tablets to place tablet in buccal pouch and refrain from mixing it with saliva, eating, or drinking, until tablet is absorbed.

Nursing Implications
1. Be alert to complaints of dyspnea and tightness in chest after injection, indications of an allergic reaction. Discontinue medication and promptly treat with epinephrine, oxygen, and corticosteroids.
2. Assess patient for reduction of edema.
3. Assess patient for reduction of inflammation.

AZATHIOPRINE IMURAN

Remarks Antimetabolite. Purine antagonist that interferes with the normal utilization of purine by the cell. Readily absorbed from the GI tract.

Uses Prevents rejection of transplanted organs (i.e., kidney); rheumatoid arthritis.

Drug Interactions

Interactant	Interaction
Allopurinol	Allopurinol ↑ pharmacologic effect of azathioprine
Corticosteroids	With azathioprine, it may cause muscle wasting after prolonged therapy

Dosage *Kidney transplantation,* **PO, IV:** *individualized,* **Initial** (*usual dose*), 3–5 mg/kg daily. **Maintenance:** 1–2 mg/kg daily.

Additional Nursing Implications
1. Observe for liver dysfunction. Drug may have to be discontinued if jaundice appears.
2. Measure intake and output of fluids.
3. Report oliguria.
4. Encourage increased fluid intake.
5. Weigh daily.
6. Watch for signs of rejection of the transplant. For kidney transplant, decrease in urine volume and creatinine clearance means larger dose is necessary. If rejection persists, removal of kidney should be considered rather than increasing drug to toxic levels.

BETA-CAROTENE SOLATENE

Classification Vitamin A precursor.

General Statement Beta-Carotene eliminates the photo-sensitivity reaction (burning sensation, edema, erythema, pruritus, and/or cutaneous lesions) in patients suffering from erythropoietic protoporphyria (edema produced by exposure to sunlight). Patients receiving beta-carotene develop yellowing of the skin, but not of the sclera. The protective effect of the drug becomes apparent 2 to 6 weeks after initial administration and persists 1 to 2 weeks after discontinuation.

Uses   Erythropoietic protoporphyria (EPP).

Contraindications   Hypersensitivity to drug, pregnancy. Use with caution in patients with impaired renal and hepatic function.

Untoward Reactions   Yellowing of skin starting with palms of hands, soles of feet and face. Loose stools.

Dosage   **PO:** *individualized*, 30–300 mg daily as single or divided dose; **children under 14 years:** 30–150 mg daily.

Administration   1. Administer with meals.
2. Mix contents of capsule with orange juice or tomato juice for those unable to swallow capsules.

Nursing Implications   Teach patient:

1. Not to ingest additional vitamin preparations of vitamin A, since beta-carotene fills normal vitamin A requirements.
2. Not to increase exposure to sun for 2 to 6 weeks after initiation of therapy (until palms and soles turn yellow, indicating that patient becomes carotemic).
3. To expose himself/herself to the sun gradually, because protective effect is not complete, and each individual must establish limits of exposure.

BROMOCRIPTINE MESYLATE PARLODEL

Classification   Prolactin secretion inhibitor; dopamine receptor agonist.

General Statement   Bromocriptine is a nonhormonal agent that inhibits the release of the hormone prolactin by the pituitary. The drug should be used only when prolactin production by pituitary tumors has been ruled out. The mechanism of action is due to the fact that the drug has been shown to be a dopamine-receptor agonist.

Uses   Short-term treatment of amenorrhea/galactorrhea associated with hyperprolactinemia. Not to be used in management of infertility.

Contraindications   Sensitivity to ergot alkaloids. Safe use of the drug during pregnancy and childhood has not been established. The drug must be discontinued immediately if pregnancy occurs.

Untoward Reactions   High incidence (68%) of mild adverse effects: nausea (51%), headaches (18%), dizziness (16%), fatigue (8%), abdominal cramps (7%), light headedness (6%), vomiting (5%), nasal congestion (5%), constipation

(3%), slight hypotension. Side effects warranted discontinuation of drug in 6% of cases.

Dosage **PO:** 2.5 mg b.i.d. or t.i.d. for maximum of 6 months.

Administration
1. To reduce side effects, start with 2.5 mg daily and increase to the full dose within 1 week.
2. Give with meals.

Nursing Implications
1. Advise use of contraceptive measures other than "the pill" while patient is receiving bromocriptine because safety of the drug during pregnancy has not been established.
2. Schedule for pregnancy tests every 4 weeks during period of amenorrhea and after resumption of menses when a menstrual period is missed.
3. Alert patient to signs and symptoms of pregnancy and advise withholding drug and reporting to medical supervision, should these occur, since pregnancy tests may fail to diagnose early pregnancy, and the medication may harm the fetus.

CROMOLYN SODIUM AARANE, INTAL

Classification Respiratory inhalant for bronchial asthma.

General Statement Cromolyn sodium appears to act locally on the lung mucosa, preventing the release of histamine and other allergy-triggering substances. When effective, it reduces the number of asthmatic attacks and the intensity of the disease and permits decrease in corticosteroid dosage. Improvement usually becomes apparent within a matter of 4 weeks after initiation of therapy. It has no anti-histaminic, anti-inflammatory, or bronchodilation effects and has no role in terminating an acute attack of asthma. Care should be exercised when cromolyn sodium is withdrawn in patients in whom the drug has permitted decrease of corticosteroids. Dosage of these may have to be increased after withdrawal.

Uses Prophylactic and adjunct in the management of severe bronchial asthma in selected patients.

Contraindications Hypersensitivity. Children under 5 years of age. Safe use in pregnancy not established. Acute attacks and status asthmaticus. Use with caution for long periods of time or in the presence of renal or hepatic disease.

Untoward Reactions Bronchospasm, cough, laryngeal edema (rare), nasal congestion, pharyngeal irritation, wheezing; also, angioedema, dizziness, dysuria, urinary frequency, joint swelling and pain, lacrimation, nausea, headaches, rash, swollen parotid gland, urticaria.

Dosage **Capsules for inhalation; adults and children over 5 years: initial,** 20 mg q.i.d. at regular intervals. Dosage can be decreased slowly to minimal effective levels, usually 20 mg t.i.d. Improvement will usually occur within first 4 weeks of use.

Administration/ Storage

1. Institute only after acute episode is over when airway is clear and patient can inhale adequately.
2. Teach patient to use special inhaler and not to swallow capsule.

Nursing Implications

Teach patient to:

1. Load capsule into inhaler.
2. Inhale fully and introduce mouthpiece between lips.
3. Tilt head back and inhale deeply and rapidly through inhaler to cause propeller to turn rapidly and supply more medication in one breath.
4. Remove inhaler, hold breath a few seconds, and exhale slowly.
5. Repeat procedure until powder is completely administered.
6. Not to wet powder with breath while exhaling.
7. Continue self-administration of medication as ordered, because it may take up to 4 weeks for frequency of asthmatic attacks to decrease.
8. Consult with medical supervision if he/she wishes to discontinue medication because discontinuation may precipitate an asthmatic attack, and concomitant corticosteroid therapy may require adjustment.

DISULFIRAM ANTABUSE, RO-SULFIRAM

Classification

Miscellaneous—treatment of alcoholism.

General Statement

Disulfiram (Antabuse) produces severe hypersensitivity to alcohol. It is used as an adjunct in the treatment of alcoholism. The toxic reaction to disulfiram appears to be due to the inhibition of liver enzymes that participate in the normal degradation of alcohol. When alcohol and disulfiram are both present, acetaldehyde accumulates in the blood. High levels of this chemical produce flushing, fall in blood pressure, palpitations, rapid pulse, dizziness, dyspnea, hyperventilation, anorexia, nausea, and vomiting. Convulsions, unconsciousness, cardiac arrhythmias, and myocardial infarctions have also been reported. The symptoms are so characteristic for acetaldehyde toxicity that, when applicable, one talks of a "disulfiram-type reaction."

Symptoms vary individually and are dose dependent, both with respect to alcohol and disulfiram. Symptoms persist for 30 minutes to several hours, and a single dose of disulfiram may be effective for 1 to 2 weeks. Treatment of severe toxic reactions is largely symptomatic and includes oxygen inhalation, ephedrine or another pressor agent, and IV administration of antihistamine.

Uses

Alcoholism.

Contraindications Alcohol intoxication; severe myocardial or occlusive coronary disease. Use with caution in narcotic addicts or patients with diabetes, goiter, epilepsy, psychosis, hepatic cirrhosis or nephritis. Use of paraldehyde.

Untoward Reactions Disulfiram should only be given to cooperating patients fully aware of the consequences of alcohol ingestion. In the absence of alcohol the drug may produce drowsiness, fatigue, impotence, headache, and peripheral neuritis. Symptoms usually subside with treatment.

Disulfiram-alcohol reaction is characterized by flushing, throbbing in head and neck, throbbing headaches, respiratory difficulties, nausea, copious vomiting, sweating, thirst, chest pain, palpitations, dyspnea, hyperventilation, tachycardia, hypotension, syncope, marked uneasiness, weakness, vertigo, blurred vision, and confusion. In severe reactions there may be respiratory depression, cardiovascular collapse, arrhythmias, myocardial infarctions, acute congestive heart failure, unconsciousness, convulsions, and death.

Drug Interactions

Interactant	Interaction
Anticoagulants, oral	↑ Effect of anticoagulants by ↑ hypoprothrombinemia
Barbiturates	↑ Effect of barbiturates due to ↓ breakdown by liver
Izoniazid	↑ Side effects of isoniazid (especially CNS)
Metronidazole (Flagyl)	Additive effect
Paraldehyde	Concomitant use produces "Antabuse-like" effect
Phenytoin (Dilantin)	↑ Effect of phenytoin due to ↓ breakdown by liver

Dosage **Initial** (after alcohol-free interval of 12 to 48 hr): 500 mg daily for 2 to 3 weeks. **Maintenance:** *usual,* 250 mg daily.

Nursing Implications
1. Be prepared to treat disulfiram-alcohol reactions symptomatically with oxygen, pressor agents, and antihistamines.
2. Emphasize to family that disulfiram must never be given to the patient without his/her knowledge.
3. Teach patient:
   a. The effects of disulfiram and insure he/she understands the necessity for close medical and psychiatric treatment when on disulfiram.
   b. That as little as 30 ml of 100-proof alcohol taken while he/she is on therapy with disulfiram may cause severe symptoms and possibly death.
   c. Not to take or use alcohol in disguised forms such as in foods, sauces, or vinegar; medications: paregoric, cough syrups, tonics; liniments or lotions—aftershave lotion.
   d. That side effects of disulfiram, such as drowsiness, fatigue, impotence, headache, peripheral neuritis, and a metallic or garliclike taste tend to subside after about 2 weeks of therapy.

e. To report skin eruptions should they occur since physician may order antihistamines.

f. To carry an identification card stating that he/she is on disulfiram therapy and describing the symptoms and their treatment should an antabuse-alcohol reaction occur. The name of his/her physician should also be on the card. Cards may be obtained from the Ayerst Laboratories, 685 Third Avenue, New York, N.Y. 10017.

GUANIDINE HYDROCHLORIDE

Classification   Miscellaneous—cholinergic muscle stimulant.

General Statement   This compound increases the release of acetylcholine at the synapses following nerve impulse transmission; it slows rate of depolarization and repolarization of muscle cell membrane. It is ineffective for the treatment of myasthenia gravis.

Uses   Reduction of muscle weakness and relief of fatigue associated with Eaton-Lambert Syndrome.

Contraindications   Hypersensitivity to and intolerance of drug. Safe use in pregnancy or in children not established.

Untoward Reactions   Anemia, leukopenia, thrombocytopenia. (The bone marrow depressant effects of the drug can be fatal.) Also, sore throat, rash, fever, various neurological, gastrointestinal, dermatologic, and cardiac manifestations. Increase in blood creatinine levels, uremia, abnormal liver function tests.

Dosage   **PO:** *individualized*, **initial,** 10–15 mg/kg/day in 3 or 4 divided doses. Increase dose gradually to 35 mg/kg/day or up to the development of side effects.

Nursing Implications
1. Verify that baseline blood, renal, and liver function tests are performed prior to initiation of therapy and then periodically while patient is receiving the drug because damage may be dose-related.
2. Assess for anorexia, increased peristalsis, or diarrhea, which are early warnings that suggest the drug should be discontinued.
3. Be alert to signs of intoxication manifested by hyperirritability, tremors, and convulsive contractions of muscles, salivation, vomiting, diarrhea, and hypoglycemia.
4. Have calcium gluconate available to control neuromuscular and convulsive symptoms.
5. Have atropine available to reduce GI symptoms, circulatory disturbances, and changes in blood sugar level.
6. Assess patient who has had primary neoplastic lesion removed for improvement of symptoms that would permit discontinuance of drug, since the latter is highly toxic and treatment should continue only as long as necessary.

HYALURONIDASE ALIDASE, WYDASE

Classification   Enzyme, miscellaneous.

General   Hyaluronidase is an enzyme that degrades collagen, the main constitu-
Statement   ent of connective tissue. It acts as a spreading factor when administered
as an adjunct to promote the diffusion of injected liquids. The purified
enzyme has no effect on blood pressure, respiration, temperature and
kidney function. It will not result in spread of localized infection as long
as it is not injected into the infected area.

Uses   Adjunct to promote absorption and dispersion of liquids and drugs, for
hypodermoclysis, adjunct in urography to improve resorption of radi-
opaque agents, administration of local anesthetics. (Hyaluronidase can
be added to primary drug solution or injected prior to administration of
primary drug solution.)

Contraindications   Do not inject into acutely infected or cancerous areas.

Untoward   Rarely, sensitivity reactions.
Reactions

Dosage   *Drug and fluid dispersion* **(usual), adults and older children:** 150 units
(this facilitates absorption of 1,000 ml fluid). *Subcutaneous urography*
(when IV injection cannot be used) *with patient in prone position:* 75
units **SC** over each scapula, followed by contrast medium in same site.

Administration   1. Conduct a preliminary skin test for sensitivity by injecting 0.02 ml of
the solution intradermally. A positive reaction occurs within 5
minutes when a wheal with pseudopods appears and persists for 20
to 30 minutes and is accompanied by localized itching. The appearance of erythema alone is not a positive reaction.
2. Methods for administering hyaluronidase:
a. Inject hyaluronidase under skin before clysis is started.
b. After the clysis has been started, inject solution of hyaluronidase
into rubber tubing close to needle.
3. Limit clysis for child under 3 years of age to 200 ml; in neonates or
premature infants, volume should not exceed 25 ml/kg/day. Rate of
infusion for infants: no more than 2 ml/minute.
4. Control rate and volume of fluid for the older patient so that it will
not exceed those used for IV administration.

Nursing   1. Do not inject hyaluronidase into an area that is infected or can-
Implications   cerous.
2. Check doctor's orders for dosage of hyaluronidase, type and amount
of parenteral solution, rate of flow, and site of injection.
3. Monitor area receiving clysis for pale color, coldness, hardness, and
pain. Should untoward signs occur, reduce rate of flow and check
with doctor.

LACTULOSE CEPHULAC, DUPHALAC

Classification Ammonia detoxicant.

General Statement Lactulose contains both lactose and galactose. It causes a decrease in the blood concentration of ammonia in patients suffering from portal-systemic encephalopathy. The mechanism involved is attributed to the bacteria-induced degradation of lactulose in the colon, resulting in an acid medium. Ammonia will then migrate from the blood to the colon to form ammonium ion, which is trapped and can not be absorbed. A laxative action then expels the trapped ammonium. The decrease in blood ammonia concentration improves the mental state, EEG tracing and diet protein tolerance of patients. The drug is partly absorbed from the GI tract.

Uses Prevention and treatment of portal-systemic encephalopathy (PSE), including hepatic and prehepatic coma, cirrhosis. Investigationally as laxative, after hemorrhoidectomy, and in the elderly, to correct barium meal retention.

Contraindications Patients on galactose-restricted diets. Use with caution in presence of diabetes mellitus. Safe use in pregnancy not established.

Untoward Reaction Gaseous distention, flatulence, belching, cramping (20%), diarrhea. Rarely, nausea and vomiting.

Drug Interaction

Interactant	Interaction
Neomycin	↓ Degradation of lactulose due to neomycin induced ↑ in elimination of certain bacteria in colon

Dosage **PO: usual,** 20–30 gm (30–45 ml of syrup) t.i.d.–q.i.d. Adjust q 2 to 3 days, according to response (2 or 3 soft stools daily) or acidity of colon (pH about 5). *During acute episodes:* 20–30 gm q 1 to 2 hrs. to induce rapid initial laxation. *Retention enema, investigational:* 200 gm (diluted to 1000 ml with water) q hr. *Chronic constipation, investigational;* **adults and children:** 2–30 gm/day as single dose after breakfast. *Hemorrhoidectomy, investigational:* 10 gm b.i.d. day before and for 5 days after surgery. *Barium meal retention, investigational:* 3.3–6.7 gm b.i.d. for 1 to 4 weeks.

Administration 1. To minimize sweet taste, dilute with water, fruit juice or add to desserts.
2. When given by gastric tube, dilute well to prevent vomiting and the possibility of aspiration pneumonia.
3. Store below 30°C (86°F). Avoid freezing.

Nursing Implications 1. Report GI distress which may subside as therapy is continued but may necessitate a dose reduction.

2. Monitor serum potassium levels of patients with portal systemic encephalopathy to evaluate whether drug is causing further potassium loss that will intensify symptoms of PSE.
3. Observe for dry flushed skin, dry mouth, intense thirst, abdominal pain, fruity breath, and low blood pressure, symptoms of hyperglycemia more likely to occur in diabetic patients because the medication contains carbohydrates.

MORRHUATE SODIUM

Classification   Sclerosing agent.

General Statement   Morrhuate sodium is derived from cod liver oil. When injected into a vein, it initiates the formation of a thrombus, which then obliterates the particular blood vessel. After injection, 2 to 4 inches of the vein harden immediately. The entire vein becomes hard and firm within 24 hrs. Injection is followed by a mild feeling of stiffness, which persists for 48 hrs. The skin above the vein assumes a bronze discoloration that disappears gradually. It usually does not cause cramping pain.

Uses   Obliteration of primary varicose veins.

Contraindications   Hypersensitivity to drug. Obliteration of superficial veins in patients suffering from deep varicose veins. Superficial thrombophlebitis or underlying arterial disease, serious systemic disorders. Safe use in pregnancy not established.

Use with particular caution in patient previously treated with morrhuate sodium.

Untoward Reactions   Occasional hypersensitivity reactions characterized by dizziness, weakness, vascular collapse, respiratory depression, GI disturbances, and urticaria.

Dosage   **IV** *small or medium veins:* 50–100 mg (1–2 ml of 5% solution); *large veins:* 150–250 mg (3–5 ml of 5% solution). Treatment may be repeated after 5 to 7 days.

Administration
1. To test sensitivity of patient, injection of test dose (0.25–1 ml of 5% solution) may be requested by medical supervision 24 hours prior to treatment.
2. Morrhuate sodium is usually administered by physician familiar with injection technique.
3. Assist in emptying vein for injection by elevating limb and applying digital pressure or a tourniquet for *only 2 to 3 minutes* after injection to prevent dilution of drug by backflow of blood.
4. The normal coloration of injection is yellow to light brown. Only use clear solution for injection.
5. Submerge ampule in hot water to warm medication, if ampule is cold, contains solid matter, or if medication is to be injected into a small vein.

6. Solution froths easily. Use large bore needle to fill syringe but change to small bore needle for actual injection by doctor.
7. Place a dry sterile dressing over site of injection.
8. Examine site of injection before patient leaves office for allergic reaction, sloughing, bleeding, or other untoward reaction.

Nursing Implications

1. Observe patient for several hours after the sensitivity test is done and assess for allergic reaction.
2. Be especially vigilant when patient has received therapy previously because sensitivity to morrhuate sodium may have developed in interval.
3. Be alert to symptoms of anaphylactoid reactions (see *Untoward Reactions*) when drug is administered and have pressor drugs (epinephrine 1 : 1,000), antihistamines, and corticosteroids available.

PIGMENTING AGENTS—PSORALENS

General Statement

The appearance of areas of skin discoloration, characteristic of vitiligo, is associated with a defect in the formation of the dark pigment melanin from a precursor. Special drugs (pigmenting agents) can initiate the formation of melanin. The transformation is enhanced by ultraviolet radiation from natural or artificial sources.

Two substances, methoxsalen and trioxsalen, collectively referred to as psoralens, are used to promote color development and sun protection in affected skin areas. The agents are also useful for selected patients with unusually low tolerance to sun exposure. Methoxsalen is for both topical and systemic use; trioxsalen is for systemic use only. The psoralens have been used on an investigational basis for the treatment of psoriasis and mycosis fungoides.

The agents are more rapidly effective on fleshy areas, such as the face, abdomen and buttocks, then on bony areas, such as the dorsum of the hands and feet. The drugs are only effective in conjunction with functioning pigment-producing cells (melanocytes). Use of pigmenting agents is difficult. Excess exposure to ultraviolet radiation results in erythema and severe burns; overdosage results in blistering and serious burning.

Uses

Vitiligo. Investigational: psoriasis, mycosis fungoides.

Contraindications

Hepatic insufficiency, familial sun sensitivity, diseases associated with photosensitivity (porphyria, systemic lupus erythematosus, hydroa [a seasonally recurring rash triggered by exposure to sunlight], polymorphic light eruptions), leukoderma of infectious origin, albinism, children under 12 years of age.

Untoward Reactions

Burning, blistering, erythema. Others: gastric discomfort, nausea, nervousness, insomnia, depression. Rarely: basal cell carcinoma, cataracts, changes in eye pigmentation, pigmentary glaucoma.

Treatment of Overdosage   In acute oral overdosage, discontinue therapy, empty stomach by inducing emesis. Place patient in dark room for 8 hours or until cutaneous reaction subsides. Supportive measures for treatment of burns should be instituted.

Nursing Implications

1. Read package insert with information supplied by manufacturer before assisting doctor or instructing patient about psoralens.
2. Administration of psoralens is to be performed by an experienced physician in his office.
3. Ascertain that liver function tests are performed before initiation of therapy, and then for the first few months of treatment.
4. Be prepared to provide burn therapy for patient who has had an overdose or overexposure to sun.
5. Teach patient:
   a. The need to maintain dosage schedule.
   b. Procedure for measured exposure to sun after treatment to prevent severe burns.
      1. After oral therapy, protect skin from sun for at least 8 hours, except for metered exposure time instituted 2 hours after ingestion of medication.
      2. After topical therapy, protect skin from sun for 12 to 48 hours, except for metered exposure time instituted 2 hours after application of unguentine. To determine sun-exposure time, use guide provided by the manufacturer of the medication.
   c. To wear sunglasses during exposure to the sun.
   d. To protect lips with a light screening lipstick during exposure to the sun.
   e. That sunlamp exposure should be carried out under the direction of an experienced physician. Inform doctor what type of sunlamp the patient has at home, so that approprite recommendations can be made.
   f. That results may be delayed, beginning anywhere between a few weeks or 6 to 9 months.
   g. That periodic treatments may be required to maintain pigmentation.
   h. To check with doctor about any medication taken concomitantly because these may increase susceptibility to burns. If this medication also causes photosensitivity, the susceptibility to burns may be greater.
   i. Not to ingest the chemical substance furocoumarin contained in certain foods, such as limes, figs, parsley, parsnips, mustard, carrots or celery, because more severe reactions to the sun may occur.

METHOXSALEN: TOPICAL   OXSORALEN

Remarks   Topical administration produces more intensive photosensitivity reactions than systemic administration. Topical usage is only indicated for small well-defined lesions (less than 10 sq cm).

Dosage   1% suspension, applied once a week.

Administration
1. Lotion is applied to well-defined vitiligous lesions only by physician. Never give to patient for home application.
2. Expose after application to natural sunlight as follows: 1 minute initially, increase exposure time with caution. Decrease exposure time to half when light source is artificial.
3. Decrease frequency of treatment if marked erythema is produced.
4. Keep treated areas protected from light with bandages or a sun screening agent.

METHOXSALEN: ORAL OXSORALEN

Dosage   *Vitiligo:* 20 mg/day or 40 mg 3 times/week. *Increased tolerance to sun:* 20 mg/day for 14 days. For *psoriasis and mycosis fungoides* (both investigational), follow dosage for trioxsalen. Should not exceed 30 days when patient receives 3 capsules/day on a continuous or interrupted regimen.

Administration
1. Administer oral preparation with milk or meals to prevent gastric distress.
2. Administer 2 hours before measured exposure time to sun or ultraviolet irradiation.
3. Follow light exposure times indicated in guide provided by manufacturer. In general, it is 2 to 2.5 hours after administration.

TRIOXSALEN TRISORALEN

Remarks   Produces fewer side effects than methoxsalen.

Dosage   *Systemic.* **PO:** *Vitiligo,* 10 mg/day. *To increase tolerance to sun:* 10 mg/day for 14 days. Should not exceed 28 tablets. *Psoriasis* (*investigational*), **50 kg or less:** 20 mg; **51 to 65 kg:** 30 mg; **66 to 80 kg:** 40 mg; **81 to 90 kg:** 50 mg; **over 90 kg:** 60 mg. Daily for 30 treatments. **Maintenance:** as above 2 times/week. *Mycosis fungoides:* 30–50 mg 3 times/week.

Administration   See *Methoxsalen, oral.*

PRALIDOXIME CHLORIDE 2-PAM CHLORIDE, PROTOPAM CHLORIDE

Classification   Miscellaneous—cholinesterase inhibitor antidote.

General Statement   This drug reactivates the enzyme cholinesterase, which is inhibited by certain anticholinesterase agents, mainly phosphate esters, such as, insecticides (like sarin, parathion). The agent is used as an antidote and is also sometimes given prophylactically to persons regularly exposed to insecticides and to correct overdosage with cholinergic drugs. Pralidoxime is less effective in antagonizing carbamate type cholinesterase inhibitors (e.g., neostigmine); it may even aggravate symptoms of carbamate pesticide poisoning.

Pralidoxime competes with cholinesterase for the carbamate or phosphorus group of the inhibitor. When displaced, the enzyme reassumes its physiological role.

The drug should be administered immediately after poisoning. It is ineffective when given more than 36 hours after exposure. Administration as antidote should be combined with gastric lavage (after PO ingestion) and (after skin contamination) thorough washing of skin with alcohol or sodium bicarbonate.

Since GI absorption of the poison is slow, and possible fatal relapses may occur, patient should be watched for 48 to 72 hours after poisoning. Barbiturates can be given cautiously to combat convulsions.

Laboratory determinations of RBC (depressed to 50% of normal), plasma cholinesterase and urinary paranitrophenol (parathion poisoning only) measurements are desirable to confirm diagnosis and follow progress of the patient.

Uses

Parathion and other organophosphate poisoning, prophylaxis of agricultural workers. Overdosage in treatment of myasthenia gravis.

Untoward Reactions

Dizziness, diplopia, impaired accommodation, headache, drowsiness, nausea, tachycardia, increased blood pressure, hyperventilation, and muscle weakness in patients not exposed to cholinesterase poisoning. Use at reduced dosage in patients with impaired renal function.

Dosage

Organophosphate poisoning, **IV**: 1–2 gm; if response is poor, repeat after 1 hr; **pediatric:** 20–40 mg/kg. May be increased to 25–60 mg/kg if response is poor. *Prophylaxis*, **PO**: 3 gm maximum for 4 to 5 doses. *Myasthenia gravis*, **IV (overdosage with cholinergics):** 50 mg initially; repeat cautiously every 4 minutes until muscle strength improves or 1 gm has been given.

Administration

In case of severe poisoning, establish patent airway before initiating therapy. Also pretreat patient with atropine sulfate (adults, IV 2–4 mg atropine sulfate; pediatric, IV or IM: 0.5–1 mg atropine sulfate. These doses are repeated every 10 to 15 minutes until signs of atropine toxicity appear.) Pralidoxime is infused in adults in 100 ml NaCl injection over 30 minutes or injected at rate of 200 mg/min. Pediatric—give as 5% solution.

Nursing Implications

1. Observe the patient closely for desired and undesired response to therapy. Desired effects—reduction of muscle weakness, cramps and paralysis. Undesired effects—dizziness, headaches, hypertension, drowsiness.
2. Make every effort to determine what insecticide the patient was exposed to since pralidoxime is ineffective or contraindicated in the treatment of poisoning by carbamate insecticides.

3. Report any history of asthma or peptic ulcer to the physician since these conditions contraindicate the use of cholinergic drugs.
4. Have atropine available to use in conjunction with pralidoxime.
5. Be alert to signs of atropine poisoning such as flushing, tachycardia, dry mouth, blurred vision or "atropine jag" demonstrated by excitement, delirium, and hallucinations.
6. Check that respirator, tracheostomy set, and other supportive measures are available when patient is being treated for insecticide poisoning.
7. Alert the public to the possible hazards of using insecticides and caution adherence to instructions on container.
8. Caution the patient to avoid contact with insecticides for several weeks after poisoning.
9. Observe patients with myasthenia gravis being treated for overdose of cholinergic drugs, as they may rapidly weaken and pass from a cholinergic crisis to a myasthenic crisis when they will require more cholinergic drugs to treat myasthenia. Call the physician immediately should a patient weaken rapidly. Have edrophonium (Tensilon) on hand to use for diagnostic purposes in such a situation.

SODIUM TETRADECYL SULFATE SOTRADECOL

Classification Sclerosing agent.

General Statement On injection, this surface-active agent (detergent) causes sufficient irritation to the intima of the vein to result in a thrombus, which causes obliteration.

Uses Obliteration of primary varicose veins of legs. Disinfectant solution for topical antisepsis.

Contraindications Hypersensitivity to drug. Obliteration of superficial varicose veins in patients suffering from deep varicose veins. Acute superficial thrombophlebitis, underlying arterial disease, varicosities resulting from tumors, serious systemic disease. Safe use in pregnancy not established. Valvular and deep vein patency should be established prior to treatment. Bedridden patients.

Untoward Reactions Sensitivity reactions (rarely) characterized by pulmonary edema, cyanosis, coma, anaphylactic shock. Allergic reactions. Also, hemolysis, faintness with palpitations and generalized rash. Postoperative sloughing. Small permanent discoloration at injection site.

Dosage IV, *small veins:* 5–20 mg (0.5–2 ml of 1% injection). *Medium-large veins:* 15–60 mg (0.5–2 ml of 3% injection). Treatment may be repeated after 5 to 7 days.

Administration 1. To test sensitivity of patient, injection of test dose (0.2–0.5 ml of 1% injection) may be requested by medical supervision several hours prior to treatment.

2. Sodium tetradecyl sulfate is usually administered by a physician familiar with injection technique.
3. Inject only small amounts (2 ml maximum in a single varicose vein) and no more than 10 ml of 3% injection during 1 treatment.
4. Inject very slowly.
5. Avoid extravasation.
6. Do not use if product is precipitated.

Nursing Implications
1. Observe injection site for allergic reaction for several hours after administration of test dose.
2. Have available epinephrine 1 : 1,000 solution for treatment of allergic reaction.

STREPTOKINASE-STREPTODORNASE VARIDASE

Classification Enzyme.

General Statement Streptokinase-Streptodornase is a 4-to-1 mixture of enzymes that help in the liquefaction and drainage of clotted blood, fibrinogen, and purulent exudates and waste materials that accumulate as a result of trauma, infections, and inflammation. The enzymes are most effective when injected into affected cavities or applied topically as a wet dressing. Beneficial effects are seen 2 days after initiation of therapy. Streptokinase-Streptodornase comes prepared for topical and intracavital, PO, and IM use.

Uses Topical: Ulcerations and abscesses, radiation necrosis, infected wounds, burns, chronic suppurations, purulent pericarditis, skin grafts, to dissolve clots in urinary bladder and drainage tubes, hemothorax, thoracic empyema, and purulent nontuberculous meningitis. PO and IM: edema associated with infections and trauma, phlebitis, epididymitis, cellulitis, hematomas, thrombophlebitis, contusions, varicose or statis ulcers, chronic bronchitis, and bronchiectasis.

Contraindicatiosn Active hemorrhage, acute cellulitis without suppuration, active tuberculosis. IM: depressed liver function, blood coagulation defects. *Never Administer IV.*

Untoward Reactions Allergic reactions, fever, nausea, vomiting, diarrhea, skin rash, urticaria.

Dosage **Topical:** *highly individualized.* Depending on size of cavity or surface to be treated, 10,000–200,000 units streptokinase and 2,500–50,000 units streptodornase. **PO:** 1 tablet (10,000 units streptokinase and 2,500 units streptodornase) q.i.d. for 4 to 6 days. **IM:** 0.5 ml of prepared solution (5,000 units streptokinase and 1,250 units streptodornase) b.i.d.

Administration/ Storage
1. Follow directions of manufacturer for dilution.
2. Reconstituted solution is stable for 24 hours at room temperature and for 2 weeks at 2–8°C (35.6°–46.4°F).

3. Use only in areas with adequate drainage or possibility of aspiration of exudate.
4. To obtain maximum benefit from topical use, preparation must stay in intimate contact with treated area. To achieve this, manufacturer supplies carboxymethylcellulose jelly to which enzyme mixture can be added.

Nursing Implications

1. Anticipate that streptokinase-streptodornase will be used as an adjunct to other suitable therapeutic measures, such as antibiotic administration and surgery.
2. Reduce pyrogenic reaction to drug by removing exudate frequently by drainage or by aspiration of exudate, especially during the first 24 hours of therapy.

APPENDICES

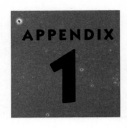

commonly used normal physiological values

Hematology	Red blood cells (erythrocytes)	4,500,000–5,000,000/cu mm
	White blood cells (leukocytes)	5,000–10,000/cμ mm
	Polymorphonuclear neutrophils	60%–70%
	Lymphocytes	25%–30%
	Monocytes	2%–6%
	Eosinophils	1%–3%
	Basophils	0.25%–0.5%
	Platelets	200,000–300,000/cu mm
	Hemoglobin (men & women)	14–16 gm/100 ml blood
	Hematocrit	
	Men	40%–54%
	Women	37%–47%
	Bleeding Time	1–3 min (Duke); 1–5 min (Ivy)
	Coagulation Time	6–12 min
	Prothrombin Time (Quick)	10–15 sec
	Sedimentation Rate (Wintrobe)	
	Men	0–9 mm/hr
	Women	0–20 mm/hr
	Thrombin Time	Within 5 sec of control
Blood Chemistry	Electrolytes (serum)	
	Bicarbonate	24–31 mEq/L
	Calcium	4.5–5.5 mEq/L
	Chloride	95–106 mEq/L
	Magnesium	1.5–3.0 mEq/L
	Phosphorus	1–1.5 mEq/L
	Potassium	3.6–5.5 mEq/L
	Sodium	136–145 mEq/L
	Enzymes (serum)	
	Amylase	80–180 Somogyi units/100 ml
	Lipase	less than 1.5 units (ml of n/20 NaOH)
	Acid Phosphatase	0.5–2.0 Bodansky units
	Alkaline Phosphatase	2–4.5 Bodansky units
	SGOT	5–40 units/ml
	SGPT	5–35 units/ml
	Proteins (serum)	
	Total	6.2–8.5 gm/100 ml
	Albumin	3.5–5.5 gm/100 ml
	Fibrinogen (Plasma)	0.2–0.4 gm/100 ml
	Globulin	1.5–3.0 gm/100 ml

Nonprotein nitrogenous
substances (serum except where
noted)

Bilirubin	0.3– 1.1 mg/100 ml
Blood urea nitrogen (BUN)	10– 20 mg/100 ml
Creatinine	0.7– 1.5 mg/100 ml
Nonprotein Nitrogen (NPN)	15– 35 mg/100 ml
Uric Acid	
Male	2.1– 7.8 mg/100 ml
Female	2.0– 6.4 mg/100 ml

Other (serum, except where
noted)

Cholesterol, total	158– 230 mg/100 ml
Cholesterol, esterified	100– 180 mg/100 ml (70% of total)
Icterus index (jaundice)	3– 8 units
Iron	75– 175 μg/100 ml
Glucose (blood, plasma)	80– 120 mg/100 ml
Lipids, total (serum, plasma)	450– 1000 mg/100 ml
Protein bound iodine	3.5– 8 μg/100 ml
pH, arterial (plasma)	7.35– 7.45

Blood Gases

Whole blood O_2 capacity	17– 21 vol %
Arterial	
pCO_2	35– 45 mm Hg
pO_2	75– 100 mm Hg
pH	7.38– 7.44
Venous	
pCO_2	40– 54 mm Hg
pO_2	20– 50 mm Hg
pH	7.36– 7.41
HCO_3, normal range	22– 28 mEq/L

Urinalysis

General

Specific gravity	1.005– 1.025
pH	6.0 (av 4.7– 8.0)
Volume	600– 2500 ml/24 hours
Total solids	55– 70 gm/24 hours (elderly 30 gm/24 hours)

Electrolytes (per 24 hours)

Calcium	7.4 mEq
Chloride	70– 250 mEq
Magnesium	15– 300 mg
Phosphorus, inorganic	0.9– 1.3 gm
Potassium	25– 100 mEq
Sodium	130– 260 mEq

Urinalysis (con't)	Nitrogenous constituents (per 24 hours)	
	Ammonia	30–50 mEq
	Creatinine	
	Men	1.0–1.9 gm
	Women	0.8–1.7 gm
	Protein	10–50 mg (up to 100 mg)
	Urea	6–17 gm
	Uric Acid	0.25–0.75 gm
	Steroids (per 24 hours)	
	17-Hydroxycorticosteroids	4.9–14.5 mg
	17-Ketosteroids	
	Men	8–21 mg
	Women	4–14 mg

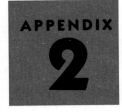

APPENDIX
2

drug therapy for antibiotics and other drugs commonly administered intravenously

Each hospital or other health care facility will have guidelines for the preparation and administration of intravenous drugs or other solutions. These guidelines must be fully known and understood by the nurse.

The chart on the following pages lists drugs that are commonly administered by intravenous infusion. Information provided for these drugs includes stability at room temperature when dissolved in either D5W or saline and compatibilities and incompatibilities with other drugs. If a particular drug combination is not listed, it must *not* be assumed the combination is safe to administer. Often, additional information on compatibilities and incompatibilities of drugs for intravenous use can be obtained from the pharmacy drug information service located in most larger hospitals.

There are several additional points which can be made about drugs administered by intravenous infusion:

1. Often the chance for incompatibilities of drugs for intravenous infusion increases with time.
2. Solutions to which a drug or drugs have been added must always be visually inspected to ensure that there is no precipitate, cloudiness,

(*Continued on p. 801*)

INFORMATION ON DRUG THERAPY FOR ANTIBIOTICS AND OTHER DRUGS COMMONLY ADMINISTERED INTRAVENOUSLY (Compatibilities and incompatibilities are for drugs mixed in infusion bottle **only** and **not** in same syringe.)

Drug	*Stability (hr at room temp) in IV Solutions* D_5W	*Saline*	*Compatibility with Following Drugs*	*Incompatibility with Following Drugs*
Amikacin Sulfate (Amikin)	24	24	*No Other Drug Should Be Physically Combined—Administer Separately*	
Aminophylline	24	24	Amobarbital, Ascorbic Acid, Ca gluconate, Cephapirin Na*, Chloramphenicol Na Succ., Chlortetracycline Na, Corticotropin*, Dimenhydrinate, Erythromycin lactobionate, Heparin Na, Hydrocortisone Na Succ., Lidocaine HCl, Methicillin Na, Methyldopate HCl, Nafcillin Na*, Novobiocin Na, Oxytetracycline HCl*, Phenobarbital Na, KCl, Procaine HCl*, Secobarbital Na, Na bicarbonate, Sulfadiazine Na, Vancomycin HCl*	Anileridine HCl, Cephalothin Na, Chlorpromazine HCl, Clindamycin Phos., Codeine Phos., Epinephrine HCl, Erythromycin gluceptate, Hydralazine HCl, Hydroxyzine HCl, Regular Insulin, Isoproterenol HCl, Levarterenol bitart., Levorphanol bitart., Meperidine HCl, Methadone HCl, Methylprednisolone Na Succ., Morphine Sulf., Penicillin G Potass., Pentazocine lactate, Prochlorperazine edisylate and mesylate, Promazine HCl, Propiomazine HCl, Sulfisoxazole diolamine, Tetracycline HCl, Vit. B Complex with C
Amphotericin B (Fungizone IV)	24		Heparin Na, Hydrocortisone Na Succinate	Ca chloride and gluconate, Carbenacillin Disod., Chlorpromazine HCl, Chlortetracycline Na, Diphenhydramine HCl, Dopamine HCl, Gentamicin Sulf., Kanamycin Sulf., Lidocaine HCl, Metaraminol bitart., Methyldopate HCl, Nitrofurantoin Na, Oxytetracycline HCl, Penicillin G Potass. and Sod., Phytonadione, KCl, Procaine HCl, Prochlorperazine mesylate, Streptomycin Sulf., Tetracycline HCl, Viomycin Sulf.

See footnote on p. 800.

(Continued)

INFORMATION ON DRUG THERAPY FOR ANTIBIOTICS AND OTHER DRUGS COMMONLY ADMINISTERED INTRAVENOUSLY ***(Continued)***

Drug	*Stability (hr at room temp) in IV Solutions*		*Compatibility with Following Drugs*	*Incompatibility with Following Drugs*
	D_5W	*Saline*		
Ampicillin Sodium (Omnipen-N, Penbritin-S, Polycillin-N)	4	8	*No Other Drugs Should Be Added to IV Solution*	
Calcium Chloride			Ascorbic Acid, Cephapirin Na, Chloramphenicol Na Succ., Hydrocortisone Na Succ., Isoproterenol HCl, Levarterenol bitart., Lidocaine HCl, Methicillin Na, Penicillin G pot and sod., Pentobarbital Na, Phenobarbital Na, Oxytetracycline HCl*, Tetracycline HCl*, Vit B Complex with C	Amphotericin B, Cephalothin Na, Cephradine, Chlorpheniramine maleate, Chlortetracycline HCl, Streptomycin Sulf., Tobramycin Sulf.
Calcium Gluceptate	+	+	Ascorbic Acid, Isoproterenol HCl, Levarterenol bitart., Lidocaine HCl, Menadione Na bisulf., Phytonadione	Cephalothin Na, Cephradine, Mg Sulf., Novobiocin Na, Prednisolone Na phos., Prochlorperazine edisylate, Streptomycin Sulf., Tobramycin Sulf.
Calcium Gluconate	+	+	Aminophylline, Ascorbic Acid, Cephapirin Na, Chloramphenicol Na Succ., Corticotropin, Dimenhydrinate, Erythromycin gluceptate, Heparin Na, Hydrocortisone Na Succ., Levarterenol bitart., Methicillin Na, Novobiocin Na*, Oxytetracycline HCl*, Penicillin G Pot. and Sod., KCl, Prochlorperazine edisylate, Sulfadiazine Na, Sulfisoxazole diolamine, Tetracycline HCl*, Vancomycin HCl, Vit. B Complex with C	Amphotericin B, Cephalothin Na, Cefazolin Na, Cephradine, Mg Sulf., Streptomycin Sulf., Tobramycin Sulf.
Carbenicillin Disod. (Geopen, Pyopen)	24	24	Clindamycin Phos., Dopamine HCl, Hydrocortisone Na Succ*, KCl, Sod. bicarb., Vit B Complex/C*	Amphotericin B, Gentamicin Sulf.*, Oxytetracycline HCl, Tetracycline HCl

Drug			
Cefazolin Sodium	24	24	Amikacin Sulf., Amobarbital Na, Ca gluceptate and gluconate, Chlortetracycline HCl, Colistimethate Na, Erythromycin gluceptate, Kanamycin Sulf., Oxytetracycline HCl, Pentobarbital Na, Polymyxin B sulfate, Tetracycline HCl
Cephaloridine (Loridine)	24	24	*Mixing with Other Antibiotics Is Not Recommended. Usually Administered Into Tubing of IV Infusion*
Cephalothin Sodium (Keflin, Keflin Neutral)	24	24	Usually administered into tubing of IV Infusion or by Y-Tube (Discontinue other infusion while this drug being given).
Cephapirin Sodium (Cefadyl)	24	24	Usually administered into tubing of IV Infusion or by Y-Tube (Discontinue other infusion while this drug being given).
Cephradine (Velosef)	2–8	2–8	Calcium ions, Epinephrine HCl, Lidocaine HCl, Tetracycline HCl
Chloramphenical Sodium Succinate (Chloromycetin Sodium Succinate)	24	24	Aminophylline, Ascorbic Acid*, Ca chloride and gluconate, Cephalothin Na, Cephapirin Na, Chlortetracycline HCl, Colistimethate Na, Corticotropin, Cyanocobalamin, Dimenhydrinate, Dopamine HCl, Ephedrine sulf., Heparin Na, Hydrocortisone Na Succ., Kanamycin Sulf., Metaraminol bitart., Methicillin Na*, Methyldopate HCl, Nafcillin Na, Nitrofurantoin Na*, Oxacillin Na, Oxytetracycline HCl*, Oxytocin, Penicillin G Pot and Sod., Pentobarbital Na, Phenylephrine HCl, Phytonadione, Potass. Chloride, Promazine HCl*, Sod. bicarb., Sulfadiazine Na*, Sulfisoxazole diolamine*, Tetracycline HCl*, Thiopental Na, Vit B Complex/C* / Chlorpromazine HCl, Gentamicin Sulf., Hydroxyzine HCl, Novobiocin Na, Polymyxin B Sulfate, Prochlorperazine edisylate and mesylate, Promethazine HCl, Vancomycin HCl

See footnote on p. 800.

(*Continued*)

INFORMATION ON DRUG THERAPY FOR ANTIBIOTICS AND OTHER DRUGS COMMONLY ADMINISTERED INTRAVENOUSLY (*Continued*)

Drug	Stability (hr at room temp) in IV Solutions		Compatibility with Following Drugs	Incompatibility with Following Drugs
	D₅W	Saline		
Chlorpromazine HCL (Thorazine, others)		+	Ascorbic acid Inj, Ethacrynate Na, Vit B Complex/C	Aminophylline, Amphotericin B, Ampicillin Na, Barbiturates, Chloramphenicol Na Succ., Chlorothiazide Na, Methicillin Na, Methohexital Na, Nitrofurantoin Na, Penicillin G Pot and Sod., Sulfadiazine Na
Chlortetracycline HCL (Aureomycin)	+	+	Aminophylline, Chloramphenicol Na Succ., Corticotropin, Dimenhydrinate, Erythromycin gluceptate, Heparin Na, Hydrocortisone Na Succ., Methicillin Na, Oxytetracycline HCl, Sulfadiazine Na, Sulfisoxazole diolamine, Tetracycline HCl, Thiopental Na, Vancomycin HCl, Vit B Complex/C	Amikacin Sulf., Calcium Chloride, Cefazolin Na, Cephaloridine, Cephalothin Na, Cephapirin Na, Colistimethate Na, Penicillin G Pot, Polymyxin B Sulf., Promazine HCl
Clindamycin Phos. (Cleocin Phos.)	24	24	Carbenicillin disod., Cephalothin Na, Gentamicin Sulf., Heparin Na, Hydrocortisone Na Succ., Kanamycin Sulf., Methylprednisolone Na Succ., Penicillin G, Pot. Chl., Sod. Bicarb., Vit B Complex/C	Aminophylline, Ampicillin, Barbiturates, Ca gluconate, Mg Sulf., Phenytoin Na
Colistimethate Sod. (Coly-Mycin M Parenteral)	+		Ascorbic acid inj., Chloramphenicol Na Succ., Diphenhydramine HCl, Heparin Na, Methicillin Na, Oxytetracycline HCl, Penicillin G Pot and Sod., Phenobarbital Na, Polymyxin B Sulf., Tetracycline HCl, Vitamin B Complex/C	Cefazolin Na, Cephalothin Na, Cephaloridine, Chlortetracycline HCl, Erythromycin lactobionate, Hydrocortisone Na Succ., Kanamycin Sulf., Lincomycin HCl

Drug				
Dexamethasone Sod. Phos. (Decadron)	+	+	Lidocaine HCl, Nafcillin Na, Prochlorperazine edisylate*	Amikacin Sulf., Metaraminol bitart., Vancomycin HCl
Doxorubicin HCl (Adriamycin)	+	+	Should be administered into tubing of IV Infusion	
Ephedrine Sulfate	+	+	Chloramphenicol Na Succ., Lidocaine HCl, Metaraminol bitart., Nafcillin Na, Penicillin G Pot, Tetracycline HCl, Thiopental Na*	Hydrocortisone Na Succ.*, Pentobarbital Na, Phenobarbital Na, Secobarbital Na
Ergonovine Maleate (Ergotrate Maleate)			*Is Usually Recommended That Ergonovine Maleate Not Be Mixed with IV Infusions—Can Be Given Through a Y-Tube Set*	
Erythromycin Gluceptate (Ilotycin Gluceptate)	+	+	Ca gluconate, Cephapirin Na*, Chlortetracycline HCl, Corticotropin, Dimenhydrinate, Heparin Na*, Hydrocortisone Na Succ., Methicillin Na, Penicillin G Pot., KCl, Sulfadiazine Na, Sulfisoxazole diolamine	Amikacin Sulf., Aminophylline, Cefazolin Na, Cephalothin Na, Cephaloridine, Metaraminol bitart., Novobiocin Na, Oxytetracycline HCl, Pentobarbital Na, Secobarbital Na, Streptomycin Sulf., Tetracycline HCl
Erythromycin Lactobionate (Erythrocin Lactobionate I.V.)	24	Do not use for initial reconstitution	Aminophylline, Ascorbic acid inj.*, Diphenhydramine HCl, Hydrocortisone Na Succ., Lidocaine HCl, Methicillin Na, Nitrofurantoin Na, Penicillin G Pot and Sod., Pentobarbital Na, Polymyxin B Sulf., KCl, Prednisolone Na Phos., Prochlorperazine edisylate, Promazine HCl, Sod. bicarb., Sod. iodide, Sulfisoxazole diolamine	*Some Recommend That No Drugs Be Added to Solutions of Erythromycin Lactobionate*
Fluorouracil	+	+	Cephalothin Na, Prednisolone Na Phos., Vincristine Sulf.	Cytarbine, Doxorubicin HCl, Methotrexate Na
Gentamicin Sulfate (Garamycin)	24	24	*Should Not Be Mixed with Other Drugs in Same IV Bottle*	

See footnote on p. 800.

(Continued)

INFORMATION ON DRUG THERAPY FOR ANTIBIOTICS AND OTHER DRUGS COMMONLY ADMINISTERED INTRAVENOUSLY (*Continued*)

Drug	Stability (hr at room temp) in IV Solutions		Compatibility with Following Drugs	Incompatibility with Following Drugs
	D₅W	*Saline*		
	D_5W	Saline		
Heparin Sodium	24	24	Aminophylline, Amphotericin B, Ampicillin Na*, Ascorbic acid inj., Ca gluconate, Cephaloridine*, Cephalothin Na*, Cephapirin Na, Chloramphenicol Na Succ., Chlortetracycline HCl, Clindamycin Phos., Colistimethate Na, Dimenhydrinate*, Erythromycin gluceptate*, Hydrocortisone Na Succ.*, Isoproterenol HCl, Levarterenol bitart., Lidocaine HCl, Methicillin Na*, Methyldopate HCl, Nafcillin Na, Nitrofurantoin Na, Oxytetracycline HCl*, Penicillin G Pot and Sod.*, KCl, Prednisolone Na Phos., Promazine HCl*, Sulfadiazine Na, Sulfisoxazole diolamine*, Tetracycline HCl*, Vit B Complex/C	Amikacin Sulf., Anileridine HCl, Codeine Phos., Daunomycin HCl, Erythromycin lactobionate, Hyaluronidase, Kanamycin Sulf., Levorphanol bitart., Meperidine HCl, Methadone HCl, Morphine Sulf., Novobiocin Na, Polymyxin B Sulf., Promethazine HCl, Streptomycin Sulf., Tobramycin Sulf., Vancomycin HCl*, Viomycin Sulf.
Hydrocortisone Sodium Succinate (Solu-Cortef)	48	48	Aminophylline, Amobarbital Na*, Ampicillin Na*, Amphotericin B, Ca chloride and gluconate, Cephalothin, Cephapirin Na, Chloramphenicol Na Succ., Chlortetracycline HCl, Clindamycin Phos., Corticotropin, Dimenhydrinate*, Erythromycin gluceptate and lactobionate, Heparin Na*, Kanamycin Sulf.*, Levarterenol bitart., Lidocaine HCl, Metaraminol bitart.*, Methicillin Na*, Oxytetracycline HCl*, Penicillin G Pot.* and Sod., Polymxin B sulf., KCl, Sulfadiazine Na, Sulfisoxazole diolamine, Thiopental Na, Vancomycin HCl*, Vit B Complex/C*	Aminophylline with cephalothin Na, Colistimethate Na, Diphenhydramine HCl, Nafcillin Na, Novobiocin Na, Pentobarbital Na, Phenobarbital Na, Prochlorperazine edisylate, Promethazine HCl, Secobarbital Na, Tetracycline HCl

Isoproterenol HCl (Isuprel)	24	24	Ca chloride and gluceptate, Cephalothin Na, Heparin Na, Mg Sulf., Multiple Vit. Infus., Oxytetracycline HCl, KCl, Succinylcholine Cl, Tetracycline HCl, Vit B Complex/C	Aminophylline, Antibiotics buffered alkaline, Barbiturates, Lidocaine HCl, Sod. bicarb.
Kanamycin Sulfate	24	24	Ascorbic acid inj., Dopamine HCl, Hydrocortisone Na Succ.*, Sod. bicarb., Vit B Complex/C	*Should Not Be Mixed with Other Antibacterial Agents*, Chlorpheniramine maleate, Colistimethate Na, Heparin Na, Hydrocortisone Na Succ.*, Methohexital Na
Levarterenol Bitartrate (Levophed)	+	Not Rec.	Ca chloride, gluceptate, and gluconate, Cephalothin Na*, Corticotropin, Dimenhydrinate, Heparin Na, Hydrocortisone Na Succ., Mg Sulf., Multiple Vit. Infus., Oxytetracycline HCl, Pot. Chlor., Succinylcholine Cl, Tetracycline HCl, Vit B Complex/C	Aminophylline, Amobarbital Na, Antibiotics Buffered Alkaline, Cephapirin Na, Chlorothiazide Na, Chlorpheniramine maleate, Lidocaine, Nitrofurantoin Na, Pentobarbital Na, Phenobarbital Na, Phenytoin Na, Sod. bicarb., Sod. Iodide, Streptomycin Sulf., Sulfadiazine Na, Sulfisoxazole diolamine, Thiopental Na
Lidocaine HCL (Xylocaine HCl I.V.)	24	24	Aminophylline, Ca chloride and gluceptate, Chloramphenical Na Succ., Chlorothiazide Na, Dexamethasone Na, Diphenhydramine HCl, Ephedrine Sulf., Erythromycin lactobionate, Heparin Na, Hydrocortisone Na Succ, Hydroxyzine HCl, Mephentermine Sulf., Metaraminol Bitart., Nitrofurantoin Na, Oxytetracycline HCl, Penicillin G Pot., Pentobarbital Na, Phenylephrine HCl, KCl, Prochlorperazine edisylate, Promazine HCl, Sod. bicarb., Sod. lactate, Sulfisoxazole diolamine, Tetracycline HCl, Vit B Complex/C	Methohexital Na, Sulfadiazine Na

See footnote on p. 800.

(Continued)

INFORMATION ON DRUG THERAPY FOR ANTIBIOTICS AND OTHER DRUGS COMMONLY ADMINISTERED INTRAVENOUSLY (Continued)

Drug	Stability (hr at room temp) in IV Solutions		Compatibility with Following Drugs	Incompatibility with Following Drugs
	D_5W	Saline		
Lincomycin HCl (Lincocin)	24	24	Ampicillin Na*, Cephaloridine, Cephalothin Na, Chloramphenicol Na Succ, Heparin Na, Methicillin Na*, Penicillin G Pot* and Sod*, Polymyxin B Sulf., Tetracycline HCl, Vit B Complex/C	Colistimethate Na, Kanamycin Sulf., Novobiocin Na, Phenytoin Na, Sulfadiazine Na
Metaraminol Bitartrate (Aramine)	24–48	24–48	Cephalothin Na, Cephapirin Na, Chloramphenicol Na Succ, Cyanocobalamin, Ephedrine Sulf., Epinephrine HCl, Hydrocortisone Sod. Phos. and Succ.*, Lidocaine HCl, Nitrofurantoin Na*, Oxytocin, KCl, Promazine HCl, Sod. Bicarb., Sulfisoxazole diolamine, Tetracycline HCl	Acid-labile drugs, Amphotericin B, Dexamethasone Na Phos., Erythromycin Lactobion., Fibrinogen, Methicillin Na, Methylprednisolone Na Succ, Nafcillin Na, Penicillin G Pot, Prednisolone Na Phos., Sulfadiazine Na, Thiopental Na, Warfarin Na
Methicillin Sodium (Celbenin, Staphcillin)	8–24	8–24	*Should Not Be Mixed with Other Drugs in Same IV Bottle*	
Methotrexate Sodium	7 days	7 days	Cephalothin Na, Cytarbine, 6-Mercaptopurine Na, Vincristine Sulf.	Fluorouracil, Prednisolone Na Phos.
Methyldopate HCl (Aldomet Ester HCl)	24	24	Aminophylline, Ascorbic acid Inj., Chloramphenicol Na Succ, Diphenhydramine HCl, Heparin Na, Mg Sulf, Oxytetracycline HCl, Pot. Chlor., Promazine HCl, Sod. Bicarb., Succinylcholine Cl, Tetracycline HCl*, Vit B Complex/C	Acid-labile drugs, Amphotericin B, Methohexital Na, Sulfadiazine Na

Drug			
Methylprednisolone Sodium Succinate (Solu-Medrol)	+	Amphotericin B, Clindamycin Phos	Aminophylline, Cephalothin Na, Metaraminol Bitart.
Mithramycin (Mithracin)	4–6		
Nafcillin Sodium (Unipen)	24	Aminophylline*, Chloramphenicol Na Succ., Chlorothiazide Na, Dexamethasome Na Phos., Diphenhydramine HCl, Ephedrine Sulf, Heparin Na, Hydroxyzine HCl, Nitrofurantoin Na, KCl, Prochlorperazine edisylate, Sod. Bicarb., Sod. Lactate, Sulfisoxazole diolamine, Vit B Complex/C*	Ascorbic Acid Inj, Gentamicin Sulf., Hydrocortisone Na Succ., Metaraminol Bitart., Penicillins, Promazine HCl, Succinylcholine Cl, Tetracyclines
Novobiocin Sodium (Albamycin Sodium)	24	Aminophylline, Ca gluconate*, Cephapirin Na, Chlortetracycline HCl, Methicillin Na, Penicillin G Pot, KCl, Sulfadiazine Na, Sulfisoxazole diolamine	Amikacin Sulf, Anileridine HCl, Ca gluceptate, Chloramphenicol Na Succ, Codeine Phos., Corticotropin, Dimenhydrinate, Epinephrine HCl, Erythromycin gluceptate, Heparin Na, Hydrocortisone Na Succ, Levarterenol Bitart, Levorphanol Bitart, Mg Sulf, Kanamycin Sulf, Lincomycin HCl, Methadone HCl, Morphine Sulf, Neomycin, Oxytetracycline HCl, Procaine HCl, Streptomycin Sulf., Tetracycline HCl, Vancomycin HCl, Vit B Complex/C
Oxacillin Sodium (Prostaphlin)	6–24	Cephapirin Na, Chloramphenicol Na Succ, Pot. Chloride	Amikacin Sulf*, Oxytetracycline, Tetracycline HCl
Oxytetracycline HCl (Terramycin IV)	24	Aminophylline, Ca Chloride* and gluconate*, Chloramphenicol Na Succ*, Chlortetracycline HCl, Corticotropin, Colistimethate Na, Dimenhydrinate, Heparin Na*, Hydrocortisone Na Succ*, Isoproterenol HCl, Levarterenol Bitart, Lidocaine HCl, Methyldopate HCl, Polymyxin B Sulf, Pot. Chlor., Tetracycline HCl, Vit B Complex/C*	Amikacin Sulf, Amphotericin B Carbenicillin Disod, Cefazolin Na, Cephalothin Na, Cephaloridine, Erythromycin gluceptate, Methicillin Na, Methohexital Na, Novobiocin Na, Oxacillin Na, Penicillin G Pot and Sod, Sod Bicarb., Sulfadiazine Na

See footnote on p. 800.

(Continued)

INFORMATION ON DRUG THERAPY FOR ANTIBIOTICS AND OTHER DRUGS COMMONLY ADMINISTERED INTRAVENOUSLY (Continued)

Drug	Stability (hr at room temp) in IV Solutions		Compatibility with Following Drugs	Incompatibility with Following Drugs
	D₅W	Saline		
Oxytocin (Pitocin)	+	+	Chloramphenicol Na Succ, Metaraminol Bitart, Tetracycline HCl, Thiopental Na	Fibrinolysin (Human), Warfarin Na
Penicillin G Potassium	48	24–48	Ascorbic Acid Inj, Ca chloride and gluconate, Cephalothin Na* Cephapirin Na, Chloramphenicol Na Succ, Clindamycin Phos, Colistimethate Na, Corticotropin, Dimenhydrinate, Diphenhydramine HCl, Ephedrine Sulf, Erythromycin glucep and lactobion, Heparin Na*, Hydrocortisone Na Succ* Kanamycin Sulf, Lidocaine HCl, Lincomycin HCl*, Methicillin Na, Nitrofurantoin Na, Novobiocin Na, Polymyxin B Sulf, Pot. Chlor., Prednisolone Na Phos, Procaine HCl*, Prochlorperazine edisylate*, Promethazine HCl*, Sod. Iodide, Sulfisoxazole diolamine*, Vit B Complex/C*,	Amikacin Sulf, Aminophylline, Amphotericin B, Chlorpromazine HCl, Chlortetracycline HCl, Dopamine HCl, Hydroxyzine HCl, Metaraminol Bitart, Oxytetracycline HCl, Pentobarbital Na, Prochlorperazine mesylate* Promazine HCl, Sod. Bicarb, Tetracycline HCl, Thiopental Na, Vancomycin HCl
Penicillin G Sodium	12–24	12–24	Ca Chloride and gluconate, Chloramphenicol Na Succ, Clindamycin Phos, Colistimethate Na, Diphenhydramine HCl, Erythromycin lactobion, Gentamicin Sulf, Heparin Na*, Hydrocortisone Na Succ, Kanamycin Sulf, Lincomycin HCl*, Methicillin Na, Nitrofurantoin Na, Polymyxin B Sulf, Pot. Chlor.*, Prednisolone Na Phos, Procaine HCl*, Vit B Complex/C	Amphotericin B, Cephalothin Na, Chlorpromazine HCl, Hydroxyzine HCl, Metaraminol Bitart, Oxytetracycline HCl, Prochlorperazine mesylate, Promethazine HCl, Tetracycline HCl, Vancomycin HCl

(Continued)

Drug				
Phenylephrine HCl (Neo-Synephrine)	+		Chloramphenicol Na Succ, Lidocaine HCl, Pot. Chlor.,	
Polymyxin B Sulfate	+	+	Ascorbic Acid Inj, Colistimethate Na, Diphenhydramine HCl, Erythromycin Lactobion, Hydrocortisone Na Succ, Kanamycin Sulf, Methicillin Na, Oxytetracycline HCl, Penicillin G Pot* and Sod*, Phenobarbital Na, Vit B Complex/C	Amphotericin B, Cefazolin Na, Cephlothin Na, Chloramphenicol Na Succ, Chlorothiazide Na, Chlortetracycline HCl, Heparin Na, Mg Sulf, Nitrofurantoin Na, Prednisolone Na Succ, Tetracycline HCl
Potassium Chloride	+		Aminophylline, Ca gluconate, Carbenicillin Disod, Cephalothin Na, Cephapirin Na, Chloramphenicol Na Succ, Clindamycin Phos, Corticotropin, Dimenhydrinate, Erythromycin gluceptate and lactobionate, Heparin Na, Hydrocortisone Na Succ, Isoproterenol HCl, Levarterenol Bitart, Lidocaine HCl, Metaraminol Bitart, Methicillin Na, Methyldopate HCl, Nafcillin Na, Novobiocin Na, Oxacillin Na, Oxytetracycline HCl, Penicillin G Pot and Sod*, Phenylephrine HCl, Sulfadiazine Na, Sulfisoxazole diolamine, Tetracycline HCl, Thiopental Na, Vancomycin HCl, Vit B Complex C	Amikacin Sulf, Amphotericin B, Streptomycin Sulf
Prednisolone Sodium Phosphate (Hydeltrasol)	+	+	Ascorbic Acid Inj, Cephalothin Na, Cytarbine, Erythromycin Lactobion, Fluorouracil, Heparin Na, Methicillin Na, Penicillin G Pot and Sod, Tetracycline HCl, Vit B Complex/C	Ca gluceptate, Metaraminol Bitart, Methotrexate Na, Polymyxin B Sulf
Prednisolone Sodium Succinate (Meticortelone Soluble) *See footnote on p. 800.*	48	48		Allopurinol Na, 6-Mercaptopurine Na

See footnote on p. 800.

Drug	Stability (hr at room temp) in IV Solutions		Compatibility with Following Drugs	Incompatibility with Following Drugs
	D_5W	Saline		
Prochlorperazine Edisylate (Compazine)	+	+	Ascorbic Acid Inj, Ca gluconate*, Dexamethasone Na Phos*, Dimenhydrinate*, Erythromycin lactobion, Ethacrynate Na, Lidocaine HCl, Nafcillin Na, Nitrofurantoin Na*, Penicillin G Pot*, Vit B Complex/C*	Aminophylline, Ca Glucceptate, Cephalothin Na, Chloramphenicol Na Succ, Chlorothiazide Na, Hydrocortisone Na Succ, Thiopental Na
Promethazine HCl (Phenergan)	+	+	Ascorbic Acid Inj, Penicillin G Pot*, Vit B Complex/C*	Aminophylline, Chloramphenicol Na Succ, Chlorothiazide Na, Heparin Na, Hydrocortisone Na Succ, Methicillin Na, Methohexital Na, Nitrofurantoin Na, Penicillin G Pot* and Sod, Pentobarbital Na*, Phenobarbital Na, Thiopental Na
Sodium Bicarbonate	+	+	Aminophylline, Carbenicillin Disod, Cephalothin Na, Cephapirin Na, Chloramphenicol Na Succ, Clindamycin Phos, Erythromycin lactobion, Kanamycin Sulf, Lidocaine HCl, Metaraminol Bitart, Methicillin Na*, Methyldopate HCl, Nafcillin Na, Phenylephrine HCl, Thiopental Na	Anileridine HCl, Ascorbic Acid Inj, Codeine Phos, Corticotropin, Hydromorphone HCl, Levarterenol Bitart, Mg Sulf, Meperidine HCl, Methadone HCl, Morphine Sulf, Oxytetracycline HCl, Pentazocine Lactate, Pentobarbital Na, Penicillin G Pot, Procaine HCl, Promazine HCl, Secobarbital Na, Streptomycin Sulf, Tetracycline HCl, Vancomycin HCl, Vit B Complex/C
Sodium Lactate	+	+	Lidocaine HCl, Nafcillin Na	Novobiocin Na, Oxytetracycline HCl, Sod. Bicarb., Sulfadiazine Na
Succinylcholine Chloride (Anectine, Quelicin)	+	+	Cephapirin Na, Isoproterenol HCl, Levarterenol Bitart, Meperidine HCl, Methyldopate HCl, Morphine Sulf, Pentobarbital Na*, Scopolamine HBr	Barbiturates*, Nafcillin Na, Methohexital Na, Thiopental Na*

798

Drug			Compatible in Same IV Bottle	Should Not Be Mixed in Same IV Bottle
Sulfisoxazole Diolamine (Gantrisin)	+	+ Dilute the 40% ampule to 5% with sterile water for injection	Ca gluconate, Cephapirin Na, Chloramphenicol Na Succ*, Chlortetracycline HCl, Corticotropin, Dimenhydrinate, Erythromycin gluceptate and lactobionate, Heparin Na*, Hydrocortisone Na Succ, Kanamycin Sulf*, Lidocaine HCl, Metaraminol Bitart, Methicillin Na, Nafcillin Na, Novobiocin Na, Penicillin G Pot*, Pot. Chlor., Sulfadiazine Na, Tetracycline HCl*	Amikacin Sulf, Aminophylline, Anileridine HCl, Ascorbic Acid Inj, Cephalothin Na, Chloramphenicol Na Succ*, Codeine Phos, Heparin Na* Levarterenol Bitart, Levorphanol Bitart, Meperidine HCl, Methadone HCl, Morphine Sulf, Procaine HCl, Promazine HCl, Streptomycin Sulf, Thiopental Na, Vancomycin HCl, Vit B Complex/C
Tetracycline HCl (Achromycin IV)	24	24	Ascorbic Acid Inj, Ca Chloride*, Ca gluconate*, Chloramphenicol Na Succ*, Chlortetracycline HCl, Colistimethate Na, Corticotropin, Diphenhydramine HCl, Dopamine HCl, Ephedrine Sulf, Heparin Na*, Isoproterenol HCl, Kanamycin Sulf, Levarterenol Bitart, Methyldopate HCl*, Oxytetracycline HCl, Oxytocin, Pentobarbital Na*, Phenobarbital Na*, Pot. Chl., Prednisolone Na Phos, Procaine HCl, Promazine HCl, Sulfisoxazole diolamine*, Vit B Complex/C	Amikacin Sulf, Aminophylline, Amphotericin B, Barbiturates, Carbenicillin Disod, Cefazolin Na, Cephaloridine, Cephalothin Na, Cephapirin Na, Chlorothiazide Na, Dimenhydrinate, Erythromycin gluceptate and lactobionate, Hydrocortisone Na Succ, Methicillin Na, Methohexital Na, Nafcillin Na, Novobiocin Na, Oxacillin Na, Penicillin G Pot, Polymyxin B Sulf, Sod Bicarb, Thiopental Na, Warfarin Na
Ticarcillin Disodium (Ticar)	72	72		
Tobramycin Sulfate (Nebcin)	48	48	*Other Drugs Should Not Be Mixed in Same IV Bottle*	
Vancomycin Hydrochloride (Vancocin HCl)	7 days	7 days	Aminophylline*, Ca gluconate, Corticotropin, Dimenhydrinate, Hydrocortisone Na Succ*, Pot. Chlor., Sulfadiazine Na*, Vit B Complex/C*	Amobarbital Na, Chloramphenicol Na Succ, Chlorothiazide Na, Heparin Na*, Methicillin Na, Nitrofurantoin Na, Novobiocin Na, Penicillin G, Pentobarbital Na, Phenobarbital Na, Secobarbital Na, Sod. Bicarb.*, Sulfisoxazole diolamine, Warfarin Na

See footnote on p. 800.

(Continued)

INFORMATION ON DRUG THERAPY FOR ANTIBIOTICS AND OTHER DRUGS COMMONLY ADMINISTERED INTRA-VENOUSLY (Continued)

| Drug | Stability (hr at room temp) in IV Solutions | | Compatibility with Following Drugs | Incompatibility with Following Drugs |
	D₅W	Saline		
Vinblastine Sulfate (Velban)	+	+	May Be Given Into Tubing of IV Infusion	
Vincristine Sulfate	+	+	May Be Given Into Tubing of IV Infusion	
Vitamin B Complex With C (Berocca-C, Folbesyn, Solu-B with Ascorbic Acid)	24	24	Ca Chloride and gluconate, Carbenicillin Disod*, Cephalothin Na, Cephapirin Na, Chloramphenicol Na Succ*, Chlorpromazine HCl, Chlortetracycline HCl, Clindamycin Phos, Corticotropin, Cyanocobalamin, Dimenhydrinate, Diphenhydramine HCl, Heparin Na, Hydrocortisone Na Succ*, Isoproterenol HCl, Kanamycin Sulf, Levarterenol Bitart, Lidocaine HCl, Methyldopate HCl, Nafcillin Na*, Oxytetracycline HCl*, Penicillin G Pot*, Polymyxin B Sulf, Pot. Chl., Prednisolone Na Phos, Procaine HCl, Prochlorperazine edisylate*, Promethazine HCl*, Tetracycline HCl*, Vancomycin HCl*	Amakacin Sulf, Aminophylline, Chlorothiazide Na, Erythromycin Lactobionate, Gentamicin Sulf, Methicillin Na, Nitrofurantoin Na, Novobiocin Na, Sod Bicarb., Sulfisoxazole diolamine, Warfarin Na

* Conflicting compatibility data available. Use caution and judgment in mixing.

+ Means no data on stability of solution is available, but drugs can be mixed with solution as indicated.

Note: Incompatibilities with drugs often are time dependent.

change in color (unless the solution is normally colored), or gas formation.

3. Drugs in solution may undergo degradation, the products of which may be toxic or have no therapeutic activity. These changes may or may not be visible, although most often such changes are manifested by changes in pH of the solution.

4. Whenever two or more drugs are mixed together, there is always the possibility that the combination may produce a pharmacological response in the patient which was not intended or expected.

5. Although not common, it has been found that certain drugs may interact with the delivery system being utilized (e.g., the drug may bind to the glass or plastic surface of the system, resulting in less than the expected quantity of drug being received by the patient).

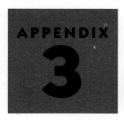

APPENDIX

3 poisoning

General Measures

1. Remove as much of the poison as possible by appropriate means, such as gastric lavage, induced emesis, washing of eyes, or skin.

   Never induce emesis if patient is unconscious, comatose, if poison is corrosive, a petroleum distillate (e.g., kerosone), or a convulsant.

   Emesis can often be induced by giving a glass of milk and then placing tongue depressor at back of patient's throat. Emesis can also be induced by ipecac syrup.

   When vomiting begins, place patient face down, with head lower than hips so that vomitus does not become aspirated.

2. If poison has been injected (insect, snake) retard absorption of poison by
   a. applying a constricting bandage between injection site and heart. Bandage should not be so tight that it suppresses pulse in affected area completely; remove for 1 minute every 15 minutes.
   b. applying ice pack to affected area.
   c. sucking out poison by suction cup.

3. Administer specific antidote if available.

4. Administer a suitable nonspecific antidote listed in following Table.

5. Institute supportive measures to maintain patient's vital functions.

Poisoning

For immediate information on the content of toxic ingredients of commercial preparations and their antidotes, record the telephone number of your regional poison control center:

Poison Control Center _____

TOXIC AGENTS AND THEIR ANTAGONISTS

Agent or Toxic Reaction	Symptoms	Antagonist or Treatment
Acids	GI symptoms: nausea, vomiting, diarrhea	Milk of magnesia or lime water, followed by milk and demulcents. Do not induce vomiting.
Alcohol, wood (Methyl alcohol)	Blurred vision	Gastric lavage within 3 hours; Ethyl alcohol (grain alcohol) **IV** 0.75–1.0 ml/kg, then 0.5 ml/kg q 4 hours; Sodium bicarbonate PO.
Alkali (lye)	GI symptoms: nausea, vomiting, diarrhea	Acetic acid, dilute vinegar, tartaric acid **PO.** Do not induce vomiting.
Anaphylaxis	Circulatory collapse, asphyxia	Epinephrine **SC** 1 : 1000 aqueous (0.01 ml/kg), repeated for total of 3 doses.
Anesthetics	Respiratory depression, coma	See *CNS Depressants*
Antidepressants, tricyclic	Arrhythmias, convulsions, coma	Physostigmine **IM or IV:** 0.5–2.0 mg, repeated at intervals if life-threatening symptoms persist.
Amphetamines	Tachycardia, convulsions, delirium	Chlorpromazine **IM or IV:** 1 mg/kg
Anticoagulants, coumarin type	Hemorrhage	Vitamin K **IM** 5–10 mg/kg
Arsenic	*See Heavy Metals below*	Dimercaprol **IM** (BAL in oil): 2.5 mg/kg or more
Aspirin	Hyperventilation, auditory and visual disturbance	Give 2 to 3 glasses of water, induce vomiting; institute gastric lavage.
Atropine	Dilated pupils, blurred vision, delirium	Activated charcoal
Peripheral poisoning		Pilocarpine
Systemic poisoning		Physostigmine; See *Antidepressants*

TOXIC AGENTS AND THEIR ANTAGONISTS (*Continued*)

Agent or Toxic Reaction	Symptoms	Antagonist or Treatment
Barbiturates	Respiratory depression, coma	See *CNS Depressants*
Black widow spider bites	Hypocalcemic tetany	Calcium gluconate **IV:** 10–20 ml of 10% solution.
Carbon monoxide	Respiratory depression and coma	Oxygen (100% O_2 for 30 minutes), artificial respiration, rest.
Carbon tetrachloride	Coma, oliguria, jaundice, abdominal pain, decrease in blood pressure	Remove by gastric lavage or emesis; artificial respiration; maintain blood pressure. **Do not give stimulants.**
CNS depressants	Respiratory depression and coma	Artificial respiration; supportive measures; use of CNS stimulants is usually not recommended.
CNS stimulants	Tachycardia, delirium	Short-acting barbiturates (for dosage See *Drug Entries*).
Cocaine	Dilated pupils, blurred vision, delirium, hallucinations.	Anti-anxiety Agent.
Codeine	Respiratory depression, coma	See *Narcotics*.
Cough medication containing narcotics	Respiratory depression	If containing codeine, see *Narcotics*.
Cyanide	Respiratory depression, cyanosis	Sodium nitrite **IV:** 3% solution at 2.5–5.0 ml/min; followed by sodium thiosulfate **IV:** 50 ml of a 25% solution at 2.5–5.0 ml/min.
Heavy metals (lead, mercury)	GI symptoms: Nausea, vomiting, and diarrhea; discoloration of gums; increased salivation	Chelating agents, such as EDTA; **IM or IV:** 50–75 mg/kg daily in 4 divided doses; or BAL, **IM:** 12–24 mg/kg/24 hours in 6 divided doses; or penicillamine (see p. 764).

(*Continued*)

TOXIC AGENTS AND THEIR ANTAGONISTS (*Continued*)

Agent or Toxic Reaction	Symptoms	Antagonist or Treatment
Heroin	See *Narcotics*, below	See *Narcotics*.
Insecticide (Organic phosphate ester type)	Convulsions, GI symptoms: nausea, vomiting, and diarrhea	Atropine **IV:** 1–4 mg with repeated doses of 2 mg q 15–30 minutes and/or pralidoxime chloride (2-PAM, Protopan chloride) **IV:** 1–2 gm, followed by 250 mg increments q 5 min.
Iron	Gastritis (may be severe), cyanosis, pallor, diarrhea, drowsiness, shock, acidosis	Deferoxamine **IM:** 1–2 gm or 20 mg/kg q 4 to 6 hours.
Kerosene	Irritation of mouth, throat, stomach; vomiting, pulmonary irritation; CNS depression	Depending on amount ingested, emesis with ipecac syrup may be indicated. Supportive treatment including artificial respiration.
Lead	Convulsions, also see *Heavy Metal Poisoning*, above.	See *Heavy Metal Poisoning*, above.
LSD (Lysergic acid diethylamide)	Dilated pupils, hallucinations.	Sedatives or antianxiety agents. Do not give chlorpromazine.
Methemoglobinemia	Cyanosis	Methylene blue **IV:** 1–2 mg/kg as a 1% solution repeated after 4 hours.
Narcotics	Respiratory depression, constricted pupils	Narcotic antagonists: Levallorphan or Naloxone; See *Drug Entries*.
Nicotine	Respiratory stimulation; GI hyperactivity, convulsions; increased blood pressure.	Emesis or lavage; activated charcoal; atropine (**IM:** 2 mg every 3–8 minutes until atropinization occurs) or phentolamine (1–5 mg **IM or IV**)

TOXIC AGENTS AND THEIR ANTAGONISTS (*Continued*)

Agent or Toxic Reaction	Symptoms	Antagonist or Treatment
Nitrites	Cyanosis	See *Methemoglobinemia,* above.
Petroleum distillates	See Kerosene	See Kerosene
Phenothiazines	Extrapyramidal symptoms	Diphenhydramine **IV:** 1–2 mg/kg
Sleeping pills	Respiratory depression, coma	See *CNS Depressants,* above.
Strychnine	Convulsions	Short-acting barbiturates or diazepam, muscle relaxants; keep patient very quiet

GENERAL AGENTS USEFUL IN TREATING OVERDOSAGE OR POISONING

Agent	Use
Acids (vinegar, dilute tartaric acid)	To counteract all types of alkali
Alkali (lime water, milk of magnesia)	To counteract all types of acids
Apomorphine	To induce emesis
Calcium Salts	Treatment of hypocalcemic tetany
Charcoal, Activated	General adsorbant for most chemicals but not cyanide or corrosive acids or alkali
Chlorpromazine (Thorazine)	General CNS depressant
Epsom Salts	For rapid evacuation of bowel
Ipecac, Syrup of	To induce emesis
Methylene Blue	To counteract cyanosis, methemoglobinemia
Milk	General adsorbant and demulcent
Narcotic Antagonists	Narcotic overdosage
Oils (olive)	Demulcent
Potassium Permanganate	To counteract cyanosis, methemoglobinemia, phosphorus poisoning
Pralidoxime Chloride	To counteract organic phosphate insecticides
Saline Cathartics	For rapid evacuation of bowel

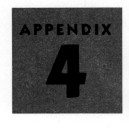

selected clinically important drug interactions (alphabetical)

SELECTED CLINICALLY IMPORTANT DRUG INTERACTIONS (ALPHA-BETICAL)

Interactants	*Interaction*
Alcohol	
Anesthetics, Antianxiety drugs, Antihistamines, Narcotics, Phenothiazines, Sedative-Hypnotics	Potentiation or addition of CNS depressant effects. Concomitant use may lead to drowsiness, lethargy, stupor, respiratory collapse, coma, or death.
Disulfiram	Acetaldehyde accumulation → mild to severe "Antabuse" reaction
Hypoglycemics, oral	Additive hypoglycemia
Tricyclic Antidepressants	See *Tricyclic Antidepressants*
Allopurinol	
Azathioprine	Allopurinol inhibits xanthine oxidase allowing toxic amounts of azathioprine metabolite, mercaptopurine, to accumulate
Aminoglycoside Antibiotics	
Ethacrynic Acid	↑ Risk of ototoxicity
Skeletal Muscle Relaxants	↑ Skeletal muscle relaxation
Amphotericin B	
Digitalis	↑ Hypokalemia → heart block and cardiac arrhythmias
Anesthetics	See *Alcohol*
Antacids	↓ Rate of absorption from GI tract of each of the drugs listed due to antacid-induced pH changes
Anticoagulants (oral), Aspirin, Nalidixic Acid, Nitrofurantoin, Pentobarbital, Phenylbutazone, Sulfonamides	

SELECTED CLINICALLY IMPORTANT DRUG INTERACTIONS (ALPHA-BETICAL) (*Continued*)

Interactants	*Interaction*
Anticholinergics, Barbiturates, Chlorpromazine, Digoxin, Isoniazid, Quinidine Tetracyclines	Antacids can adsorb the drugs listed → inhibition of absorption from GI tract
Antianxiety Agents	See *Alcohol*
Anticoagulants, Oral	
Anabolic Steroids	↑ Bleeding or hemorrhage due to ↓ synthesis of clotting factors
Antacids	See *Antacids*
Barbiturates	↓ Effect of anticoagulant due to ↑ breakdown by liver
Chloramphenicol	Potentiates pharmacological effects of anticoagulants
Clofibrate	↑ Effect of anticoagulant due to ↓ plasma protein binding
Disulfiram	↑ Effect of anticoagulant due to ↓ breakdown by liver
Glutethimide	↓ Effect of anticoagulant due to ↑ breakdown by liver
Hypoglycemics, Oral	↑ Effect of anticoagulant due to ↓ breakdown by liver
Indomethacin	↑ Effect of anticoagulant by ↓ plasma protein binding; also, indomethacin is ulcerogenic and may inhibit platelet function → hemorrhage
Nalidixic Acid	↑ Effect of anticoagulant by ↓ plasma protein binding
Oral Contraceptives	↓ Effect of anticoagulant by ↑ synthesis of certain clotting factors
Oxyphenbutazone	↑ Effect of anticoagulant by ↓ plasma protein binding; oxyphenbutazone may also produce GI ulceration → ↑ chance of bleeding
Phenylbutazone	See *Oxyphenbutazone*, above
Phenytoin	↑ Effect of phenytoin due to ↓ breakdown by liver; also, possible ↑ in anticoagulant effect by ↓ plasma protein binding
Salicylates	↑ Effect of anticoagulant by ↓ plasma protein binding, ↓ platelet aggregation, and ↓ plasma prothrombin
Sulfonamides	↑ Effect of anticoagulant by ↓ plasma protein binding
Thyroid Preparations	↑ Effect of anticoagulant by ↑ hypoprothrombinemia

(*Continued*)

SELECTED CLINICALLY IMPORTANT DRUG INTERACTIONS (ALPHABETICAL) (*Continued*)

Interactants	*Interaction*
Anticholinergics	
Antacids	See *Antacids*
Tricyclic Antidepressants	See *Tricyclic Antidepressants*
Antihistamines	See *Alcohol*
Azathioprine	See *Allopurinol*
Barbiturates	See *Alcohol*
	See *Anticoagulants, Oral*
	See *Monoamine oxidase inhibitors*
Carbamazepine	
Propoxyphene	↑ Effect of carbamazepine due to ↓ breakdown by liver
Cephalosporins	
Furosemide	↑ Risk of renal toxicity from cephalosporins
Chloramphenicol	See *Anticoagulants, Oral*
Chlorpromazine	See *Antacids*
Cholestyramine	
Anticoagulants, oral	Binds to drugs listed preventing absorption from GI tract
Digitalis glycosides	
Thiazide diuretics	
Thyroxine	
Clofibrate	See *Anticoagulants, oral*
CNS Depressants	See *Alcohol*
Colistin	
Skeletal Muscle Relaxants	↑ Skeletal muscle relaxation
Digitalis Glycosides	
Amphotericin B	See *Amphotericin B*
Antacids	See *Antacids*
Cholestyramine	See *Cholestyramine*
Ethacrynic Acid, Furosemide, Thiazide Diuretics	Drugs listed produce ↑ K and Mg loss with ↑ chance of digitalis-induced heart block or cardiac arrhythmias
Digoxin	See *Antacids*
Disulfiram	
Alcohol	Acetaldehyde accumulation → mild to severe "Antabuse" reaction
Anticoagulants, oral	See *Anticoagulants, oral*
Phenytoin	↑ Effect of phenytoin due to ↓ breakdown by liver
Ethacrynic Acid	
Aminoglycoside Antibiotics	See *Aminoglycoside Antibiotics*
Digitalis Glycosides	See *Digitalis glycosides*
Lithium	See *Lithium*

SELECTED CLINICALLY IMPORTANT DRUG INTERACTIONS (ALPHA-BETICAL) *(Continued)*

Interactants	*Interaction*
Furosemide	
Cephalosporins	See *Cephalosporins*
Digitalis Glycosides	See *Digitalis Glycosides*
Lithium	See *Lithium*
Glutethimide	See *Anticoagulants, oral*
Guanethidine	See *Tricyclic Antidepressants*
Hypoglycemics, oral	
Alcohol	Additive hypoglycemia
Anticoagulants, oral	↑ Effect of anticoagulant due to ↓ breakdown by liver
Monoamine oxidase inhibitors	MAO inhibitors ↑ and prolong hypoglycemic response
Phenylbutazone	↑ Effect of oral hypoglycemics due to ↓ breakdown by liver and ↓ plasma protein binding
Salicylates	↑ Effect of hypoglycemics due to ↓ plasma protein binding
Indomethacin	See *Anticoagulants, oral*
Insulin	
MAO Inhibitors	MAO Inhibitors ↑ and prolong hypoglycemic response to insulin
Propranolol	Propranolol inhibits the rebound of blood glucose following insulin-induced hypoglycemia
Iron Preparations	See *Tetracyclines*
Isoniazid	
Antacids	See *Antacids*
Phenytoin	↑ Effect of phenytoin due to ↓ breakdown by liver
Kaolin-Pectin	
Digoxin, Alkaloids, Lincomycin	Kaolin-pectin adsorbs drugs listed ↓ absorption from the GI tract
Levodopa	
Monoamine Oxidase Inhibitors	See *MAO Inhibitors*
Pyridoxine	Pyridoxine-induced acceleration of dopamine formation from levodopa → ↑ amount levodopa available to brain
Lincomycin	See *Kaolin-pectin*
Lithium	
Ethacrynic Acid, Furosemide, Thiazide Diuretics	↑ Lithium effect due to ↓ excretion of drugs listed by kidney
Methadone	
Rifampin	Narcotic withdrawal possibly due to ↓ plasma levels of methadone since rifampin ↑ breakdown by liver

(Continued)

SELECTED CLINICALLY IMPORTANT DRUG INTERACTIONS (ALPHA-BETICAL) (*Continued*)

Interactants	*Interaction*
Methotrexate	
Salicylates	↑ Effect of methotrexate by ↓ plasma protein binding; also, salicylates block renal excretion of methotrexate
Sulfonamides	↑ Effect of methotrexate by ↓ plasma protein binding
Methoxyflurane	See *Tetracyclines*
Monoamine Oxidase Inhibitors	
Barbiturates	↑ Effect of barbiturates due to ↓ breakdown by liver
Hypoglycemics, oral	See *Hypoglycemics, oral*
Insulin	See *Insulin*
Levodopa	↑ Storage and release of dopamine and NE → hypertension, flushing, light headedness
Narcotic Analgesics	Possible potentiation of either MAO inhibitors (excitation, muscle rigidity, hypertension) or narcotic (hypotension, coma) effects
Phenothiazines	↑ Effects of phenothiazines due to ↓ breakdown by liver; also, ↑ chance of severe extrapyramidal effects and hypertensive crisis.
Sympathomimetic Drugs (amphetamine, ephedrine, metaraminol, methoxamine, methylphenidate, phenylephrine, phenylpropanolamine)	All peripheral metabolic, cardiac, and central effects of sympathomimetic drugs are potentiated. Symptoms include acute hypertensive crisis with possible cardiac arrhythmias, intracranial hemorrhage, hyperthermia, convulsions, coma. Death may occur.
Tricyclic Antidepressants	Concomitant use may result in excitation, ↑ body temperature, delirium, tremors, convulsions
Nalidixic Acid	See *Anticoagulants, oral*
Narcotic Analgesics	
Alcohol	See *Alcohol*
MAO Inhibitors	See *MAO Inhibitors*
Oral Contraceptives	See *Anticoagulants, oral*
Oxyphenbutazone	See *Anticoagulants, oral*
Phenothiazines	
Alcohol	See *Alcohol*
MAO Inhibitors	See *MAO Inhibitors*
Phenylbutazone	
Anticoagulants, oral	↑ Effect of anticoagulant by ↓ plasma protein binding; phenylbutazone may also produce GI ulceration → ↑ chance of bleeding
MAO Inhibitors	See *MAO Inhibitors*
Phenytoin	See *Phenytoin*

SELECTED CLINICALLY IMPORTANT DRUG INTERACTIONS (ALPHA-BETICAL) (*Continued*)

Interactants	*Interaction*
Phenytoin	
Anticoagulants, oral	See *Anticoagulants, oral*
Disulfiram	See *Disulfiram*
Isoniazid	See *Isoniazid*
Phenylbutazone	↑ Effect of phenytoin due to ↓ breakdown by liver
Potassium Salts	
Spironolactone	See *Spironolactone*
Triamterene	See *Triamterene*
Probenecid	
Salicylates	Salicylates inhibit the uricosuric action of probenecid
Propoxyphene	See *Carbamazepine*
Propranolol	See *Insulin*
Pyridoxine	See *Levodopa*
Quinidine	
Antacids	See *Antacids*
Skeletal Muscle Relaxants	↑ Skeletal muscle relaxation
Rifampin	See *Methadone*
Salicylates	
Anticoagulants, oral	See *Anticoagulants, oral*
Hypoglycemics, oral	See *Hypoglycemics, oral*
Methotrexate	See *Methotrexate*
Probenecid	See *Probenecid*
Sulfinpyrazone	Salicylates inhibit the uricosuric action of sulfinpyrazone
Sedative-Hypnotics	See *Alcohol*
Skeletal Muscle Relaxants	
Aminoglycoside Antibiotics	See *Aminoglycoside Antibiotics*
Colistin	See *Colistin*
Quinidine	See *Quinidine*
Spironolactone	
Potassium Salts	Accumulation of potassium → serious hyperkalemia
Sulfinpyrazone	See *Salicylates*
Sulfonamides	
Anticoagulants, oral	See *Anticoagulants, oral*
Methotrexate	See *Methotrexate*
Sympathomimetic Drugs	
MAO Inhibitors	See *MAO Inhibitors*
Tricyclic Antidepressants	Potentiation of sympathomimetic effects → hypertension or cardiac arrhythmias

(*Continued*)

SELECTED CLINICALLY IMPORTANT DRUG INTERACTIONS (ALPHABETICAL) (*Continued*)

Interactants	Interaction
Tetracyclines	
Antacids	See *Antacids*
Iron Preparations	↓ Effect of tetracyclines due to ↓ absorption from GI tract
Methoxyflurane	↑ Risk of kidney toxicity
Thiazide Diuretics	
Cholestyramine	See *Cholestyramine*
Digitalis Glycosides	See *Digitalis Glycosides*
Lithium	See *Lithium*
Thyroid Preparations	
Anticoagulants, oral	See *Anticoagulants, oral*
Cholestyramine	See *Cholestyramine*
Triamterene	
Potassium Salts	Accumulation of potassium → serious hyperkalemia
Tricyclic Antidepressants	
Alcohol	↑ Risk of impaired performance
Anticholinergics	Additive anticholinergic side effects
Guanethidine	Tricyclics ↓ effect of guanethidine by preventing uptake to its site of action
Monoamine Oxidase Inhibitors	See *MAO Inhibitors*
Sympathomimetics	See *Sympathomimetics*

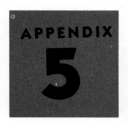

APPENDIX 5

effects of drugs on laboratory test values

See table on page 813.

EFFECTS OF DRUGS ON LABORATORY TEST VALUES*

	Hepato-toxicity	Ne-phro-tox-icity	In-test. Malabs.	Cre-ati-nine	BUN	Uric Acid	Bili-rubin	SGOT/ SGPT	Serum Glu-cose	Cho-les-terol	Pro-throm-bin time	Urine Color	Urine Glu-cose	Comments
Acetazolamide						I								
Acetohexamide (sulfonylurea)	X			I										
ACTH						D			I					
Allopurinol	X					D								
Aminosalicylic acid (PAS)	X	X											+	
Amphotericin B	X	X												
Ampicillin		X												
Anabolic steroids and androgens	X													
Antihistamines											D			
Antimony compounds	X	X												
Arsenicals	X	X												
Ascorbic acid				I		I	I	I	I				+	
Caffeine		X					D		I					
Cephaloridine		X											+	
Cephalothin													+	
Chloral hydrate					I						D		+	
Chloramphenicol (Chloromycetin)	X				X								+	* Direction depends on method
Chlordiazepoxide (Librium)	X													
Chlorpromazine (Thorazine)	X					D			I					
Chlorpropamide (Diabenese)	X													May cause + pregnancy test

See footnote on p. 816.

(Continued)

813

EFFECTS OF DRUGS ON LABORATORY TEST VALUES*

	Hepato-toxicity	Ne-phro-tox-icity	In-test. Malabs.	Cre-ati-nine	BUN	Uric Acid	Bili-rubin	SGOT/SGPT	Serum Glu-cose	Cho-les-terol	Pro-throm-bin time	Urine Color	Urine Glu-cose	Comments
Chlorprothixene (Taractan)	X					D								
Chlorthalidone (Hygroton)		X							I		I			
Cholinergics							I	I						I – BSP. Changes due to spasm, sphincter of Oddi
Clofibrate (Atromid-S)	X					D				D	I			D – triglycerides, total lipids, LDH
Codeine							I	I						
Colchicine	X		X								D			On coumarins
Colistin		X												
Corticosteroids						D			I	I			+	
Coumarins	X					D					I			
Cyclophosphamide	X													
Dextran					I	I	I		I					
D-Thyroxine									I	D	I			
Erythromycin	X							I				•		• Colorimetric method
Estrogens	X								I	D			+	
Ethacrynic acid (Edecrin)	X	X				I			I		I		+	
Furosemide (Lasix)					I	I			I					
Gentamicin	X	X												
Gold	X	X												
Griseofulvin	X	X												
Guanethidine analogs					I				I	D	I			

Drug							Remarks
Heparin						I	
Hydralazine	X						
Imipramine (Tofranil)	X			I	I	I	+
Indomethacin (Indocin)	X					I	I X
Isoniazid	X	X			I		+
Kanamycin	X	X	X			I	
Levodopa	X			I			X +
Lincomycin	X						
MAO inhibitors	X		X				
Meperidine (Demerol)				I	I		
Methicillin	X	X					
Methotrexate	X			I*			In gout
Methyldopa (Aldomet)	X		I	I		I	X +
Nalidixic acid (Neg Gram)	X	*			I**		+ *Nitrogen retention **Copper reduction method
Neomycin	X	X					
Nicotonic acid (large doses)	X			I			+
Nitrofurantoin (Furadantin)	X	X					X
Novobiocin	X						
Oleandomycin	X						
Oral contraceptives	X					D	
Oxacillin	X	X					
Penicillin							+* *Large doses. PSP-D with massive doses
Phenobarbital						D	
Phenylbutazone (Butazolidin)	X					I	

Alters turbidity tests (e.g., thymol) and lipoprotein electrophoresis pattern. May interfere with BSP and calcium.

See footnote on p. 816.

(Continued)

815

EFFECTS OF DRUGS ON LABORATORY TEST VALUES* (Continued)

	Hepatotoxicity	Nephrotoxicity	Intest. Malabs.	Creatinine	BUN	Uric Acid	Bilirubin	SGOT/ SGPT	Serum Glucose	Cholesterol	Prothrombin time	Urine Color	Urine Glucose	Comments
Polymyxin B		X												
Phenytoin sodium (Dilantin)	X		X						I			X		
Probenecid (Benemid)	X	X				D							+	
Procainamide	X													
Propylthiouracil	X					I					I			
Quinacrine	X											X		
Quinine, quinidine											I	X		
Radiopaque contrast media		X				D	X						+	I – BSP and protein. Serum protein electrophoresis pattern cannot be interpreted
Reserpine									I					
Rifampin	X	X										X		
Salicylates	X	X				I*							+	*High doses decrease uric acid
Streptomycin		X			D								+	
Sulfonamides	X	X			I							X	+	
Tetracyclines	X	X											+	
Theophylline						I	I							I – ESR
Thiazides	X					I			I				+	D – PSP and creatinine tolerance
Thiothixene	X													
Tolbutamide (Orinase)	X							I						
Vitamin A							I			I				
Vitamin D		*								I				*With hypervitaminosis D
Vitamin K									D					

* Chart includes both toxic reactions and methodological interference. Tests cited are incomplete. Hepatotoxicity refers to liver damage which can be reflected in the alteration of one or more tests including alkaline phosphatase, bilirubin, transaminases, cephalin flocculation, thymol turbidity, BSP retention. Nephrotoxicity refers to renal damage causing changes in BUN, creatinine, presence of urine protein casts or cells. X refers to change in laboratory tests, + refers to positive, including false positives, I refers to increase and D to decrease.

Source: Table adapted with permission from Interpretation of Diagnostic Tests, (Little Brown & Co.) by Jacques Wallach.

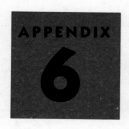

APPENDIX

6 commonly prescribed combination drugs

See table on page 818.

COMMONLY PRESCRIBED COMBINATION DRUGS

Trade Name	Generic Name(s)	Amount (mg)	Pharmacological Classification	Use	Dose/Other Information	Location in Text (p)
Actified (Syrup, Tablets)	Pseudoephedrine HCl Triprolidine HCl	1.25–2.5 30–60	Sympathomimetic Antihistamine	Upper Respiratory Problems	**Adults and children over 12 years:** 1 tablet or 10 ml syrup t.i.d.–q.i.d.; **pediatric:** 1.25–5 ml syrup t.i.d.–q.i.d.	482 687
Actifed-C Expectorant	Pseudoephedrine HCl Triprolidine HCl Codeine Phosphate Guaifenesin	30 2 10 100	Sympathomimetic Antihistamine Narcotic antitussive Expectorant	Antitussive/Expectorant	**Adults and children over 12 years:** 10 ml q.i.d.; **7–12 years:** 5 ml q.i.d.; **2–6 years:** 2.5 ml q.i.d.	482 687 357 714
Aldactazide	Spironolactone Hydrochlorothiazide	25 25	Diuretic Diuretic	Diuretic/Antihypertensive	**Adults:** 2–4 tablets/day.	651 636
Aldoril	Hydrochlorothiazide Methyl-DOPA	15–50 250–500	Diuretic Antihypertensive	Antihypertensive	**Adults:** 1 tablet b.i.d.–t.i.d. for 48 hrs; **then,** adjust dose to desired response.	636 268
Azo-Gantrisin	Sulfisoxazole Phenazopyridine HCl	500 50	Sulfonamide Urinary antiseptic	Urinary Antiinfective	**Adults:** 4–6 tablets initially; **then,** 2 q.i.d. for up to 3 days.	119 *
Bactrim (Oral Suspension, Tablets) Bactrim DS (Double Strength) contains 160 mg Trimethoprim and 800 mg Sulfamethoxazole	Trimethoprim Sulfamethoxazole	40–80 200–400	Anti-infective Sulfonamide	Anti-infective	*Urinary tract infections, shigellosis, acute otitis media:* 2 tablets q 12 hr for 14 days. *Pneumocytitis carinii pneumonitis,* **adults:** 20 mg/kg trimethoprim and 100 mg/kg sulfamethoxazole/day in divided doses for 14 days.	118 *
Bendectin	Doxylamine succinate Pyridoxine HCl	10 10	Antihistamine Vitamin	Antiemetic	2 tablets at bedtime; *severe nausea:* 1 additional tablet in AM and PM	686 699
Butazolidine Alka	Phenylbutazone Dried Aluminum Hydroxide Gel Magnesium Trisilicate	100 100 150	Anti-inflammatory Antacid Antacid	Antirheumatic/Anti-inflammatory	**Initial, adults:** 300–600 mg/day in divided doses. **Maintenance:** not to exceed 400 mg/day.	426 718 723
Chlor-Trimeton Tablets	Chlorpheniramine Maleate Pseudoephedrine Sulfate	4 60	Antihistamine Decongestant	Upper Respiratory Tract Problems	**Adults:** 1 tablet q 4 hr not to exceed 6 tabs/day; **children 6 to 11 yrs:** ½ tab q 4 hr not to exceed 3 whole tabs/day; **2 to 5 years:** ¼ tab q 4 hr not to exceed 1½ tabs/day.	684 482

Product	Ingredient	Amount	Classification	Use	Directions	
Chlor-Trimeton Expectorant	Chlorpheniramine Maleate	2	Antihistamine	Upper Respiratory Tract Problems	**Adults:** 5 ml q.i.d.; **children, 6 to 12 years:** 2.5 ml q.i.d.	684
	Phenylephrine HCl	10	Decongestant			487
	Ammonium Chloride	100	Expectorant			*
	Sodium Citrate	50	Expectorant			*
	Guaifenesin	50	Expectorant			714
Combid	Isopropamide Iodide	5	Anticholinergic	GI problems	*Sustained release*, **adults and children over 12 years:** 1 capsule b.i.d.	514
	Prochlorperazine Maleate	10	Antiemetic/sedative			377
Darvocet-N	Acetaminophen	325–650	Non-narcotic analgesic	Analgesic	1 tablet q 4 hr	415
	Propoxyphene Napsylate	50–100	Analgesic			418
Darvon Compound-65	Aspirin	227	Non-narcotic analgesic	Analgesic	1 capsule q 4 hr. This is a C–IV Scheduled drug.	410
	Propoxyphene HCl	65	Analgesic			418
	Caffeine	32	Stimulant			399
	Phenacetin	162	Non-narcotic analgesic			415
Dimetane Expectorant	Brompheniramine Maleate	2	Antihistamine	Expectorant/Decongestant	**Adult:** 5–10 ml q.i.d.; **children:** 2.5–5 ml t.i.d.–q.i.d.	684
	Guaifenesin	100	Expectorant			714
	Phenylephrine HCl	5	Decongestant			487
	Phenylpropanolamine HCl	5	Decongestant			481
Dimetane Expectorant DC	Brompheniramine Maleate	2	Antihistamine	Antitussive/Decongestant/Expectorant	**Adult:** 5–10 ml q.i.d.; **children:** 2.5–5 ml t.i.d.–q.i.d.	684
	Codeine phosphate	10	Narcotic antitussive			357
	Guaifenesin	100	Expectorant			714
	Phenylephrine HCl	5	Decongestant			487
	Phenylpropanolamine HCl	5	Decongestant			481
Dimetapp Tablets	Brompheniramine maleate	12	Antihistamine	Decongestant	**Adult:** 1 tablet b.i.d. *Elixir*, **adults:** 5–10 ml t.i.d.–q.i.d.; **children 4 to 12 years:** 5 ml; **2 to 4 years:** 3.75 ml; **7 months to 2 years:** 2.5 ml; **1 to 6 months:** 1.25 ml. Pediatric dose given t.i.d.–q.i.d.	684
	Phenylephrine HCl	15	Decongestant			487
	Phenylpropanolamine HCl	15	Decongestant			481

Elixir contains ⅓ amount of tablet/5 ml.

Product	Ingredient	Amount	Classification	Use	Directions	
Diupres	Chlorothiazide	250–500	Diuretic	Antihypertensive	1–2 tablets 1 to 2 times/day. Not indicated for initial therapy.	635
	Reserpine	0.125	Antihypertensive			258
Donnatal (Capsules, Tablets, Elixir)	Atropine Sulfate	0.0194	Anticholinergic	GI problems	*Tablets, Capsules:* **adult:** 1–2 t.i.d.–q.i.d. *Elixir:* 5–10 ml t.i.d.–q.i.d., **pediatric:** Give elixir. Dose depends on weight.	510
	Hyoscine HBr	0.0065	Anticholinergic			516
	Hyoscyamine HBr	0.1037	Anticholinergic			513
	Phenobarbital	16	Sedative			306

(See footnote on p. 823)

(Continued)

COMMONLY PRESCRIBED COMBINATION DRUGS

Trade Name	Generic Name(s)	Amount (mg)	Pharmacological Classification	Use	Dose/Other Information	Location in Text (p)
Drixoral	Dexbrompheniramine maleate	6	Antihistamine	Upper Respiratory Problems	1 tablet b.i.d.	
	Pseudoephedrine SO$_4$	120	Decongestant			482
Dyazide	Hydrochlorothiazide	25	Diuretic	Diuretic/ Antihypertensive	1 to 2 capsules b.i.d.	636
	Triamterene	50	Diuretic			653
Empirin compound with Codeine	Aspirin	227	Non-narcotic analgesic	Analgesic	*Usual*, **adult:** 1–2 tablets q 4 hr. Depends on severity of pain. This is a C-III Scheduled drug.	410
No. 1, 7.5 mg*	Caffeine	32	Stimulant			399
No. 2, 15 mg*	Codeine phosphate	7.5–60	Narcotic analgesic			357
No. 3, 30 mg*	Phenacetin	162	Non-narcotic analgesic			415
No. 4, 60 mg*						
* Codeine phosphate						
Equagesic	Aspirin	250	Non-narcotic analgesic	Analgesic	1–2 tablets t.i.d.–q.i.d. **Not recommended for children 12 years and younger.**	410
	Ethoheptazine citrate	75	Non-narcotic analgesic			416
	Meprobamate	150	Anti-anxiety agent			326
Fiorinal (Capsules, Tablets)	Aspirin	200	Non-narcotic analgesic	Analgesic	1–2 tablets or capsules q 4 hr. Daily dose should not exceed 6 tablets or capsules	410
	Butalbital	50	Sedative Barbiturate			304
	Caffeine	40	Stimulant			399
	Phenacetin	130	Non-narcotic analgesic			415
Fiorinal/ Codeine	Aspirin	200	Non-narcotic analgesic	Analgesic	1–2 capsules up to 6 capsules/day as required. This is a C-III Scheduled drug.	410
No. 1, 7.5 mg*	Butalbital	50	Sedative Barbiturate			304
No. 2, 15 mg*	Caffeine	40	Stimulant			399
No. 3, 30 mg*	Codeine phosphate	7.5–30	Narcotic analgesic			357
	Phenacetin	130	Non-narcotic analgesic			415
* Codeine phosphate						
Hydropres	Hydrochlorothiazide	25–50	Diuretic	Antihypertensive	1 tablet 1 to 4 times/day	636
	Reserpine	0.125	Antihypertensive			258

Librax	Chlordiazepoxide HCl	5	Anti-anxiety agent	GI problems	Usual: 1-2 capsules t.i.d.-q.i.d. before meals and at bedtime	324
	Clidinium Bromide	2.5	Anticholinergic			511
Lomotil (Liquid, Tablets)	Diphenoxylate HCl	2.5	Narcotic antidiarrheal	Antidiarrheal	**Adult:** 5 mg diphenoxylate q.i.d.; **children 2 to 12 years:** 0.3-0.4 mg/kg/day in divided doses. Use liquid only. Do not use in children under 2 years.	740
	Atropine sulfate	0.025	Anticholinergic			510
Marax	Ephedrine Sulfate	25	Sympathomimetic	Antiasthmatic	**Adult:** 1 tablet b.i.d.-q.i.d.	470
	Hydroxyzine HCl	10	Anti-anxiety agent			328
	Theophylline	130	Sympathomimetic			486
Naldecon (Syrup, Tablet, Pediatric)	Chlorpheniramine Maleate	1.66-5	Antihistamine	Upper Respiratory Tract Problems	**Adult:** 1 tablet t.i.d.; *Syrup;* 5 ml q 3-4 hr; **pediatric:** 2.5-10 ml q 3 to 4 hr.	684
	Phenylephrine HCl	1.25-10	Decongestant			487
	Phenylpropanolamine HCl	5-40	Decongestant			487
	Phenyltoloxamine Citrate	2-15	Antihistamine			*
Norgesic & Norgesic Forte	Aspirin	225-450	Non-narcotic analgesic	Skeletal Muscle Relaxant	**Adult:** 1-2 Norgesic tabs t.i.d.-q.i.d. *Forte:* ½-1 tab t.i.d.-q.i.d.	410
	Caffeine	30-60	Stimulant			399
	Phenacetin	160-320	Non-narcotic analgesic			415
	Orphenadrine Citrate	25-50	Skeletal muscle relaxant			443
Ornade	Chlorpheniramine	8	Antihistamine	Upper Respiratory tract Problems	Sustained release. **Adults and children over 6 years:** 1 capsule b.i.d. **Not indicated in children less than 6 years.**	684
	Isopropamide Iodide	2.5	Anticholinergic			514
	Phenylpropanolamine	50	Decongestant			481
Parafon Forte	Acetaminophen	300	Non-narcotic analgesic	Skeletal Muscle Relaxant	2 tablets q.i.d.	415
	Chlorzoxazone	250	Skeletal muscle relaxant			332
Phenaphen/ Codeine No. 2, 15 mg* No. 3, 30 mg* No. 4, 60 mg*	Acetaminophen	325	Non-narcotic analgesic	Analgesic	Adjust dose for severity of pain and response of patient. *Usual:* **No. 2 or No. 3:** 1-2 capsules q 4 hr. **No. 4:** 1 cap. q 4 hr. This is a C-III Scheduled drug.	415
	Codeine Phosphate	15-60	Narcotic analgesic			357
*Codeine Phosphate						
Phenergan Expectorant Plain	Citric Acid	60	Expectorant	Expectorant	**Adult:** 5 ml q 4 to 6 hr.	*
	Pot. Guaiacolsulfonate	44	Expectorant			*
	Promethazine HCl	5	Antihistamine			686
	Sodium Citrate	197	Expectorant			*

(See footnote on p. 823)

(Continued)

COMMONLY PRESCRIBED COMBINATION DRUGS

Trade Name	Generic Name(s)	Amount (mg)	Pharmacological Classification	Use	Dose/Other Information	Location in Text (p)
Phenergan Expectorant/Codeine	Citric Acid Codeine Phosphate Pot. Guaiacolsulfonate Promethazine HCl Sodium Citrate	60 10 44 5 197	Expectorant Narcotic antitussive Expectorant Antihistamine Expectorant	Antitussive/ Expectorant	**Adult:** 5 ml q 4 to 6 hr. This is a C-V Scheduled drug.	* 357 * 686 *
Phenergan VC Expectorant Plain	Citric Acid Phenylephrine HCl Pot. Guaiacolsulfonate Promethazine HCl Sodium Citrate	60 5 44 5 197	Expectorant Decongestant Expectorant Antihistamine Expectorant	Expectorant/ Decongestant	**Adult:** 5 ml q 4 to 6 hr.	* 487 * 686 *
Phenergan VC Expectorant/Codeine	Citric Acid Codeine Phosphate Phenylephrine HCl Pot. Guaiacolsulfonate Promethazine HCl Sodium Citrate	60 10 5 44 5 197	Expectorant Narcotic antitussive Decongestant Expectorant Antihistamine Expectorant	Antitussive/ Expectorant/ Decongestant	**Adult:** 5 ml q 4 to 6 hr. This is a C-V Scheduled drug.	* 357 487 * 686 *
Quibron (Capsules, Elixir)	Guaifenesin Theophylline	90–180 150–300	Expectorant Sympathomimetic	Anti-asthmatic	1–2 capsules q 6 to 8 hr. *Elixir:* 15–30 ml q 6 hr.	714 328
Regroton	Chlorthalidone Reserpine	50 0.25	Diuretic Antihypertensive	Antihypertensive	*Usual:* 1 tab/day in AM with food.	635 258
Salutensin	Hydroflumethiazide Reserpine	50 0.25	Diuretic Antihypertensive	Antihypertensive	*Individualized, usual* **adult:** 1 tablet 1 to 2 times/day.	* 258
Ser-Ap-Es	Hydralazine HCl Hydrochlorothiazide Reserpine	25 15 0.1	Antihypertensive Diuretic Antihypertensive	Antihypertensive	*Individualized, usual,* **adult:** 1–2 tablets t.i.d..	274 636 258

Product	Ingredient	Amount (mg)	Action	Class	Dosage	Page
Synalogos-DC	Aspirin	194	Non-narcotic analgesic	Analgesic	Dose individualized according to severity of pain and response of patient. *Usual,* **adult:** 2 caps q 4 hr. This is a C-III Scheduled drug.	410
	Caffeine	30	Stimulant			399*
	Dihydrocodeine Bitartrate	16	Narcotic analgesic			
	Promethazine HCl	6.25	Antihistamine			686
	Phenacetin	162	Non-narcotic analgesic			415
Tedral *Tablets*	Ephedrine HCl	24	Sympathomimetic	Anti-Asthmatic	**Adults:** 1–2 tabs q 4 hr; **children over 60 pounds:** ½ adult dose.	470
	Phenobarbital	8	Sedative			306
	Theophylline	130	Sympathomimetic			486

Elixir: 5 ml. is equivalent to one-quarter Tedral Tablet

Adults: 15–30 ml q 4 hr; **children:** 5 ml/30 lb body weight q 4 to 6 hr.

Suspension: 5 ml. is equivalent to one-half Tedral Tablet

Adults: 10–20 ml q 4 hr.; **children:** 5 ml/60 lb body wt. q 4 to 6 hr.

Expectorant: 1 tab is equivalent to 1 Tedral Tablet plus 100 mg guaifenesin

Adults: 1–2 tablets q.i.d. Not recommended for children under 12 years.

Product	Ingredient	Amount (mg)	Action	Class	Dosage	Page
Triavil	Amitriptyline HCl	10–50	Antidepressant	Psychotherapeutic	*Initial,* 2–8 mg perphenazine and 25–50 mg amitriptyline t.i.d.–q.i.d. Then adjust dose to response.	390
	Perphenazine	2–4	Antipsychotic			376
Tuss-Ornade (Liquid, Capsules)	Caramiphen edisylate	5–20	Antitussive	Antitussive/Decongestant	**Adult:** *liquid.* 5–10 ml t.i.d.–q.i.d.; **children over 25 pounds:** 5 ml t.i.d.–q.i.d.; **15–25 pounds,** 2.5 ml t.i.d.–q.i.d. *Sustained release capsule:* 1 q 12 hr. (Age 12 years and older only)	*
	Chlorpheniramine Maleate	2–8	Antihistamine			684
	Isopropamide Iodide	0.75–2.5	Anticholinergic			514
	Phenylpropanolamine HCl	15–50	Decongestant			481
Tylenol/Codeine Tabs No. 1, 7.5 mg*; No. 2, 15 mg*; No. 3, 30 mg*; No. 4, 60 mg*	Acetaminophen	300	Non-narcotic analgesic	Analgesic	**Adults: Tablets, no. 1, no. 2, no. 3:** 1–2 q 4 hr; **No. 4:** 1 q 4 hr. *Elixir,* **adults:** 15 ml q 4 hr; **pediatric 7 to 12 years:** 10 ml t.i.d.–q.i.d.; **3 to 6 years:** 5 ml t.i.d.–q.i.d.	415
	Codeine Phosphate	7.5–60	Narcotic analgesic			357

*Codeine Phosphate

The Elixir contains 12 mg codeine phosphate and 120 mg acetaminophen/5 ml.

* Available only in combination products.

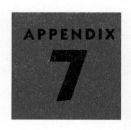

federal controlled substances act

Federal Controlled Substances Act

The Federal Controlled Substances Act of 1970 placed drugs controlled by the Act into five categories or schedules.

Schedule I
Includes substances for which there is a high abuse potential and no current approved medical use. Substances in this category include heroin, marihuana, LSD, peyote, mescaline, psilocybin, tetrahydrocannabinols, certain opiates, opium derivatives, and hallucinogens.

Schedule II
Includes drugs which have a high abuse potential, high ability to produce physical and/or psychological dependence, and a current approved or acceptable medical use. Drugs in this category include narcotics, such as morphine, codeine, hydromorphone, methadone, meperidine, oxycodone, anileridine, and oxymorphine; stimulants, such as cocaine, amphetamine, methylphenidate, and phenmetrazine; depressants, such as amobarbital, pentobarbital, and secobarbital, and methaqualone; and, phencyclidine.

Schedule III
Includes drugs for which there is less potential for abuse than drugs in Schedule II and for which there is a current approved medical use. Certain drugs in this category are preparations containing limited quantities of codeine, such as Empirin Compound with Codeine, Tylenol with Codeine, and Phenaphen with Codeine. Other drugs include depressants, such as the barbiturates not listed in other schedules, glutethimide, methyprylon, and other sedative-hypnotics; stimulants, such as benzphetamine, chlorphentermine, clortermine, mazindol, and phendimetrazine; and, the narcotic Paregoric.

Schedule IV
Includes drugs for which there is a relatively low abuse potential and for which there is a current approved medical use. Drugs in this category include depressants, such as chloral hydrate, ethchlorvynol, ethinimate, meprobamate, methohexital, chlordiazepoxide, diazepam, oxazepam, chlorazepate, flurazepam, clonazepam, prazepam, loraze-

pam, and mebutamate; stimulants, such as fenfluramine, diethylpropion, and phentermine; and, dextropropoxyphene.

Schedule V
Drugs in this category consist mainly of preparations containing limited amounts of certain narcotic drugs for use as antitussives and
antidiarrheals.

medic alert system

WHO NEEDS MEDIC ALERT? Persons with any medical problem or condition that cannot be easily seen or recognized need the protection of Medic Alert. Heart conditions, diabetes, severe allergies and epilepsy are common problems. Others are listed on the application form under this page. About one in every five persons has some special medical problem.

WHY MEDIC ALERT? Tragic or even fatal mistakes can be made in emergency medical treatment unless the special problem of the person is known. A diabetic could be neglected and die because he was thought to be intoxicated. A shot of penicillin could end the life of one who is allergic to it. Persons dependent on medications must continue to receive them at all times.

WHEN IS MEDIC ALERT IMPORTANT? Whenever a person cannot speak for himself — because of unconsciousness, shock, delirium, hysteria, loss of speech, etc. — the Medic Alert emblem speaks for him.

HOW DOES MEDIC ALERT WORK? The Medic Alert emblem —worn on the wrist or neck — is recognized the world over. On the back of the emblem is engraved the medical problem and the file number of the wearer, and the telephone number of Medic Alert's Central File. Doctors, police, or anyone giving aid can immediately get vital information — addresses of the personal physician and nearest relative, etc. — via collect telephone call (24 hours a day) to the Central File.

WHAT IS MEDIC ALERT? It is a charitable, nonprofit organization. Its services are maintained by a one-time-only membership fee and by voluntary contributions from friends, corporations and foundations. Additional services such as replacement of lost emblems and up-dating of records are charged to members at cost. Membership is tax deductible as a medical expense, and contributions are always deductible on income tax returns.

WHERE IS MEDIC ALERT? Medic Alert Foundation International was founded in Turlock, California in 1956, after a doctor's daughter almost died from reaction to a sensitivity test for tetanus antitoxin. The Foundation is endorsed by over 100 organizations including the American Academy of General Practice (and many more national and state medical organizations) the International Associations of Fire Chiefs, Police Chiefs, the National Sheriffs' Association, and the National Association of Life Underwriters.

For further information, write to:

Medic Alert Foundation International
Turlock, CA 95380
Phone (209) 632-2371.

John D. McPherson, President

Produced internally by Medic Alert Foundation

MEDIC ALERT EMBLEMS ARE SHOWN IN ACTUAL SIZE

BRACELETS:

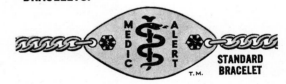

STANDARD BRACELET
T.M.

SMALL BRACELET
T.M. (Children's and Ladies')

DISC:

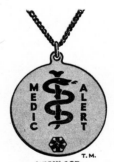

NECKLACE
With 26" Chain

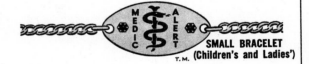

Phone (209) 634-4917
Allergic To PENICILLIN
101546

EXAMPLE OF REVERSE SIDE
OF MEDIC ALERT
EMBLEM

ALL MEMBERSHIP FEES AND DONATIONS ARE TAX-DEDUCTIBLE

glossary

ACHLORHYDRIA	Absence of hydrochloric acid in the stomach
ACROCYANOSIS	Symmetrical cyanosis (blueness) of extremities
ACROPARESTHESIA	Tingling and numbness of the extremities
ADAMS-STOKES SYNDROME	Condition caused by heart block characterized by sudden attacks of unconsciousness
ADDISON'S DISEASE	Condition caused by insufficiency or deficiency of adrenal glands
ADH	Vasopression
ADRENERGIC	Acting like epinephrine, pertaining to the sympathetic portion of the autonomic nervous system
AGRANULOCYTOSIS	Acute febrile disease characterized by high fever, ulceration of mucous membranes, and a reduction in the number of granular leukocytes
AKATHISIA	Extreme restlessness, mental turbulence, increased motor activity
AKINESIA	Impaired or absence of motor function
ALOPECIA	Hair loss
AMBLYOPIA	Dimness of vision
AMYLOIDOSIS	Deposition of complex protein material in various organs and tissues of the body
ANABOLISM	Building up of body tissues
ANALEPETIC	Drug acting as stimulant of CNS especially respiration and wakefulness

ANAPHYLACTOID REACTION	Shock; unusual or exaggerated reaction to drug protein or other foreign substance
ANDROGENIC	Producing masculine characteristics
ANGINA, ANGINAL	Any disease marked by attacks of choking as suffocation. Spasmotic, cramplike pain
ANGIO	Pertaining to blood vessel
ANGIONEUROTIC EDEMA	Large hives often accompanied by itching, fever, nausea, and general malaise
ANOXIA	Lack of oxygen
ANTABUSE REACTION	Interaction of two agents—one of which is often alcohol—resulting in fall in BP, palpitations, rapid pulse, dizziness, anorexia, nausea and vomiting. Also called *Disulfiram Reaction*
ANTINUCLEAR ANTIBODY TEST (ANA)	Test indicating the presence of antibodies to DNA that are characteristic of some auto-immune diseases. A positive test can be drug-induced
APHASIA	Loss or impairment of speech
APLASTIC ANEMIA	Anemia due to impairment of the bone marrow
APNEA	To be without breath
ARTHRALGIA	Joint pain
ASCITES	Accumulation of fluid in peritoneal cavity
ASTHENIA	Weakness, loss of strength
ASYSTOLE	Faulty or imperfect contraction of the ventricles of the heart
ATAXIA	Impairment of muscle coordination
ATONIC	Lack of normal tone, especially of muscles
ATOPIC	Atypical, out of place
AZOTEMIA	Presence of urea or nitrogen in blood
BACTERIOSTATIC	Prevention of multiplication (reproduction) or growth of bacteria
BACTERICIDAL	Killing of bacteria

BALANITIS	Inflammation of the glans penis
BIGEMINAL PULSE	Characterized by paired heart beats in close proximity with longer intervals between pairs
BIOAVAILABILITY	Amount of a drug that is physiologically available to the patient
BLEPHARITIS	Inflammation of the eyelids
BONE RESORPTION	Loss of bone through physiological or pathological means
BRADYCARDIA	Slowness of the heart (less than 60 beats per minute)
BRUIT	Heart sound or murmur usually abnormal
BUERGER'S DISEASE	(Thromboangiitis obliterans) inflammation of the blood vessels of the extremities, especially the legs, often resulting in gangrene
BURSITIS	Inflammation of a bursa
CACHEXIA	Weakness and emaciation usually caused by disease
CARDIOSPASM	Spasm of cardiac sphincter of stomach
CATABOLISM	Breaking down by the body of complex compounds
CATATONIA	Phase of schizophrenia during which a patient is unresponsive
CELLULITIS	Diffuse inflammation of connective tissue
CERVICOTHORACIC	Pertaining to neck and thorax
CHEILITIS	Inflammation of the lips
CHEILOSIS	Disorder of the lips due to avitaminosis
CHLOASMA	Deposit of pigment in the skin
CHOLANGITIS	Inflammation of the biliary ducts
CHOLECYSTITIS	Inflammation of the gallbladder
CHOLECYSTOGRAPHY	X-ray of the gallbladder after it has been visualized by administration of a radiopaque substance
CHOLINERGIC	Acting like acetylcholine, pertaining to the parasympathetic portion of the autonomic nervous system
CHOREIFORM	Jerky, ticlike twitching of face and body

CHOROIDITIS	Inflammation of the middle "coat" (choroid) of the eye
CLAUDICATION	Lameness. Loss of function temporarily due to spasm
COARCTATION	A stricture. Compression of the walls of a vessel or canal, narrowing or closing the lumen
COLITIS	Inflammation of the colon
COLOSTOMY	Formation of an artificial opening in the abdominal wall for evacuation of feces
CONJUNCTIVITIS	Inflammation of the conjunctiva of the eye
CRETINISM	Inborn deficiency of thyroid gland resulting in arrested physical and mental development
CRYSTALLURIA	Formation of crystals in urine producing irritation of kidneys
CURARIFORM	Producing muscle paralysis like the poison curare
CUSHINOID	Resembling characteristics of Cushing's Disease, i.e. obesity of face, neck, and trunk, decreased sexual activity, hairiness, abdominal pain, weakness
CYCLOPLEGIA	Paralysis of the ciliary muscles of the eye
CYLINDURIA	The presence of casts in the urine
CYSTITIS	Inflammation of bladder
CYTOTOXIC	Poisonous to cells
DELIRIUM TREMENS	Form of alcoholic psychosis characterized by trembling, hallucinations, excitement, anxiety, exhaustion
DIAPHORESIS	Heavy perspiration
DIATHESIS	A state or condition in an individual causing susceptibility to a particular disease
DIPLOPIA	Double vision
DISULFIRAM REACTION	See *Antabuse Reaction*
DIVERTICULITIS	Inflammation of a diverticulum (a small pouch or sac in lining or wall of intestine)

DNA	Short for deoxyribonucleic acid. The nucleic acid "blueprint" essential for transmittal of genetic information and protein synthesis
DYSARTHRIA	Impairment of articulation; stammering
DYSCRASIA	Abnormal state of body—usually means abnormal condition of blood elements or constituents for clotting
DYSKINESIA	Impairment of voluntary muscle movement, spasms
DYSPEPSIA	Disturbed digestion
DYSPHAGIA	Difficulty or inability to swallow
DYSPHORIA	Impatience, restlessness, mental anxiety
DYSPNEA	Difficult or labored breathing
DYSTONIA	Involuntary movements
DYSURIA	Difficult or painful urination
EATON-LAMBERT SYNDROME	Muscle weakness (Myasthenic) syndrome, often involving a single nerve
ECCHYMOSIS	Escape of blood under skin producing a large blotchy area of superficial discoloration
ECLAMPSIA	Complication of pregnancy manifested by increase in blood pressure, edema, proteinuria, convulsions, or coma
ECTOPIC	At a site other than normal. For example, a cardiac rhythm originating outside the sinoatrial node.
ECTOPIC PREGNANCY	Embryo implanted outside the uterus
ELIXIR	Sweetened, aromatic solution, usually hydroalcoholic, containing medication
EMESIS	Vomiting
EMULSION	A product consisting of minute globules of one liquid dispersed throughout the body of a second liquid
ENCEPHALITIS	Inflammation of the brain
ENTERITIS	Acute or chronic inflammation of the intestine

ENURESIS	Incontinence of urine
EOSINOPHILIA	Increase in the normal number of circulating eosinophils
EPIPHYSEAL JUNCTION	Junction between long bones
EPISTAXIS	Bleeding from the nose
ERUCTATION	Belching
ERYTHEMA	Any redness (rash) of skin
ERYTHEMA MULTIFORME	A skin rash characterized by dark red papules, vesicles and bullae usually on the extremities
EXACERBATION	Increase in severity
EXANTHEMA	An eruption on the skin
EXTRAPYRAMIDAL	Outside of the pyramidal tracts of the CNS—usually results in excess stimulation
EXFOLIATIVE DERMATITIS	Itchy, scaling, and flaking of skin frequently accompanied by loss of hair and nails
EXTRAVASATION	Also called infiltration: leakage of fluid into surrounding tissue; may occur during IV administration of drugs
FIBROSIS	Growth of white fibrous connective tissue in excess of that normally present in the tissue
FIBROSITIS	Inflammation of the white fibrous tissue
FURUNCULOSIS	Presence of numerous boils
GASTRITIS	Acute or chronic inflammation of the stomach
GILLES DE LA TOURETTE'S DISEASE	Special form of motor incoordination characterized by patient uttering repetitive sounds and obscene words
GLAUCOMA	Group of diseases characterized by increased intraocular pressure
GLOSSITIS	Inflammation of the tongue
GLYCOSURIA	The presence of glucose in urine
GYNECOMASTIA	Enlargement of the mammary gland in the male
HEMATEMESIS	Vomiting of blood
HEMATOPOIETIC	Pertaining to formation and development of blood cells

HEMATOMA	Extravasation of blood that forms a solid mass and appears as a visible swelling or bruise
HEMOCHROMATOSIS	Excess deposition of iron in tissues
HEMOGLOBINEMIA	Abnormal presence of hemoglobin in the serum
HEMOGLOBINURIA	Presence of hemoglobin in urine
HEMOLYTIC	Causing hemolysis, i.e. destruction of red blood cells
HEMOPTYSIS	Coughing and spitting of blood caused by bleeding in respiratory tract
HEMOSIDEROSIS	See *Hemochromatosis*
HEPA-	Referring to liver
HEPATITIS	Inflammation of the liver
HIRSUTISM	Abnormal hairiness
HYPER-	Above normal
HYPERCALCEMIA	Excessive amount of calcium in the blood
HYPEREMIA	An increased content of blood in a portion of the body
HYPERGLYCEMIA	Excess of sugar in the blood
HYPERHIDROSIS	Excessive sweating
HYPERKALEMIA	Abnormally high potassium in the blood
HYPERNATREMIA	Abnormally high sodium in the blood
HYPERPLASIA	Overgrowth of normal tissue
HYPERPYREXIA	Excessively high fever
HYPERREFLEXIA	Exaggeration of reflexes
HYPERSENSITIVITY REACTION	Allergic response to an allergen. The allergen may be a medication
HYPERURICEMIA	Abnormally high uric acid level in the blood
HYPERVENTILATION	An increase in the quantity of air breathed as a result of an increase in the rate and/or depth of respiration
HYPERVOLEMIA	Too large a blood volume
HYPO-	Below normal
HYPOCHROMIC ANEMIA	Red blood cells with hemoglobin deficiency comparatively less than normal

HYPOGLYCEMIA	Low level of sugar in the blood
HYPOKALEMIA	Abnormally low serum potassium
HYPONATREMIA	Abnormally low sodium in the blood
HYPOPROTHROMBINEMIA	Deficient supply of prothrombin in the blood
HYPOXIA	Oxygen deficiency in a tissue or organ
IDIOPATHY, IDEOPATHIC	Spontaneous disease state of unknown origin
ILEOSTOMY	Formation of a fistula or artificial opening through the abdominal wall into the ileum
INTERMITTANT CLAUDICA-TION	Cramps and weakness in the legs, induced by walking
INTRATHECAL	Introduction of a therapeutic agent into spinal subarachnoid space
INVOLUTIONAL PSYCHOSIS	Severe mental disorder, of late middle age, characterized by depression, and sometimes paranoid ideas, excessive worry, severe insomnia, and anxiety.
ISCHEMIA	Reduction of the blood supply to an organ or tissue
KERATOSIS	Any disease of the skin characterized by an overgrowth of cornified epithelium
KERNICTERUS	Bile pigmentation of brain and other nerve structure; can cause nerve and brain damage
KETOSIS	Excessive amount of ketones present in the body
KRAUROSIS	Progressive shriveling process of the skin
KYPHOSCOLIOSIS	Backward and lateral curvature of spine
LEUKOPENIA	Too few leukocytes in the peripheral blood
LIBIDO	Sexual desire
LITHIASIS	Formation of calculi in the body
LOADING DOSE	Initial dose to establish certain level of drug in blood; usually higher than subsequent doses

LOCHIA	Discharge from the uterus and vagina after childbirth
MEGOBLAST	A large, nucleated red blood cell
MELASMA	Black pigmentation of the skin
MELENA	Blood found in the stools
MENORRHAGIC	Abnormally heavy menses
METHEMOGLOBINEMIA	Condition in which hemoglobin is converted to methemoglobin, which cannot carry O_2
MICROCYTIC ANEMIA	Red blood cells smaller than normal
MIOSIS	Constriction of pupils of the eye
MIOTIC, MYOTIC	Drug that causes the pupils to constrict
MOON FACE	Fat deposits and swelling of face usually associated with corticosteroid treatment
MYALGIA	Muscle pain
MYASTHENIA GRAVIS	Disorder at the myoneural junction, characterized by extreme weakness of the muscles
MYCOSIS	Any disease caused by fungus
MYDRIASIS	Dilation of the pupils of the eye
MYDRIATIC	Drug causing pupil of eye to dilate
MYOSITIS	Inflammation of voluntary muscle
MYOTONIA	Transitory rigidity after muscle spasms. Increased irritability and/or tonic spasms of muscles
MYXEDEMA	Reaction to lack of thyroid hormone in adults including dry, thickened edematous skin, especially around eyelids, enlarged tongue, hair loss (scalp, eyebrows), mental apathy, deepening of voice, constipation
NARCOLEPSY	Uncontrollable attacks of desire to sleep
NEPHRITIS	Inflammation of the kidney
NEPHROTOXICITY	Damage to kidneys
NEUROPATHY	Any pathological change involving the nervous system
NEUTROPENIA	Decrease below normal of the number of neutrophils in the blood

NOCTURIA	Frequency of urination at night
NYSTAGMUS	Involuntary oscillatory movement of the eyeballs
OLIGURIA	Marked decrease in amount of urine excreted
OPHTHALMIC	Pertaining to the eyes
ORCHITIS	Inflammation of the testes
ORTHOSTATIC HYPOTEN- SION	Low blood pressure when standing up quickly from a reclining position or during prolonged standing
OSTEOMALACIA	Weakened, "soft" bones caused by failure of deposition of calcium salts
OTIC	Pertaining to the ear
OTITIS	Inflammation of the ear
PALLIATIVE	Affording relief without curing
PANCREATITIS	Inflammation of the pancreas
PANCYTOPENIA	Reduction of erythrocytes, leukocytes, and platelets in the blood
PAPILLA	Nipple, any small nipple-like growth
PARALYTIC ILEUS	Absence of peristalis. Paralysis of the intestinal wall resulting in distention and intestinal obstruction. May occur after surgery
PARESTHESIA	Abnormal sensation, burning, prickling of the skin
PAROXYSM	Sudden return or intensification of symptoms of a disease
PEMPHIGUS	An acute or chronic disease of the skin characterized by the appearance of blisters
PERIPHERAL NEURITIS	Inflammation of nerve endings
-PENIA	Meaning too few
PETECHIA	Purplish red spot on a surface such as the skin caused by intradermal or submucosal bleeding
PHEOCHROMOCYTOMA	Tumor of adrenal gland often resulting in hypertension
PHOTOPHOBIA	Intolerance or fear of light
PHOTOSENSITIVITY	Excess response to sunlight
POLYARTHRALGIA	Pain or arthritis, or both, in many joints

POLYDIPSIA	Excessive thirst
POLYURIA	Passage of large amounts of urine
PORPHYRIA	Disorder of porphyrin metabolism characterized by abdominal pain and GI, psychological and neurological disturbances
POSTURAL HYPOTENSION	See *Orthostatic Hypotension*
PRECORDIAL PAIN	Pain in the region over heart and stomach
PRESSOR EFFECT	Tending to increase blood pressure
PROPTOSIS, OCULAR	Bulging of the eyeballs
PROSTAGLANDINS	Hormone-like substances that play a key role in many processes including inflammation, pain, fever, muscle contractility, and platelet aggregation
PROSTATIC	Referring to the prostate gland
PRURITUS	Itching
PSEUDOPARKINSONISM	Muscle tremors, rigidity
PUNCTATE	Dotted, full of small points
PURPURA	Hemorrhage occurring in skin and mucous membrane
PYELITIS	Inflammation of the pelvis of the kidney
PYROSIS	Heartburn
PYURIA	Presence of pus in the urine
RAYNAUD'S PHENOMENA	Cold, cyanotic, painful fingers and hands caused by disturbance in blood circulation
RDA	Recommended Dietary Allowance (of key nutrients) for persons over 4 years, also called USRDA
REFRACTORY PERIOD	Time interval during which a nerve cannot be stimulated
RESISTANT STRAIN	Microorganisms no longer susceptible to particular pharmacologic agent
RETICULAR ACTIVATING SYSTEM	Portion of the brain involved in initiating and maintaining wakefulness
REVERSE ISOLATION	Protection of patient from pathological organisms
RHINITIS	Inflammation of the nasal mucosal membranes

SCLERODERMA	Disease characterized by induration of the skin in localized or diffuse areas
SCORBUTIC	Having scurvy or vitamin C deficiency
SEBORRHEIC	Referring to glands that secrete fatty (sebaceous) matter
SEPSIS	A febrile reaction due to the action of bacteria
SEPTICEMIA	Systemic disease produced by microorganisms and their poisons in the blood
SIALORRHEA	Salivation
SIDEROSIS	Chronic inflammation of the lungs due to prolonged inhalation of dust of iron salts
SPASMOLYTIC	Relieving spasms
SPASMOPHILIA	A tendency toward convulsions or tonic spasms as in tetany
SPRUE	Chronic disease characterized by sore mouth and tongue, impairment of fat metabolism, and passage of voluminous, mushy stools
STEATORRHEA	Fatty stools
STENOSIS, STENOSING	Narrowing of any canal or duct
STEVENS-JOHNSON SYNDROME	Extreme inflammatory eruption of skin and mucosa of mouth, pharynx, anogenital region, and conjunctiva
STOMATITIS	Inflammation of the soft tissues of the mouth
SUPERINFECTION	Overgrowth by bacteria different from those causing original infection
SUSPENSION	Dispersion of solid particles throughout the body of a liquid
SYNCOPE	Fainting
SYMOGYI EFFECT	Hyperglycemia following a hypoglycemic reaction that triggers the counterregulation with release of epinephrine, glucocorticoids and growth hormone. These stimulate glucogenesis by the liver and require reduction in insulin dosage

SYSTEMIC LUPUS ERYTHE-MATOSUS	A collagen type of disease characterized by an abnormal response of the immune system, joint pain, fever, and a characteristic rash. A transitory lupus-like syndrome can be drug-induced
TACHYCARDIA	Increased heart beat (usually pulse rate of more than 130 beats/minute)
TACHYPNEA	Abnormal frequency of respiration
TERATOGENIC	May induce birth defects; monster producing
VESICANT DRUG	Drug that causes blistering and irritation of tissue

APPENDIX 10

bibliography

Albanese JA: *Nurses' Drug Reference.* New York, McGraw-Hill Book Co, 1979.

AMA Drug Evaluations. Littleton, Mass., Publishing Science Group, ed. 3, 1977.

American Hospital Formulary Service, American Society of Hospital Pharmacists. Current.

Bergersen BS, Krug EE: *Pharmacology in Nursing.* St. Louis, Mo, CV Mosby Company, 1979.

Brunner LS, Suddarth DM: *Textbook of Medical-Surgical Nursing.* Philadelphia, Pa, JB Lippincott Co, 1975.

Burnside IM: *Nursing and the Aged.* New York, McGraw-Hill Book Co, 1974.

Cape R: *Aging: Its Complex Management.* New York, Harper & Row, 1978.

Daniels L: How can you improve patient compliance? *Nursing '78*, May 1978, pp 39–47.

Eliopoulos C: *Gerontological Nursing.* New York, Harper & Row, 1979.

Falconer MW, Normal MR, Patterson HR, Gustafson EA: *The Drug, The Nurse, The Patient.* Philadelphia, Pa, WB Saunders Co, 1970.

Fuerst EV, Wolff L: *Fundamentals of Nursing.* Philadelphia, Pa, JB Lippincott Co, 1969.

Garb S, Crim BJ, Garf T: *Pharmacology and Patient Care.* New York, Springer Publishing Company, 1970.

Goodman LS, Gilman A: *The Pharmacological Basis of Therapeutics.* New York, Macmillan, 1975.

Govoni LE, and Hayes JE: *Drugs and Nursing Implications.* New York, Appleton-Century-Crofts, 1979.

Graef JW: *Manual of Pediatric Therapeutics.* Boston, Little Brown & Co, 1974.

Grant J: "The Nurses' Role in Parenteral Hyperalimentation," *RN* July 1973, pp 28–33.

Greenwald E: *Cancer Chemotherapy.* Garden City, NY, Medical Examination Publishing Co Inc, 1973.

Hansen PD: *Drug Interactions.* Philadelphia, Pa, Lea and Febinger, 4th ed, 1979.

Jones D, Dunbar C, Jirovec M: *Medical Surgical Nursing.* New York, McGraw-Hill Book Co, 1978.

Kastrup EK, Boyd JR: *Facts and Comparisons, Inc*, Current.

Kee J: *Fluids and Electrolytes With Clinical Applications.* New York, John Wiley & Sons Inc, 1978.

Leifer G: *Principles and Techniques in Pediatric Nursing.* Philadelphia, Pa, WB Saunders Co, 1972.

Marlow D: *Textbook of Pediatric Nursing.* Philadelphia, Pa, WB Saunders Co, 1973.

Martin EW: *Hazards of Medication.* Philadelphia, Pa, JB Lippincott Co, 1978.

Martin L: *Health Care of Women.* Philadelphia, Pa, JB Lippincott Co, 1978.

McNall L, Galeener: *Current Practice in Obstetrics and Gynecological Nursing.* St Louis, Mo, CV Mosby Co, 1976.

Myers FH, Jawetz E, Goldfien A: *A Review of Medical Pharmacology*. Los Altos, Calif, Lange Medical Publications, 6th ed, 1978.

Physicians Desk Reference. Medical Economics. Oradell, NJ, Litton Industries, 1979.

Reeder S, Mastroianni L, Fitzpatrick E. *Maternity Nursing*. Philadelphia, Pa, JB Lippincott Co, 1976.

Rodman MJ, Smith DW: *Clinical Pharmacology in Nursing*. Philadelphia, Pa, JB Lippincott Co, 1979.

Shafer K, Sawyer J, McCluskey A, Beck E, Phipps W: *Medical Surgical Nursing*. St Louis, Mo, CV Mosby Co, 1975.

Smith B: Safeguarding Your Patient After Anesthesia, *Nursing '78*. October 1978, pp 53–56.

Strand M, Elmer L: *Clinical Laboratory Tests*. St Louis, Mo, CV Mosby Co, 1976.

Wallach, Jacques: *Interpretation of Diagnostic Tests*. Boston, Little Brown & Co, 1974.

Williams S: *Nutrition and Diet Therapy*. St Louis, Mo, CV Mosby Co, 1977.

Woods D: *The TPN Lifeline*, Nurses' Drug Alert, (1) #9/77.

Wyeth Laboratories, *Intramuscular Injections*, 1968.

Yura H, Walsh M: *The Nursing Process*. New York, Appleton-Century-Crofts, 1978.

Ziegel E, Van Blarcom CC: *Obstetric Nursing*. New York, Macmillan, 1972.

INDEX*

*Generic drug names and subject headings of particular importance are set in bold type; trade drug names are set in regular type.

A

G

H